Gastrointestinal Medicine

Gastrointestinal Medicine

Edited by Ronald Graves

hayle medical

New York

Hayle Medical,
750 Third Avenue, 9th Floor,
New York, NY 10017, USA

Visit us on the World Wide Web at:
www.haylemedical.com

ISBN: 978-1-63241-613-1

Printed in China.

Cataloging-in-Publication Data

Gastrointestinal medicine / edited by Ronald Graves.
p. cm.
Includes bibliographical references and index.
ISBN 978-1-63241-613-1
1. Gastrointestinal system--Diseases. 2. Gastrointestinal system--Diseases--Diagnosis.
3. Gastrointestinal system--Diseases--Treatment. 4. Gastroenterology. I. Graves, Ronald.
RC801 .G37 2019
616.33--dc23

Table of Contents

Preface

This book aims to highlight the current researches and provides a platform to further the scope of innovations in this area. This book is a product of the combined efforts of many researchers and scientists, after going through thorough studies and analysis from different parts of the world. The objective of this book is to provide the readers with the latest information of the field.

All diseases related to the gastrointestinal tract and the accessory organs of digestion are known as gastrointestinal diseases. The gastrointestinal tract comprises of the stomach, esophagus, small intestine, large intestine and rectum. The accessory organs of digestion include the tongue, salivary glands, liver, gallbladder and pancreas. Oral diseases related to the GI tract include gingivitis, acid erosion, periodontitis, mouth ulcers, dental caries and angular cheilitis. Gastroesophageal reflux disease and Barrett's oesophagus are some of the oesophageal diseases. Gastric diseases include gastroenteritis and peptic ulcers. Enterocolitis and ulcerative colitis are two common intestinal diseases. Fatty liver diseases, non-alcoholic fatty liver diseases and hepatitis are examples of common liver diseases. The topics included in this book on gastrointestinal medicine are of utmost significance and bound to provide incredible insights to readers. It presents researches and studies performed by experts across the globe. This book will prove to be immensely beneficial to students, doctors and researchers in this field.

I would like to express my sincere thanks to the authors for their dedicated efforts in the completion of this book. I acknowledge the efforts of the publisher for providing constant support. Lastly, I would like to thank my family for their support in all academic endeavors.

Editor

1

Rapid Progression of Primary Sclerosing Cholangitis Complicated with Ulcerative Colitis

Piotr Pardak,[1] Ewa Walczak,[1] and Rafał S. Filip[2,3]

[1]*Department of Internal Medicine, Institute of Rural Health, 20-090 Lublin, Poland*
[2]*Department of Clinical Endoscopy, Institute of Rural Health, 20-090 Lublin, Poland*
[3]*Department of Public Health and Social Medicine, University of Rzeszów, 35-959 Rzeszów, Poland*

Correspondence should be addressed to Piotr Pardak; piotrpardak@mp.pl

Academic Editor: Hideto Kawaratani

Primary sclerosing cholangitis is a cholestatic condition with unknown etiology and long-standing, progressive course, leading to cirrhosis and requiring orthotropic liver transplant. In approximately 80%, primary sclerosing cholangitis is accompanied by inflammatory bowel disease, and in most cases the recognition of bowel disease precedes the diagnosis of primary sclerosing cholangitis. We describe a case of 22-year-old male diagnosed simultaneously with primary sclerosing cholangitis and ulcerative colitis, with a medical history suggesting uncommon prior development of the liver disease. Five months after the initial diagnosis, we observed advanced lesions of bile tree due to progression of primary sclerosing cholangitis, which led to the unusually fast necessity for the orthotopic liver transplant.

1. Introduction

Primary sclerosing cholangitis (PSC) is a chronic cholestatic condition with unknown etiology. The outcome of the progressive fibrosis and destruction of bile ducts is a persistent cholestasis leading to the development of liver cirrhosis. It is estimated that, in approximately 80%, PSC is accompanied by inflammatory bowel disease (IBD), mostly ulcerative colitis (UC). However, UC may remain clinically silent; therefore, the course of PSC usually does not correlate with intestinal activity. In most cases, the recognition of IBD precedes the PSC diagnosis by several years. The natural history of PSC is long-standing and variable and frequently progressive, leading to cirrhosis, requiring orthotropic liver transplant (OLT). The most ominous adverse event of PSC is the development of cholangiocarcinoma (CC) [1–6].

2. Case Report

A 22-year-old male was referred to the Department of Internal Medicine due to periodic abdominal pain accompanied by loose stools and rectal bleeding lasting for a couple of weeks. General weakness, pruritus, and weight loss were also noticeable. He had no noteworthy medical or family history, including IBD and liver diseases; however, abnormal liver function tests were first noted approximately 1 year earlier. He had no history of drug abuse or significant alcohol consumption prior to admission. Physical examination showed grey-sallow colour of the skin, yellowness of the sclera, singular mutilations in the skin area of the abdominal cavity and thighs, and hepatomegaly. Laboratory tests showed anaemia as well as elevated levels of total bilirubin and hepatobiliary enzymes. Other clinical tests, including those for infectious diseases, were normal (Table 1).

Abdominal ultrasound examination showed hepatosplenomegaly and slight dilatations of bile ducts in the area of the left liver lobe. Enhanced computerized tomography (CT) demonstrated hepatomegaly and splenomegaly, lymphadenopathy, and changes suggesting the presence of inflammation in the area of intrahepatic bile ducts. Magnetic resonance cholangiopancreatography (MRCP) revealed the presence of irregular dilatations and constrictions of the intrahepatic bile ducts (especially in the area of left liver lobe), suggesting the recognition of PSC (Figures 1(a)–1(c)).

Endoscopic examination of the large bowel showed erythema and friability of the mucosa and loss of vascular pattern

TABLE 1: Laboratory tests results on PSC diagnosis and on OLT qualification.

Laboratory parameter	PSC diagnosis (02.2013)	OLT qualification (07.2013)
WBC [$\times 10^3$/uL]	9.86	13.5
RBC [$\times 10^6$/uL]	4.24	4.8
HGB [g/dL]	10.3	14.1
PLT [$\times 10^3$/uL]	342	287
ALP [U/L]	1,097	354
GGTP [U/L]	677	378
Bil. tot. [mg/dL]	1.6	1.0
ALT [U/L]	104	38
AST [U/L]	50	22
Albumin [g/dL]	3.4	4.1
INR	1.04	0.9
Fibrinogen [g/L]	472	443

WBC: white blood cells, RBC: red blood cells, HGB: haemoglobin, and INR: International Normalized Ratio.

in the whole colon. More intensive inflammatory changes with additional superficial erosions and ulcers were visible within the sigmoid colon (Mayo UC score: 2/3). Histology confirmed inflammatory changes of the mucosa which are characteristic for UC. The presence of the hiatus hernia and slight superficial inflammation of the antral mucosa was diagnosed during esophagogastroduodenoscopy. The patient received typical treatment with glucocorticosteroids p.o. (prednisone 30 mg/day) and mesalazine p.o. (3 g/day) and p.r. (4 g/day) with good tolerance and satisfactory clinical response.

Three months later, the patient was hospitalized due to elevation of aminotransferases, total bilirubin, alkaline phosphatase (ALP), and gamma-glutamyl transpeptidase (GGTP). Endoscopic retrograde cholangiopancreatography (ERCP) showed significant constrictions of bile ducts (intrahepatic bile ducts did not contrast virtually, only partially in the right liver lobe), a sphincterotomy was performed, and a plastic stent was implanted in the common bile duct. During hospitalization, PSC-AIH (autoimmune hepatitis) overlap syndrome was also considered; however, on the basis of all available clinical data, its probability was estimated as very low. It is important to note that abdominal ultrasound, due to parietal solid lesion of uncertain etiology in the gallbladder, raised the suspicion of malignancy, which was subsequently excluded. However, given rapidly progressing PSC which would require transplantation in the future, the patient was transferred to the hepatology referential centre for cholecystectomy. UC was in remission and none of the intestinal symptoms were present at the time.

Five months later, the patient was once more referred to the transplantology centre. The general condition of the patient was poor, and laboratory tests showed impaired liver function (with cholestasis and jaundice), additionally complicated by local symptoms suggesting bacterial inflammation. ECPW was performed, and further exacerbation of lesions characteristic for PSC combined with the inflammatory changes was seen. A common bile duct free passage was restored by the reimplantation of a new stent (the previous stent was expelled prior to admission). After completion of all the tests included in the OLT qualification protocol, the patient was enrolled on the liver recipient's waiting list.

OLT was performed three months later. Histopathological examination of excised liver showed preserved architecture of the organ and severe fibrosis in the majority of the portobiliary sinuses, with bands of connective tissue penetrating into the parenchyma and separating more clearly demarcated nodules. Within the portobiliary sinuses and in some bands of connective tissue were found mainly chronic inflammatory infiltration and multifocally devastation of the wall of the bile canaliculus. Multifocally, within the walls of large interlobular and hilum bile ducts, massive inflammatory infiltrations, almost complete disappearance of the epithelium, and numerous mucosal ulceration were found. In addition, locally, in the portobiliary sinuses exacerbated growth of neocholangioli was present. Characteristic periductal fibrosis was found around the walls of some bile ducts. Hepatocytes were without significant abnormalities; in the gallbladder, chronic inflammation was found. The above result supported the diagnosis of PSC.

The patient's postoperative course was complicated by bleeding from the vascular anastomosis approximately one month after OLT and provided with surgical treatment. The patient is well 15 months after transplantation.

3. Discussion

It is commonly believed that the PSC has a long-standing course; however, the dynamics of the destruction of the biliary duct system is highly variable, although usually leading to liver-related morbidity, mortality, and the need for liver transplantation [1, 4–7]. Usually, IBD symptoms precede the occurrence of PSC, even by several years, and PSC is often identified during follow-up in patients treated for IBD. The scenario in which liver symptoms appear before the development of IBD is rare [1–4, 8–13]. In the presented case of a 22-year-old male, PSC and UC were diagnosed simultaneously, although the medical data indicated prior development of the liver disease. However, the possibility that nonspecific inflammatory lesions in the colon mucosa were present without any clinical symptoms of UC cannot be excluded. Such a possibility was observed among patients with PSC combined with UC, as described later by Swedish authors [14].

Clinical symptoms of PSC usually develop together with progression of the inflammation, fibrosis, and strictures of the biliary tree [1, 4, 6]. The average time from the PSC diagnosis to liver transplant or death ranges between 9 and 18 years; however, it is strongly dependent on specific patient characteristics and the overall number of performed liver transplants. The average life span of PSC patients before liver transplant introduction was approximately 9.6–18 years and extended by OLT up to 25.5 years [5–7]. The major indications for OLT in PSC are hepatic failure, suspicion of CC, major advancement of destructive lesions in the bile ducts, and recurrent bacterial cholangitis [2, 11, 15].

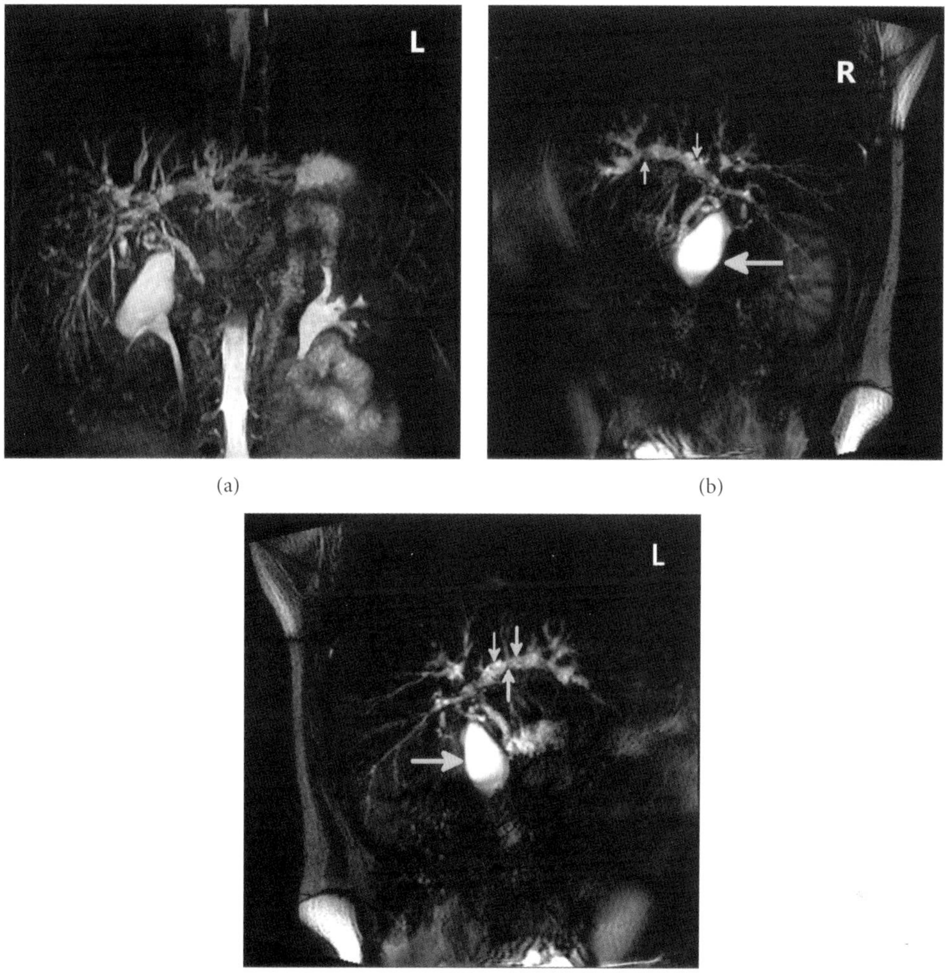

(a) (b) (c)

Figure 1: Irregular dilatations and constrictions of bile ducts (small arrows) diagnosed in MRCP (gall bladder, large arrows).

Patients with PSC are at increased risk for malignancy of the gallbladder; therefore, any change within the gallbladder found on imaging studies should be an indication for an urgent cholecystectomy [16, 17].

In the presented case, 5 months after the initial diagnosis, very fast progression of bile tree destruction due to PSC was noted, with bacterial cholangitis, chronic symptoms (general weakness, pruritus), and lesion of uncertain etiology within the gallbladder, which raised the suspicion of malignancy. The coexistence of these factors with poor efficacy of the endoscopic treatment resulted in the unusually fast necessity for the OLT which, in fact, shortened the natural history of PSC in this patient to less than 12 months.

To the best of our knowledge, this is only description of a very rapid course of PSC which finally led to the OLT. However, in the cited case the OLT was performed 3 years after the initial diagnosis, mainly due to the suspicion of CC (which was subsequently confirmed) [18].

4. Conclusion

We describe an example of a particularly rare and fast progression of PSC, which led to the OLT in less than 12 months from establishing the initial diagnosis. Moreover, PSC was diagnosed simultaneously with UC and the patient's medical history suggested uncommon, previous to UC, development of the liver disease. This report highlights that patients with an atypical course of the PSC may benefit from early referral to the hepatology referential centre.

Consent

The patient, whose identity is protected, has granted permission to publish the features of his case.

Authors' Contribution

All authors have read the paper and have approved its submission.

References

[1] T. H. Karlsen, E. Schrumpf, and K. M. Boberg, "Primary sclerosing cholangitis," *Best Practice and Research: Clinical Gastroenterology*, vol. 24, no. 5, pp. 655–666, 2010.

[2] European Association for the Study of the Liver, "EASL Clinical Practice Guidelines: management of cholestatic liver diseases," *Journal of Hepatology*, vol. 51, no. 2, pp. 237–267, 2009.

[3] J. Fevery, L. Henckaerts, R. van Oirbeek et al., "Malignancies and mortality in 200 patients with primary sclerosering cholangitis: a long-term single-centre study," *Liver International*, vol. 32, no. 2, pp. 214–222, 2012.

[4] N. F. LaRusso, B. L. Shneider, D. Black et al., "Primary sclerosing cholangitis: summary of a workshop," *Hepatology*, vol. 44, no. 3, pp. 746–764, 2006.

[5] J. J. W. Tischendorf, H. Hecker, M. Krüger, M. P. Manns, and P. N. Meier, "Characterization, outcome, and prognosis in 273 patients with primary sclerosing cholangitis: a single center study," *The American Journal of Gastroenterology*, vol. 102, no. 1, pp. 107–114, 2007.

[6] U. Broomé, R. Olsson, L. Lööf et al., "Natural history and prognostic factors in 305 Swedish patients with primary sclerosing cholangitis," *Gut*, vol. 38, no. 4, pp. 610–615, 1996.

[7] C. Y. Ponsioen, S. M. E. Vrouenraets, W. Prawirodirdjo et al., "Natural history of primary sclerosing cholangitis and prognostic value of cholangiography in a Dutch population," *Gut*, vol. 51, no. 4, pp. 562–566, 2002.

[8] U. Navaneethan, P. G. K. Venkatesh, B. A. Lashner, B. Shen, and R. P. Kiran, "The impact of ulcerative colitis on the long-term outcome of patients with primary sclerosing cholangitis," *Alimentary Pharmacology and Therapeutics*, vol. 35, no. 9, pp. 1045–1053, 2012.

[9] A. Bergquist, H. Glaumann, B. Lindberg, and U. Broomé, "Primary sclerosing cholangitis can present with acute liver failure: report of two cases," *Journal of Hepatology*, vol. 44, no. 5, pp. 1005–1008, 2006.

[10] X. P. Miao, X. N. Sun, H. Wei, and Q. Ouyang, "Crohn's disease and primary sclerosing cholangitis: a case report and review of the literature," *Internal Medicine*, vol. 51, no. 16, pp. 2077–2081, 2012.

[11] H. E. Vargas, "A difficult case of primary sclerosing cholangitis," *Liver Transplantation*, vol. 12, no. 11, pp. S65–S67, 2006.

[12] M. Seo, M. Okada, S. Osamura et al., "Colonic cancer in a patient with primary sclerosing cholangitis and long-standing ulcerative colitis," *Journal of Gastroenterology*, vol. 32, no. 1, pp. 83–88, 1997.

[13] J. C. Ong, E. V. O'Loughlin, K. R. Kamath, S. F. Dorney, M. de Silva, and K. J. Gaskin, "Sclerosing cholangitis in children with inflammatory bowel disease.," *Australian and New Zealand Journal of Medicine*, vol. 24, no. 2, pp. 149–153, 1994.

[14] U. Broomé, R. Löfberg, K. Lundqvist, and B. Veress, "Subclinical time span of inflammatory bowel disease in patients with primary sclerosing cholangitis," *Diseases of the Colon & Rectum*, vol. 38, no. 12, pp. 1301–1305, 1995.

[15] W. Andraus, L. Haddad, L. S. Nacif, F. D. Silva, R. Blasbalg, and L. A. C. D'Albuquerque, "The best approach for diagnosing primary sclerosing cholangitis," *Clinics*, vol. 66, no. 11, pp. 1987–1989, 2011.

[16] G. Vázquez-Elizondo, J. Muciño-Bermejo, and N. Méndez-Sánchez, "Gallbladder disease in patients with primary sclerosing cholangitis," *Annals of Hepatology*, vol. 7, no. 2, pp. 182–183, 2008.

[17] U. C. Leung, P. Y. Wong, R. H. Roberts, and J. B. Koea, "Gall bladder polyps in sclerosing cholangitis: does the 1-cm rule apply?" *ANZ Journal of Surgery*, vol. 77, no. 5, pp. 355–357, 2007.

[18] M. Deneau, D. G. Adler, J. J. Schwartz et al., "Cholangiocarcinoma in a 17-year-old boy with primary sclerosing cholangitis and inflammatory bowel disease," *Journal of Pediatric Gastroenterology and Nutrition*, vol. 52, no. 5, pp. 617–620, 2011.

2

Liver Injury Secondary to Anti-TNF-Alpha Therapy in Inflammatory Bowel Disease: A Case Series and Review of the Literature

Ravish Parekh and Nirmal Kaur

Inflammatory Bowel Disease Center, Henry Ford Health System, 39450 West Twelve Mile Roud, Novi, MI 48377, USA

Correspondence should be addressed to Nirmal Kaur; nkaur1@hfhs.org

Academic Editors: T. Hirata, H. Kawaratani, M. Neri, and I. Siddique

Background. Biologic therapy to inhibit tumor necrosis factor-alpha (TNF-α) is an effective, safe treatment for patients with inflammatory bowel disease (IBD). All TNF-α inhibitors have been associated with liver toxicity, but many of these cases have been reported in patients receiving therapy for rheumatologic disease. Herein we report the first single-center case series of TNF-α antagonist related liver injury in patients with IBD. *Methods.* A retrospective case series was performed at the Henry Ford Inflammatory Bowel Diseases Center. IRB approval was obtained. *Results.* 2 patients were treated with infliximab, whereas the 3rd patient was treated with adalimumab for IBD. All 3 patients had negative viral markers, normal autoimmune serologies, and normal biliary imaging studies. Liver biopsy was performed in all 3 patients, and evidence of portal inflammation was seen. Liver enzymes normalized after discontinuation of therapy in all patients, and no long term effects have been observed. One patient was successfully transitioned from infliximab to adalimumab without relapse of either IBD or liver injury. *Conclusion.* Liver injury secondary to TNF-α antagonist is an underrecognized, important clinical entity with potentially serious consequences. The mechanism of drug-induced injury is idiosyncratic. Larger cohort studies are needed to establish risk factors and injury patterns related to hepatotoxicity in these patients.

1. Introduction

Biologic therapy to inhibit tumor necrosis factor-alpha (TNF-α), a proinflammatory cytokine, has become a widely used, safe, and effective treatment for patients with inflammatory bowel disease (IBD) [1]. Since 2008, the number of patients treated with TNF-α antagonists has rapidly increased, and as of 2011 more than 1,500,000 people have been exposed to infliximab therapy [2]. However, the side effect profile of these medications is still being established. TNF-α antagonists have been associated with the reactivation of latent tuberculosis, reactivation of hepatitis B, demyelinating neurologic disease, and congestive heart failure, among other adverse effects [3]. Cases of TNF-α antagonist-induced liver toxicity have been reported, but mainly in patients receiving therapy for rheumatologic disease [4–8]. Little has been reported about anti-TNF-α related hepatotoxicity in patients with IBD [2, 4, 9–12]. Clinician awareness of the adverse effects of commonly used therapies is paramount for safe administration of treatment. Herein we report the first single-center case series of anti-TNF-α related liver injury in patients with IBD.

2. Methods and Materials

The Henry Ford Health System Institutional Review Board approved this retrospective case series. All patients were seen at the Henry Ford Health System Inflammatory Bowel Disease Center in Novi, Michigan. Patient charts were reviewed and clinical information was extracted.

3. Ethical Considerations

Since this study required only chart review and no patient intervention, ethical considerations were minimal. Patient privacy was maintained with de-identification of all study documents.

4. Results

All results are listed in Table 1.

4.1. Subject 1. A 49-year-old female with a 15-year history of ulcerative pancolitis was initially treated with 5-aminosalicylic acid (5-ASA) derivatives, with good control for 12 years. Due to an increase in symptoms as well as moderately severe colitis seen on endoscopy, infliximab was added at 5 milligrams per kilogram (mg/kg) at weeks 0, 2, 6, and then every 8 weeks. After 6 months, due to persistent symptoms as well as persistent endoscopic disease severity, the infliximab dose was escalated to 10 mg/kg every 8 weeks. Prior to infliximab initiation, liver function tests were normal. After 18 months of infliximab therapy, liver enzymes were found to be elevated on routine serologic check: alanine aminotransferase (ALT) elevated to 85; aspartame aminotransferase (AST) was 104, alkaline phosphatase (ALP) elevated to 518, and bilirubin remained normal. The patient remained asymptomatic, with no features of compromised hepatic function, both subjectively and objectively. Autoimmune liver panel, including antinuclear antibody (ANA), antismooth muscle antibody (ASMA), and anti-liver-kidney-mitochondrial antibody (anti-LKM), was negative. Serologic markers for Hepatitis A, B, and C were also negative, including Hepatitis A Immunoglobulin M (IgM), Hepatitis B surface antigen (HBsAg), Hepatitis B core antibody (cAb) IgM, Hepatitis C antibody (HCV Ab), and Hepatitis C RNA (HCV RNA). The patient underwent magnetic resonance cholangiopancreatography (MRCP), which showed no evidence of primary sclerosing cholangitis. She ultimately underwent a liver biopsy, which showed minimal chronic portal inflammation with lack of any autoimmune features or fibrosis. After three months of persistent liver enzyme abnormalities, infliximab was discontinued. Twenty weeks after discontinuation of infliximab, ALT normalized to 21 and AST trended down to 37 and ALP to 142. Despite our discussion of adalimumab therapy or colectomy, the patient elected to avoid all medication except oral mesalamine. She has remained minimally symptomatic, with minimal mucosal activity on follow-up colonoscopy at 6 months.

4.2. Subject 2. A 34-year-old female with a 9-year history of mild ulcerative pancolitis developed worsening disease both symptomatically as well as endoscopically. Therapy with infliximab 5 mg/kg, at standard induction dosing and maintenance every 8 weeks, was prescribed, with good symptomatic response. Prior to initiation of infliximab, liver enzymes were within the normal range. After 2 infusions, liver enzymes elevated: ALT was 173 and AST was 160. Following the 3rd infusion at week 6, the patient's liver enzymes elevated even further: ALT was 300 and AST was 259. Autoimmune serologies including ANA, ASMA, and anti-LKM antibody and viral hepatitis panel including hepatitis A IgM, HBsAg, HBcAb IgM, HCV Ab, and HCV RNA were all negative. Alpha-1-antitrypsin levels were also normal. MRCP was unrevealing. Liver biopsy demonstrated chronic periportal inflammation with presence of eosinophils and focal stage 1 fibrosis. No autoimmune features were seen. Given the extent and persistence of enzyme elevation, infliximab was

Table 1

Patient	Patient 1	Patient 2	Patient 3
Age	49	34	19
Sex	Female	Female	Female
Disease	UC	UC	Crohn's
Concomitant drugs	Mesalamine, synthroid	Mesalamine, synthroid, sertraline	None
TNF-α-antagonist	Infliximab	Infliximab	Adalimumab
Time to liver toxicity	18 months	3 months	1 month
Peak ALT	104	300	184
Peak AST	85	259	167
Total bilirubin	0.4	0.4	1.7
Direct bilirubin	0.1	0.1	1
Peak ALP	518	77	527
Albumin	3.3	4	3.2
INR	1.07	0.98	1.14
ANA	Negative	Negative	Negative
Anti-LKM	Negative	Negative	Negative
ASMA	N/A	Negative	Negative
Hep A IgM	Negative	Negative	Negative
Hep B sAg	Negative	Negative	Negative
Hep B core IgM	Negative	Negative	Negative
Hep C Ab	Negative	Negative	Negative
MRCP	Normal biliary system	Normal biliary system	Normal biliary system
Liver Biopsy	Chronic portal inflammation	Chronic portal inflammation	Lobular and chronic portal inflammation with microgranulomas
Outcome	Infliximab discontinued. Liver recovery in 8 weeks. In clinical and endoscopic remission on ASA monotherapy	Switched to Adalimumab. Liver recovery in 8 weeks. In clinical and endoscopic remission	Adalimumab discontinued. Liver recovery in 6 weeks. In clinical remission on no therapy

Ulcerative colitis (UC), Crohn's disease (CD), aspartate aminotransferase (AST), alanine aminotransferase (ALT), alkaline phosphatase (ALP), international normalized ratio (INR), antinuclear antibody (ANA), antismooth muscle antibody (ASMA), antiliver-kidney-mitochondrial antibody (anti-LKM), Hepatitis A immunoglobulin M (IgM), Hepatitis B surface antigen (HBsAg), Hepatitis B core antibody (cAb) IgM, Hepatitis C antibody (HCV Ab), and magnetic resonance cholangiopancreatography (MRCP).

discontinued after 3 infusions. Liver enzymes improved after discontinuation of infliximab. The patient was started on adalimumab therapy after 8 weeks of discontinuation of infliximab. Liver enzymes continued to improve even after discontinuation of infliximab and subsequent initiation of adalimumab. After 6 months of treatment with adalimumab, with concomitant ASA therapy, this patient has continued to be in clinical and endoscopic remission, with liver enzymes being in the normal range.

4.3. Subject 3. A 19-year-old female with a 7-year history of severe, fistulizing, ileocolonic, and perianal Crohn's disease was initially treated with ASA, azathioprine, and infliximab. Her disease was refractory to medical management and she underwent total colectomy and permanent end-ileostomy. Given the patient's young age of disease onset and severity of disease, therapy with adalimumab at standard induction dosing (160 mg at week 0, 80 mg at week 2, and 40 mg every other week thereafter) was initiated three months postoperatively to prevent postoperative recurrence of Crohn's disease [13]. Liver enzymes prior to initiation of adalimumab were normal. Four weeks after drug initiation, the patient was hospitalized with complaints of nausea, abdominal pain, and diarrhea. She was found to have elevated liver enzymes, with ALT 184 and AST 167 (Figure 1). Viral hepatitis panel including Hepatitis A Ab IgM, HBsAg, HBcAb IgM, HCV Ab, and HCV RNA was negative. Autoimmune workup with ANA, ASMA, AMA, and Anti LKM Ab was negative as well. MRCP showed an unremarkable biliary system. The patient underwent liver biopsy, which showed lobular and chronic portal inflammation with microgranulomas. The infiltrate included lymphocytes and plasma cells with rare eosinophils and neutrophils. Also, histologically, occasional lymphocytic infiltrates of the bile duct epithelium were seen, focally resembling a florid ductal lesion (Figures 2 and 3). Given the temporal relationship of liver injury to the initiation of adalimumab, as well as the degree of symptomatic involvement, adalimumab therapy was discontinued. After six weeks of drug discontinuation, liver enzymes normalized (Figure 1). This patient has not initiated any further therapy. At 6 months of follow-up, her disease has remained quiescent symptomatically. A discussion regarding azathioprine initiation with close liver monitoring is planned for her follow-up visit.

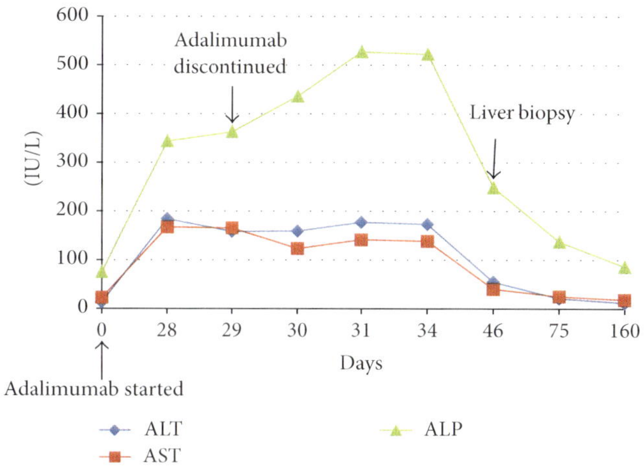

FIGURE 1: Graphic summary of biochemical liver injury with administration of adalimumab in Subject 3. Aspartate aminotransferase (AST), alanine aminotransferase (ALT), and alkaline phosphatase (ALP).

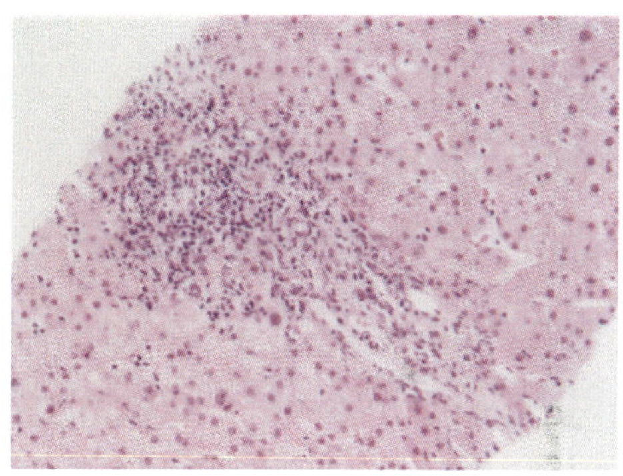

FIGURE 2: Liver biopsy showing portal inflammation in Subject 3 (hematoxylin and eosin stain, magnification ×200).

5. Discussion

Our study reports the largest, single-center case series of anti-TNF-α drug-induced liver injury in patients with IBD. A recent case series by Ghabril and colleagues [2] reported 6 cases of anti-TNF-α drug-induced liver injury from United States Drug Induced Liver Injury Network database, over 8 years, between 2003 and 2011. Our experience of three such cases, seen in one region, over the course of one year, suggests that the incidence of this adverse effect may be more prevalent than is currently recognized. Furthermore, because biologic agents have been utilized for rheumatologic conditions with much more frequency than that of IBD, much of the safety data pertaining to biologic therapy is published in the rheumatology literature. Clinician awareness of this adverse effect is likely lower amongst gastroenterologists.

Liver injury secondary to TNF-α antagonist can present with either a hepatocellular pattern or an autoimmune pattern. Several reported cases of TNF-α antagonist related liver injury describe a predominantly hepatocellular pattern [2, 4, 5, 10, 14, 15]. Autoimmune injury with positive autoantibodies, including ANA, ASMA, and Anti-LKM antibody, along with classic histologic features of autoimmune hepatitis such as interface hepatitis, lymphoplasmacytic infiltrate, and bridging fibrosis has been reported as well [7–9, 12, 16–19]. In the case series reported by Ghabril and colleagues, patients with autoimmune features experienced longer latency times and higher peak ALT levels compared to those lacking autoimmune features [2]. Cholestatic hepatitis secondary to anti-TNF-α agents has been reported [2, 6, 10, 20] and in one case report, hepatic necrosis resulted in fulminant liver failure requiring urgent liver transplantation [11]. There has also been a case report of hepatocellular carcinoma in a patient treated with a TNF-α antagonist in combination with

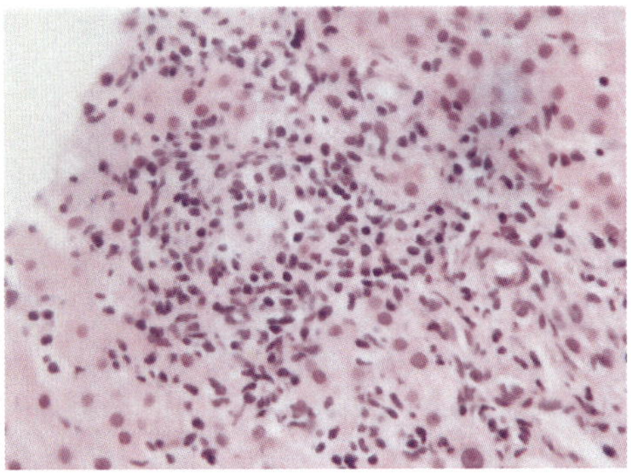

Figure 3: Liver biopsy showing lymphocytic and plasma cell infiltrate in Subject 3 (hematoxylin and eosin stain, magnification ×400).

azathioprine [21]. In our series, all three patients experienced hepatocellular injury both biochemically as well as histologically, with negative autoimmune serologies. Our patients did exhibit microscopic features of hepatitis, without interface hepatitis or lymphoplasmacytic infiltration. This pattern of injury is more consistent with drug-induced injury rather than acute autoimmune hepatitis, as evidenced by histology as well as resolution after discontinuation of the offending agent. The hepatitis was not fatal and no serious injury was reported.

We initially postulated that the variation in injury pattern could be secondary to variables such as concomitant medications or dosage of medications. However, review of our cases and the existing literature showed no such relationship. Dosage of TNF-α antagonists did not correlate with liver injury in our case series. Amongst our patients, Subject 1 received therapy with high dose infliximab (10 mg/kg every 8 weeks) when hepatotoxicity was documented. However, Subjects 2 and 3 received standard doses of infliximab (5 mg/kg every 8 weeks) and standard induction dosing of adalimumab (160 mg at week 0, 80 mg at week 2, and 40 mg every other week thereafter), respectively, when liver injury was noticed. Review of previously reported cases revealed that the onset of hepatitis has been noticed with single administration of infliximab in one case [10], but after prolonged administration of the medication in other cases.

Latency time to the development of liver toxicity was also variable. In our case series, Subject 1 developed liver toxicity after 18 months of infliximab, whereas toxicity developed within 3 months in Subjects 2 and 3. Hepatotoxicity was not related to any particular TNF-α antagonist, and patient age also varied among our three patients. The variability of histology, dosage, time to toxicity, and presence of concomitant medications, in our patients as well as in review of published cases, highlights the idiosyncratic nature of this drug-induced liver injury. As clinician awareness of this entity increases, and more cases are detected, hopefully distinct patterns of injury will be delineated so that early detection can take place and fulminant liver failure can be prevented [17, 22, 23].

The lack of cross-reactivity between the TNF-α-antagonist-related liver injury, as seen in multiple case reports [2, 4, 14, 15, 18, 19, 24, 25], is likely due to the difference in molecular structure of these agents. Since infliximab is a chimeric IgG1 monoclonal antibody and adalimumab is a fully humanized IgG1 monoclonal antibody and etanercept is a fusion of recombinant soluble TNF-a receptor type 2 with an Fc domain of human IgG1, antibody formation and immune-mediated reactions are more likely to develop against infliximab rather than the latter two molecules. This phenomenon is supported by the above-referenced case studies, in which patients with infliximab-induced hepatitis have successfully transitioned to therapy with etanercept and adalimumab. In our case series, Subject 2 experienced infliximab-induced hepatocellular injury, which resolved after discontinuation of the drug. Therapy was successfully transitioned to adalimumab with no evidence of hepatocellular injury on follow-up laboratory testing, and the patient's disease remained in clinical and endoscopic remission. Thus, in the setting of infliximab-related liver injury, transitioning to an alternate TNF-α antagonist is a reasonable therapeutic strategy.

One clear limitation of our study is the lack of formal causality assessments. However, given the thorough clinical evaluation pursued in each of the three patients, the strong temporal relationship between the drug and liver injury, the lack of other causal factors such as acetaminophen, alcohol, nonalcoholic fatty liver disease, or metabolic syndrome, and, most importantly, the resolution of injury after discontinuation of the offending agent, the authors determined that suspicion for drug-induced injury was sufficient. A second limitation of the study is the small number of patients. However, given the retrospective, observational nature of this study, we believe that our case series is indicative of a larger, underrecognized clinical entity.

In conclusion, TNF-α antagonist-related liver injury is an underrecognized, important clinical entity with potentially serious consequences, such as liver failure. The mechanism of drug-induced injury can be either hepatocellular or autoimmune, and injury can occur irrespective of dose, number of infusions or injections, or time. Given the increasing utilization of TNF-α antagonists, many more patients will be at risk for hepatotoxicity in the future. Larger cohort studies are needed to establish the risk factors and injury patterns related to hepatotoxicity in these patients. Currently, most IBD clinics do not utilize protocols to monitor liver function in patients receiving therapy with TNF-α antagonists, but perhaps this practice should be considered.

Disclosure

Dr. Kaur has received honoraria from UCB Pharmaceuticals and previously served on the speaker's bureau for AbbVie Pharmaceuticals. Dr. Parekh has no relationships to disclose.

References

[1] A. C. Ford, W. J. Sandborn, K. J. Khan, S. B. Hanauer, N. J. Talley, and P. Moayyedi, "Efficacy of biological therapies in inflammatory bowel disease: systematic review and meta-analysis," *American Journal of Gastroenterology*, vol. 106, no. 4, pp. 644–659, 2011.

[2] M. Ghabril, H. L. Bonkovsky, C. Kum et al., "Liver injury from tumor necrosis factor-alpha antagonists: analysis of thirty-four cases," *Clinical Gastroenterology and Hepatology*, vol. 11, no. 5, pp. 558.e3–564.e3, 2013.

[3] O. H. Nielsen and M. A. Ainsworth, "Tumor necrosis factor inhibitors for inflammatory bowel disease," *The New England Journal of Medicine*, vol. 369, no. 8, pp. 754–762, 2013.

[4] S. Mancini, E. Amorotti, S. Vecchio, M. P. de Leon, and L. Roncucci, "Infliximab-related hepatitis: discussion of a case and review of the literature," *Internal and Emergency Medicine*, vol. 5, no. 3, pp. 193–200, 2010.

[5] G. J. Tobon, C. Cañas, J.-J. Jaller, J.-C. Restrepo, and J.-M. Anaya, "Serious liver disease induced by infliximab," *Clinical Rheumatology*, vol. 26, no. 4, pp. 578–581, 2007.

[6] V. V. Menghini and A. S. Arora, "Infliximab-associated reversible cholestatic liver disease," *Mayo Clinic Proceedings*, vol. 76, no. 1, pp. 84–86, 2001.

[7] V. Germano, A. P. Diamanti, G. Baccano et al., "Autoimmune hepatitis associated with infliximab in a patient with psoriatic arthritis," *Annals of the Rheumatic Diseases*, vol. 64, no. 10, pp. 1519–1520, 2005.

[8] G. Ozorio, B. McGarity, H. Bak, A. A. Jordan, H. Lau, and C. Marshall, "Autoimmune hepatitis following infliximab therapy for ankylosing spondylitis," *Medical Journal of Australia*, vol. 187, no. 9, pp. 524–526, 2007.

[9] A. Doyle, G. Forbes, and N. Kontorinis, "Autoimmune hepatitis during infliximab therapy for Crohn's disease: a case report," *Journal of Crohn's and Colitis*, vol. 5, no. 3, pp. 253–255, 2011.

[10] E. Ierardi, N. Della Valle, M. C. Nacchiero, V. De Francesco, G. Stoppino, and C. Panella, "Onset of liver damage after a single administration of infliximab in a patient with refractory ulcerative colitis," *Clinical Drug Investigation*, vol. 26, no. 11, pp. 673–676, 2006.

[11] U. Kinnunen, M. Färkkilä, and H. Mäkisalo, "A case report: ulcerative colitis, treatment with an antibody against tumor necrosis factor (infliximab), and subsequent liver necrosis," *Journal of Crohn's and Colitis*, vol. 6, no. 6, pp. 724–727, 2012.

[12] K. Subramaniam, S. Chitturi, M. Brown, and P. Pavli, "Infliximab-induced autoimmune hepatitis in Crohn's disease treated with budesonide and mycophenolate," *Inflammatory Bowel Diseases*, vol. 17, no. 11, pp. e149–e150, 2011.

[13] M. Regueiro, W. Schraut, L. Baidoo et al., "Infliximab prevents Crohn's disease recurrence after ileal resection," *Gastroenterology*, vol. 136, no. 2, pp. 441.e1–450.e1, 2009.

[14] K. M. Carlsen, L. Riis, and O. R. Madsen, "Toxic hepatitis induced by infliximab in a patient with rheumatoid arthritis with no relapse after switching to etanercept," *Clinical Rheumatology*, vol. 28, no. 8, pp. 1001–1003, 2009.

[15] A. Haennig, D. Bonnet, S. Thebault, and L. Alric, "Infliximab-induced acute hepatitis during Crohn's disease therapy: absence of cross-toxicity with adalimumab," *Gastroenterologie Clinique et Biologique*, vol. 34, no. 8-9, pp. e7–e8, 2010.

[16] T. Adar, M. Mizrahi, O. Pappo, A. Scheiman-Elazary, and O. Shibolet, "Adalimumab-induced autoimmune hepatitis," *Journal of Clinical Gastroenterology*, vol. 44, no. 1, pp. e20–e22, 2010.

[17] C. S. Coffin, H. F. Fraser, R. Panaccione, and S. Ghosh, "Liver diseases associated with anti-tumor necrosis factor-alpha (TNF-α) use for inflammatory bowel disease," *Inflammatory Bowel Diseases*, vol. 17, no. 1, pp. 479–484, 2011.

[18] M. Cravo, R. Silva, and M. Serrano, "Autoimmune hepatitis induced by infliximab in a patient with crohn's disease with no relapse after switching to adalimumab," *BioDrugs*, vol. 24, supplement 1, pp. 25–27, 2010.

[19] D. A. Goldfeld, E. C. Verna, J. Lefkowitch, and A. Swaminath, "Infliximab-induced autoimmune hepatitis with successful switch to adalimumab in a patient with Crohn's disease: the index case," *Digestive Diseases and Sciences*, vol. 56, no. 11, pp. 3386–3388, 2011.

[20] Administration, U.S.F.a.D, "Remicaide Label and Approval History," 2009.

[21] S. C. Chen, O. W. Cummings, M. P. Hartley, C. A. Filomena, and W. K. Cho, "Hepatocellular carcinoma occurring in a patient with Crohn's disease treated with both azathioprine and infliximab," *Digestive Diseases and Sciences*, vol. 51, no. 5, pp. 952–955, 2006.

[22] T. Davern, Drug Induced Liver Disease, 2007: Informa Healthcare, 2007.

[23] O. S. Khokhar and J. H. Lewis, "Hepatotoxicity of agents used in the management of inflammatory bowel disease," *Digestive Diseases*, vol. 28, no. 3, pp. 508–518, 2010.

[24] A. M. García Aparicio, J. R. Rey, A. H. Sanz, and J. S. Alvarez, "Successful treatment with etanercept in a patient with hepatotoxicity closely related to infliximab," *Clinical Rheumatology*, vol. 26, no. 5, pp. 811–813, 2007.

[25] M. Massarotti and B. Marasini, "Successful treatment with etanercept of a patient with psoriatic arthritis after adalimumab-related hepatotoxicity," *International Journal of Immunopathology and Pharmacology*, vol. 22, no. 2, pp. 547–549, 2009.

3

Postoperative Megarectum in an Adult Patient with Imperforate Anus and Rectourethral Fistula

Yoshifumi Nakayama,[1,2] Toshihito Uehara,[1,2] Masaki Akiyama,[1,2] Noritaka Minagawa,[1] Takayuki Torigoe,[1] and Naohiro Fujimoto[3]

[1]*Department of Surgery 1, School of Medicine, University of Occupational and Environmental Health, 1-1 Iseigaoka, Yahata-nishi-ku, Kitakyushu 807-8555, Japan*
[2]*Department of Gastroenterological and General Surgery, Wakamatsu Hospital of University of Occupational and Environmental Health, 1-17-1 Hamamachi, Wakamatsu-ku, Kitakyushu 808-0024, Japan*
[3]*Department of Urology, School of Medicine, University of Occupational and Environmental Health, 1-1 Iseigaoka, Yahata-nishi-ku, Kitakyushu 807-8555, Japan*

Correspondence should be addressed to Yoshifumi Nakayama; nakayama@med.uoeh-u.ac.jp

Academic Editor: Fadi H. Mourad

This report presents a surgical case of postoperative megarectum in an adult patient with imperforate anus/anorectal malformations. A 71-year-old Japanese male presented with a mass in the lower abdomen which was 15 × 12 × 8 cm in diameter, edema in the right lower extremity, and frequent urination. He had undergone sigmoid loop colostomy for an imperforate anus as a newborn infant. At 28 years of age, the sigmoid loop colostomy was changed to sigmoid divided colostomy in the left lower abdomen. Computed tomography revealed a large cystic mass in the lower abdomen. Retrograde urethrography indicated a rectourethral fistula and megarectum with stones. A small laparotomy incision was created in the right lower abdomen, and the wall of the megarectum was identified. Approximately 2,300 mL of gray muddy fluid was identified and drained. A mucous fistula of the upper rectum was created in the right lower abdomen. This is an extremely rare case of postoperative megarectum in an adult patient with an imperforate anus and rectourethral fistula.

1. Introduction

Imperforate anus/anorectal malformations occur in approximately 1 in 5000 births [1, 2]. This rare anomaly is usually detected and repaired by pediatric surgeons during the neonatal period or early infancy. Imperforate anus is conventionally classified into three main types [3, 4]. In patients with a high imperforate anus, the bowel ends above the pelvic floor, typically with a fistula to the prostatic urethra in males or the posterior vaginal fornix in females. In patients with an intermediate imperforate anus, the bowel traverses the pelvic floor with its crucial puborectalis sling but fails to migrate back to the normal anal site. A low imperforate anus involves a covered anus or anal stenosis [3].

Megarectum is a rare condition defined as follows. Patients with idiopathic megarectum have a bowel diameter greater than 6.5 cm at the pelvic brim on a lateral X-ray of the abdomen [5]. The *Principles of Surgery* textbook describes a rectum that can hold more than 1,500 cc of fluid as a megarectum. The term megarectum is also used to describe large rectal masses detected on rectal examinations.

This report presents an extremely rare surgical case of postoperative megarectum in an adult patient with an imperforate anus.

2. Case Report

A 71-year-old Japanese male presented with an increasing lower abdominal mass and frequent urination. He had undergone sigmoid loop colostomy for an imperforate anus as a newborn. At 28 years of age, he underwent an operation for which the details are unclear. At that time, the

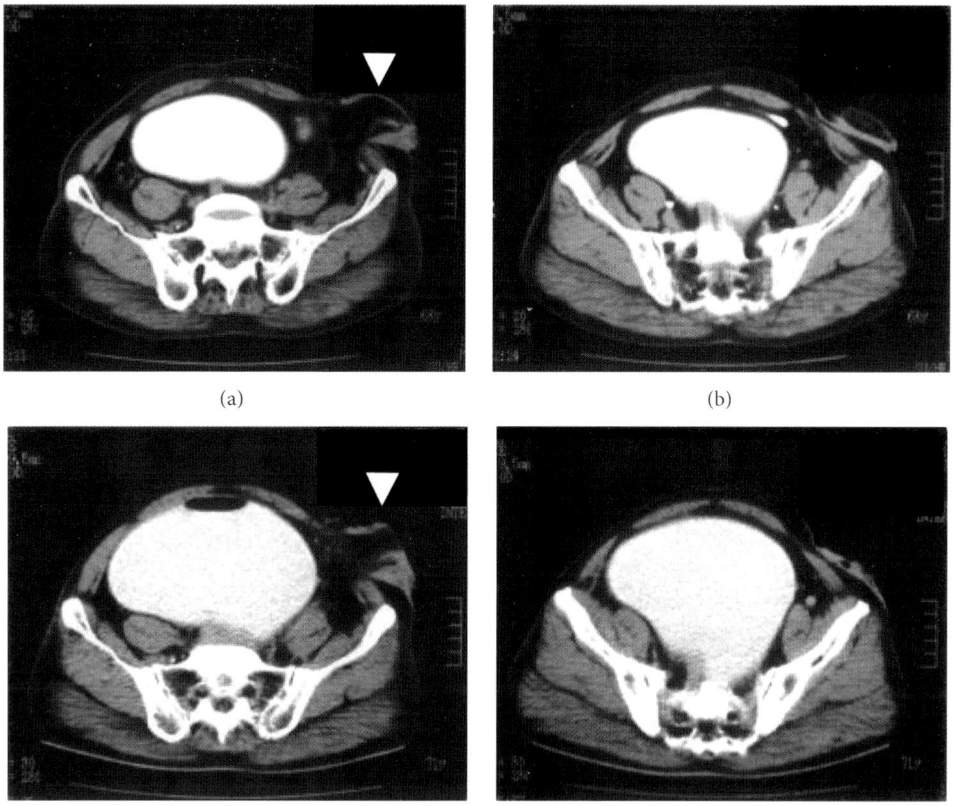

(a) (b) (c) (d)

FIGURE 1: Computed tomography (CT) revealed a large cystic mass in the pelvic cavity at our surgical outpatient clinic ((c), (d)) and at another hospital two years previously ((a), (b)). A sigmoid divided colostomy was created in the left lower abdomen (arrow head).

sigmoid loop colostomy was changed to sigmoid divided colostomy in the left lower abdomen. The patient had not used the colostomy pouch before arriving at our hospital. He was referred to the surgical outpatient clinic for a detailed examination and surgical treatment of an increasing lower abdominal mass, edema of the right lower extremity, and frequent urination. Computed tomography (CT) revealed a large cystic mass measuring 15 × 12 × 8 cm in diameter in the lower abdomen (Figures 1(c) and 1(d)). CT performed two years previously at the other hospital showed a smaller cystic mass measuring 11 cm × 8 cm in diameter in the lower abdomen (Figures 1(a) and 1(b)). Retrograde urethrography indicated a rectourethral fistula and megarectum with stones (Figure 2(a)). Moreover, magnetic resonance imaging (MRI) revealed a megarectum with stones (Figure 2(b)).

A physical examination revealed a mass in the lower abdomen which was 15 × 12 × 8 cm in diameter and edema of the right lower extremity. A sigmoid colostomy incision was created in the patient's left lower abdomen. Laboratory investigations revealed a white blood cell count of 6,700/mm^3, a hemoglobin level of 13.9 g/dL with a hematocrit value of 40.9%, and a platelet count of 205,000/mm^3. The renal and liver function test results were all within the normal limits. Coagulation studies revealed prothrombin time of 12.3 seconds and activated partial thromboplastin time of 25.6 seconds.

A small laparotomy incision was created in the right lower abdomen, and a wall of the megarectum was identified. Approximately 2,300 mL of gray muddy fluid was identified and drained. A mucous fistula of the upper rectum was created in the right lower abdomen.

The patient had an uneventful recovery. He was discharged from the hospital on the fourteenth day after the operation and was followed up in the outpatient clinic without recurrence of the lower abdominal mass (Figure 3), edema of the right lower extremity, or frequent urination.

3. Discussion

Imperforate anus/anorectal malformations are classified into three main groups high (supralevator), intermediate, and low (translevator) according to the relationship between the end of the bowel and pelvic floor [3]. In addition, high and intermediate malformations are subdivided into those with and without fistulas [3]. In the present case, a retrograde urethrography indicated a rectourethral fistula between the prostate urethra and lower rectum, and the distal end of the rectum was located beyond the pelvic floor (Figure 2(a)). Therefore, the patient was diagnosed with a high imperforate anus and rectourethral fistula.

In the present case, the diameter of the expanded rectum was 15 × 12 cm, and the rectum contained 2,300 mL of

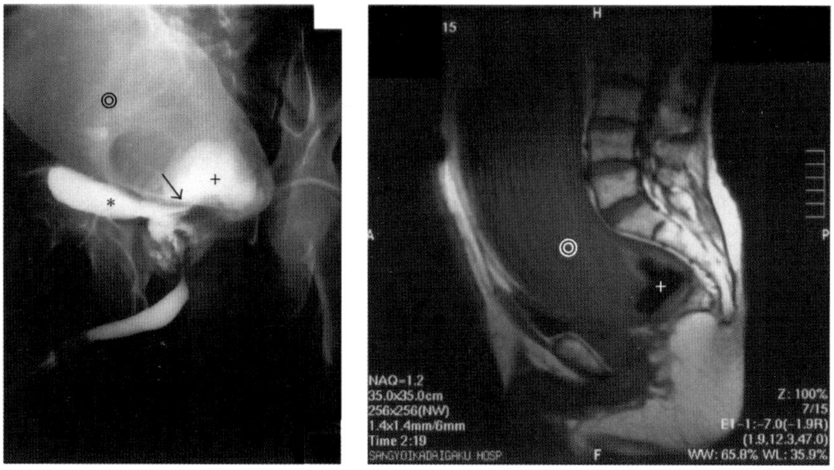

(a) (b)

FIGURE 2: (a) Retrograde urethrography indicated a dilated rectum (black double concentric circles), urinary bladder (black star), and rectourethral fistula between the prostate urethra and lower rectum (black arrow) with stones (black cross). (b) Magnetic resonance imaging (MRI) revealed a megarectum (white double open circles) with stones (white cross).

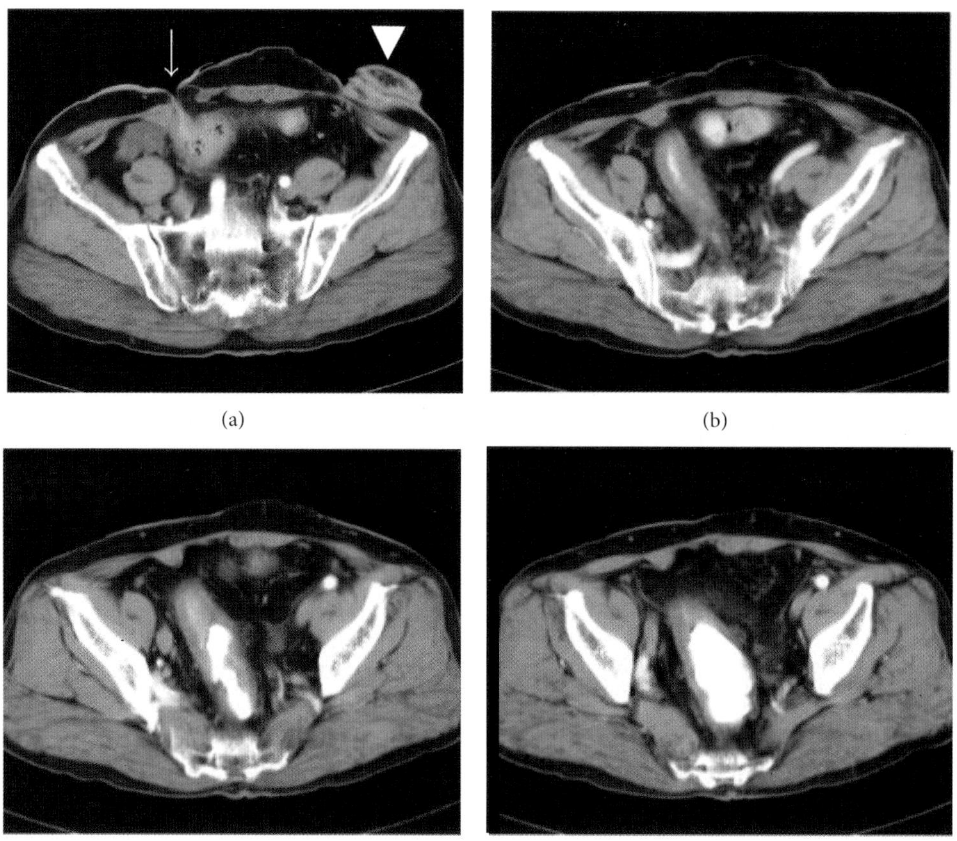

(a) (b)

(c) (d)

FIGURE 3: CT performed after surgery indicated that the rectal dilation had resolved ((a), (b), (c), and (d)). A mucous fistula of the upper rectum was created in the right lower abdomen (arrow). A sigmoid divided colostomy was created in the left lower abdomen (arrow head).

gray muddy fluid. Therefore, the patient was diagnosed with megarectum. Megarectum is caused by several factors, including severe constipation [6], Hirschsprung's disease, anorectal obstruction, and disorders of the endocrine and central nervous systems [7]. Idiopathic megarectum is an unusual cause of intractable constipation [8, 9], presenting with a chronically dilated rectum alone or in combination with the colon with a morphologically normal small intestine. However, the cause of megarectum in the present case has not been previously reported. We speculate that the cause of the megarectum in this case reflected closure of the anal stump of the sigmoid loop colostomy and rectourethral fistula. The semiclosed cavity of the rectum between the rectosigmoid region and anus may have resulted from the previous operation and then was gradually dilated by the urine due to the rectourethral fistula between the prostate urethra and lower rectum.

Surgical cases of imperforate anus with rectourethral fistulas in adulthood are extremely rare [10, 11]. Odaka et al. reported an unusual case of anorectal agenesis with a rectourethral fistula in a 48-years-old male who was treated with end colostomy and resection of the rectourethral fistula, dilated rectum, and sigmoid colon [10]. Resection of the megarectum and repair of the rectourethral fistula could have been performed in this case. However, a mucous fistula of the upper rectum was created in the right lower abdomen because the patient rejected major surgery.

In conclusion, this report presented a rare surgical case of postoperative megarectum in an adult patient with an imperforate anus and rectourethral fistula.

Authors' Contribution

Yoshifumi Nakayama contributed to the drafting and the editing of the paper. Toshihito Uehara contributed to obtain the clinical details. Masaki Akiyama contributed to literature search. Noritaka Minagawa and Takayuki Torigoe helped in drafting the paper. Naohiro Fujimoto edited the paper.

References

[1] F. D. Stephen and E. D. Smith, "Anatomy and function of the normal rectum and anus; individual deformities in the female; operative management of anal deformities," in *Anorectal Malformations in Children*, F. D. Stephen, Ed., pp. 212–273, Year Book, Chicago, Ill, USA, 1971.

[2] E. D. Smith, "Incidencem frequency of type, and etiology of anrectal malformations," in *Anorectal Malformations in Children*, F. D. Stephens and E. D. Smith, Eds., pp. 231–246, 1988.

[3] H. H. Nixon, "Anorectal anomalies: with an international proposed classification," *Postgraduate Medical Journal*, vol. 48, no. 562, pp. 465–470, 1972.

[4] F. D. Stephens and E. D. Smith, "Classification, identification, and assessment of surgical treatment of anorectal anomalies," *Pediatric Surgery International*, vol. 1, no. 4, pp. 200–205, 1986.

[5] D. M. Preston, J. E. Lennard-Jones, and B. M. Thomas, "Towards a radiologic definition of idiopathic megacolon," *Gastrointestinal Radiology*, vol. 10, no. 2, pp. 167–169, 1985.

[6] R. N. van der Plas, M. A. Benninga, C. R. Staalman et al., "Megarectum in constipation," *Archives of Disease in Childhood*, vol. 83, no. 1, pp. 52–58, 2000.

[7] T. Ehrenpreis, "Megacolon and megarectum in older children and young adults: classification and terminology," *Proceedings of the Royal Society of Medicine*, vol. 60, no. 8, pp. 799–801, 1967.

[8] P. Belliveau, S. M. Goldberg, D. A. Rothenberger, and S. Nivatvongs, "Idiopathic acquired megacolon: the value of subtotal colectomy," *Diseases of the Colon & Rectum*, vol. 25, no. 2, pp. 118–121, 1982.

[9] M. A. Kamm and G. Stabile, "Management of idiopathic megarectum and megacolon," *British Journal of Surgery*, vol. 78, no. 8, pp. 899–900, 1991.

[10] A. Odaka, S. Takahashi, T. Tanimizu et al., "Anorectal agenesis with a rectourethral fistula diagnosed in an adult: report of a case," *Surgery Today*, vol. 34, no. 2, pp. 170–172, 2004.

[11] K. Hirano, K. Watanabe, H. Nakamura, I. Iwasaki, and K. Yanagida, "A case of imperforate anus (ano-rectal agenesis with recto-urethral fistula) in adult," *Japanese Journal of Pediatric Surgery*, vol. 29, pp. 661–668, 1997 (Japanese).

4

Acute on Chronic Pancreatitis Causing a Highway to the Colon with Subsequent Road Closure: Pancreatic Colonic Fistula Presenting as a Large Bowel Obstruction Treated with Pancreatic Duct Stenting

Justin Cochrane[1] and Greg Schlepp

[1]*Junior Faculty Spokane Teaching Health Center (Internal Medicine Residency), Providence Sacred Heart Medical Center, Spokane, WA 99204, USA*
[2]*Spokane Digestive Disease Center, Spokane, WA 99204, USA*

Correspondence should be addressed to Justin Cochrane; justin.cochrane@providence.org

Academic Editor: Hideto Kawaratani

Context. Colonic complications associated with acute pancreatitis have a low incidence but carry an increased risk of mortality with delayed diagnosis and treatment. Pancreatic colonic fistula is most commonly associated with walled off pancreatic necrosis or abscess formation and rarely forms spontaneously. Classic clinical manifestations for pancreatic colonic fistula include diarrhea, hematochezia, and fever. Uncommonly pancreatic colonic fistula presents as large bowel obstruction. *Case.* We report a case of a woman with a history of recurrent episodes of acute pancreatitis who presented with large bowel obstruction secondary to pancreatic colonic fistula. Resolution of large bowel obstruction and pancreatic colonic fistula was achieved with pancreatic duct stenting. *Conclusion.* Pancreatic colonic fistula can present as large bowel obstruction. Patients with resolved acute pancreatitis who have radiographic evidence of splenic flexure obstruction, but without evidence of mechanical obstruction on colonoscopy, should be considered for ERCP to evaluate for PCF. PCF not associated with walled off pancreatic necrosis or peritoneal abscess can be treated conservatively with pancreatic duct stenting.

1. Introduction

Pancreatic colonic fistula (PCF) occurs in 0.4 to 5% of patients with acute pancreatitis [1, 2]. Most cases of PCF formation occur secondary to percutaneous drainage or surgical debridement of pancreatic necrosis. Typical clinical manifestations are diarrhea, hematochezia, and fever [3]. Rarely does PCF present as large bowel obstruction. A 73-year-old female with acute on chronic pancreatitis developed large bowel obstruction secondary to spontaneous PCF formation.

2. Case

Mrs. L is a 73-year-old female with a history of chronic pancreatitis secondary to chronic alcohol abuse who presented to an outside hospital with worsening abdominal pain and distention. At the outside hospital she was diagnosed with pancreatitis. She received pain medication, intravenous fluids, and bowel rest. She demonstrated no signs of clinical improvement with conservative medical management over the next 48 hours. CT imaging of the abdomen/pelvis demonstrated inflammatory stranding around the splenic flexure of the colon and two small fluid collections (3.6 cm and 4.7 cm) adjacent to pancreatic tail and splenic flexure (Figures 1–3). No mechanical obstruction was noted on colonoscopy. Abdominal pain and distention improved after colonoscopy but returned over the next 24 hours. Repeat CT imaging 4 days later demonstrated high grade obstruction of the large bowel with stricture at the splenic flexure with fluid collections remaining stable and resolution of the colonic inflammatory stranding (Figure 4).

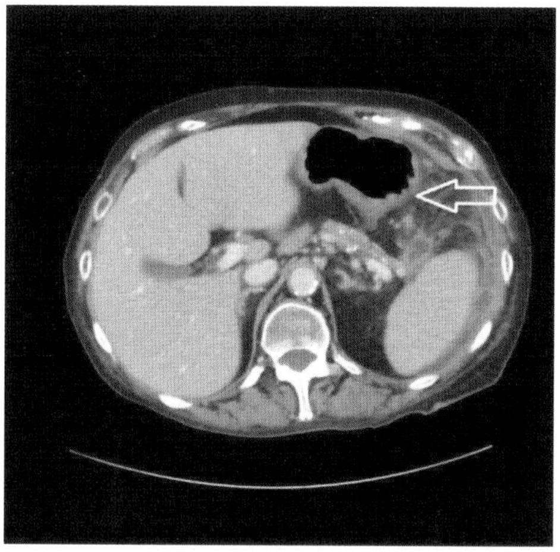

Figure 1: CT abdomen/pelvis done at time of admission to outside hospital showing colonic thickening at the splenic flexure.

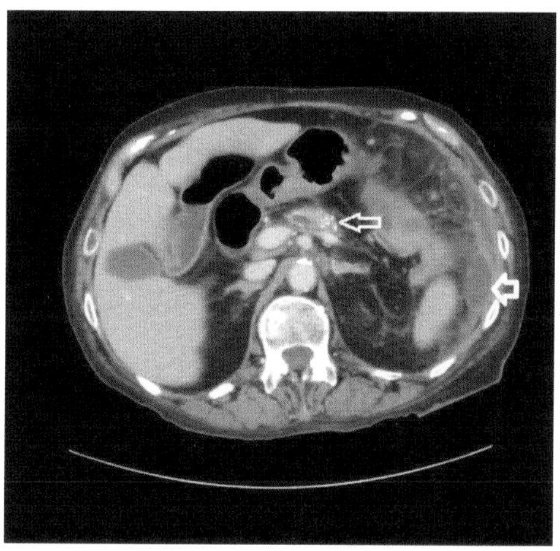

Figure 2: CT abdomen/pelvis done at outside hospital at time of admission: Fat arrow indicates fluid collection near the pancreatic tail and splenic flexure 3.5 cm. Skinny arrow calcification of the pancreas suggesting chronic pancreatitis.

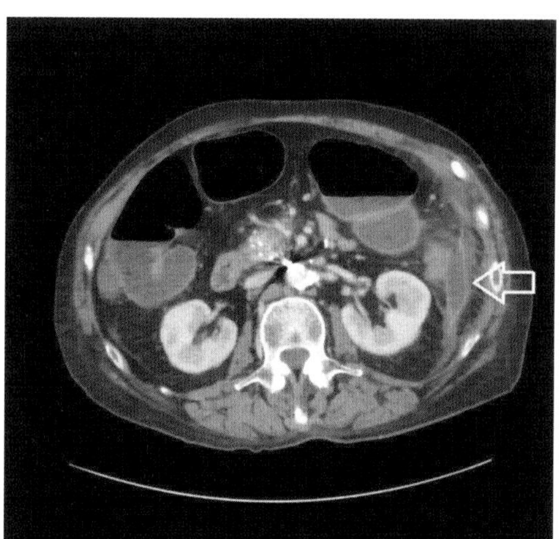

Figure 3: CT abdomen/pelvis done at outside hospital at time of admission showing fluid collection around the pancreatic tail and splenic flexure 4.7 cm.

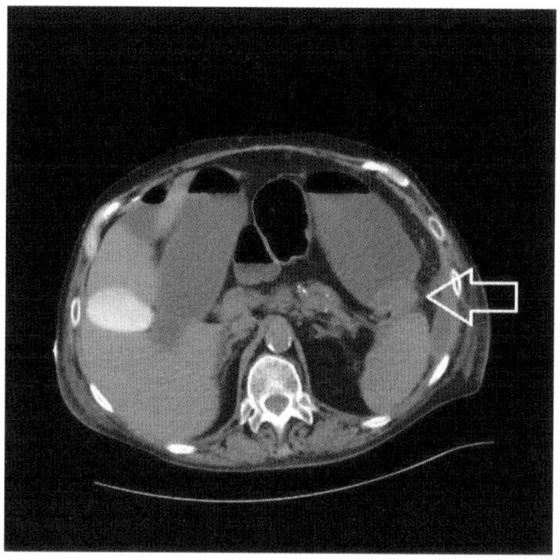

Figure 4: CT abdomen/pelvis done at admission to tertiary medical center demonstrating cut-off sign at the splenic flexure with distended transverse colon.

She was transferred to a tertiary medical center for surgical evaluation. She continued to have 10/10 diffuse abdominal pain and distention. Physical exam showed normal vitals with diffuse abdominal pain, no rebounding or guarding, and diffuse abdominal distention with no obvious fluid wave or shifting dullness. Laboratory tests showed total bilirubin 0.7 mg/dL, INR 1.2, and albumin 3.0 g/dL, liver enzymes ALP 143 U/L, AST 20 IU/L, ALT 6 IU/L, lipase 469 units/mg, hemoglobin 11.5 g/dL, WBC 19×10^9/L, and PLT 265×10^9/L.

Colorectal surgery was consulted and identified neither pericolonic abscesses nor an intraluminal obstruction. A repeat colonoscopy was performed at our institution for colonic decompression and inspection of the splenic flexure for possible intraluminal obstruction. Colonoscopy demonstrated increased luminal diameter in the descending and sigmoid colon without visible signs of mechanical obstruction or fistula near the splenic flexure. Several pedunculated polyps and serrated polyps were identified, but no evidence of colorectal cancer was present. After colonoscopy she again reported decrease in abdominal pain and distention but returned 48 hours after colonoscopy.

Secondary to CT imaging showing fluid collections at the tail of the pancreas with extension near the splenic flexure endoscopic retrograde cholangiopancreatography (ERCP) was performed to further evaluate the pancreatic duct (Figure 5). The pancreatogram demonstrated tortuosity of the pancreatic duct with extravasation of contrast from the tail of the pancreas into the colon confirming a pancreatic colonic fistula (Figure 6). A single 7-French 12 cm plastic stent was placed in the pancreatic duct with subsequent improvement of abdominal pain and abdominal distention. She continued to improve and had return of her bowel function. On follow-up at 3 months she continued to have no abdominal pain or distention. Repeat ERCP at 3 months confirmed resolution of the pancreatic colonic fistula (Figure 7).

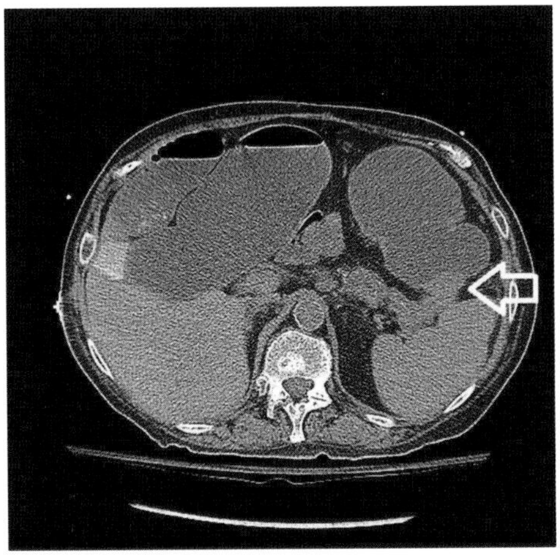

FIGURE 5: CT abdominal/pelvis obtained after repeat colonoscopy negative for intraluminal obstruction and return of abdominal distention and increase of abdominal pain. Question of pancreatic colonic fistula.

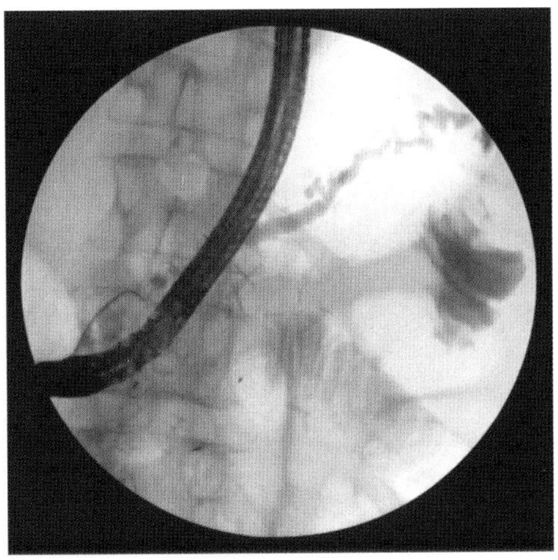

FIGURE 6: Pancreatogram demonstrating pancreatic colonic fistula.

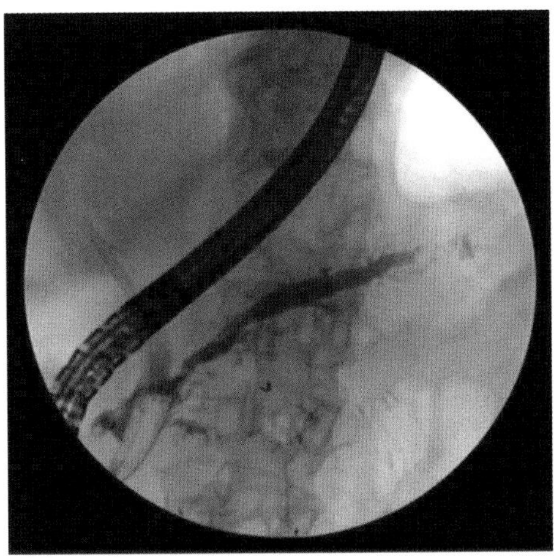

FIGURE 7: Pancreatogram after removal of 7F × 12 cm pigtail plastic stent in place for 3 months with resolution of the pancreatic colonic fistula.

3. Discussion

PCF incidence ranges 0.4–5% with symptoms typically including diarrhea, hematochezia, fever, and abdominal pain [1, 2]. Hematochezia is the most common clinical manifestation found in 60% of patients and is associated with mortality rate of 77% [3]. Obstruction accounts for less than 1% [1].

Majority of PCF formation occurs in association with walled off pancreatic necrosis or abscess. WOPN or abscess causes destruction of the pancreatic parenchyma with release of digestive enzymes into the surrounding peritoneum causing fistula tract formation. Formation occurs days to month after acute pancreatitis. Discovery of PCF is usually after percutaneous catheter placement for drainage of WOPN or abscess with "tube checking" via fluoroscopy demonstrating contrast flow into the colon via the fistula tract. Surgical debridement of WOPN with subsequent identification has also been described. PCF not associated with WOPN or abscess is believed to be secondary to extension of necrosis into the transverse colon or pseudocyst that expands and applies pressure to the transverse colon causing erosion with tract formation.

In a study from Mayo [4] clinic 8 patients were identified with PCF formation of which 1 (12%) was spontaneous and 7 formed after debridement of pancreatic necrosis at 4 to 60 days. Identification can be difficult due to nonspecific symptoms (nausea, vomiting, and abdominal pain) and the insidious nature of PCF leading to diagnosis several months after initial episode of pancreatitis. Enhanced CT Imaging may show air fluid levels in a necrotic pancreas or directly visualize a fistula tract to the colon. However, CT may demonstrate obstruction or bowel wall thickening which may be interpreted as mechanical obstruction or colitis. High clinical suspicion for PCF warrants an investigation with ERCP to evaluate contrast extravasation into the colon along a fistula tract. Kochhar et al. [1] identified 4 patients with PCF via ERCP or colonoscopy 12 to 20 days after an episode of pancreatitis. Only 1 of these 4 patients presented with large bowel obstruction identified via CT imaging with dilated ascending colon.

Conservative treatment for PCF with bowel rest and antibiotics is associated with a 50% mortality if sepsis or hemorrhagic transformation occurs [5]. Surgical treatment with laparotomy or open repair improves mortality to 15%. Heeter et al. [3] identified 20 patients with PCF treated with antibiotics, percutaneous drainage, and pancreatic duct stent, but this was associated with abscess or WOPN as the source of PCF. Several other small case series have data showing resolution of spontaneous PCF with endoscopic clips being placed in the pancreatic duct or in the colon [6–8]. Limited case reports of treatment of PCF with pancreatic stents alone are effective [5].

Mrs. L case was unique in that her PCF was secondary to recurrent pancreatitis and extension of a pseudocyst in the tail of the pancreas into the transverse colon causing erosion and fistula tract formation. Lacking association with WOPN or abscess allowed conservative treatment with pancreatic stent placement. Resolution of the fistula at 3 months was demonstrated with no-hemorrhagic or septic conversion.

PCF can present as large bowel obstruction. Patients with resolved acute pancreatitis who have radiographic evidence of splenic flexure obstruction, but without evidence of mechanical obstruction on colonoscopy, should be considered for ERCP to evaluate for PCF. PCF not associated with WOPN or peritoneal abscess can be treated conservatively with pancreatic duct stenting.

References

[1] R. Kochhar, K. Jain, V. Gupta et al., "Fistulization in the GI tract in acute pancreatitis," *Gastrointestinal Endoscopy*, vol. 75, no. 2, pp. 436–440, 2012.

[2] R. Rerknimitr, N. Lakananurak, P. Prueksapanich et al., "A fatal case of a colonic fistula communicating with a walled-off area of pancreatic necrosis," *Endoscopy*, vol. 46, no. 1, pp. E30–E31, 2014.

[3] Z. R. Heeter, E. Hauptmann, R. Crane et al., "Pancreaticocolonic fistulas secondary to severe acute pancreatitis treated by percutaneous drainage: successful nonsurgical outcomes in a single-center case series," *Journal of Vascular and Interventional Radiology*, vol. 24, no. 1, pp. 122–129, 2013.

[4] G. G. Tsiotos, C. D. Smith, and M. G. Sarr, "Incidence and management of pancreatic and enteric fistulas after surgical management of severe necrotizing pancreatitis," *Archives of Surgery*, vol. 130, no. 1, pp. 48–52, 1995.

[5] C. T. Thomas, P. J. Hinton, and E. Thomas, "Spontaneous pancreatic duct-colon fistula," *Journal of Clinical Gastroenterology*, vol. 8, no. 1, pp. 69–73, 1986.

[6] Y. Igarashi, T. Mimura, Y. Kishimoto et al., "Severe acute pancreatitis with complicating colonic fistula successfully closed using the over-the-scope clip system," *Case Reports in Gastroenterology*, vol. 7, no. 2, pp. 314–321, 2013.

[7] K. Fujii, K. Suzuki, A. Goto et al., "Pancreatic-colonic fistula successfully treated with endoscopic transpapillary nasopancreatic drainage," *Endoscopy*, vol. 43, supplement 2, pp. E154–E155, 2011.

[8] A. Kirschniak, N. Subotova, D. Zieker, A. Königsrainer, and T. Kratt, "The Over-The-Scope Clip (OTSC) for the treatment of gastrointestinal bleeding, perforations, and fistulas," *Surgical Endoscopy*, vol. 25, no. 9, pp. 2901–2905, 2011.

5

Deciphering Autoimmune Pancreatitis, a Great Mimicker: Case Report and Review of the Literature

Satya Allaparthi, Mohammed Sageer, and Mark J. Sterling

Lahey Clinic, Burlington, MA 01805, USA

Correspondence should be addressed to Satya Allaparthi; surgsatya@yahoo.com

Academic Editor: Haruhiko Sugimura

Background. Autoimmune pancreatitis (AIP) is an atypical chronic inflammatory pancreatic disease that appears to involve autoimmune mechanisms. In recent years, AIP has presented as a new clinical entity with its protean pancreaticobiliary and systemic presentations. Its unique pathology and overlap of clinical and radiological features and absence of serological markers foster the disease's unique position. We report a case of diffuse type 1 autoimmune pancreatitis with obstructive jaundice managed with biliary sphincterotomy, stent placement, and corticosteroids. A 50-year-old Caucasian woman presented to our hospital with epigastric pain, nausea, vomiting, and jaundice. Workup showed elevated liver function tests (LFT) suggestive of obstructive jaundice, MRCP done showed diffusely enlarged abnormal appearing pancreas with loss of normal lobulated contours, and IgG4 antibody level was 765 mg/dL. EUS revealed a diffusely hypoechoic and rounded pancreatic parenchyma with distal common bile duct (CBD) stricture and dilated proximal CBD and common hepatic duct (CHD). ERCP showed tight mid to distal CBD stricture that needed dilatation, sphincterotomy, and placement of stent that led to significant improvement in the symptoms and bilirubin level. Based on clinical, radiological, and immunological findings, a definitive diagnosis of AIP was made. Patient was started on prednisone 40 mg/day and she clinically responded in 4 weeks.

1. Introduction

In 1961, Sarles et al. [1] first described a case series of unusual pancreatitis associated with obstructive jaundice and hyper-g globulinemia. However, it was not until 1995 that Yoshida et al. [2] termed autoimmune pancreatitis to describe a case of diffusely enlarged pancreas with irregularly narrowing pancreatic duct that was serologically associated with hyper-g-globulinemia, anti-nuclear antibody positivity, and responsivity to steroid treatment.

Clinically, AIP is characterized by protean symptoms that have many features in common with pancreatic cancer. These symptoms include abdominal pain, obstructive jaundice, weight loss, steatorrhea, new-onset diabetes mellitus (DM), and elevated levels of serum tumor markers. Hardacre et al. in their single institutional study reported that about 2.5% of pancreatoduodenectomies were performed in AIP patients following a mistaken diagnosis of pancreatic cancer [3]. Since AIP responds extremely well to steroid therapy, it is of utmost importance that it be differentiated from pancreatic cancer to avoid unnecessary laparotomy or pancreatic resection. AIP is frequently associated with other systemic autoimmune diseases, such as rheumatoid arthritis, Sjogren's syndrome, sarcoidosis, and inflammatory bowel diseases.

The diagnosis of AIP is challenging as it closely mimics pancreatic cancer. We further report a case of a 50-year-old Caucasian woman who presented with epigastric pain, nausea, vomiting, and jaundice. Subsequent workup revealed AIP as the etiology of her symptoms, and she was treated effectively with steroids.

2. Case Presentation and Management

A 50-year-old Caucasian woman presented to our hospital with 2-day duration of epigastric pain, nausea, vomiting, and jaundice. Her physical examination was unremarkable except for scleral icterus. An abdominal examination revealed epigastric tenderness without rebound. Laboratory investigations revealed hemoglobin 12.9 g/dL, white blood cell count 9.6/μL, serum lipase 109 U/L, serum amylase

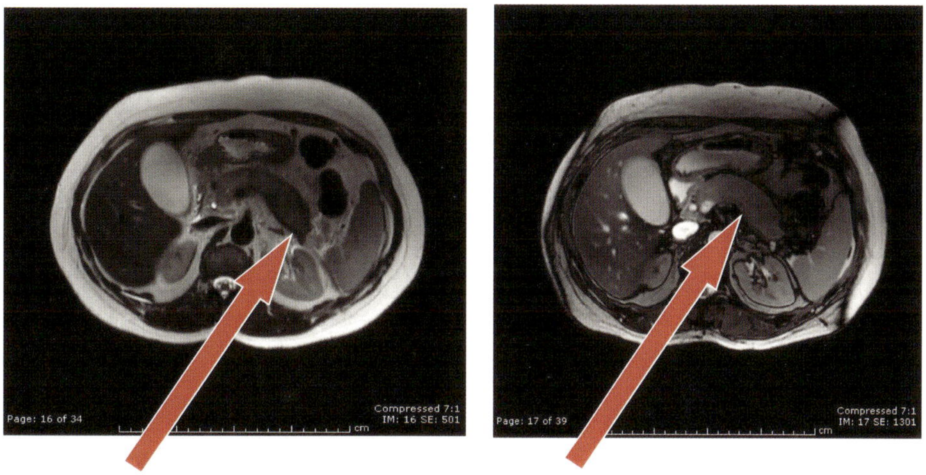

FIGURE 1: MRCP images arrow showing sausage-like pancreas in delayed phase.

10 U/L, and total bilirubin 10.6 mg/dL (direct and indirect fractions 8 mg/dL and 2.6 mg/dL, resp.). Her liver enzymes were elevated (aspartate aminotransferase 110 U/L, alanine aminotransferase 131 U/L, and alkaline phosphatase 389 U/L). Tests for hepatitis A, B, and C are negative and found to have elevated immunoglobulin IgG Ab level of 765 mg/dl. Given these lab findings and clinical presentation, MRCP was further ordered which showed diffusely enlarged abnormal appearing pancreas with loss of normal lobulated contours. The pancreatic parenchyma is diffusely hypoenhancing, with focal hypoenhancement within pancreatic head, distal body, and tail (Figure 1). In view of her clinical presentation with worsening jaundice and MRCP findings, an endoscopic ultrasound (EUS) was done that revealed a diffusely hypoechoic and rounded pancreatic parenchyma with distal common bile duct (CBD) stricture and dilated proximal CBD and common hepatic duct (CHD) (Figure 2). Endoscopic retrograde cholangiopancreatography (ERCP) showed tight mid to distal CBD stricture that needed dilatation, sphincterotomy, and placement of stent that significantly improved her clinical symptoms and bilirubin level (Figure 3). She was started on tapering dose of prednisone 40 mg/day and 4 weeks after treatment she improved clinically and radiologically. Our ability to recognize AIP and differentiate it from pancreatic adenocarcinoma is aided by the use of international consensus criteria.

3. Discussion

Autoimmune pancreatitis is rare disease with a much lower rate of incidence than its principal differential diagnosis, pancreatic cancer. The overall incidence and prevalence are still unclear owing to lack of prospective natural history studies. Study series from Japan have reported the prevalence of autoimmune pancreatitis in a range between 5 and 6% of all patients with chronic pancreatitis of which 6–8% (0.82 per 100,000) had pancreatic resections performed for presumed pancreatic cancer [4, 5]. Moreover, in the last two decades, there has been an increase in the number of reports of autoimmune pancreatitis in the medical literature; however, the overall number of patients is still relatively small. Though this clinical entity was well described initially in Japan, a growing awareness of the condition has led to reports around the world. Hamano et al. [6] reported that serum IgG4 levels are specifically elevated in Japanese patients with AIP; however, in further reported case series by Hirano et al. [7] and Pezzilli and Corinaldesi [8], an increase of IgG4 levels in AIP cohorts has been also confirmed in Western and Eastern countries. Although the pathogenesis of the disease is unknown, current evidence strongly suggests that an autoimmune process has been implicated [9, 10]. Unlike most autoimmune conditions, AIP has a male predominance, with a male : female ratio of 2 : 1. The peak age of onset is the sixth and seventh decades [5, 9, 11].

The histopathological hallmark findings in patients with AIP include dense infiltration of T lymphocytes, IgG4-positive plasma cells, storiform fibrosis, and obliterative phlebitis in the pancreas; this form is termed lymphoplasmacytic sclerosing pancreatitis (LPSP) [12–14]. Of late, recent studies have provided evidence that there is another subtype of AIP with different histological findings named as idiopathic duct-centric pancreatitis (IDCP) that is more prevalent in Europe and the United States [15, 16]. Recent studies showed consensus that LPSP and IDCP are regarded as two distinct subtypes of AIP, and it has been proposed that LPSP be called "type 1 AIP" and IDCP "type 2 AIP" [17, 18].

In 2011, an international panel of experts met during the 14th Congress of the International Association of Pancreatology held in Fukuoka, Japan, and an international consensus diagnostic criterion for AIP was proposed [19]. According to these, AIP is classified into type 1 and 2. Five cardinal features of AIP are used: imaging of pancreatic parenchyma and ducts; serology; other organ involvement; pancreatic histology; and an optional criterion of response to steroid therapy. Each feature is categorized as a level 1 or 2 finding, depending on the diagnostic reliability (as shown in Table 1).

AIP should always be included in the differential diagnosis particularly in elderly presenting with obstructive

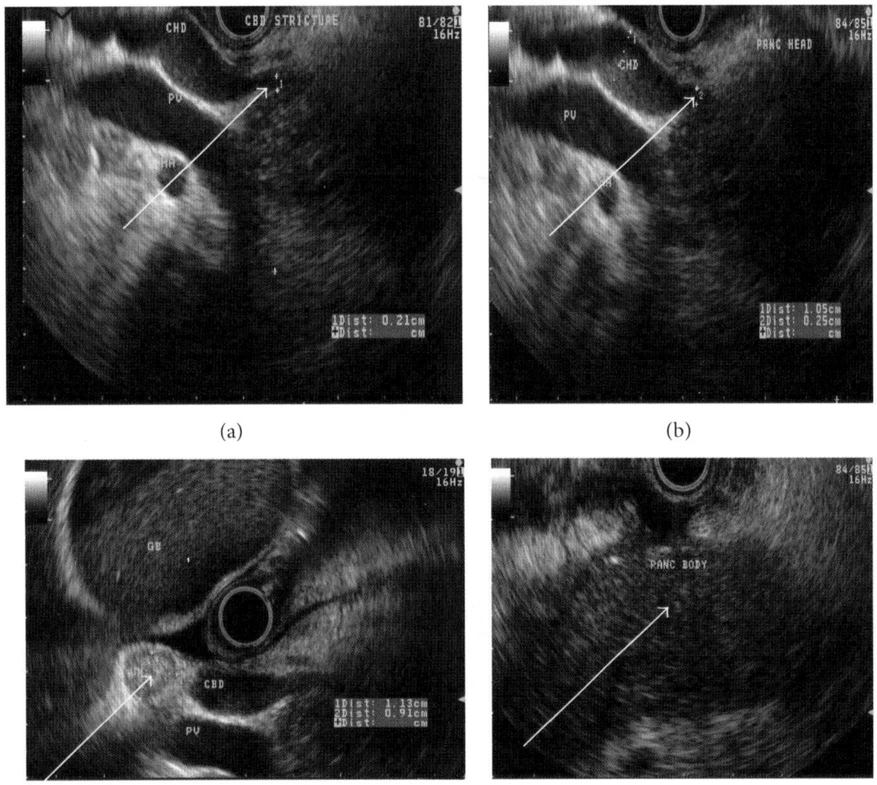

(a) (b) (c) (d)

FIGURE 2: Endoscopic ultrasound images arrows showing (clockwise) (a) CBD stricture, (b) dilated CHD, (c) reactive lymph node, and (d) homogenous pancreatic body.

jaundice and a pancreatic mass. Prior to initiation of therapy, it is of paramount importance to differentiate AIP from pancreatic cancer. Various strategies help differentiate the clinical, immunological, and radiological presentations in between AIP and pancreatic cancer. Obstructive jaundice induced by bile duct stenosis secondary to pancreatic cancer typically progresses steadily, whereas the jaundice of AIP in IgG4-related sclerosing disease sometimes fluctuates or, in rare cases, improves spontaneously [13, 20]. Elevated serum levels of IgG4 (>135 mg/dL) are seen in more than 90% of patients with AIP [6]. This is the most sensitive and specific diagnostic test for type I AIP, with 95% sensitivity, 97% specificity, and 97% accuracy for discrimination from pancreatic cancer [6]. Ghazale et al [21] in their study series of pancreatic cancer patients 13/135 (10%) noted that elevation of serum IgG4 levels alone cannot rule out pancreatic cancer, as only 1% of the above patients had elevated IgG4 levels >280 mg/dL, compared with 53% of AIP patients. Presence of other organ involvements such as bilateral salivary gland swelling, retroperitoneal fibrosis, and hilar or intrahepatic sclerosing cholangitis is highly suggestive of AIP rather than pancreatic cancer.

Radiological studies aid in differentiation based on the characteristic features on computed tomography (CT) and magnetic resonance imaging (MRI) that include diffuse or focal pancreatic enlargement, a peripancreatic capsule-like rim, enhancement at the late phase of contrast-enhanced images, and abnormal signal intensity on MRI. Diffuse enlargement of the pancreas and effacement of the lobular contour of the pancreas, the so-called "sausage-like" appearance, are a typical finding in AIP and are rarely seen in pancreatic cancer. On delayed phase of dynamic CT and MRI, enhancement of an enlarged pancreas is characteristic of AIP. As fibroinflammatory changes involve the peripancreatic adipose tissue, a capsule-like rim surrounding the pancreas is specifically detected in some AIP patients [22, 23]. The role of transabdominal ultrasonography in the diagnosis of autoimmune pancreatitis is not well established. Ultrasonographic images of the pancreas, obtained transabdominally, are rarely diagnostic of autoimmune pancreatitis. Furthermore, findings on ultrasonography may be similar for autoimmune pancreatitis and for other forms of acute and chronic pancreatitis.

The hallmark finding on endoscopic retrograde cholangiopancreatography (ERCP) in patients with autoimmune pancreatitis is diffuse or segmental attenuation of the main pancreatic duct (MPD), in contrast to the segmental stenoses often encountered with pancreatic adenocarcinoma. The other common findings are narrowing of the intrapancreatic portion of the common bile duct, irregular narrowing of extrahepatic bile ducts, and, less frequently, enlarged intrahepatic bile ducts [24]. It is of paramount importance

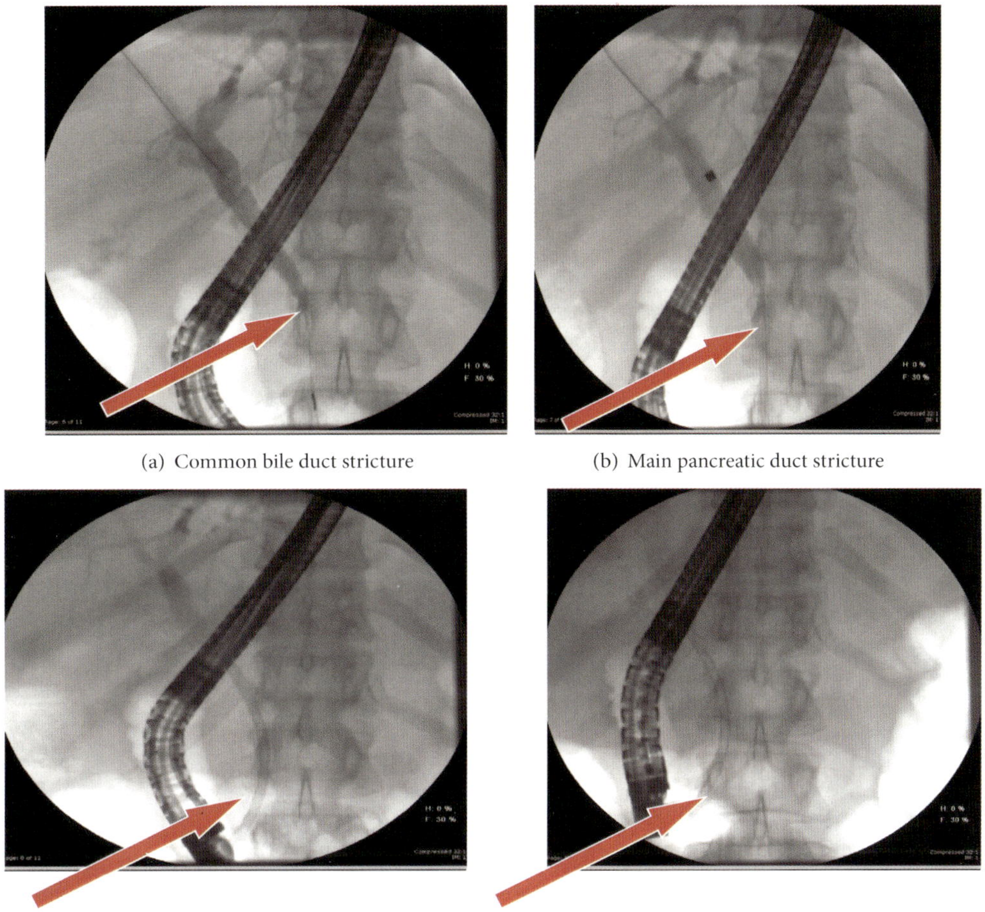

(a) Common bile duct stricture

(b) Main pancreatic duct stricture

(c) Stent in common bile duct

(d) Stent in main pancreatic duct

Figure 3: ERCP arrows showing CBD and MPD strictures pre stent insertion (a) and (b); post stent insertion (c) and (d) (clockwise).

to reliably distinguish AIP from PSC as making a reliable diagnosis is critical due to the often dramatic response of AIP related biliary strictures to steroid therapy in contrast to equivocal response seen in primary sclerosing cholangitis (PSC) and cholangiocarcinoma. The presence of a long, monomorphic stenosis of the intrapancreatic bile duct is suggestive of AIP, while band-like strictures, beading, or prune-tree appearance is most often found in PSC. Magnetic resonance cholangiopancreatography (MRCP) has become popular as a noninvasive method and it is becoming preferable to diagnostic ERCP. However, the narrowest MPD seen on ERCP cannot be visualized by MRCP due to the inferior resolution of MRCP compared with ERCP, so distinguishing between narrowing of the MPD in AIP and stenosis of the MPD in pancreatic cancer is not possible [25].

Endoscopic ultrasonography (EUS) emerged as a particularly important pancreatic imaging tool due to its ability to provide high-resolution imaging along with short working distances for transluminal pancreatic interventions. Though nonspecific, most common finding on EUS is diffuse or focal pancreatic enlargement inhomogeneous echo pattern, stranding and calcification [26]. EUS guided fine-needle aspiration or core biopsy of the pancreas may aid in the cytologic or histologic diagnosis; however, this approach to tissue acquisition was generally proven inadequate in providing a definitive diagnosis of AIP owing to a small sample size and lack of preserved tissue architecture and has not been evaluated in larger trials [26, 27].

4. Conclusion

In summary, we further report another case of AIP that reemphasizes the importance and various strategies of distinguishing it from pancreatic adenocarcinoma in order to avoid unnecessary surgical intervention. The concept of a "great mimicker" may be invoked and a heightened vigilance of AIP in one's differential diagnosis must be emphasized. As it is sometimes difficult to obtain adequate biopsy material from the pancreas, AIP is currently diagnosed based on careful consideration of a combination of characteristic clinical, serological, morphological, and histopathological features. More widespread use of pancreatic biopsy will aid in the diagnosis of autoimmune pancreatitis and provide a secure basis for the treatment with corticosteroids. Combined with a lack of prospectively validated clinical criteria that reliably establish the diagnosis, it is expected that the endoscopist

Table 1: Level 1 and level 2 criteria for type 1 AIP.

Criterion	Level 1	Level 2
Parenchymal imaging	Typical: diffuse enlargement with delayed enhancement (sometimes associated with rim-like enhancement)	Indeterminate (including atypical): segmental/focal enlargement with delayed enhancement
Ductal imaging (ERP)	Long (>1/3 length of the main pancreatic duct) or multiple strictures without marked upstream dilatation	Segmental/focal narrowing without marked upstream dilatation (duct size, <5 mm)
Serology	IgG4, >2x_upper limit of normal value	IgG4, 1-2x_upper limit of normal value
Other organ involvement (OOI)	a or b (a) Histology of extrapancreatic organs Any three of the following: (1) Marked lymphoplasmacytic infiltration with fibrosis and without granulocytic infiltration (2) Storiform fibrosis granulocytic infiltration (3) Obliterative phlebitis (4) Abundant (>10 cells/HPF) IgG4-positive cells (b) Typical radiological evidence At least one of the following: (1) Segmental/multiple proximal (hilar/intrahepatic) or proximal and distal bile duct stricture (2) Retroperitoneal fibrosis	a or b (a) Histology of extrapancreatic organs including endoscopic biopsy of bile duct Both of the following: (1) Marked lymphoplasmacytic infiltration with fibrosis without granulocytic infiltration (2) Abundant (>10 cells/HPF) IgG4-positive cells (b) Physical or radiological evidence At least one of the following: (1) Symmetrically enlarged salivary/lacrimal glands (2) Radiological evidence of renal involvement described in association with AIP
Histology of the pancreas	LPSP (core biopsy/resection) At least 3 of the following: (1) Periductal lymphoplasmacytic infiltrate without granulocytic infiltration (2) Obliterative phlebitis (3) Storiform fibrosis (4) Abundant (>10 cells/HPF) IgG4-positive cells	LPSP (core biopsy) Any 2 of the following: (1) Periductal lymphoplasmacytic infiltrate without granulocytic infiltration (2) Obliterative phlebitis (3) Storiform fibrosis (4) Abundant (>10 cells/HPF) IgG4-positive cells

Reproduced with permission from 2012 Kamisawa, Tabata, Hara, Kuruma, Chiba, Kanno, Masamune, and Shimosegawa.

will continue to play a central role in the diagnosis and management of AIP in the future.

Abbreviations

AIP: Autoimmune pancreatitis
MPD: Main pancreatic duct
CBD: Common bile duct
CHD: Common hepatic duct
LPSP: Lymphoplasmacytic sclerosing pancreatitis
IDCP: Idiopathic duct-centric pancreatitis
CT: Computer tomography
MRI: Magnetic resonance imaging
MRCP: Magnetic resonance cholangiopancreatography
ERCP: Endoscopic retrograde cholangiopancreatography
EUS: Endoscopic ultrasound-guided fine needle aspiration.

Authors' Contribution

Satya Allaparthi, Mohammed Sageer, and Mark J. Sterling reviewed, designed, edited, and organized the report; Mark J. Sterling served as the attending doctor for the patient and performed the ERCP; Satya Allaparthi performed the literature review and wrote the paper.

References

[1] H. Sarles, J.-C. Sarles, R. Muratore, and C. Guien, "Chronic inflammatory sclerosis of the pancreas—an autonomous pancreatic disease?" *The American Journal of Digestive Diseases*, vol. 6, no. 7, pp. 688–698, 1961.

[2] K. Yoshida, F. Toki, T. Takeuchi, S.-I. Watanabe, K. Shiratori, and N. Hayashi, "Chronic pancreatitis caused by an autoimmune abnormality. Proposal of the concept of autoimmune pancreatitis," *Digestive Diseases and Sciences*, vol. 40, no. 7, pp. 1561–1568, 1995.

[3] J. M. Hardacre, C. A. Iacobuzio-Donahue, T. A. Sohn et al., "Results of pancreaticoduodenectomy for lymphoplasmacytic sclerosing pancreatitis," *Annals of Surgery*, vol. 237, no. 6, pp. 853–858, 2003.

[4] K. P. Kim, M. H. Kim, M. H. Song, S. S. Lee, D. W. Seo, and S. K. Lee, "Autoimmune chronic pancreatitis," *The American Journal of Gastroenterology*, vol. 99, no. 8, pp. 1605–1616, 2004.

[5] I. Nishimori, A. Tamakoshi, and M. Otsuki, "Prevalence of autoimmune pancreatitis in Japan from a nationwide survey in 2002," *Journal of Gastroenterology*, vol. 42, no. 18, supplement, pp. 6–8, 2007.

[6] H. Hamano, S. Kawa, A. Horiuchi et al., "High serum IgG4 concentrations in patients with sclerosing pancreatitis," *New England Journal of Medicine*, vol. 344, no. 10, pp. 732–738, 2001.

[7] K. Hirano, Y. Komatsu, N. Yamamoto et al., "Pancreatic mass lesions associated with raised concentration of IgG4," *American Journal of Gastroenterology*, vol. 99, no. 10, pp. 2038–2040, 2004.

[8] R. Pezzilli and R. Corinaldesi, "IgG4 as a serological marker of autoimmune pancreatitis: the latest news," *Journal of the Pancreas*, vol. 5, no. 6, pp. 531–533, 2004.

[9] K. Okazaki, K. Uchida, M. Ohana et al., "Autoimmune-related pancreatitis is associated with autoantibodies and a Th1/Th2-type cellular immune response," *Gastroenterology*, vol. 118, no. 3, pp. 573–581, 2000.

[10] T. S. Davidson, D. S. Longnecker, and W. F. Hickey, "An experimental model of autoimmune pancreatitis in the rat," *American Journal of Pathology*, vol. 166, no. 3, pp. 729–736, 2005.

[11] K. Notohara, L. J. Burgart, D. Yadav, S. Chari, and T. C. Smyrk, "Idiopathic chronic pancreatitis with periductal lymphoplasmacytic infiltration: clinicopathologic features of 35 cases," *The American Journal of Surgical Pathology*, vol. 27, no. 8, pp. 1119–1127, 2003.

[12] K. Okazaki, S. Kawa, T. Kamisawa et al., "Japanese clinical guidelines for autoimmune pancreatitis," *Pancreas*, vol. 38, no. 8, pp. 849–866, 2009.

[13] T. Kamisawa, K. Takuma, N. Egawa, K. Tsuruta, and T. Sasaki, "Autoimmune pancreatitis and IgG4-related sclerosing disease," *Nature Reviews Gastroenterology and Hepatology*, vol. 7, no. 7, pp. 401–409, 2010.

[14] K. Kawaguchi, M. Koike, K. Tsuruta, A. Okamoto, I. Tabata, and N. Fujita, "Lymphoplasmacytic sclerosing pancreatitis with cholangitis: a variant of primary sclerosing cholangitis extensively involving pancreas," *Human Pathology*, vol. 22, no. 4, pp. 387–395, 1991.

[15] D. H. Park, M.-H. Kim, and S. T. Chari, "Recent advances in autoimmune pancreatitis," *Gut*, vol. 58, no. 12, pp. 1680–1689, 2009.

[16] G. Zamboni, J. Lüttges, P. Capelli et al., "Histopathological features of diagnostic and clinical relevance in autoimmune pancreatitis: a study on 53 resection specimens and 9 biopsy specimens," *Virchows Archiv*, vol. 445, no. 6, pp. 552–563, 2004.

[17] T. Kamisawa, K. Notohara, and T. Shimosegawa, "Two clinicopathologic subtypes of autoimmune pancreatitis: LPSP and IDCP," *Gastroenterology*, vol. 139, no. 1, pp. 22–25, 2010.

[18] R. P. Sah, S. T. Chari, R. Pannala et al., "Differences in clinical profile and relapse rate of type 1 versus type 2 autoimmune pancreatitis," *Gastroenterology*, vol. 139, no. 1, pp. 140–148, 2010.

[19] T. Shimosegawa, S. T. Chari, L. Frulloni et al., "International consensus diagnostic criteria for autoimmune pancreatitis: guidelines of the international association of pancreatology," *Pancreas*, vol. 40, no. 3, pp. 352–358, 2011.

[20] T. Kamisawa, N. Egawa, and H. Nakajima, "Autoimmune pancreatitis is a systemic autoimmune disease," *The American Journal of Gastroenterology*, vol. 98, no. 12, pp. 2811–2812, 2003.

[21] A. Ghazale, S. T. Chari, T. C. Smyrk et al., "Value of serum IgG4 in the diagnosis of autoimmune pancreatitis and in distinguishing it from pancreatic cancer," *The American Journal of Gastroenterology*, vol. 102, no. 8, pp. 1646–1653, 2007.

[22] K. D. Bodily, N. Takahashi, J. G. Fletcher et al., "Autoimmune pancreatitis: pancreatic and extrapancreatic imaging findings," *American Journal of Roentgenology*, vol. 192, no. 2, pp. 431–437, 2009.

[23] T. Kamisawa, N. Egawa, H. Nakajima, K. Tsuruta, A. Okamoto, and N. Kamata, "Clinical difficulties in the differentiation of autoimmune pancreatitis and pancreatic carcinoma," *The American Journal of Gastroenterology*, vol. 98, no. 12, pp. 2694–2699, 2003.

[24] D. V. Sahani, S. P. Kalva, J. Farrell et al., "Autoimmune pancreatitis: imaging features," *Radiology*, vol. 233, no. 2, pp. 345–352, 2004.

[25] K. Takuma, T. Kamisawa, R. Gopalakrishna et al., "Strategy to differentiate autoimmune pancreatitis from pancreas cancer," *World Journal of Gastroenterology*, vol. 18, no. 10, pp. 1015–1020, 2012.

[26] J. J. Farrell, J. Garber, D. Sahani, and W. R. Brugge, "EUS findings in patients with autoimmune pancreatitis," *Gastrointestinal Endoscopy*, vol. 60, no. 6, pp. 927–936, 2004.

[27] M. J. Levy, R. P. Reddy, M. J. Wiersema et al., "EUS-guided trucut biopsy in establishing autoimmune pancreatitis as the cause of obstructive jaundice," *Gastrointestinal Endoscopy*, vol. 61, no. 3, pp. 467–472, 2005.

6

Eosinophilic Gastroenteritis: Case Report and Review in Search for Diagnostic Key Points

Guillermo López-Medina,[1] Manuel Gallo,[1] Alejandro Prado,[1] Iliana Vicuña-Honorato,[1] and Roxana Castillo Díaz de León[2]

[1] *Hospital Angeles Clinica Londres, Durango No. 50, Roma Norte, Cuauhtémoc, 06700 Ciudad de México, DF, Mexico*
[2] *Hospital Angeles Mocel, Gregorio V. Gelati No. 29, San Miguel Chapultepec, Miguel Hidalgo, 11850 Ciudad de México, DF, Mexico*

Correspondence should be addressed to Guillermo López-Medina; mosca_mtv@hotmail.com

Academic Editor: Matteo Neri

Eosinophilic gastroenteritis is considered an uncommon disease with a low incidence rate that remains as a diagnostic challenge for the clinician, in spite of the fact that seventy years have passed since its original description. Hereby we present the case of a 29-year-old male without history of allergies who was evaluated for unspecific gastrointestinal symptoms, without relevant findings on physical examination and presenting an initial complete blood count (CBC) with severe eosinophilia. The patient was evaluated and the diagnosis of eosinophilic gastroenteritis was confirmed by histopathological findings. The relevance of the case resides in highlighting the lack of guidelines or consensus for histological diagnosis being virtually the only one available. To a similar extent, treatment evidence is based on case series with a reasonable number of patients and case reports.

1. Introduction

Primary eosinophilic gastrointestinal diseases include five variants according to their localization on the gastrointestinal tract: esophagitis, gastritis, gastroenteritis, enteritis, and eosinophilic colitis. As to gastroenteritis, stomach and small bowel are the most affected segments by 26% to 81% and 28% to 100%, respectively, often associated with simultaneous infiltration of the esophagus, colon, and rectum with a minor intensity. Reports of localized infiltration to the biliary tract come to emphasize that clinical spectrum may vary to a large extent, in accordance with the affected site and depth of the infiltration [1–4].

2. Case Description

We present a 29-year-old male, resident of an urban area, single, and without relevant family background, who consumes alcoholic beverages once a weak, denies smoking, allergies or previous transfusions. History of acute viral hepatitis type A during his childhood, pneumococcal, and flu vaccines were applied two weeks prior to his admission. Surgical history of amygdalectomy, appendectomy, renal lithotomy, and installation of double J stent secondary to renal lithiasis, all without noticed complications. He arrived to the emergency department with a chief complaint of three days prior to his admission with liquid depositions without blood or mucus, in 10 occasions approximately, along with vomit of gastric content. Within the next 48 hrs, moderate intensity, acute epigastric pain appeared. Fever was not reported. At the initial physical examination, he presented stable vital signs with palpable cervical lymph nodes, which were painless, mobile, without features suggesting malignancy and abdominal pain were discovered at palpation of the inferior quadrants, rest of the examination ended without further findings. The CBC resulted in a white blood cell count of $13.1 \times 10^3/\text{mm}^3$ and $3{,}537/\text{mm}^3$ (27%) corresponding to eosinophils, and the rest of cell count was within normal range. Parasitoscopic fecal analysis was positive for *Entamoeba histolytica* trophozoites and cysts, metronidazole plus iodoquinol were initiated. The parasitic infestation did not explain the severe eosinophilia; therefore, an abdominal ultrasonogram was performed and

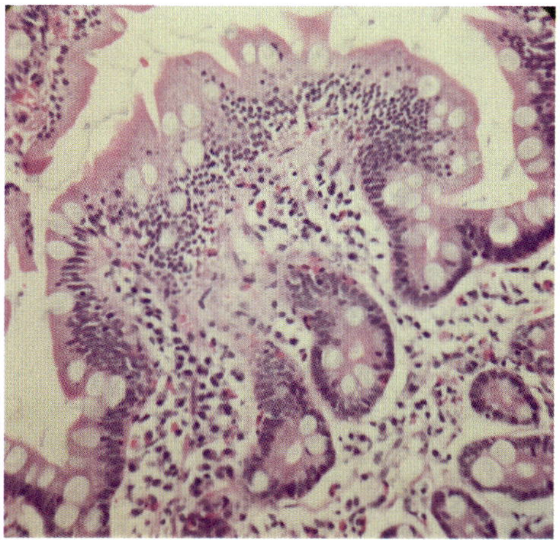

FIGURE 1: Photomicrography of a duodenal mucosal biopsy specimen (40x) shows a villous surface with hypercellular lamina propria and eosinophilic infiltrates.

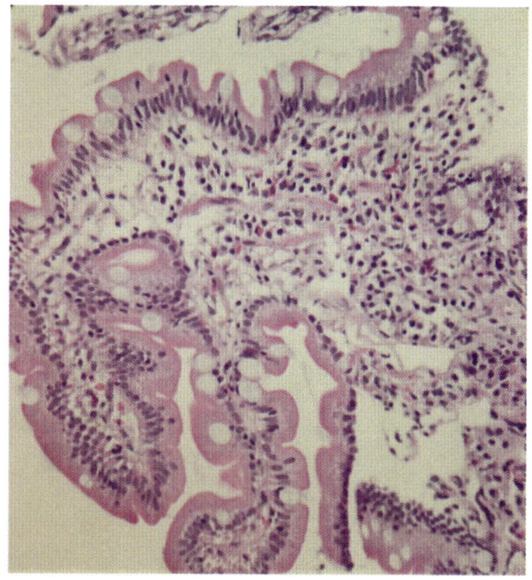

FIGURE 2: Photomicrography of a duodenal mucosal biopsy specimen (40x) depicts predominant eosinophilic inflammation within the lamina propria, and the glands appeared normal.

evidenced free fluid in both iliac fossae and pelvis, and an image compatible with a calculus within the inferior pole of left kidney was also observed. Abdominal fluid was obtained via an ultrasound guided puncture resulting in albumin of 1.7 d/dL, proteins 3.3 gr/dL, glucose 65 mg/dL, total cells of 4400/mm^3, 70% corresponding to eosinophils, and cultures tested negative for bacterial or fungi growth. Following the assessment of the ascites a contrast computed tomography confirmed free fluid in the right parietocolic gutter from epigastrium to pelvis, and a calculus on the inferior pole of the left kidney and thickening of the wall of the terminal ileum, enlarged pelvic, and inguinal lymph nodes were observed as well. Under the suspicion of intestinal malignancy a superior endoscopy revealed a redundant esophagus with generalized, moderate epithelium thickening, diffuse, moderate inflammatory process of the gastric mucous, normal antrum, and pylorus and duodenum, and urease test was negative for *Helicobacter pylori*. Samples from the esophagus and stomach were not taken. Colonoscopy reported normal perianal structures, spastic and redundant rectumsigmoid with normal mucosa, and the rest of colon without alterations. Biopsies of duodenum and colon were taken and the histopathologic study concluded unspecific mild chronic duodenitis without atrophy of vellus and moderate eosinophilia (mean 30 eosinophils/high power field), and no microorganisms by routine tinctions nor histopathological findings suggestive of intestinal malabsorption were identified (Figures 1 and 2) and mild chronic colitis with moderate eosinophilia (mean of 24 eosinophils/high power field) for the colon specimens (Figures 3 and 4). Microscope slides from both biopsies were revised with the maximum magnification (40x) in the form of "sweeping," that is, downwards then upwards and from left to right. Because of the small sized samples and the limited amount of tissue available, a "skipped" overview was not considered an option. The number of eosinophils in each field was counted and the total was divided by the absolute number of fields, in this way obtaining an average number of eosinophils. Serum IgE concentration was normal.

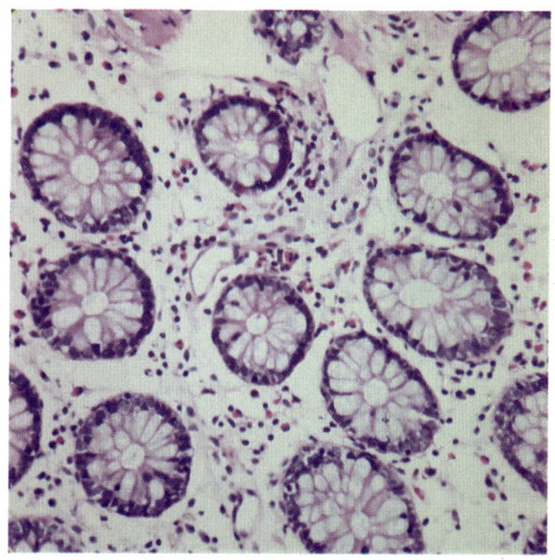

FIGURE 3: Photomicrography of a colonic mucosal biopsy specimen (40x) with chronic lymphoid inflammation, accentuating the gross number of eosinophils: the glands appeared normal.

Given the histopathological findings, ascites with a marked eosinophil predominance in the absence of an infectious or neoplastic disease, supported by high serum eosinophil concentration, the diagnosis of eosinophilic gastroenteritis was concluded. While no attributed allergenic source was evident, he received inpatient treatment base on a gluten and dairy free diet, minimum seasoning, and well-cooked poultry and beef, without administration of steroids, being effective by inducing remission in this patient. At the time of discharge the patient persisted with an elevated count of eosinophils of 3,002/mm^3. A couple of months after discharge under the same dietary regimen, the patient showed sustained clinical remission.

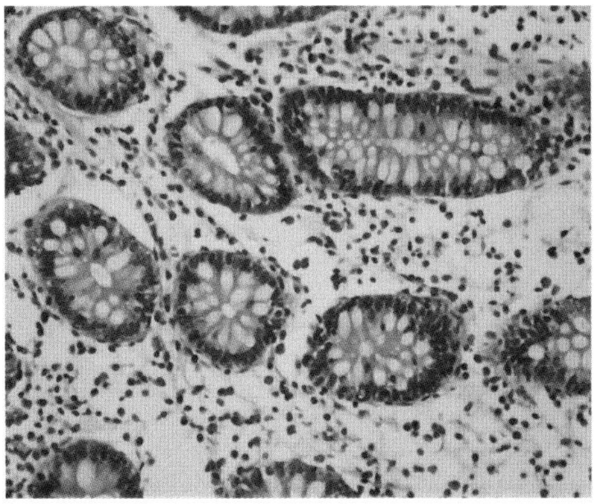

Figure 4: Photomicrography of a colonic mucosal biopsy specimen (40x) showing oedema of the lamina propria and chronic inflammatory infiltrate along with abundant eosinophils.

3. Discussion

Eosinophilic gastroenteritis is a nonfrequent primary gastrointestinal disease of which its etiology is not fully understood and characterized by histopathologic eosinophilic infiltrates in one or more segments from de stomach to the rectum [5]. Since its initial description by Kaijser in 1937 reports has shown that it may affect adults as well as pediatric population, preponderance within the male gender has been suggested [6]. It is important to differentiate it from secondary diseases associated with eosinophilia of which eosinophilic accumulation has an identifiable cause, like hypereosinophilic syndrome, inflammatory intestinal diseases, infections particularly by helminthes, vasculitis such as Churg-Strauss or polyarteritis nodosa, connective tissue diseases such as systemic lupus erythematosus, scleroderma, dermatomyositis, neoplasms, graft versus host disease in bone marrow transplant recipient patients, secondary reactions to nonsteroidal anti-inflammatory drugs, interferon, enalapril, carbamazepine, trimethoprim/sulfamethoxazole, clopidogrel, food allergies, *Helicobacter Pylori* infection, all of the above considered as differential diagnosis [7, 8].

The estimated prevalence reported for eosinophilic gastroenteritis is 1/100 000; however given the rarity of the diagnosis it is yet underestimated [5]. Six series have been published with a significant number of cases worldwide, and Talley et al. gathered 40 cases during a period from 1950 to 1986, Chang et al. gathered 59 new cases from 1987 to 2010, de Chambrun et al. presented 49 cases from 1988 to 2009, and Chen et al. from 1984 to 2002 described 15 patients, just to name a few [5, 9], highlighting the scarcity of this entity.

All ethnic groups may be affected, between 20 and 50 years of age, commonly around the third decade of life, 70% of the cases have personal and/or family history of allergies such as atopia, eczema, asthma, or allergic rhinitis. Unlike eosinophilic colitis most patients with gastroenteritis variant present elevated total serum IgE concentration [2, 8, 10].

The pathophysiology of eosinophilic gastroenteritis remains not fully comprehended. A hypersensitivity response is strongly suggested by clinical improvement reported in patients managed with corticosteroids. As part of the innate defense system, the presence of eosinophils in the intestinal lamina propria is a normal finding; however infiltration to deeper layers is considered abnormal. It is known that peripheral eosinophil concentration greater than 1.5×10^9/L can produce tissular damage regardless of the underlying cause [11, 12]. The main cytokines involved in the pathogenesis of this condition are IL-3, IL-5, granulocytes, and macrophages colony stimulating factors (GM-CSF); IL-5 plays a major role being the most potent, selective, chemotactic factor along with eotaxin (CCL11) for the migration of eosinophils towards the intestinal mucosa, promoting degranulation and inhibiting their apoptosis, remaining highly activated for any event that alters the intestinal mucosa, even in noninflammatory states [4, 11].

Eosinophils dwelling within the intestinal mucosa participate in the innate immune response mainly against helminthic infections and those caused by Mycobacteria spp., *Isospora belli*, *Sarcocystis coccidiomycosis*, *Dientamoeba fragilis*, and HIV infection; hence, gastrointestinal eosinophilia is usually not associated with infections of common bacteria, viruses, or fungus. Other agents like intestinal protozoa including giardiasis and amebiasis do not course with eosinophilia [4, 13].

Clinical manifestations thoroughly vary depending on their location within the gastrointestinal tract and depth through the intestinal wall; dysphagia, abdominal pain, and diarrhea are the most frequent symptoms in adults, and other symptoms are stenosis, hemorrhage, ulcers, and a wide range of motility alterations. Up to 80% manifest symptoms for several years, rarely presenting as an acute abdomen or intestinal perforation, all of the above should raise suspicion of a tumor which must be ruled out [10, 11].

The classification proposed in 1970 by Klein et al. has been the most employed, based on the depth of the eosinophilic infiltration; it can be divided according to mucous, muscular o serous involvement [2]. The mucous variant is the most common ranging from 25% to 100%, however this is not reliable due to diagnosis bias, being serous samples the least obtained for histopathological assessment. The key manifestations in mucous variant include protein-losing enteropathy, bleeding or malabsorption, nausea, vomit, diarrhea, and dyspepsia that do not respond to antisecretory therapy; the above symptoms can be confused with irritable bowel syndrome, pancreatitis, dyspepsia, appendicitis, or inflammatory intestinal disease. Muscular affection comprehends 13% to 70% of cases, manifested as thickening of the wall and obstructive symptoms such as colic pain, nausea, and vomit; it is rare to find true stenosis and, if present, jejunum is the most common site and less frequent as a cecal mass. Affection of the serosa exists in 14% to 40%, and ascites with predominance of eosinophils are the typical manifestation, along with abdominal distention and a large peripheral blood count of eosinophils, characteristically with good response to corticosteroid therapy [2, 11].

The initial workup comprehends a complete medical history and exhaustive physical examination, a CBC and chemistry panel. The hemogram will typically show eosinophilia in 20% to 80% of the cases, with a mean serum count of 2000 eos/μL when the mucosa is involved, 1000 eos/μL and 8000 eos/μL for the muscular wall, and the serosa, respectively. It is possible to find sideropenic anemia and hypoalbuminemia especially in association with the mucous variant and a case has been reported of hypercholesterolemia as a manifestation of gastroenteritis within the duodenal muscularis mucosae as part of a protein-losing enteropathy [11, 14]. The production of eosinophils is moderated by a net of cytokines that maintain their normal peripheral blood count between 0.05 and 0.5×10^9/L and their concentration in bone marrow aspiration between 1% and 6%. It is not normal to find eosinophils in the rest of the human economy, except for the thymus, spleen, lymphatic nodules, uterus, and gastrointestinal tract from stomach to rectum as mentioned above; however, it is important to notice that the normal count has not been yet determined [15]. Efforts have been made into establishing the normal eosinophil count throughout different segments of the gastrointestinal tract; nevertheless, it may not be widespread since the evidence is limited to small samples and including just a few ethnic groups in the same way as for pediatric population [16, 17].

According to the "2011 Year Working Conference on Eosinophil Disorders and Syndromes" the term hypereosinophilia is defined as a blood count of eosinophils greater than 1.5×10^9/L in two samples, taken 1 month apart and/or hypereosinophilia in tissues defined by (1) eosinophils greater than 20% of all nucleated cell in bone marrow and/or (2) eosinophilic infiltration cataloged as extensive according to pathologist opinion and/or (3) marked deposition of protein granules of eosinophils in presence or absence of important tissue infiltration. Hypereosinophilia must fulfill the above criteria plus evidence of specific organ damage. However eosinophilic gastroenteritis is excluded and categorized as an organ-restricted condition accompanied by hypereosinophilia, reason by which no definitive criteria have been determined for this entity [15]; therefore peripheral eosinophilia is not an universal phenomenon in the context of eosinophilic gastroenteritis [11, 15].

The stool analysis will show up to 30% of patients, mild to moderate steatorrhea. In relation to image studies, nodular or irregular thickening of the stomach or small bowel folds can be found on computed tomography [11]. Ultrasonogram is useful in the search for ascites in the variation affecting the serosa and guided paracentesis will result in being sterile with eosinophilic cellular predominance. Endoscopy is poorly specific showing a friable mucosa, nodular changes or ulcers, occasionally diffuse inflammation with vellus atrophy, submucosa oedema, or fibrosis. Technetium (99mc) exametazime labeled leukocytes single photon emission computed tomography (SPECT/CT) can be useful for evaluating extension but not for establishing the diagnosis [8, 11].

In the histopathological study of 6 samples from normal and abnormal areas, the diagnosis is suggested by the presence of eosinophilic infiltrates in intestinal crypts of gastric glands, extracellular deposition of eosinophilic remnants such as mayor basic protein or cationic protein, and incremented infiltration by mastocytes, keeping in mind that even the processing of samples may activate eosinophil degranulation [8, 10, 11]. For the muscular variant full thickness biopsy is required via laparoscopy since endoscopic biopsy is useless in the absence of compromise of the mucosa. The infiltration of the colon may be diffuse affecting the lamina propria with focal aggregates reaching the muscularis mucosae preserving the underlying submucosa [8].

In sum, in order to reach a diagnosis the following are required: (1) gastrointestinal symptoms, (2) eosinophilic infiltration in one or more segments of the gastrointestinal tract, by measuring the number of eosinophils under high power field view, without established threshold ranging from more than 20 to even more than 50 eosinophils, and (3) exclusion of other causes that course with eosinophilic intestinal infiltration [11, 18, 19].

Once the diagnosis of gastroenteritis is established, an evaluation by an allergologist is helpful in practicing environmental allergen detection, food allergy testing, food specific IgE by immuno-CAP and atopy patch test (APT), since triggers mediated by IgE make diet modifications poorly effective [8].

The first step of treatment includes withdraw of common allergens in the diet; nevertheless the therapeutic response is highly variable. The treatment with steroids shows an improvement in up to 90% of cases; however, the duration is not specified, and relapse is not uncommon; hence, treatment tends to extend. There is no consensus about the optimal type or dose of steroid; however, budesonide has the advantage of a local effect and a first step metabolism which entails less risk for adrenal suppression; prednisolone at 20 to 40 mg/day, for 6 to 8 weeks including the tapering, has been the most utilized regimen. Sodium cromoglicate, ketotifen, and montelukast have been proposed as therapeutic measures with inconclusive results. Surgery becomes useful in cases of obstructive symptoms lacking improvement with medical treatment. Parental nutrition will be useful in cases where patient comorbidities exclude the enteral route [11, 18, 19].

Not much is known about the natural evolution and prognosis of this disease, and it is possible that different segments are affected in the course of time or even progress to a complete hypereosinophilic syndrome which entails extraintestinal involvement for which endoscopic and cardiopulmonary follow-up is recommended [8].

4. Conclusions

Since its initial description more than 70 years ago, the efforts for characterizing the pathophysiology process and establishing standard diagnostic criteria for eosinophilic gastroenteritis have been scarce. A nondespicable number of cases have been reported, which indicates that clinical suspicion is increasing despite its low incidence.

This entity emphasizes the importance of an invasive approach along with a thorough medical history; findings on physical examination are not useful for reaching the diagnosis, hence being fundamentally histological.

Unlike other forms of primary eosinophilic gastrointestinal diseases such as eosinophilic esophagitis, there are no clinical guidelines available for eosinophilic gastroenteritis; therefore, it will remain underdiagnosed, with uncertain prognosis, and as for the patient we can only offer low evidence-based therapeutic options.

Authors' Contribution

All authors have contributed material, images, and revision of the final document.

References

[1] J. A. Elliott, O. McCormack, N. Tchrakian et al., "Eosinophilic ascites with marked peripheral eosinophilia: a diagnostic challenge," *European Journal of Gastroenterology & Hepatology*, vol. 26, no. 4, pp. 478–484, 2014.

[2] S. Khan and S. R. Orenstein, "Eosinophilic gastroenteritis," *Gastroenterology Clinics of North America*, vol. 37, no. 2, pp. 333–348, 2008.

[3] M. E. Rothenberg, "Eosinophilic gastrointestinal disorders (EGID)," *Journal of Allergy and Clinical Immunology*, vol. 113, no. 1, pp. 11–29, 2004.

[4] N. Powell, M. M. Walker, and N. J. Talley, "Gastrointestinal eosinophils in health, disease and functional disorders," *Nature Reviews Gastroenterology and Hepatology*, vol. 7, no. 3, pp. 146–156, 2010.

[5] G. P. de Chambrun, F. Gonzalez, J.-Y. Canva et al., "Natural history of eosinophilic gastroenteritis," *Clinical Gastroenterology and Hepatology*, vol. 9, no. 11, pp. 950–956.e1, 2011.

[6] A. Mori, C. Enweluzo, D. Grier, and M. Badireddy, "Eosinophilic gastroenteritis: review of a rare and treatable disease of the gastrointestinal tract," *Case Reports in Gastroenterology*, vol. 7, no. 2, pp. 293–298, 2013.

[7] F. Wang and J. Han, "Delayed eosinophilic gastroenteritis, a possible side effect of clopidogrel?" *International Journal of Cardiology*, vol. 165, no. 3, pp. e53–e54, 2013.

[8] D. M. Fleischer and D. Atkins, "Evaluation of the patient with suspected eosinophilic gastrointestinal disease," *Immunology and Allergy Clinics of North America*, vol. 29, no. 1, pp. 53–63, 2009.

[9] M.-J. Chen, C.-H. Chu, S.-C. Lin, S.-C. Shih, and T.-E. Wang, "Eosinophilic gastroenteritis: clinical experience with 15 patients," *World Journal of Gastroenterology*, vol. 9, no. 12, pp. 2813–2816, 2003.

[10] S. Mueller, "Classification of eosinophilic gastrointestinal diseases," *Best Practice and Research: Clinical Gastroenterology*, vol. 22, no. 3, pp. 425–440, 2008.

[11] S. B. Ingle and C. R. Hinge Ingle, "Eosinophilic gastroenteritis: an unusual type of gastroenteritis," *World Journal of Gastroenterology*, vol. 19, no. 31, pp. 5061–5066, 2013.

[12] F. Roufosse and P. F. Weller, "Practical approach to the patient with hypereosinophilia," *Journal of Allergy and Clinical Immunology*, vol. 126, no. 1, pp. 39–44, 2010.

[13] T. Löscher and E. Saathoff, "Eosinophilia during intestinal infection," *Best Practice and Research: Clinical Gastroenterology*, vol. 22, no. 3, pp. 511–536, 2008.

[14] S. Gonnelli, L. Tanzilli, L. Burroni, and C. Caffarelli, "New-onset hypercholesterolemia as an unusual presenting manifestation of eosinophilic gastroenteritis," *Journal of Clinical Lipidology*, vol. 7, no. 3, pp. 229–233, 2013.

[15] P. Valent, A. D. Klion, H.-P. Horny et al., "Contemporary consensus proposal on criteria and classification of eosinophilic disorders and related syndromes," *Journal of Allergy and Clinical Immunology*, vol. 130, no. 3, pp. 607–612.e9, 2012.

[16] C. W. DeBrosse, J. W. Case, P. E. Putnam, M. H. Collins, and M. E. Rothenberg, "Quantity and distribution of eosinophils in the gastrointestinal tract of children," *Pediatric and Developmental Pathology*, vol. 9, no. 3, pp. 210–218, 2006.

[17] T. Matsushita, R. Maruyama, N. Ishikawa et al., "The number and distribution of eosinophils in the adult human gastrointestinal tract: a study and comparison of racial and environmental factors," *The American Journal of Surgical Pathology*, vol. 39, no. 4, pp. 521–527, 2015.

[18] L. Santarpia, R. Cuomo, L. Camera, L. Alfonsi, F. Contaldo, and F. Pasanisi, "A patient with oeosinophilic gastroenteritis and severe malnutrition improved with home parenteral nutrition," *BMJ Case Reports*, 2010.

[19] H. E. Oh and R. Chetty, "Eosinophilic gastroenteritis: a review," *Journal of Gastroenterology*, vol. 43, no. 10, pp. 741–750, 2008.

7

Ascites in a Young Woman: A Rare Presentation of Eosinophilic Gastroenteritis

Carina Santos, Francisco Morgado, Celestina Blanco, João Parreira, João Costa, Lara Rodrigues, Luís Marfull, and Patrícia Cardoso

Department of Internal Medicine, Radiology, University Hospital Center "Sousa Martins", Guarda, Portugal

Correspondence should be addressed to Carina Santos; a18518@fcsaude.ubi.pt

Academic Editor: Ken Haruma

Introduction. Eosinophilic gastroenteritis (EGE) is a rare idiopathic disease that can affect one or more organs of the digestive tract. It has an estimated incidence of 1–20 cases per 100,000 patients. Klein et al. classified EGE into 3 subtypes: predominant mucosal, muscular, or subserosal. *Clinical Case.* We report a case of a 32-year-old woman, who presented with diffuse abdominal pain, nausea, postprandial infarction, diarrhea, and moderate ascites of three-week evolution. The rest of physical examination did not show alterations. The past medical history was unremarkable. Laboratory test results revealed peripheral blood eosinophilia. Abdominal CT scan revealed diffuse and concentric parietal thickening of the distal 2/3 of esophagus, moderate volume ascites, and small bowel wall thickening and distension on the left quadrants. The paracentesis revealed 93.3% of eosinophils. The colon biopsies evidenced an increase in the number of eosinophils. Secondary causes of eosinophilia were excluded. The patient was treated with oral prednisolone 40 mg/day with immediate clinical and analytical improvement. *Conclusion.* Eosinophilic gastroenteritis is a rare condition with a nonspecific and highly variable clinical presentation, which requires a high level of clinical suspicion. It is a diagnosis of exclusion. Secondary causes of eosinophilia such as intestinal tuberculosis, parasitosis, and malignant neoplasms should be excluded.

1. Introduction

Eosinophilic gastroenteritis (EGE) is a rare idiopathic disease which can affect one or more organs of the digestive tract, including the stomach, small intestine, and less often the colon. Only 280 cases were described between 1937 and 2006 [1]. The estimated incidence of EGE remains relatively rare with 1–20 cases per 100,000 patients.

Although it may manifest from childhood to adulthood, the peak incidence occurs between the 3rd and 5th decades of life, with a slight predominance in males (3 : 2) [2]. The etiology and pathogenesis of EGE have not yet been established. The mechanisms responsible for GI tract infiltration by eosinophils remains controversial. However, several studies have shown that half of the patients with EGE presented a previous history of atopy. In addition, Immunoglobulin E (IgE) levels are elevated in some patients [3]. The diagnosis is suggested by clinical history and peripheral eosinophilia and confirmed by eosinophilic infiltration of the wall of the digestive tract [4], in the absence of known causes of eosinophilia [5].

In 1970, Klein et al. classified EGE into three types depending on the depth of eosinophilic infiltration: predominant mucosal, muscular, and subserosal.

The mucosal layer disease is the most frequent subtype and presents with nonspecific symptoms such as a general abdominal pain, nausea, diarrhea and vomiting which may mimic other gastrointestinal diseases; in the most severe form patients may present with blood loss in stools, iron deficiency anemia, or protein-losing enteropathy. The muscular subtype, the second most frequently reported, is characterized by infiltration of eosinophils predominantly in the muscle layer, causing bowel wall thickening and, consequently, symptoms of intestinal obstruction [2]. The subserosal subtype occurs in only 10% of the cases [5]; it presents typically with isolated abdominal ascites or ascites accompanied by symptoms of the mucosal or muscular forms; the hallmark of this subtype is marked eosinophilia in the ascitic fluid; frequently, this subtype has the best response to corticosteroids [2]; according to the guideline published in 2014 by the Japanese Ministry of Health, Labor and Welfare, as negative endoscopic mucosal biopsies do not definitively rule out muscular or subserosal EGE, laparoscopic full-thickness biopsy is necessary to establish the diagnosis [6].

Matsushita et al. studied a Japanese, a Japanese American, and a Caucasian group living in Hawaii, in what concerns the normal number of eosinophils in the gastrointestinal tract. Their results on the Japanese surgical biopsy samples showed a significant increase in the number of eosinophils from the esophagus to the right colon (mean ± SD/mm: 0.07 ± 0.43 for the esophagus, 12.18 ± 11.39 for the stomach, and 36.59 ± 15.50 for the right colon), compared with a decrease in the left colon (8.53 ± 7.83). Investigation using surgical samples showed that the distribution patterns in the gastrointestinal tract were very similar among the 3 ethnic groups, and there were no significant differences in the number of eosinophils among these groups, except in the esophageal epithelium. Their data suggest that a cutoff value for eosinophil counts, when rendering a diagnosis of eosinophilic gastrointestinal tract disease, should be individualized to the different biopsy sites. [7]. However, further studies needed to generalize these results among other geographic areas and ethnic groups.

Many authors agree that, in order to confirm the histological diagnosis, at least 15–20 eosinophils/high power microscopic fields are considered necessary [8].

Corticosteroids are effective in 80–100% of cases, although there are no randomized controlled trials for EGE treatment. Second-line therapies include mast cell stabilizers (sodium cromoglycate), antihistamines, leukotriene antagonists (montelukast), diet (elimination of milk, soy, wheat, eggs, peanuts, and seafood), immunotherapy (desensitization), immunomodulators (azathioprine and 6-mercaptopurine), mepolizumab, tumor necrosis factors inhibitors (e.g., infliximab), and IgE monoclonal antibody (omalizumab) [1].

The oral prednisolone dose most frequently administered is 40 mg/day for 7–14 days, followed by a progressive dose reduction. In some cases, maintenance treatment with low doses (5 to 10 mg a day) is necessary [9].

2. Clinical Case

A 32-year-old Caucasian woman, with no relevant medical history, was admitted to the Emergency Department due to generalized abdominal pain, nausea, postprandial infarction, diarrhea, and enlargement of abdominal perimeter, lasting 3 weeks. She reported an aggravation in the last 3 days. She denied other symptoms, including fever, night sweats, weight loss, arthralgia, or skin rash, as well as history of atopic diseases, food allergies, raw fishing eating, or recent medication intake.

On examination she had painful and distended abdomen. The cardiopulmonary examination was normal. Blood tests revealed leukocytosis [13360/microliter (μl)] with 36.5% of eosinophils (4880/μl). The abdomen X-ray showed levels in the upper right quadrant (Figure 1).

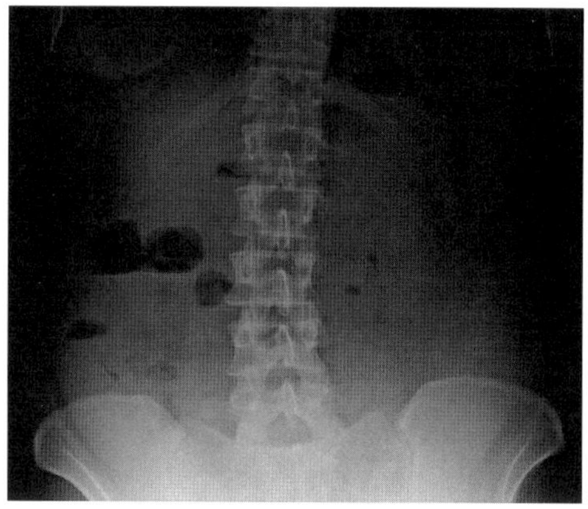

FIGURE 1: X-ray showing levels in the upper right quadrant of the abdomen.

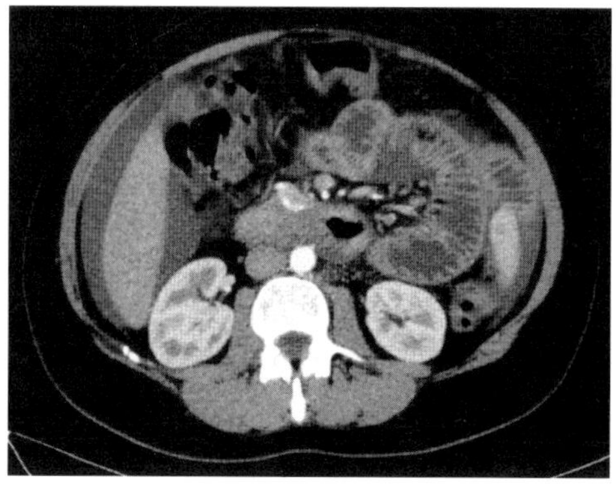

FIGURE 2: CT scan showing ascites and thickening and distension of small bowel loops.

Abdominal CT scan revealed diffuse and concentric parietal thickening of the distal two-thirds of esophagus, moderate volume ascites, and small bowel wall thickening with distension on the left quadrants (Figure 2).

The gastroscopy showed a "peptic ring at 40 cm and hyperemia of the body and antrum mucosa"; no biopsies were taken (Figures 3 and 4). She was admitted to the Internal Medicine Department for complementary study. The abdominal ultrasound showed several dilated loops in the small bowel, with significant reduction of their peristalsis, compatible with intestinal subocclusion. The parasitological stool exam was negative for eggs, cysts, and parasites. Serum IgE level was normal (83.8 KU/L).

The patient underwent an ultrasound-guided paracentesis. Results showed 6912 leukocytes/mm3, of which 93.3% were eosinophils (6450/μl), without malignancy; laboratory testing of the ascitic fluid for bacterial culture and tuberculosis was negative.

Colonoscopy showed a congestive and petechial ileocecal valve and hypotrophic mucosa with evidence of submucosal circulation, suspected of microscopic colitis. Colon biopsies showed mucosa with nodular lymphoid hyperplasia and increased number of eosinophils/high power microscopic

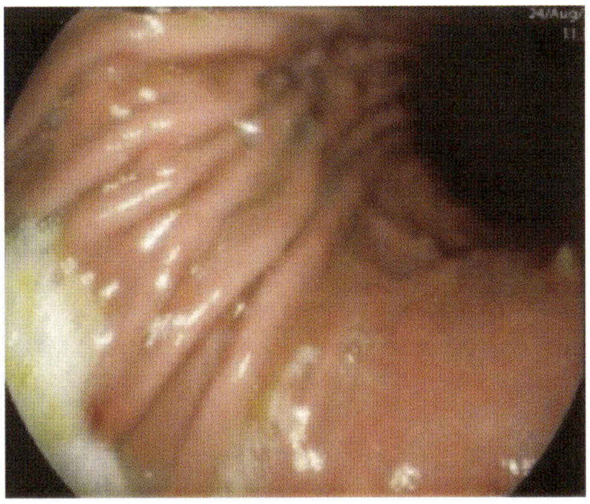

Figure 3: Greater curvature of the stomach.

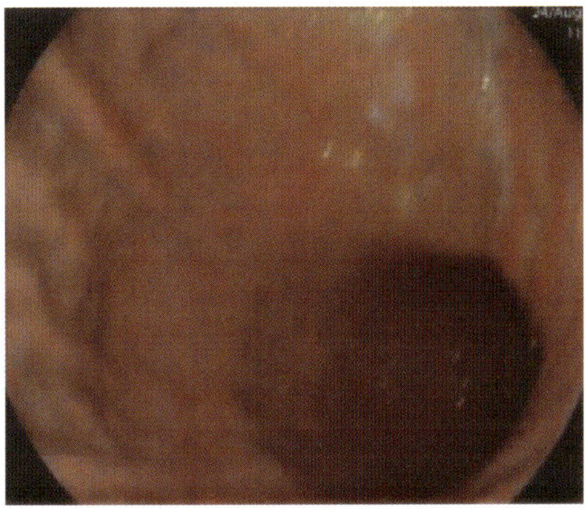

Figure 4: Gastric antrum and body.

fields in left colon (20–24/high power microscopic fields) (Figure 5).

The constellation of clinical, analytical, and histopathological results suggested the diagnosis of eosinophilic gastroenteritis.

The patient was started on 40 mg of oral prednisolone/day, with clinical and analytical rapid improvement (decrease of 5130 eosinophils/uL to 100 eosinophils/uL with 2 doses of prednisolone). To date, the patient stopped taking corticosteroids and remains asymptomatic.

3. Discussion

EGE is a rare medical condition that presents with nonspecific clinical symptoms. The diagnosis requires a high level of clinical suspicion. It is necessary to rule out other pathologies such as intestinal tuberculosis, parasitosis, and malignant neoplasms.

The clinical case presented refers to the rarest subtype of EGE which makes the diagnostic challenge even more difficult.

An early diagnosis and rapid introduction of corticosteroids may reduce the duration and severity of symptoms, thus reducing the morbidity of this disease. However, the clinician should keep in mind the possibility of a relapsing disease.

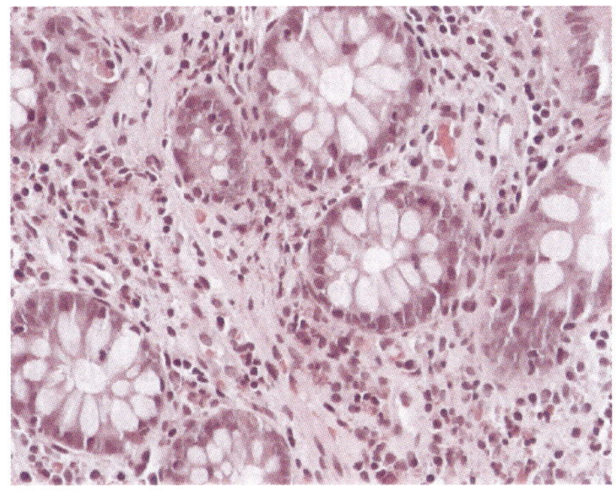

Figure 5: Colon biopsy with >20 eosinophils/field.

Given the limited number of EGE cases reported in the literature, further data are needed about the epidemiology, clinical and histological characteristics, and evolution of the disease.

References

[1] T. Alhmoud, J. A. Hanson, and G. Parasher, "Eosinophilic Gastroenteritis: An Underdiagnosed Condition," *Digestive Diseases and Sciences*, vol. 61, no. 9, pp. 2585–2592, 2016.

[2] V. Uppal, P. Kreiger, and E. Kutsch, "Eosinophilic gastroenteritis and colitis: a comprehensive review," *Clinical Reviews in Allergy & Immunology*, 2015.

[3] F. Bleibel, K. Fragoza, and G. T. Faller, "Acute Eosinophilic Ascites in a Middle-Aged Man," *Case Reports in Gastrointestinal Medicine*, vol. 2012, pp. 1–4, 2012.

[4] A. Fukuda, T. Kajiyama, H. Kishimoto et al., "Eosinophilic gastroenteritis with predominant muscular layer disease: Feature of endoscopic ultrasonography," *Digestive Endoscopy*, vol. 16, no. 4, pp. 368–371, 2004.

[5] I. Quack, L. Sellin, N. J. Buchner, D. Theegarten, L. C. Rump, and B. F. Henning, "Eosinophilic gastroenteritis in a young girl - Long term remission under Montelukast," *BMC Gastroenterology*, vol. 5, article no. 24, 2005.

[6] S. Ishihara, Y. Kinoshita, and A. Schoepfer, "Eosinophilic Esophagitis, Eosinophilic Gastroenteritis, and Eosinophilic Colitis: Common Mechanisms and Differences between East and West," *Inflammatory Intestinal Diseases*, vol. 1, no. 2, pp. 63–69, 2016.

[7] T. Matsushita, R. Maruyama, and N. Ishikawa, "The number and distribution of eosinophils in the adult human gastrointestinal tract: a study and comparison of racial and environmental factors," *The American Journal of Surgical Pathology*, vol. 39, no. 4, pp. 521–527, 2015.

[8] Y. Kinoshita, N. Ishimura, N. Oshima et al., "Recent Progress in the Research of Eosinophilic Esophagitis and Gastroenteritis," *Digestion*, vol. 93, no. 1, pp. 7–12, 2016.

[9] A. Campos Ruiz, I. Ganchegui Aguirre, L. Urtasun Arlegui et al., "Eosinophilic gastroenteritis: Three clinical cases with different presentations," *Gastroenterología y Hepatología (English Edition)*, vol. 40, no. 4, pp. 327–329, 2017.

8

Unique Presentation of Giant Metastatic Microcystic Serous Adenocarcinoma of the Pancreas

Cyriac Abby Philips,[1] Chetan Ramesh Kalal,[1] Chhagan Bihari,[2] Amrish Sahney,[1] KN Chandan Kumar,[1] and Archana Rastogi[2]

[1] *Department of Hepatology, Institute of Liver and Biliary Sciences, D-1, Vasant Kunj, New Delhi 110070, India*
[2] *Department of Pathology, Institute of Liver and Biliary Sciences, D-1, Vasant Kunj, New Delhi 110070, India*

Correspondence should be addressed to Cyriac Abby Philips; abbyphilips@gmail.com

Academic Editors: N. Courcoutsakis, H. Kawaratani, N. Koide, and J. Wig

Tumors of the pancreas that contain substantial cystic components include mainly mucinous cystic neoplasm, intraductal papillary mucinous neoplasm, solid pseudopapillary tumor, and cystadenomas (which encompass microcystic, macrocystic/oligocystic, and rare solid serous adenomas). Microcystic adenoma of the pancreas is a tumor that is benign in nature. Malignant transformation in the tumor with metastases is rare and only about 26 cases have been reported so far. Here we present a giant microcystic adenoma of the pancreas, possibly the largest ever malignant type in this group ever reported in the literature with extensive metastases to the liver and causing extensive compression and encasement on surrounding structures.

1. Introduction

Pancreatic cystic tumors fall into the serous or mucinous category. The latter most prominently shows malignant transformation in the long run, while the former is considered benign [1]. Microcystic adenoma of the pancreas is a rare tumor that presents indolently with features of slow growth and abdominal pain secondary to mass effect. These tumors are managed expectantly and surgical management is considered only when the patient becomes symptomatic [2]. The mucinous cystadenomas on the other hand, even though slow growing, have high chances of malignant transformation and hence need to be managed earlier, surgically [3]. Malignant transformation of cystic adenomas of the pancreas was first described in 1989 wherein the tumor showed invasion into surrounding structures and into the liver [4]. Afterwards, about 26 case reports and reviews have been inculcated into the literature on cystadenocarcinomas [5]. Characterization of benign cystic adenomas from cystadenocarcinomas has been extremely difficult. The presence of histological invasion is the only modality that can differentiate these two conditions [6]. One recent case report by Zhu et al. revealed for the first time carcinoma ex microcystic adenoma in which the tumor, without metastases, showed inherent malignant changes [7]. Of all the cystadenocarcinomas reported, our report is unique in three aspects. Firstly, this is the largest cystadenocarcinoma reported in the literature. Secondly, the radiological appearance of the tumor is that of a "parasite mass" that takes up extensive blood supply from the celiac axis, and lastly the tumor extensively involved surrounding structures, notably the biliary tree, producing features of obstructive jaundice, a feature never reported before.

2. Case Report

A 70-year-old woman, hailing from Kashmir in India, presented to us with progressively increasing abdominal mass since 11 years. This was associated with progressive appearance of jaundice and dull aching pain in abdomen since 3 months with pruritus for one month that worsened nocturnally. She neither complained of fever, bleeding diathesis, chest pain, cough or palpitations, and altered bowel habits nor did she suffer from anorexia. There was significant unintentional weight loss secondary to early satiety since last one year. There was no history of swelling of legs or puffiness of face during this period. There was no history of swelling over other parts of the body or associated skin changes. The patient is a known case of diabetes mellitus on oral hypoglycemic agents with adequate glycemic control since the last 20 years. Eleven years ago, the patient underwent an open laparotomy for complicated symptomatic gall stone disease and was incidentally detected to have a space occupying lesion of the head of pancreas. The lesion was highly vascular on intraoperative analysis and was left alone at that time with a fine needle aspiration cytology evaluation, which was later confirmed to be that of benign microcystic adenoma. The patient thereafter started noticing progressive enlargement of an epigastric mass which was initially seen 8 years ago. This mass progressed to involve the whole of the abdomen with associated lethargy and early satiety and difficulty in performing routine works. Multiple fine needle aspiration cytology of the mass lesion was done at various hospitals outside, before presentation to our facility. All those reports were noncontributory and confirmed the presence of only blood and cystic elements. On examination, at our center, the patient was found to be conscious and alert but emaciated with temporal hollowing and facial muscle wasting, with good performance status (ECOG-PS 0). Pallor was evident, as were icterus and scratch marks over the abdomen and arms. There was no cyanosis, clubbing, lymphadenopathy, or edema. The abdominal examination revealed the presence of a large epigastric mass, extending towards the right iliac fossa and trespassing on the left lateral aspect of umbilicus with a rough nodular surface, being firm in consistency, nontender, and without visible pulsations. A palpable bruit and a venous hum were also evident. There were areas of engorged, nontortuous veins over the stretched skin surface of the mass. No other organomegaly was appreciable and free fluid in abdomen was difficult to ascertain. The rest of the systemic examination was essentially normal. On further evaluation, the patient was found to have hemoglobin levels of 10 g/dL (normal 12–15) with normal total leukocyte and platelet counts. The ESR was 30 mm in the first hours (normal 0–2). The liver function tests revealed normal bilirubin levels with normal transaminases, in the presence of alkaline phosphatase of 326 IU/L (normal 32–92) and gamma glutamyl transpeptidase of 228 U/L (normal 7–64). The kidney function tests were normal and so were all the viral markers and autoimmune markers. The serum tumor markers, including CA19-9, CEA, AFP, tumoral Beta-HCG, Chromogranin A, and CA-125, were all within normal limits. Computed tomography imaging of the abdomen subsequently followed by angiographic studies in triple phase and magnetic resonance imaging in triple phase revealed the presence of a large lobulated heterogenous mass in the retroperitoneum extending from the undersurface of the liver to the whole of lower abdomen (Figures 1(a), 1(b), 1(c), and 1(d)). The mass measured 26 × 26 cm in size and contained hyperechoic and hypoechoic areas which were hypointense on T1 and hyperintense on T2 weighted images.

Multiple hypodense septation (which was T2 hypointense) was noted within the heterogenous mass. Contrast administration revealed moderate heterogenous enhancement with enhancing septation. Compression and displacement of structures at the porta and compression of common bile duct with upstream dilatation of the CBD and bilobar intrahepatic biliary radical dilatation were also evident. The CBD measured 2.7 cm. The inferior vena cava was compressed posteriorly with displacement of the bowel laterally. The tumor derived its supply mostly from the celiac axis with extensive tumoral angiogenesis (Figure 2). Multiple well defined T2 hyperintense and T1 hypointense lesions were noted in both lobes of the liver showing enhancement suggestive of metastases. The liver was otherwise normal and the pancreas could not be delineated. Subsequently the patient underwent a ultrasonography guided percutaneous biopsy from the SOL liver, the histopathological examination of which revealed features of a neoplastic lesion composed of cells arranged in acinar microcystic pattern around the small vessels. These acini and microcysts were lined by single cell layer of uniform cuboidal and Hobnail cells (omit type).

These cells also showed features of monomorphic round hyperchromatic nuclei and moderate amount of clear cytoplasm with inconspicuous nucleoli. The intervening stroma contained several vascular channels with hyalinised stroma. The tumor cells were positive for CK-7, SMA, CD34, and focal EMA. They were negative for focal S-100, CD10, HMB45, MUC1/2, and calretinin (Figures 3(a), 3(b), 3(c), and 3(d)). The glycogen content was documented by PAS positive reaction on histology.

With these clinical, imaging, and histopathological features, a diagnosis of microcystic adenoma was made and the carcinomatous transformation was confirmed by the presence of liver metastases. The patient was not a candidate for surgical or interventional therapy and hence was managed medically for symptom relief. According to the patient's family's wishes, she was then allowed to follow up at her hometown at a nearby center and was lost to follow-up from our side.

3. Discussion

Cystadenomas of the pancreas are mainly microcystic, oligo- or macrocystic, and solid serous in type. The cystadenomas are almost always considered benign [7]. The malignant transformation in this group of tumor is documented only in the presence of distant metastases or local invasiveness and histological features suggestive of vascular/lymphatic or neural invasion. The prevalence of carcinomatous change in microcystic adenomas has been reported to be 3% [8]. Since its first description in 1989, the few cases reported relied mostly on histological proof rather than clinical or radiological imaging. The average age range at presentation is 66 to 70 years and more than 50% of the affected patients are female [9]. The commonest presenting complaint is abdominal pain and the least common includes that of jaundice and palpable mass [10]. Our case report showcases a presentation not reported before, that of surgical obstructive jaundice and abdominal pain with a large palpable mass per abdomen. These tumors show synchronous (as in our

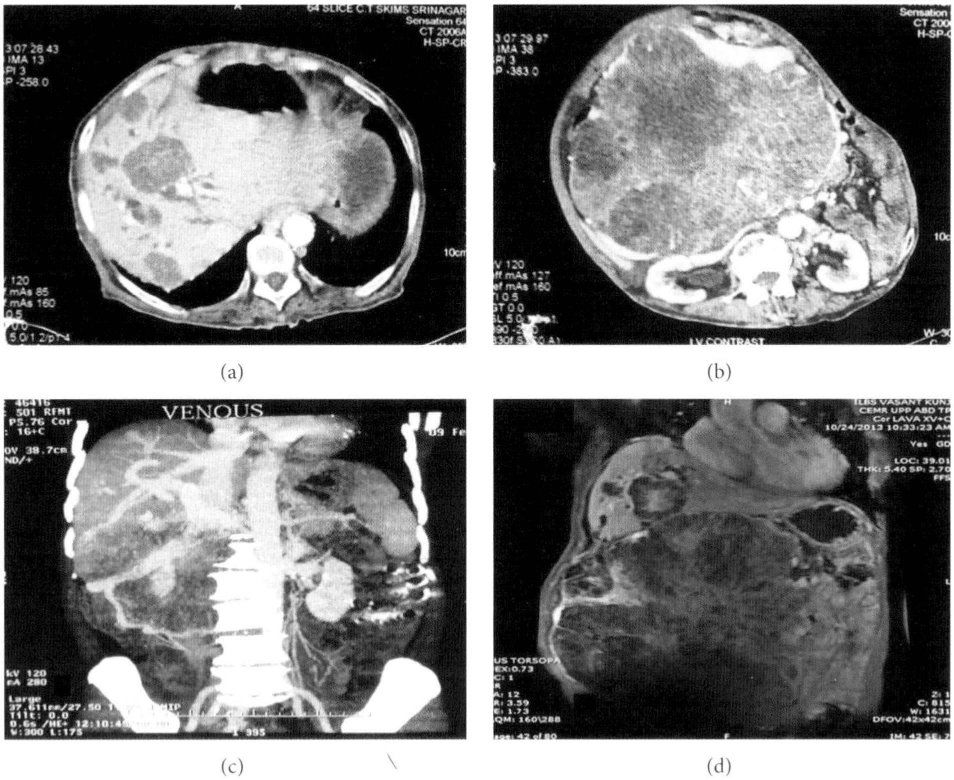

FIGURE 1: The computed tomographic ((a) to (c)) and magnetic resonance (d) imaging of the abdomen showing features of multiple metastatic lesions in the liver, predominantly in the right lobe (a); 26 cm large heterogenous retroperitoneal mass with areas of necrosis, breakdown, and calcifications involving almost the whole of the abdominal cavity producing mass effect (b); large venovenous communication between the tumor and the major venous channels on venography (c); Large lobulated heterogenous mass with internal septations and surrounding liver metastases extending from the upper to the lower part of the abdomen showing mass effect.

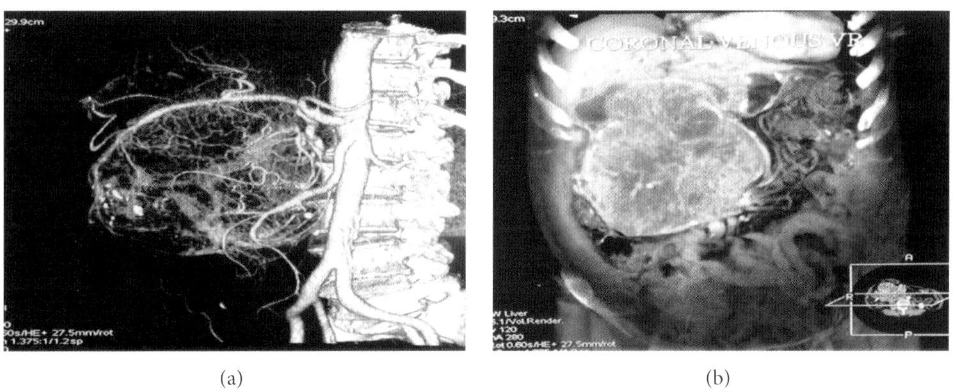

FIGURE 2: The computed angiographic images of the mass lesion in the abdomen showing features of extensive supply of the tumor derived from the celiac branches (a) and the presence of multiple dilated venous communications within and around the tumoral structure on venography (b).

case) or metachronous liver metastases. There have also been case reports where lymph nodal, splenic, neural, perineural, stomach, lung, adrenal, peritoneal, and mesenteric invasions were also documented [11]. Our case report is the first one to document involvement of the biliary tree with presentation of surgical obstructive jaundice and extensive vascular compression. Cystic tumors of the pancreas have varied behavior and histological characteristics. The serous cystadenoma (also known as microcystic adenoma of the pancreas, unless otherwise specified) is a benign tumor that is usually asymptomatic and is diagnosed incidentally during work up for other conditions. In our case, the patient underwent cholecystectomy many years before this presentation and was incidentally detected to have a mass in the head of the pancreas, which, at the time, was diagnosed as microcystic adenoma, and further management was abandoned in view

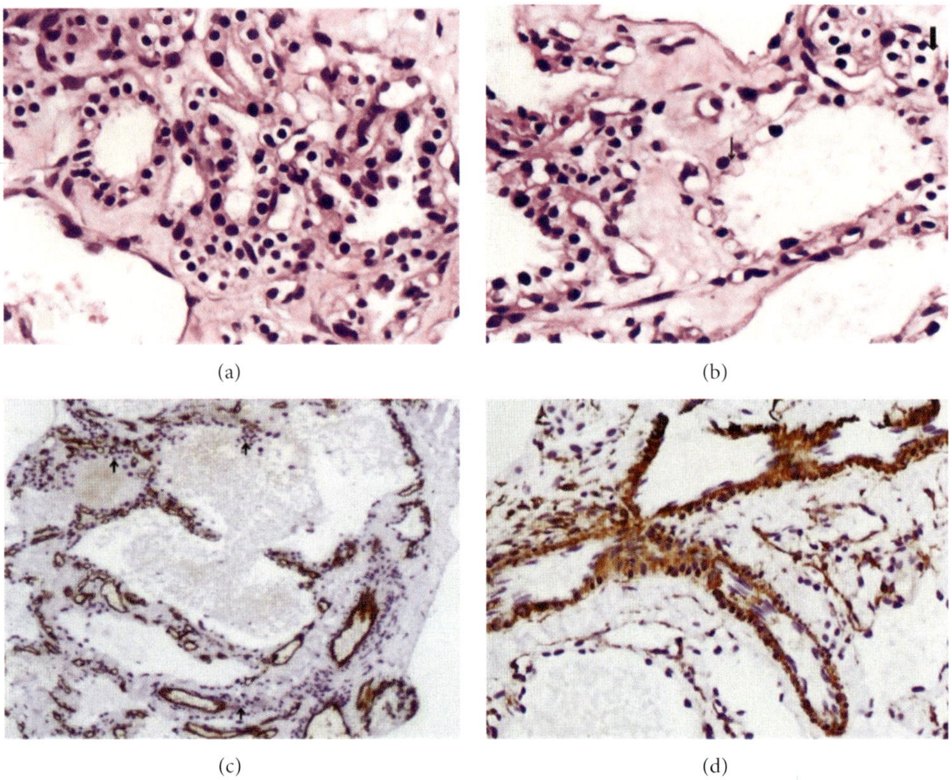

Figure 3: Histopathological evaluation of the SOL from liver. The tumoral mass comprising microcysts lined by cuboidal cells with bland looking nuclei and clear cytoplasm (200x; H&E stain) (a); tumor cells showing clear cytoplasm (thick arrow) and hobnail appearance (thin arrow) (200x; H&E) (b); tumor cells are accompanied by CD34 immunostaining positive vessels (100x) (c); Vessel wall highlighted by smooth muscle actin positivity (200x; SMA immunostaining) (d).

of benign nature and absence of symptoms. Follow-up was suggested, but the patient sought follow-up medical help only when the tumor was very large and surgical intervention was not feasible. The conclusion that surgical treatment in management of this tumor should be commenced only when the patient is symptomatic should be changed; in lieu with case reports, the malignant potential of this tumor group is getting more realized and patients, even if they are only a few, should be given the benefit of cure eventually, even though mean survival is about 36 months even with metastatic disease [1, 2]. Surgical management can be extended to a selected group of patients in whom the follow-up shows considerable growth and a change in clinical behavior. Microcystic adenomas are found throughout the pancreas with around 50% located in the head of the pancreas. These tumors have an average size of 6 cm, are well demarcated, and consist of multiple small thin walled cysts that contain straw colored fluid. In cases that reported malignant transformation, the average size ranged from 10 to 14 cm [12]. Our case was unique in that aspect. The tumor we report here is massive, being 26 cm in size, one that filled almost the whole of abdomen with extensive compression features on surrounding tissues. On computed tomography, microcystic adenomas appear well circumscribed with innumerable cysts. Sometimes, the tumor shows features of calcifications within the lesion or in the capsule and a central scar with a starburst pattern which is seen in about 30% of the cases [13]. Another unique presentation in this case was that of a huge retroperitoneal mass with solid and cystic heterogeneous components with patchy arterial enhancement with biliary tree involvement and vascular and surrounding tissue compression with angiographic findings suggestive of a "parasite" like mass lesion taking on extensive arterial supply from the celiac axis, a feature never presented in cases before. The histological findings of microcystic adenoma include the presence of single layer of small epithelial cysts lined by cuboidal cells with round to oval nuclei and pale to clear cytoplasm. Nuclear atypia is absent and mitoses are very rare. The cytoplasm is clear to pale and contains glycogen which stains positive for PAS as noticed in our case. Benign and malignant variants have identical histological features. The only distinguishing feature is presence of gross or microscopic evidence of invasiveness [14]. Immunohistochemistry normally reveals positivity for CK7, CK8, CK18, CK19, EMA, alpha-inhibin, and NSE.

Calretinin, CEA, chromogranin, MUC1, MUC2, S-100, HMB-45, CD-31, and vimentin are usually negative [15]. In our patient, the staining pattern was consistent with that of microcystic adenoma. The invasiveness was evident grossly and also microscopically with CD34 staining being positive, that is specific to vascular involvement. Treatment options in early tumor have been gladdening, but in late stages, with the development of metastases with large growth, surgical options they become moribund. Considering the age of the patient and also the associated comorbid conditions, surgical or ablative management was not provided. In conclusion, microcystic adenomas are rare tumors of the pancreas that cannot be completely judged to be benign in nature. They present variedly in patients and the choice of early surgical management should be given to the patient in the event of clinical and biological variation during follow-up which is picked up by the treating physician/surgeon.

References

[1] H. Abe, K. Kubota, M. Mori et al., "Serous cystadenoma of the pancreas with invasive growth: benign or malignant?" *American Journal of Gastroenterology*, vol. 93, no. 10, pp. 1963–1966, 1998.

[2] J. Compagno and J. E. Oertel, "Microcystic adenomas of the pancreas (glycogen-rich cystadenomas). A clinicopathologic study of 34 cases," *American Journal of Clinical Pathology*, vol. 69, no. 3, pp. 289–298, 1978.

[3] N. Yoshimi, S. Sugie, T. Tanaka et al., "A rare case of serous cystadenocarcinoma of the pancreas," *Cancer*, vol. 69, no. 10, pp. 2449–2453, 1992.

[4] D. H. George, F. Murphy, R. Michalski, and B. G. Ulmer, "Serous cystadenocarcinoma of the pancreas: a new entity?" *American Journal of Surgical Pathology*, vol. 13, no. 1, pp. 61–66, 1989.

[5] W. Kimura and M. Makuuchi, "Operative indications for cystic lesions of the pancreas with malignant potential—our experience," *Hepato-Gastroenterology*, vol. 46, no. 25, pp. 483–491, 1999.

[6] M. Shintaku, A. Arimoto, and N. Sakita, "Serous cystadenocarcinoma of the pancreas," *Pathology International*, vol. 55, no. 7, pp. 436–439, 2005.

[7] H. Zhu, L. Qin, M. Zhong et al., "Carcinoma ex microcystic adenoma of the pancreas: a report of a novel form of malignancy in serous neoplasms," *The American Journal of Surgical Pathology*, vol. 36, no. 2, pp. 305–310, 2012.

[8] K. K. Roggin, J. Chennat, A. Oto, A. Noffsinger, A. Briggs, and J. B. Matthews, "Pancreatic cystic neoplasm," *Current Problems in Surgery*, vol. 47, no. 6, pp. 459–510, 2010.

[9] J. C. King, T. T. Ng, S. C. White, G. Cortina, H. A. Reber, and O. J. Hines, "Pancreatic serous cystadenocarcinoma: a case report and review of the literature," *Journal of Gastrointestinal Surgery*, vol. 13, no. 10, pp. 1864–1868, 2009.

[10] J. le Borgne, L. de Calan, and C. Partensky, "Cystadenomas and cystadenocarcinomas of the pancreas: a multiinstitutional retrospective study of 398 cases," *Annals of Surgery*, vol. 230, no. 2, pp. 152–161, 1999.

[11] C. M. Wu, E. K. Fishman, R. K. Hruban, W. D. Schlott, and J. L. Cameron, "Serous cystic neoplasm involving the pancreas and liver: an unusual clinical entity," *Abdominal Imaging*, vol. 24, no. 1, pp. 75–77, 1999.

[12] K. Yamazaki and B. Eyden, "An immunohistochemical and ultrastructural study of pancreatic microcystic serous cyst adenoma with special reference to tumor-associated microvasculature and vascular endothelial growth factor in tumor cells," *Ultrastructural Pathology*, vol. 30, no. 1-2, pp. 119–128, 2006.

[13] K. Zirinsky, M. Abiri, and J. B. Baer, "Computed tomography demonstration of pancreatic microcystic adenoma," *American Journal of Gastroenterology*, vol. 79, no. 2, pp. 139–142, 1984.

[14] C. Galanis, A. Zamani, J. L. Cameron et al., "Resected serous cystic neoplasms of the pancreas: a review of 158 patients with recommendations for treatment," *Journal of Gastrointestinal Surgery*, vol. 11, no. 7, pp. 820–826, 2007.

[15] K. D. Horvath and J. A. Chabot, "An aggressive resectional approach to cystic neoplasms of the pancreas," *American Journal of Surgery*, vol. 178, no. 4, pp. 269–274, 1999.

An Uncommon Cause of a Small-Bowel Obstruction

Ali Zakaria, Bayan Al Share, Issam Turk, Samira Ahsan, and Waseem Farra

Department of Internal Medicine, Division of Pulmonology, Providence-Providence Park Hospital, Michigan State University College of Human Medicine, Southfield, MI, USA

Correspondence should be addressed to Ali Zakaria; alizakaria86@hotmail.com

Academic Editor: Shinji Tanaka

Sarcoidosis is a systemic granulomatous disease of unknown etiology, characterized by the formation of noncaseating granulomas. Gastrointestinal (GI) system involvement that is clinically recognizable occurs in less than 0.9% of patients with sarcoidosis, with data revealing small intestine involvement in 0.03% of the cases. A high index of suspension is required in patients presenting with small-bowel obstruction and previous history of sarcoidosis. Establishing a definitive diagnosis of GI sarcoidosis depends on biopsy evidence of noncaseating granulomas, exclusion of other causes of granulomatous disease, and evidence of sarcoidosis in at least one other organ system. Treatment of GI sarcoidosis depends on symptomatology and disease activity. Herein, we are presenting a case of 67-year-old female patient who had acute small-bowel obstruction at the level of jejunum with postoperative histopathologic evidence of noncaseating granulomatous inflammation with multinucleated giant cells, consistent with sarcoidosis.

1. Introduction

Sarcoidosis is a systemic granulomatous disease of unknown etiology, characterized by the formation of noncaseating granulomas. Gastrointestinal (GI) involvement is very rare and can occur in a patient with known sarcoidosis or as the initial manifestation of the disease. Small-bowel obstruction secondary to sarcoidosis has been described in few case reports. Herein, we are reporting a case of 67-year-old female patient who had acute small-bowel obstruction at the level of jejunum with postoperative histopathologic evidence of noncaseating granulomatous inflammation consistent with sarcoidosis.

2. Case Report

A 67-year-old female with previous medical history of inactive pulmonary sarcoidosis (Figure 1), hypertension, and impaired glucose tolerance, presented to emergency department with five-day history of nausea, vomiting, abdominal pain, and constipation. On physical examination she was alert, oriented, and not in acute distress. Her vital signs were as follows: Temp 36.7°C; pulse 93 bpm; respiratory rate 18 bpm; blood pressure 147/85 mmHg; and O_2% of 98% on room air. Her abdomen was distended and mildly tender over the epigastric area, with no evidence of organomegaly. Her bowel sounds were hyperactive. Initial imagining studies with abdominal X-ray revealed dilated small-bowel loops with multiple scattered air fluid levels suggesting partial versus early complete small-bowel obstruction. A contrasted computed tomography (CT) scan of the abdomen and pelvis demonstrated multiple dilated loops of proximal small bowel with no definitive transition point and no intraperitoneal free air or fluid identified, a picture suggestive of a high-grade small-bowel obstruction (Figure 2).

She was managed conservatively with bowel rest, nasogastric tube, and IV fluids. Her symptoms failed to improve, so gastrografin small-bowel follow-through was performed and demonstrated failure of contrast to pass into the colon (Figure 3).

General surgery was consulted and diagnostic laparoscopy was performed and revealed multiple dilated bowel loops which revealed diffuse skin tag appearing lesions on the antimesenteric surface of the midjejunum causing inflammatory adhesions to the mesentery (Figure 4). The bowel was completely viable with no additional lesions in the liver, stomach, or visible parts of the colon. Histopathologic examination of tissue biopsy revealed lymphohistiocytic noncaseating granulomatous inflammation with multinucleated giant cells, consistent with sarcoidosis (Figure 5). Further

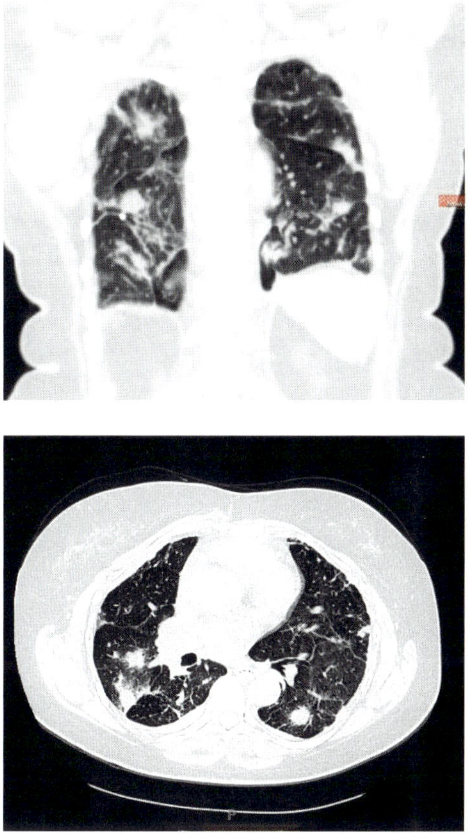

FIGURE 1: Computed tomography (CT) scan of the chest reveals diffuse parenchymal nodularity, with no honeycombing, hilar, or mediastinal adenopathy, consistent with stage III sarcoidosis.

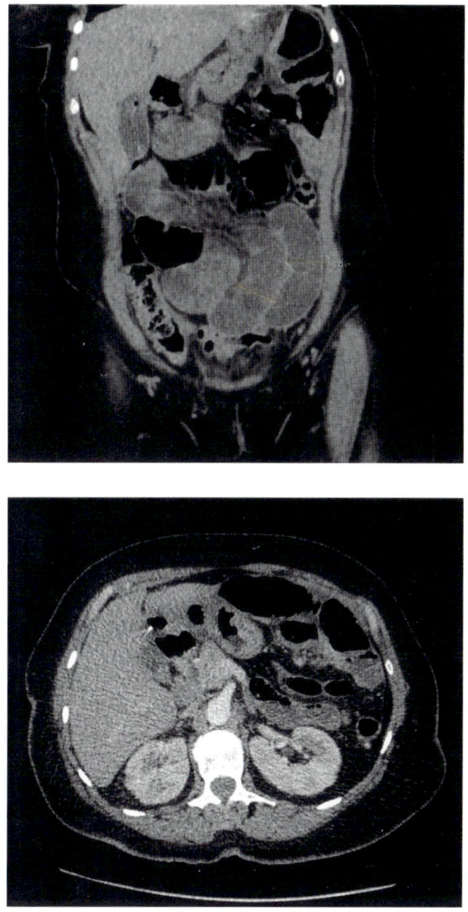

FIGURE 2: Computed tomography (CT) scan of the abdomen demonstrated early complete bowel obstruction at the level of midjejunum.

evaluation revealed negative acid-fast bacilli and fungal and viral tissue cultures. Her postoperative course was uncomplicated and she was discharged on prednisone taper dose with close outpatient follow-up.

3. Discussion

Sarcoidosis is a systemic granulomatous disease of unknown etiology, characterized by the formation of noncaseating granulomas. Gastrointestinal (GI) system involvement that is clinically recognizable occurs in 0.1–0.9% of patients with sarcoidosis, with one study revealing postmortem small intestine involvement on autopsy in 0.03% of the cases [1, 2]. It usually occurs in patients in their fifth or sixth decade of life with evidence of multisystem sarcoidosis in approximately one-half of patients. The most common manifestation is nonbloody diarrhea with colicky abdominal pain. It can also present with nonspecific constitutional symptoms, obstruction, and/or intestinal hemorrhage, a presentation that can mimic other diseases such as Crohn's disease. Other rare manifestations include mesenteric venous insufficiency due to pressure from enlarged sarcoid lymphadenopathy, megaloblastic anemia caused by terminal ilium infiltration, and protein-losing enteropathy [3–6]. Establishing a definitive diagnosis of GI sarcoidosis depends on three components: (1) biopsy evidence of noncaseating granulomas in the symptomatic or incident organ, (2) exclusion of other causes of granulomatous disease, particularly mycobacterial, fungal, and parasitic infections, and (3) clinical, radiographic, and optimally histopathologic evidence of sarcoidosis in at least one other organ system [7]. Imaging studies using computed tomography scan considered appropriate initial step in diagnosing patients who present with abdominal pain, while, in those who present with prominent diarrhea, endoscopy is more appropriate. Treatment of GI sarcoidosis depends on symptomatology and disease activity; asymptomatic patients can be monitored without active therapy, while symptomatic patients with substantial organ involvement and granulomatous inflammation on tissue biopsy should be treated with corticosteroid for six to eight weeks or until a response to therapy is noted and then gradually tapered, over a period of approximately six months [7]. The optimal duration of corticosteroid treatment for gastrointestinal sarcoidosis is not known, but experts recommend treating the initial manifestation for at least one year. Other treatments such as surgical intervention may be necessary in patients with bowel

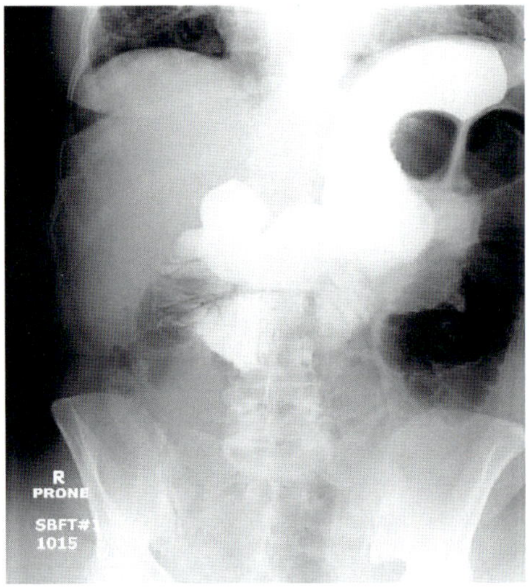

FIGURE 3: Gastrografin small-bowel follow-through demonstrated failure of contrast to pass into the colon.

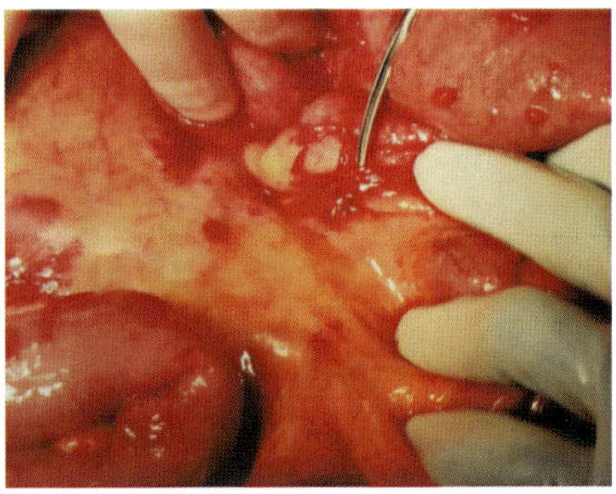

FIGURE 4: Intraoperative demonstration of the skin tag appearing lesion at the level of midjejunum causing inflammatory adhesions.

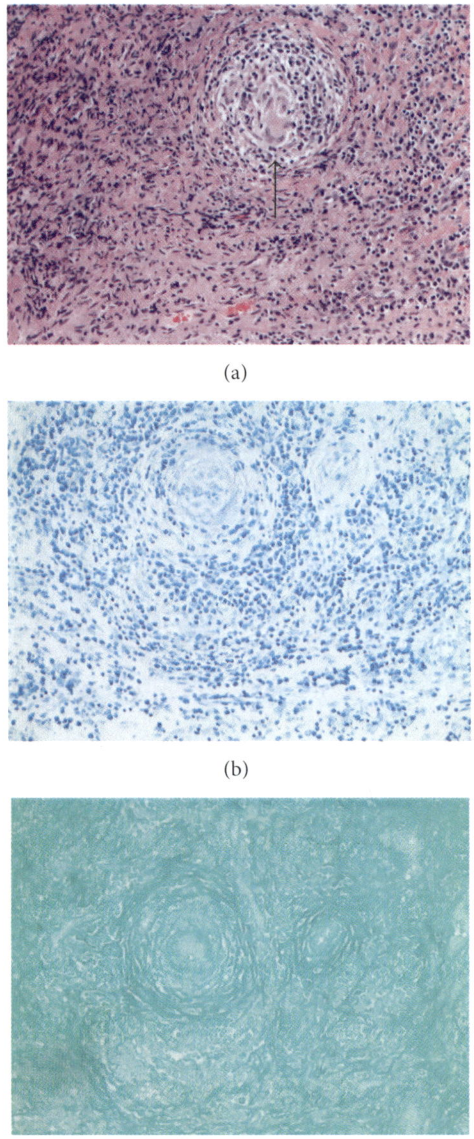

(a)

(b)

(c)

FIGURE 5: Histopathology of the resected small-bowel lesion. (a) H&E stain revealed lymphohistiocytic noncaseating granuloma with multinucleated giant cells (black arrow). (b) Negative for acid-fast bacilli (AFB) stain. (c) GMS stain negative for fungal infection.

obstruction, perforation, or massive hemorrhage. Monitoring of GI sarcoidosis is achieved clinically and radiographically, but there is no evidence for the role of serum angiotensin converting enzyme or serum interlukin-2 receptor in monitoring [8, 9].

4. Conclusion

Gastrointestinal (GI) sarcoidosis is very rare and can occur in a patient with known diagnosis or as initial presentation. A high index of suspension is required in patients presenting with small-bowel obstruction and previous history of sarcoidosis.

Acknowledgments

Authors would like to express their deepest appreciation to Dr. Juanita Evans for her valuable expertise in providing and reading the histopathology slides.

References

[1] A. M. Sharma, J. Kadakia, and O. P. Sharma, "Gastrointestinal sarcoidosis," *Seminars in Respiratory Medicine*, vol. 13, no. 6, pp. 442–449, 1992.

[2] K. Iwai, T. Takemura, M. Kitaichi, Y. Kawabata, and Y. Matsui, "Pathological studies on sarcoidosis autopsy. II. Early change,

mode of progression and death pattern," *Acta Pathologica Japonica*, vol. 43, no. 7-8, pp. 377–385, 1993.

[3] W. Schwarzschild and R. M. Myerson, "Venous insufficiency of the small intestine secondary to sarcoidosis of mesenteric lymph nodes," *American Journal of Gastroenterology*, vol. 50, no. 1, pp. 69–72, 1968.

[4] R. H. Fleming, M. Nuzek, and D. W. McFadden, "Small intestinal sarcoidosis with massive hemorrhage: report of a case," *Surgery*, vol. 115, no. 1, pp. 127–131, 1994.

[5] A. Rauf, P. Davis, and H. Levendoglu, "Sarcoidosis of the small intestine," *American Journal of Gastroenterology*, vol. 83, no. 2, pp. 187–189, 1988.

[6] O. S. Popović, S. Brkić, P. Bojić et al., "Sarcoidosis and protein losing enteropathy," *Gastroenterology*, vol. 78, pp. 119–125, 1980.

[7] E. C. Ebert, M. Kierson, and K. D. Hagspiel, "Gastrointestinal and hepatic manifestations of sarcoidosis," *The American Journal of Gastroenterology*, vol. 103, no. 12, pp. 3184–3192, 2008.

[8] J. C. Grutters, J.-M. Fellrath, L. Mulder, R. Janssen, J. M. M. Van Den Bosch, and H. Van Velzen-Blad, "Serum soluble interleukin-2 receptor measurement in patients with sarcoidosis: a clinical evaluation," *Chest*, vol. 124, no. 1, pp. 186–195, 2003.

[9] S. Miyoshi, H. Hamada, T. Kadowaki et al., "Comparative evaluation of serum markers in pulmonary sarcoidosis," *Chest*, vol. 137, no. 6, pp. 1391–1397, 2010.

10

A Novel Use of Early Radiation Therapy in the Treatment of Hyperbilirubinemia in a Patient with Primary Hepatic Lymphoma and Chronic Hepatitis C

Venkata S. Tammana,[1] Rehana Begum,[1] Patricia Oneal,[1] Hemamalini Karpurapu,[1] Amruta Muley,[1] Sri Lakshmi Hyndavi Yeruva,[1] Jacquelyn Dunmore-Griffith,[2] Eyasu Mekonen,[1] and Nabhani Hasan[3]

[1] *Department of Internal Medicine, Howard University Hospital, 2041 Georgia Avenue, NW, Washington, DC 20060, USA*
[2] *Department of Radiation Oncology, Howard University Hospital, Washington, DC, USA*
[3] *Department of Radiology, Howard University Hospital, Washington, DC, USA*

Correspondence should be addressed to Venkata S. Tammana; drtammana@yahoo.com

Academic Editor: Haruhiko Sugimura

Lymphomas arising in the liver are extremely rare. Here, we describe a case of Hepatitis C virus infection with primary hepatic lymphoma (PHL) presenting with hyperbilirubinemia. A 45-year-old African American male presented with abdominal pain, pruritus, and itching for two days. CT of abdomen and pelvis with contrast showed numerous masses in the liver. The liver biopsy was consistent with diffuse large B cell lymphoma (DLBCL). Conventional chemotherapy was avoided initially because of hyperbilirubinemia. Hence, radiation therapy was given initially to reduce his bilirubin levels and tumor size. The patient was able to complete six cycles of rituximab combined with cyclophosphamide, adriamycin, vincristine, and prednisone (R-CHOP) chemotherapy and achieved a complete response verified by positron emission tomography-computed tomography (PET-CT). PHL should be considered when there are numerous space occupying liver lesions seen on imaging. Hyperbilirubinemia may be a reason for delay in treatment for some of these patients. Hence, the role of radiation therapy prior to treatment with R-CHOP is an alternative to management for stage IV diffuse large B cell lymphoma.

1. Introduction

Lymphomas arising in liver are extremely rare. They can be primary (extranodal lymphoma arising solely in the liver without involvement of any other organ) or secondary (secondary involvement of liver in systemic non-Hodgkin's lymphoma (NHL)). Primary hepatic lymphoma (PHL) comprises only about 0.016% of all cases of non-Hodgkin's lymphoma [1]. PHL have been described in patients with Hepatitis C virus (HCV) infection [2]. Because of nonspecific clinical symptoms or imaging pattern, PHL is often misdiagnosed as hepatocellular carcinoma, metastatic tumor, or liver abscess. Here, we present a case of PHL in a patient with HCV infection presenting with significant hyperbilirubinemia and highlight his response to radiation therapy and systemic chemotherapy.

2. Case Presentation

A 45-year-old African American male with a past medical history of hypertension, HCV infection, and polysubstance abuse was admitted with epigastric and right upper quadrant abdominal pain, pruritus, and itching for two days. Symptoms are associated with nonbilious vomiting, fatigue, and a 9 kg unintentional weight loss over three months. He denied any history of Hepatitis B in the past. Ten months before, he had a similar complaint where evaluation at an outside facility showed a hepatic mass. A liver biopsy at that time showed acute inflammation suggestive of an abscess with extensive chronic inflammation and fibrosis adjacent to the necrosis, moderate to severe acute and chronic periportal inflammation with portal lymphoid aggregates. Cultures from the biopsy were negative for any organisms but the patient was treated with an empiric course of vancomycin and piperacillin/tazobactam for four weeks. His social history was significant for cigarette smoking, alcohol, and intravenous illicit drug use of heroin and cocaine. The family history was significant for a brother with gastric lymphoma, now in remission. Physical exam was significant for skin excoriations, scleral icterus without any lymphadenopathy, hepatomegaly, and tenderness along the epigastrium and right upper quadrant areas.

Initial laboratory values showed a hemoglobin of 13.0 gm/dL, hematocrit of 37.7%, white blood cell count of 4.4×10^3, and platelet count of 240×10^3. His metabolic panel showed normal renal function tests with a calcium of 9.4 mg/dL. His comprehensive metabolic panel revealed a total bilirubin of 6.1 mg/dL, direct bilirubin of 4.1 mg/dL, aspartate aminotransferase (AST) of 150 U/L, alanine aminotransferase (ALT) of 142 U/L, alkaline phosphatase (ALP) of 282 IU/L, gamma-glutamyl transferase (GGT) of 385 IU/L, total protein of 7.4 g/dL, and albumin of 3.6 g/dL. His prothrombin time was 13.7 seconds with an International Normal Ratio (INR) of 1.04. Amylase and lipase levels were within normal limits. Hepatitis B panel showed immunity to Hepatitis B. His HCV RNA viral load was 422131 IU/mL (5.63 log). HCV genotype is 1b. HIV by ELISA was negative. His alpha-fetoprotein levels (AFP) were 2.2 ng/mL. Blood cultures were negative. Triphasic computed tomography (CT) of the abdomen and pelvis with contrast showed multiple masses in the liver (largest being 8.8 cm) without any cholelithiasis or extrahepatic bile duct dilatation (Figure 1). There was no significant enhancement of the hepatic lesions on arterial phase, while on portal venous phase the lesions showed slight enhancement. The spleen, pancreas, gallbladder, kidneys, and adrenals appeared within normal limits. Over his hospital course, his bilirubin levels increased to 23.3 mg/dL on eleventh day along with aspartate transaminase (AST) of 277 U/L, alanine aminotransferase (ALT) of 197 U/L, and alkaline phosphatase (ALP) of 199 IU/L (Table 1). In spite of high bilirubin levels, the patient maintained normal coagulation parameters and showed no evidence of hepatic encephalopathy. CT chest with contrast was within normal limits. Meanwhile, both upper endoscopy and colonoscopy were negative for occult malignancy. The biopsy of the liver mass done under fluoroscopic guidance was consistent with diffuse large B cell lymphoma (DLBCL). By immunohistochemistry, the cells were positive for CD 20, CD 10, and BCL-6. The Ki-67 proliferative index was 100% (Figure 2). FISH for c-myc rearrangement was negative. Bone marrow biopsy was negative for lymphoma.

With stage IVB DLBCL and elevated bilirubin levels, there was a concern for giving full dose chemotherapy, since the liver metabolizes most of the chemotherapy agents. A decision was made to do local irradiation to the liver and reevaluate his bilirubin level to determine if chemotherapy could be administered. The patient's liver received a total dose of 6 Gy in 4 fractions of 1.5 Gy each using a 2-field 3D conformal technique with 10 MV photon beam therapy on days 1, 2, 9, and 12. Initial staging positron emission tomography- (PET-) CT showed decreased metabolic activity compared with normal adjacent liver parenchyma, suggesting a positive response to treatment and no extranodal disease. Meanwhile, total bilirubin levels fell to 3.4 mg/dL (Table 2) and allowed the first dose of R-CHOP (rituximab combined with cyclophosphamide, adriamycin, vincristine, and prednisone) chemotherapy to be administered at a 50% dose reduction. The patient subsequently received six cycles of R-CHOP. After completion, beside neutropenia, no other significant adverse effects were noted. Restaging PET-CT showed no hypermetabolic activity in the liver.

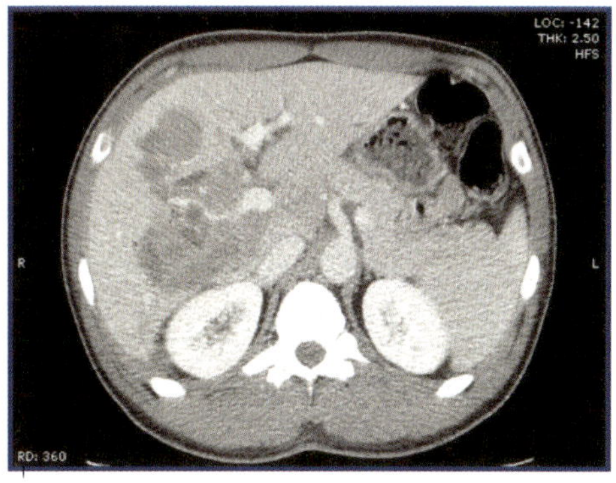

FIGURE 1: CT scan with intravenous contrast-portal venous phase showing multiple lesions in the liver.

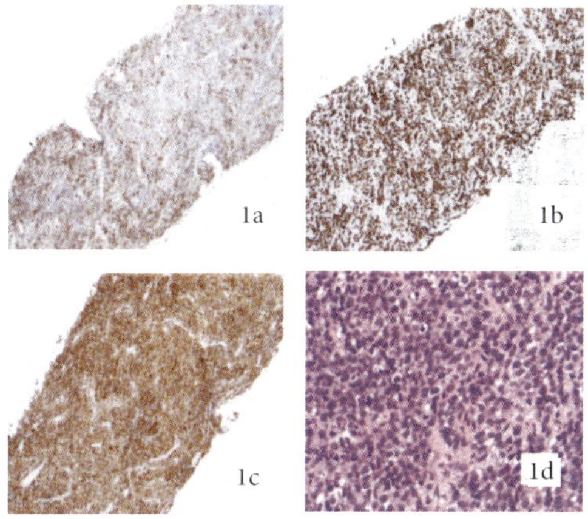

FIGURE 2: Liver Biopsy shows (1a) CD 20 positive on IHC. (1c) CD 10 positive on IHC. (1b) Ki 67 of 100% (1d) DLBCL.

3. Discussion

Caccamo et al. [9] defined PHL as a lymphoma localized and limited to the liver without extrahepatic involvement. The vast majority (67%) of PHL patients are middle aged men (median age 53 years) [10]. The male to female ratio is 2.3 : 1.0. Page et al. [2] reviewed twenty-four patients with PHL in which seventeen patients (71%) had right

Table 1: Trend of patients LFTs.

Date (month/day/year)	Total bilirubin (mg/dL)	Direct bilirubin (mg/dL)	AST	ALT	ALP
11/21/2012	0.3		56	88	68
12/12/2012	6.1	4.1	150	142	282
12/22/2012	23.3	14.9	277	197	199

Table 2: LFTs trend table after initiating radiation therapy.

Date (month/day/year)	Total bilirubin (mg/dL)	Direct bilirubin (mg/dL)	AST	ALT	ALP
12/28/2012 **(day of radiation therapy)**	19.8	10.9	147	155	176
12/30/2012	10.3	5.4	103	127	140
01/10/2013	3.8	Not done	93	151	90
05/08/2013	1.3	Not done	71	69	85

upper quadrant pain, nine patients (38%) had B symptoms (fever, night sweats), four patients (16.7%) had nausea and emesis, and three patients (12.5%) had weakness and fatigue. Hepatomegaly was present in eighteen patients (75%) and jaundice was present in only one patient (4.2%). Acute liver failure due to tumor infiltration in NHL has been reported earlier [11]. Higuchi et al. [12] reported the presence of chronic liver disease in 16 patients (31%) of the 51 cases of PHL.

It is rare for a patient with PHL to present with very high bilirubin levels. Jaundice in PHL patients can be due to the following reasons: (a) patients having a concomitant history of cirrhosis, (b) patients presenting with fulminant liver failure due to massive sinusoidal infiltration by lymphoma, and (c) lymphoma causing intra- or extrahepatic biliary obstruction. The patient that we described above had a progressive increase in total bilirubin reaching a peak value of 23.3 mg/dL. To the best of our knowledge, this is the first report described in literature where a patient with HCV infection had such a high bilirubin level due to PHL.

60% of the patients with PHL tested for HCV were positive [2]. Some of the possible theories for HCV induced lymphoma genesis include (a) continuous external stimulation of lymphocyte receptors by viral antigens and consecutive proliferation, (b) HCV replication in B cells with oncogenic effect mediated by intracellular viral proteins, (c) permanent B cell damage, for example, mutation of tumor suppressor genes, caused by a transiently intracellular virus (hit and run theory), and (d) prevention of B cell apoptosis by downregulation of caspase 1 and caspase 4 [13, 14].

Histological subtypes of PHL described in the literature include diffuse large B cell lymphoma (DLBCL), Burkitt's lymphoma, mucosa associated lymphoid tissue (MALT) lymphoma, mantle cell lymphoma, and T cell lymphoma with the most frequent one being DLBCL (96%) [10]. PHL has its own characteristic imaging features. Elsayes et al. [15] described 12 cases of PHL. Three patients (25%) presented with a single focal lesion, 8 patients (67%) presented with multiple well-defined lesions, and 1 patient (8%) presented with diffuse hepatic involvement on CT imaging. Prognosis of PHL patients with nodular infiltration of the liver is better than that of diffuse infiltrative pattern [6]. The patient that we described has nodular infiltration pattern of the liver involvement. Imaging studies in PHL can mimic that of metastatic disease, hepatocellular carcinoma, and liver abscess and hence liver biopsy is necessary to make the diagnosis. Tumor markers like AFP, carcinoembryonic antigen (CEA), and CA 19–9 are usually normal.

4. Management

The treatment of patients with PHL reported in the literature has not been consistent. Patients were treated with various modalities like surgery, combination chemotherapy, radiation therapy, or a combination of these. Localized PHL could be cured by resection, or the tumor burden could be reduced before or after surgery with chemotherapy [16]. Surgical resection was not feasible in our patient due to presence of multiple lesions.

A complete remission (CR) rate of 83.3% was achieved in PHL when systemic combination chemotherapy was used as the main modality of treatment [2]. Similarly, CR was achieved in all 4 cases of PHL in HCV patients after systemic chemotherapy. The presence of chronic active hepatitis on account of the HCV infection does not appear to influence response and tolerance to chemotherapy [17].

Adriamycin (one of the agents in CHOP regimen), an anthracycline, is predominantly excreted in bile. Patients with cholestasis have delayed clearance of doxorubicin and its metabolites and can lead to greater systemic toxicity [3, 18]. Despite reports that treatment with systemic chemotherapy can lead to complete response, it is not an option in our patient as his bilirubin is >20 mg/dl. Ma et al. [19] reported a patient with PHL whose total bilirubin was 20.87 mg/dL prior to initiation of an attenuated R-CHOP chemotherapy. Though the patient's total bilirubin improved to 1.19 mg/dL prior to the third cycle of chemotherapy, patient died from the complication of chemotherapy after fourth cycle. So patients with PHL and jaundice are a challenge in regard to the safest and best available modality of treatment. Table 3 summarizes the cases of jaundice (bilirubin >2 mg/dL) due to PHL reported in the literature and how they were managed on a Pubmed search. Cases where the management was not outlined were not included in the table. In our management,

Table 3

n = PHL + jaundice	Age, sex	Lesion	T bili mg/dL	Histology	Treatment	Outcome	Reference
1	67, M	Multiple nodules in liver	20.87	DLBCL	R-CHOP	Died after 4th cycle due to ARDS	Ma et al. [19]
1	62, M	Large solitary right hepatic lobe mass	N/M	DLBCL	None	Died 3 months after tumor diagnosis	DeMent et al. [4]
2	53, M	Diffuse	N/M	Pleiomorphic small cell*	Prednisolone and later multiagent chemotherapy	Died of disease at 18 months	Anthony et al. [5]
	76, M	Diffuse	N/M	T zone*	Prednisolone and chlorambucil	Alive and well at 3 years	
2	49, M	Nodular	N/M	B cell type	8 cycles of anthracycline containing CT#	CR at 52 months	Emile et al. [6]
1	90, F	Single mass in left lobe	2.3	DLBCL	4 cycles of attenuated CHOP	CR at 2 years	Agmon-Levin et al. [7]
1	55, F	Presented as biliary stricture with tumor in caudate lobe and left lobe of the liver invading CBD and occluding portal vein	3.4	DLBCL	Surgery followed by 6 cycles of CHOP + VP 16	Alive after 4.5 years after surgery	Yoneyama et al. [8]

N/M: not mentioned; M: male; F: female; CT: chemotherapy; DLBCL: diffuse large B cell lymphoma; *based on Kiel's classification subtype; #complete chemotherapy regimen not mentioned; CR: complete remission; VP 16: etoposide, ARDS: acute respiratory distress syndrome, T bili: total bilirubin, mg/dL: milligram/deciliter, PHL: primary hepatic lymphoma; R-CHOP: rituximab, cyclophosphamide, adriamycin, vincristine, and prednisone; CBD: common bile duct.

we have opted to give localized radiation therapy to reduce bilirubin levels, which thereby facilitated our use of R-CHOP chemotherapy. Our patient did have a complete response after six cycles of chemotherapy without any residual activity in the liver on the restaging PET scan. By administering chemotherapy, when the bilirubin was relatively mildly elevated, we think we might have prevented more serious complications from the chemotherapy. To the best of our knowledge, this is the first report in the literature where use of localized radiation therapy to the liver before systemic chemotherapy prompted a dramatic drop in bilirubin levels, thereby allowing the use of systemic chemotherapy (R-CHOP) and achieving a complete response in a PHL patient with HCV infection.

5. Conclusion

When multiple space occupying lesions are seen on imaging of the liver without any primary lesion or any other organ involvement with normal alpha fetoprotein, CA19–9, and carcinoembryonic antigen (CEA) levels, PHL should be considered in the differential diagnosis of these lesions and biopsy should be strongly considered in patients with HCV infection. PHL can cause significant hyperbilirubinemia in patients with HCV infection. If PHL is causing hyperbilirubinemia in a patient with HCV infection, localized radiation therapy can be considered to reduce bilirubin levels within an acceptable range where full dose of chemotherapy can be initiated in avoiding serious life-threatening complications.

References

[1] C. Freeman, J. W. Berg, and S. J. Cutler, "Occurrence and prognosis of extranodal lymphomas," *Cancer*, vol. 29, no. 1, pp. 252–260, 1972.

[2] R. D. Page, J. E. Romaguera, B. Osborne et al., "Primary hepatic lymphoma: favorable outcome after combination chemotherapy," *Cancer*, vol. 92, pp. 2023–2029, 2001.

[3] J. Floyd, I. Mirza, B. Sachs, and M. C. Perry, "Hepatotoxicity of chemotherapy," *Seminars in Oncology*, vol. 33, no. 1, pp. 50–67, 2006.

[4] S. H. DeMent, R. B. Mann, S. P. Staal, F. P. Kuhajda, and J. K. Boitnott, "Primary lymphomas of the liver. Report of six cases and review of the literature," *American Journal of Clinical Pathology*, vol. 88, no. 3, pp. 255–263, 1987.

[5] P. P. Anthony, P. Sarsfield, and T. Clarke, "Primary lymphoma of the liver: clinical and pathological features of 10 patients," *Journal of Clinical Pathology*, vol. 43, no. 12, pp. 1007–1013, 1990.

[6] J.-F. Emile, D. Azoulay, J.-M. Gornet et al., "Primary non-Hodgkin's lymphomas of the liver with nodular and diffuse infiltration patterns have different prognoses," *Annals of Oncology*, vol. 12, no. 7, pp. 1005–1010, 2001.

[7] N. Agmon-Levin, I. Berger, M. Shtalrid, H. Schlanger, and Z. M. Sthoeger, "Primary hepatic lymphoma: a case report and review

of the literature," *Age and Ageing*, vol. 33, no. 6, pp. 637–640, 2004.

[8] F. Yoneyama, Y. Nimura, J. Kamiya et al., "Primary lymphoma of the liver with bile duct invasion and tumoral occlusion of the portal vein: report of a case," *Journal of Hepatology*, vol. 29, no. 3, pp. 485–488, 1998.

[9] D. Caccamo, N. K. Pervez, and A. Marchevsky, "Primary lymphoma of the liver in the acquired immunodeficiency syndrome," *Archives of Pathology and Laboratory Medicine*, vol. 110, no. 6, pp. 553–555, 1986.

[10] K. I. K. Lei, "Primary non-Hodgkin's lymphoma of the liver," *Leukemia and Lymphoma*, vol. 29, no. 3-4, pp. 293–299, 1998.

[11] D. Rowbotham, J. Wendon, and R. Williams, "Acute liver failure secondary to hepatic infiltration: a single centre experience of 18 cases," *Gut*, vol. 42, no. 4, pp. 576–580, 1998.

[12] T. Higuchi, K. Nomoto, H. Mori et al., "Case report: Primary hepatic lymphoma associated with chronic liver disease," *Journal of Gastroenterology and Hepatology*, vol. 12, no. 3, pp. 237–242, 1997.

[13] J. Peveling-Oberhag, L. Arcaini, M. L. Hansmann, and S. Zeuzem, "Hepatitis C-associated B-cell non-Hodgkin lymphomas. Epidemiology, molecular signature and clinical management," *J Hepatol*, vol. 59, no. 1, pp. 169–177, 2013.

[14] C.-G. Wu, A. Budhu, S. Chen et al., "Effect of hepatitis C virus core protein on the molecular profiling of human B lymphocytes," *Molecular Medicine*, vol. 12, no. 1–3, pp. 47–53, 2006.

[15] K. M. Elsayes, C. O. Menias, J. M. Willatt, A. Pandya, and M. Wiggins, "Primary hepatic lymphoma: Imaging findings," *Journal of Medical Imaging and Radiation Oncology*, vol. 53, no. 4, pp. 373–379, 2009.

[16] V. S. Avlonitis and D. Linos, "Primary hepatic lymphoma: A review," *European Journal of Surgery*, vol. 165, no. 8, pp. 725–729, 1999.

[17] A. De Renzo, F. Perna, M. Persico et al., "Excellent prognosis and prevalence of HCV infection of primary hepatic and splenic non-Hodgkin's lymphoma," *European Journal of Haematology*, vol. 81, no. 1, pp. 51–57, 2008.

[18] P. J. Johnson, N. Dobbs, C. Kalayci et al., "Clinical efficacy and toxicity of standard dose Adriamycin in hyperbilirubinaemic patients with hepatocellular carcinoma: relation to liver tests and pharmacokinetic parameters," *British Journal of Cancer*, vol. 65, no. 5, pp. 751–755, 1992.

[19] Y. J. Ma, E. Q. Chen, X. B. Chen, J. Wang, and H. Tang, "Primary hepatic diffuse large b cell lymphoma: a case report," *Hepatitis Monthly*, vol. 11, no. 3, pp. 203–205, 2011.

11

Loss of HER2 Positivity after Trastuzumab in HER2-Positive Gastric Cancer: Is Change in HER2 Status Significantly Frequent?

Yu Ishimine,[1] Akira Goto,[1] Yoshito Watanabe,[2] Hidetaka Yajima,[3] Suguru Nakagaki,[1] Takashi Yabana,[1] Takeya Adachi,[1] Yoshihiro Kondo,[1] and Kiyoshi Kasai[4]

[1] *Department of Gastroenterology, Otaru General Hospital, 1-2-1 Wakamatu, Otaru 047-8550, Japan*
[2] *Department of Surgery, Otaru General Hospital, 1-2-1 Wakamatu, Otaru 047-8550, Japan*
[3] *Department of Gastroenterology, Rheumatology, and Clinical Immunology, Sapporo Medical University, S1W17, Chuo-ku, Sapporo 060-8556, Japan*
[4] *Department of Laboratory Medicine, Otaru General Hospital, 1-2-1 Wakamatu, Otaru 047-8550, Japan*

Correspondence should be addressed to Akira Goto; goa@sapmed.ac.jp

Academic Editor: Olga I. Giouleme

Trastuzumab has recently been introduced as a treatment for HER2-positive metastatic and/or unresectable gastric cancer (MUGC); however, compared with breast cancer, some issues concerning HER2 and trastuzumab therapy for gastric cancer remain unclear. A 74-year-old woman received trastuzumab-containing chemotherapy for HER2-positive MUGC. She had a marked response to 8 months of chemotherapy, and gastrectomy and hepatic metastasectomy with curative intent were performed. The resected specimen showed complete loss of HER2 positivity in the residual tumor. For MUGC, a change in HER2 status during the course of the disease with or without chemotherapy has rarely been reported. However, in breast cancer, a significant frequency of change in HER2 status during the course of disease has been reported, and reevaluation of HER2 positivity in metastatic/recurrent sites is recommended. The choice of trastuzumab for MUGC is currently based on the HER2 status of the primary tumor at the time of initial diagnosis, without reassessment of HER2 status during the course of disease and/or in metastatic/recurrent sites, on the assumption that HER2 status is stable. However, our case casts doubt on the stability of HER2 in gastric cancer.

1. Introduction

The primary treatment for patients with metastatic and/or unresectable gastric cancer (MUGC) is systematic chemotherapy. Although the combination of 5-fluorouracil and cisplatin has been the standard regimen for the treatment of MUGC, new cytotoxic agents such as S-1, capecitabine, paclitaxel, docetaxel, oxaliplatin, irinotecan, and their combinations have proven to be more effective and better tolerated, resulting in the improvement of median survival up to 13 months [1–3]. In addition, recent research has shown that adding trastuzumab, a humanized monoclonal antibody targeting the human epidermal growth factor receptor 2 (HER2) protein, to chemotherapy (fluoropyrimidines and cisplatin) for patients with MUGC with HER2 overexpression and/or gene amplification (the so-called HER2-positive gastric cancer) has a significant superiority to chemotherapy alone in terms of overall survival (median survival 13.8 months with trastuzumab versus 11.1 months with chemotherapy alone) [4].

We report a case in which chemotherapy containing trastuzumab made it possible to perform curative gastrectomy in a patient with HER2-positive MUGC at initial diagnosis; this case is noteworthy in that HER2 positivity in resected specimens of the residual tumor was completely lost. Loss of HER2 positivity after treatment with trastuzumab for HER2-positive MUGC has rarely been reported. HER2 status is an essential biomarker for the effectiveness of trastuzumab, and consequently, knowledge of HER2 stability during the course of disease is critical for determining the introduction, the continued use, or elimination of trastuzumab. We discuss

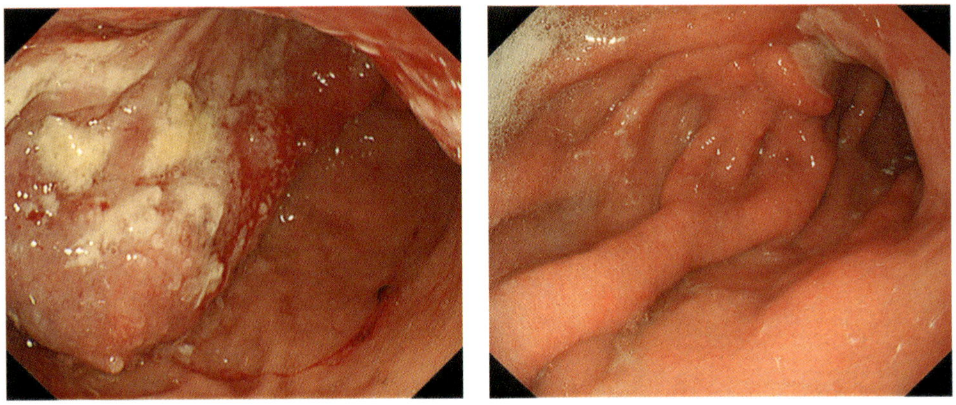

(a) (b)

Figure 1: Endoscopic findings. (a) Gastroscopy at presentation revealed an ulcerative mass with raised margins along the lesser curvature extending from the lower body of the stomach to the antrum. (b) After completion of the 11th course of chemotherapy (capecitabine + CDDP + trastuzumab), the gastric tumor is decreased remarkably.

the stability of HER2 status in gastric cancer and provide a literature review of this important topic.

2. Case Report

A 74-year-old woman with the chief complaint of palpable masses in her abdomen presented to our hospital in May 2013. Physical examination revealed one 50-mm mass in the upper central abdomen and three 20–30-mm palpable masses in the other parts of her abdomen. Esophagogastroduodenoscopy (EGD) revealed an ulcerative mass with raised margins along the lesser curvature extending from the lower body of the stomach to the antrum (Figure 1(a)). Biopsy of the lesion revealed a well-differentiated tubular adenocarcinoma (Figure 2(a)), and HER2 immunohistochemistry (IHC) scoring of the tumor in the biopsy specimen was 3+, indicating HER2-positivity (Figure 2(b)). Contrast-enhanced computed tomography (CT) demonstrated marked wall thickening of the lower part of the stomach with irregular outer borders and an increased density of the surrounding fat tissue, forming a mass that was 80 × 45 mm (Figure 3(a)). Several nodules in the liver were detected. Two of these nodules in the lateral segment of the liver were directly contiguous from the gastric mass and were considered direct invasion of the gastric cancer (Figure 3(b)). Invasion into the pancreas was suggested by obliteration of the fat plane between the gastric mass and the pancreas. CT also revealed multiple nodules in the peritoneal cavity, a few masses in the abdominal wall, and ascites. Many perigastric lymph nodes and several para-aortic lymph nodes were swollen.

With this information, this patient's gastric cancer was classified as stage IV (cT4bN3aM1) according to the 7th TNM classification of the American Joint Committee on Cancer/Union for International Cancer Control (AJCC/UICC) staging system for gastric cancer. She was treated with 3-week courses of capecitabine (2000 mg/m^2/day) orally on days 1–14, cisplatin (80 mg/m^2) intravenously on day 1, and trastuzumab (8 mg/kg loading dose followed by 6 mg/kg) intravenously on day 1. From the 3rd course, the doses of capecitabine and cisplatin were reduced to 1500 mg/m^2/day and 60 mg/m^2, respectively, due to nonhematologic toxicity (nausea, anorexia, and renal impairment). After completion of the 4th course of chemotherapy, at 3 months after diagnosis, a 76% decrease in measureable tumor burden compared to baseline according to RECIST 1.1 criteria was observed. From the 6th course, cisplatin was discontinued due to renal impairment, but treatment with capecitabine and trastuzumab continued. After completion of the 11th course, at 8 months after diagnosis, EGD showed a marked reduction of the gastric tumor (Figure 1(b)), and contrast-enhanced CT (Figures 3(c) and 3(d)) showed a 90% reduction in measureable tumor burden. No metastases were detected in the liver except for one small nodule in the lateral segment (Figure 3(d)). Ascites and metastases in the peritoneal cavity, abdominal wall, and para-aortic lymph nodes were completely resolved.

Given this response to the treatment, complete resection of the residual tumor was deemed possible, and 9 months after the diagnosis, distal gastrectomy with D2 lymphadenectomy and hepatic metastasectomy of the small nodule in the lateral segment were performed. Operative findings showed no macroscopic peritoneal metastasis and the absence of peritoneal lavage cytology. Macroscopic complete resection was possible. Pathologic findings of the 36×25 mm mass from the resected stomach revealed a moderately differentiated adenocarcinoma with subserosal invasion (Figure 2(c)) and hyalinization and fibrosis adjacent to the tumor in the lower third of the gastric wall. Eight regional lymph nodes were positive for tumor cells. Specimens of the nodule from the resected liver revealed only hyalinization and fibrosis without tumor cells. HER2 by IHC was completely negative in the residual tumor from the resected stomach (Figure 2(d)) and lymph nodes. HER2 also was negative by fluorescence in situ hybridization (FISH). The patient received adjuvant chemotherapy comprising capecitabine and trastuzumab for 6 months, and at the completion of adjuvant chemotherapy, the patient had no signs of recurrence.

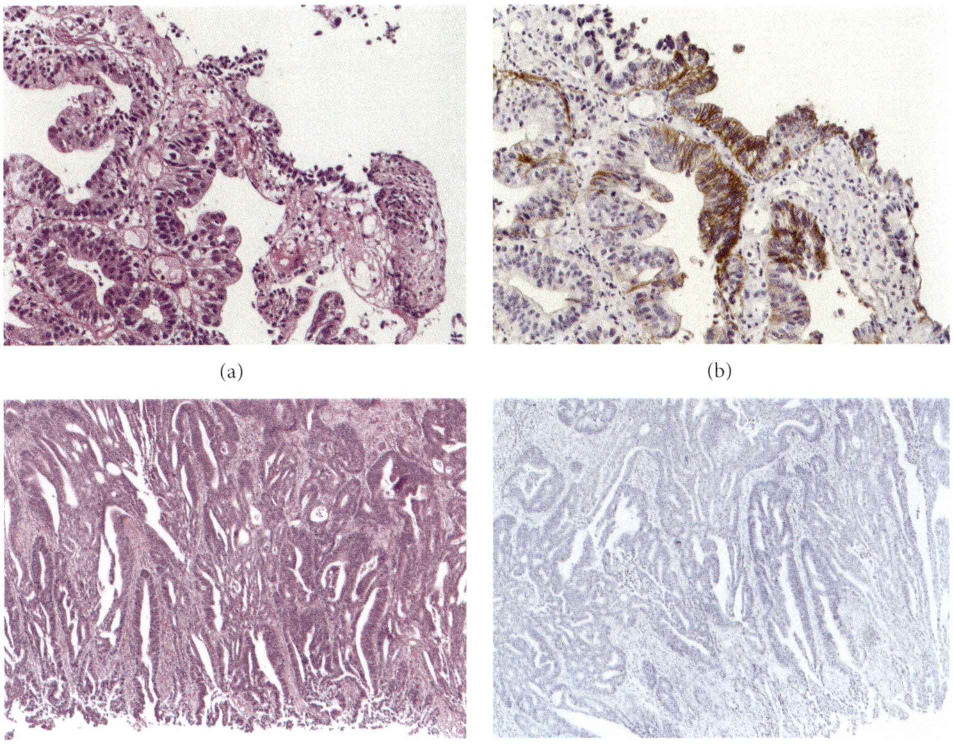

FIGURE 2: Microscopic findings of gastric cancer. (a) and (b) show biopsy specimens at presentation. (a) Histological findings show a well-differentiated tubular adenocarcinoma (hematoxylin and eosin staining, original magnification ×40). (b) Immunohistological findings of HER2 immunostaining show strong basolateral membrane reactivity with heterogeneity. The gastric cancer is scored as 3+ by HER2 immunohistochemistry scoring criteria (original magnification ×40). (c) and (d) show the resected specimen after chemotherapy including trastuzumab. (c) Histological findings show a moderately differentiated tubular adenocarcinoma invading into the subserosa (hematoxylin and eosin staining, original magnification ×40). (d) Immunohistological findings of HER2 immunostaining showed no membranous reactivity in any tumor cells (original magnification ×40).

3. Discussion

Approximately 15–20% of invasive breast cancers have HER2 overexpression and/or gene amplification [5, 6]. HER2 has been used as a molecular target for breast cancer for many years. Trastuzumab was initially approved for the treatment of patients with HER2-positive metastatic breast cancer [7]. Trastuzumab is now the standard treatment in adjuvant therapy for HER2-positive early-stage breast cancer [8] and is also recommended as part of neoadjuvant chemotherapy (NAC) [9].

In breast cancer, discordance in HER2 status between the primary tumor and the metastasis/recurrence and HER2 stability during the course of disease has been evaluated in several reports. The discordance rate of HER2 status in breast cancer has been reported to be 3–16% [10–13], with 12–19% of HER2-positive tumors in the primary site converting to HER2-negative status at the sites of metastasis/recurrence [11, 12] and 7–10% of HER2-negative tumors converting to HER2-positive status [11, 12, 14]. Conversion of the HER2 status from positive to negative may be more frequent than conversion from negative to positive. The cause of discordance of HER2 status has been attributed to changes in the molecular profile during the course of tumor progression, the differing effects of prior treatment on clonal subsets, heterogeneity of HER2 expression within the tumor, and technical errors in tissue processing and evaluation.

Several previous reports have evaluated how chemotherapy with or without anti-HER2 agents, including trastuzumab, influences HER2 expression. The discordance rate of HER2 status before and after NAC has been reported to be 0–9.5% [15–17]. In HER2-positive breast cancer, loss of HER2 positivity after NAC has been reported to be 8–32% [15, 17–19], and in HER2-negative breast cancer, gain of HER2 positivity after NAC has been reported in 0–5% of cases [15, 17]. Niikura et al. reported that the conversion rate from positive in the primary tumors to negative in the sites of metastases was significantly higher in patients with prior chemotherapy than in patients without prior chemotherapy (17% versus 10%) [20]. These previous reports have suggested that chemotherapy can be associated with a change of HER2 status in breast cancer.

In addition to studying the association between HER2 status and traditional chemotherapeutic agents, several reports have analyzed the association between change in HER2 status and trastuzumab therapy. A loss of HER2 positivity in patients treated with trastuzumab therapy has been reported in 14.7–37% of HER2-positive breast cancers [14, 18–21].

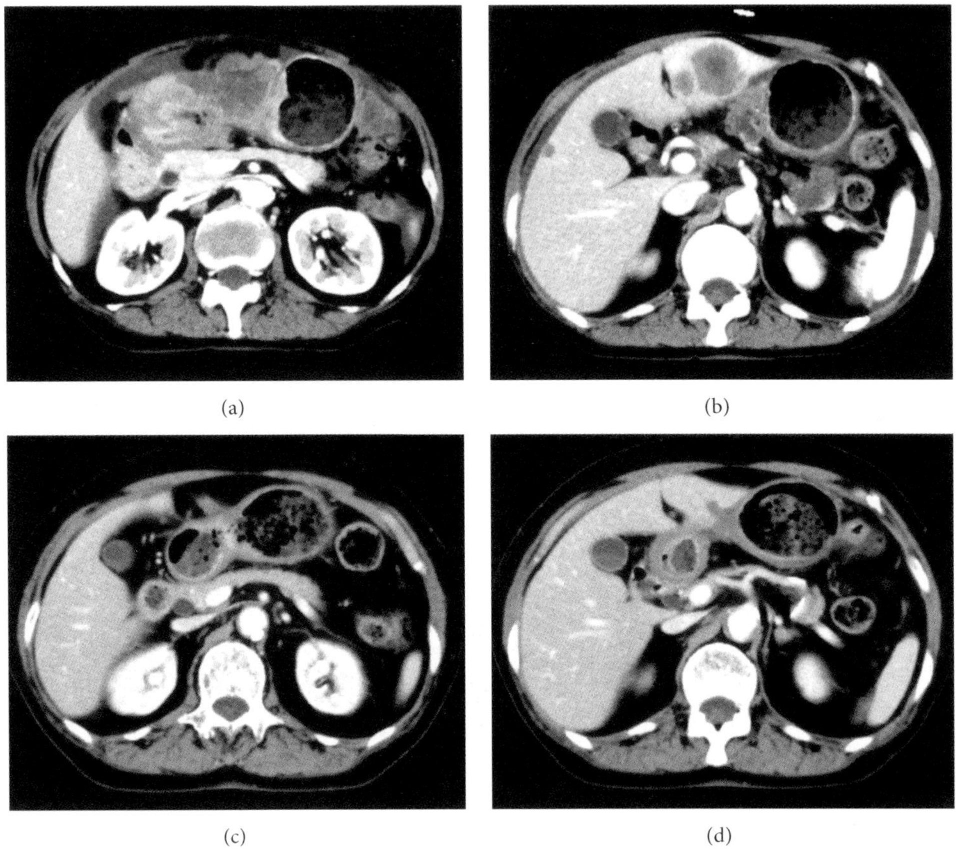

FIGURE 3: Contrast-enhanced computed tomography (CT) findings. (a) and (b) show the CT at presentation. (a) The wall of the lower part of the stomach is markedly thickened, and the density of the surrounding fat tissue is increased, forming an 80 × 45 mm mass. (b) Two nodules are detected in the lateral segment of the liver, and these are directly contiguous from the gastric mass. (c) and (d) show the CT findings after completion of the 11th course of chemotherapy (capecitabine + CDDP + trastuzumab). (c) The gastric mass is markedly decreased. (d) Only a small nodule in the lateral segment of the liver is detected.

Nakamura et al. reported that, in HER2-positive primary breast cancer, the rate of HER2 loss in the site of recurrence was significantly higher in patients treated with trastuzumab than in patients treated without trastuzumab (37% versus 6%) [11]. However, others have reported that trastuzumab therapy was not significantly associated with loss of HER2 positivity in HER2-positive primary breast cancer (13.2% with trastuzumab versus 17.9% without trastuzumab and 20% with trastuzumab versus 26% without trastuzumab) [14, 20]. In fact, some research has shown that treatment with trastuzumab is associated with a lower rate of HER2 status conversion. Guarneri et al. reported that in HER2-positive breast cancer the rate of loss of HER2 after NAC with trastuzumab was significantly lower than the rate of conversion after treatment with NAC without trastuzumab (14.7% versus 40%) [19]. It is evident that available results on the association between loss of HER2 status and trastuzumab therapy are conflicting. These conflicting results imply that loss of HER2 in HER2-positive breast cancer after trastuzumab therapy might not simply be caused by survival of trastuzumab-resistant clones and elimination of HER2-positive clones.

HER2 overexpression and/or amplification occurs in 7–34% of gastric cancer cases [22, 23]. In gastric cancer, the rate of HER2 status discordance between primary tumors and simultaneous metastasis in the liver or lymph nodes has been reported to be 0–12.5% [24–26]. However, HER2 stability during disease progression with or without chemotherapy has rarely been reported. In fact, our literature review identified only one case report similar to ours in which HER2 positivity in the resected specimen from curative surgery was lost after 12 courses of capecitabine + cisplatin + trastuzumab in a patient with HER2-positive MUGC [27]. However, the actual frequency of HER2 loss in HER2-positive MUGC remains unknown, because in MGC, reevaluation of HER2 status in primary sites and/or sites of metastases/recurrence during the course of disease is not typically performed.

When analyzing loss of HER2 in a sample obtained after treatment, we must consider the possibility of a false-negative result for HER2 expression on immunohistochemistry. A sample taken by biopsy is only part of a tumor, and a resected sample might be one of many tumors within the body; therefore, loss of HER2 might be a false-negative due to heterogeneity within the tumor or discordance between the sites of tumors. In fact, it is known that the heterogeneity of HER2 expression within gastric tumors is much more frequent than in breast cancer [22, 23]. Therefore, heterogeneity might account for a small fraction of HER2 conversion. Resolution of this issue is quite challenging, because it is difficult in practice to obtain adequate specimens to overcome the heterogeneity of HER2 within a given tumor and to evaluate the HER2 status of every tumor within the entire body. However, we believe that our particular case was not due to a false-negative result of HER2, because we carefully evaluated HER2 status in the entire residual tumor of the resected stomach and lymph nodes. Although previous studies have demonstrated that 0–10% of cases negative for HER2 by IHC were positive by FISH [24, 25, 28], we confirmed negativity of HER2 in this case by FISH as well.

Current practice guideline for the treatment of breast cancer recommended that biomarkers, including HER2 status and hormone receptors, should be evaluated not only for the primary tumor but also for the initial metastatic or recurrence tumor tissues, especially if the first determination of HER2 status is negative, in order not to lose the chance of anti-HER2 therapy [29]. Currently, the decision to use trastuzumab to treat patients with MUGC is based on the HER2 status in the primary tumor at the time of initial diagnosis without reassessment of HER2 status in primary sites and/or metastases/recurrence during the course of disease, on the assumption that HER2 status is stable. However, just as it is known that HER2 is not necessarily stable in breast cancer, our case casts some doubt on the notion of HER2 stability in gastric cancer.

Although the use of trastuzumab has been shown to be highly effective in treating HER2-positive MUCG, several issues regarding HER2 stability and trastuzumab therapy for gastric cancer remain to be elucidated. First, clinicians need to know how often HER2 status converts with tumor progression, metastasis, or treatment. If a change in HER2 status is found to be significantly frequent in gastric cancer, management strategy recommendations similar to those of breast cancer should be introduced for gastric cancer, although it will be important to consider that biopsy from metastases/recurrence or metastasectomy is invasive and burdensome for patients. If the factors that contribute to HER2 change are identified, only those patients who have such factors, rather than all patients with MUGC, would need to submit to biopsy from metastases/recurrence or metastasectomy. Second, clinicians need to evaluate whether loss of HER2 positivity in specimens obtained during the disease course in HER2-positive gastric cancer always indicates resistance to trastuzumab. As we have mentioned, HER2 status taken from samples may not always represent all tumors in the body. In the present case, although macroscopic complete resection was possible, there was still a sufficient possibility of remaining micrometastases. We decided to treat the patient with adjuvant therapy comprised of capecitabine and trastuzumab after the patient gave her informed consent. Therapy comprised of capecitabine and trastuzumab was chosen because her tumors were not resistant to these medications until resection, and trastuzumab has a significant benefit in tumor cell eradication in the event that the remaining micrometastases retain HER2-positivity. Third, clinicians need to know if the loss of HER2 positivity has a significant prognostic impact on MUGC, because some studies have shown that loss of HER2 positivity in HER2-positive breast cancer was associated with a significantly worse prognosis compared to patients with tumors that maintained HER2 expression [12, 18, 20, 21].

Even if a marked response to chemotherapy allows the possibility of curative resection in MUGC, currently, the consistent standard treatment is to continue chemotherapy. However, the survival rate in MUGC treated by chemotherapy alone is obviously insufficient. Surgical resection with curative intent after a response to chemotherapy for MUGC is called adjuvant or salvage surgery. The benefit of such surgery was recently evaluated, and a favorable prognosis was suggested, with a 3-year survival rate of 46–55% and a median survival of 29–43 months [30–32], although these studies were small and retrospective in nature. In carefully selected patients, adjuvant surgery might become the treatment of choice. To support the efficacy of adjuvant surgery, a randomized controlled study is warranted.

In conclusion, we report the case of a patient with HER2-positive MUGC at initial diagnosis who received chemotherapy including trastuzumab; following chemotherapy and surgery in this patient, a resected specimen of the stomach showed loss of HER2-positivity in the residual tumor, suggesting that HER2 status is not always stable. Treatment with trastuzumab is very effective and less toxic than traditional cytotoxic drugs. If HER2 positivity is gained during the course of disease, it is an easy judgment for clinicians to add trastuzumab to chemotherapy, thus allowing patients to benefit from trastuzumab therapy. However, when cases convert from positive HER2 status to negative HER2 status, clinicians remain uncertain as to whether the change in status is truly due to a biologic change rather than a false-negative result. Therefore, it is a more difficult and less confident judgment to remove trastuzumab from chemotherapy, even though its removal may result in avoiding unnecessary treatment. Further studies concerning HER2 status in gastric cancer are needed in order to appropriately use trastuzumab for these patients.

References

[1] E. Van Cutsem, V. M. Moiseyenko, S. Tjulandin et al., "Phase III study of docetaxel and cisplatin plus fluorouracil compared with cisplatin and fluorouracil as first-line therapy for advanced gastric cancer: a report of the V325 study group," *Journal of Clinical Oncology*, vol. 24, no. 31, pp. 4991–4997, 2006.

[2] W. Koizumi, H. Narahara, T. Hara et al., "S-1 plus cisplatin versus S-1 alone for first-line treatment of advanced gastric cancer (SPIRITS trial): a phase III trial," *The Lancet Oncology*, vol. 9, no. 3, pp. 215–221, 2008.

[3] D. Cunningham, N. Starling, S. Rao et al., "Capecitabine and oxaliplatin for advanced esophagogastric cancer," *The New England Journal of Medicine*, vol. 358, no. 1, pp. 36–46, 2008.

[4] Y.-J. Bang, E. van Cutsem, A. Feyereislova et al., "Trastuzumab in combination with chemotherapy versus chemotherapy alone

for treatment of HER2-positive advanced gastric or gastro-oesophageal junction cancer (ToGA): a phase 3, open-label, randomised controlled trial," *The Lancet*, vol. 376, no. 9742, pp. 687–697, 2010.

[5] D. J. Slamon, W. Godolphin, L. A. Jones et al., "Studies of the HER-2/neuproto-oncogene in human breast and ovarian cancer," *Science*, vol. 244, no. 4905, pp. 707–712, 1989.

[6] D. M. Reese and D. J. Slamon, "HER-2/neu signal transduction in human breast and ovarian cancer," *Stem Cells*, vol. 15, no. 1, pp. 1–8, 1997.

[7] D. J. Slamon, B. Leyland-Jones, S. Shak et al., "Use of chemotherapy plus a monoclonal antibody against her2 for metastatic breast cancer that overexpresses HER2," *The New England Journal of Medicine*, vol. 344, no. 11, pp. 783–792, 2001.

[8] L. Gianni, U. Dafni, R. D. Gelber et al., "Treatment with trastuzumab for 1 year after adjuvant chemotherapy in patients with HER2-positive early breast cancer: a 4-year follow-up of a randomised controlled trial," *The Lancet Oncology*, vol. 12, no. 3, pp. 236–244, 2011.

[9] L. Gianni, W. Eiermann, V. Semiglazov et al., "Neoadjuvant and adjuvant trastuzumab in patients with HER2-positive locally advanced breast cancer (NOAH): follow-up of a randomised controlled superiority trial with a parallel HER2-negative cohort," *The Lancet Oncology*, vol. 15, no. 6, pp. 640–647, 2014.

[10] J. Liu, H. Deng, W. Jia et al., "Comparison of ER/PR and HER2 statuses in primary and paired liver metastatic sites of breast carcinoma in patients with or without treatment," *Journal of Cancer Research and Clinical Oncology*, vol. 138, no. 5, pp. 837–842, 2012.

[11] R. Nakamura, N. Yamamoto, Y. Onai, Y. Watanabe, H. Kawana, and M. Miyazaki, "Importance of confirming HER2 overexpression of recurrence lesion in breast cancer patients," *Breast Cancer*, vol. 20, no. 4, pp. 336–341, 2013.

[12] M. V. Dieci, E. Barbieri, F. Piacentini et al., "Discordance in receptor status between primary and recurrent breast cancer has a prognostic impact: a single-institution analysis," *Annals of Oncology*, vol. 24, no. 1, Article ID mds248, pp. 101–108, 2013.

[13] E. M. de Dueñas, A. L. Hernández, Á. G. Zotano et al., "Prospective evaluation of the conversion rate in the receptor status between primary breast cancer and metastasis: results from the GEICAM 2009-03 ConvertHER study," *Breast Cancer Research and Treatment*, vol. 143, no. 3, pp. 507–515, 2014.

[14] C. Xiao, Y. Gong, E. Y. Han, A. M. Gonzalez-Angulo, and N. Sneige, "Stability of HER2-positive status in breast carcinoma: a comparison between primary and paired metastatic tumors with regard to the possible impact of intervening trastuzumab treatment," *Annals of Oncology*, vol. 22, no. 7, pp. 1547–1553, 2011.

[15] T. Shet, A. Agrawal, R. Chinoy, R. Havaldar, V. Parmar, and R. Badwe, "Changes in the tumor grade and biological markers in locally advanced breast cancer after chemotherapy—implications for a pathologist," *The Breast Journal*, vol. 13, no. 5, pp. 457–464, 2007.

[16] M. Kasami, T. Uematsu, M. Honda et al., "Comparison of estrogen receptor, progesterone receptor and Her-2 status in breast cancer pre- and post-neoadjuvant chemotherapy," *Breast*, vol. 17, no. 5, pp. 523–527, 2008.

[17] T. Hirata, C. Shimizu, K. Yonemori et al., "Change in the hormone receptor status following administration of neoadjuvant chemotherapy and its impact on the long-term outcome in patients with primary breast cancer," *British Journal of Cancer*, vol. 101, no. 9, pp. 1529–1536, 2009.

[18] E. A. Mittendorf, Y. Wu, M. Scaltriti et al., "Loss of HER2 amplification following trastuzumab-based neoadjuvant systemic therapy and survival outcomes," *Clinical Cancer Research*, vol. 15, no. 23, pp. 7381–7388, 2009.

[19] V. Guarneri, M. V. Dieci, E. Barbieri et al., "Loss of HER2 positivity and prognosis after neoadjuvant therapy in HER2-positive breast cancer patients," *Annals of Oncology*, vol. 24, no. 12, pp. 2990–2994, 2013.

[20] N. Niikura, J. Liu, N. Hayashi et al., "Loss of human epidermal growth factor receptor 2 (HER2) expression in metastatic sites of HER2-overexpressing primary breast tumors," *Journal of Clinical Oncology*, vol. 30, no. 6, pp. 593–599, 2012.

[21] D. Pectasides, A. Gaglia, P. Arapantoni-Dadioti et al., "HER-2/neu status of primary breast cancer and corresponding metastatic sites in patients with advanced breast cancer treated with trastuzumab-based therapy," *Anticancer Research*, vol. 26, no. 1, pp. 647–654, 2006.

[22] M. Hofmann, O. Stoss, D. Shi et al., "Assessment of a HER2 scoring system for gastric cancer: results from a validation study," *Histopathology*, vol. 52, no. 7, pp. 797–805, 2008.

[23] J. Rüschoff, W. Hanna, M. Bilous et al., "HER2 testing in gastric cancer: a practical approach," *Modern Pathology*, vol. 25, no. 5, pp. 637–650, 2012.

[24] A. H. Marx, L. Tharun, J. Muth et al., "HER-2 amplification is highly homogenous in gastric cancer," *Human Pathology*, vol. 40, no. 6, pp. 769–777, 2009.

[25] C. Bozzetti, F. V. Negri, C. A. Lagrasta et al., "Comparison of HER2 status in primary and paired metastatic sites of gastric carcinoma," *British Journal of Cancer*, vol. 104, no. 9, pp. 1372–1376, 2011.

[26] F. Pagni, S. Zannella, S. Ronchi, C. Garanzini, and B. E. Leone, "HER2 status of gastric carcinoma and corresponding lymph node metastasis," *Pathology and Oncology Research*, vol. 19, no. 1, pp. 103–109, 2013.

[27] N. Ikari, G. Nakajima, K. Taniguchi et al., "HER2-positive gastric cancer with paraaortic nodal metastasis successfully resected after chemotherapy with trastuzumab: a case report," *Anticancer research*, vol. 34, no. 2, pp. 867–872, 2014.

[28] H. Yoshida, N. Yamamoto, H. Taniguchi et al., "Comparison of HER2 status between surgically resected specimens and matched biopsy specimens of gastric intestinal-type adenocarcinoma," *Virchows Archiv*, vol. 465, no. 2, pp. 145–154, 2014.

[29] National Comprehensive Cancer Network, *NCCN Clinical Practice Guidelines in Oncology: Breast Cancer*, Version 3, 2014.

[30] H. Okabe, S. Ueda, K. Obama, H. Hosogi, and Y. Sakai, "Induction chemotherapy with S-1 plus cisplatin followed by surgery for treatment of gastric cancer with peritoneal dissemination," *Annals of Surgical Oncology*, vol. 16, no. 12, pp. 3227–3236, 2009.

[31] T. Suzuki, K. Tanabe, J. Taomoto et al., "Preliminary trial of adjuvant surgery for advanced gastric cancer," *Oncology Letters*, vol. 1, no. 4, pp. 743–747, 2010.

[32] T. Kanda, K. Yajima, S.-I. Kosugi, T. Ishikawa, Y. Ajioka, and K. Hatakeyama, "Gastrectomy as a secondary surgery for stage IV gastric cancer patients who underwent S-1-based chemotherapy: a multi-institute retrospective study," *Gastric Cancer*, vol. 15, no. 3, pp. 235–244, 2012.

12

Single-Operator Peroral Cholangioscopy for Extraction of Cystic Duct Stones in Postcholecystectomy Mirizzi Syndrome

Jason Deforest Jones and Rishi Pawa

Division of Gastroenterology, Department of Internal Medicine, Wake Forest School of Medicine, Winston-Salem, NC, USA

Correspondence should be addressed to Rishi Pawa; rpawa@wakehealth.edu

Academic Editor: Hideto Kawaratani

Mirizzi syndrome is an exceptionally rare diagnosis with an annual incidence of less than 1% in developed countries. In this disease process, stone burden in the cystic duct or gallbladder neck leads to common hepatic duct obstruction, either by mechanical compression or secondary inflammation. Mirizzi syndrome is classified into one of four types based on the presence and severity of cholecystobiliary fistulization. Treatment is primarily surgical in nature and largely dictated by the type of Mirizzi syndrome encountered. It is typically diagnosed in the preoperative or operative setting of cholecystectomy; however, there have been rare occurrences of postcholecystectomy diagnosis. Factors thought to predispose to postcholecystectomy disease include low insertion of the cystic duct and long remnant duct length. Few case reports exist describing this phenomenon and its management, which is made exceptionally difficult due to the presence of inflammation and surgical adhesion. We present the case of a young female with postcholecystectomy Mirizzi syndrome who underwent successful endoscopic management using peroral cholangioscopy and electrohydraulic lithotripsy. We also provide a brief overview of both Mirizzi syndrome and peroral cholangioscopy.

1. Introduction

Mirizzi syndrome is defined as common hepatic duct obstruction caused by extrinsic compression or inflammation from cystic duct or gallbladder neck stone burden. The syndrome is quite rare, especially in patients with prior cholecystectomy, in whom only a small amount of case reports have been published. The management of cystic duct stones in these patients with prior cholecystectomy can prove difficult and often requires surgical intervention. Peroral cholangioscopy using direct visualization and electrohydraulic lithotripsy (EHL) offers an alternative management solution which gives a single-operator the ability to detect strictures and remove large stones in the pancreaticobiliary system which are otherwise not amenable to endoscopic retrograde cholangiopancreatography (ERCP). We present a case of the successful use of cholangioscopy and EHL for endoscopic visualization and management of a cystic duct stone causing Mirizzi syndrome in a postcholecystectomy patient.

2. Case Presentation

A 27-year-old female with a history of cholecystectomy for symptomatic cholelithiasis three years prior to admission presented with epigastric pain radiating to the right upper quadrant and back. Initial laboratory tests on presentation were a total bilirubin (TBili) 5.5 mg/dL, alkaline phosphatase (ALP) 288 U/L, aspartate aminotransferase (AST) 316 U/L, and alanine aminotransferase (ALT) 394 U/L, and magnetic resonance cholangiopancreatography (MRCP) revealed a fluid collection in continuity with the cystic duct and a nine-millimeter stone at the confluence of the cystic and common hepatic duct, resulting in both biliary and cystic duct dilatation with adjacent inflammation (Figures 1 and 2). Using ERCP, the cystic duct was cannulated and a filling defect consistent with a nine-millimeter stone was confirmed, along with proximal cystic duct dilatation and extravasation of contrast suggestive of a contained bile leak (Figures 3 and 4). Following failed attempts at balloon-assisted stone extraction, cholangioscopy was performed. A single therapeutic

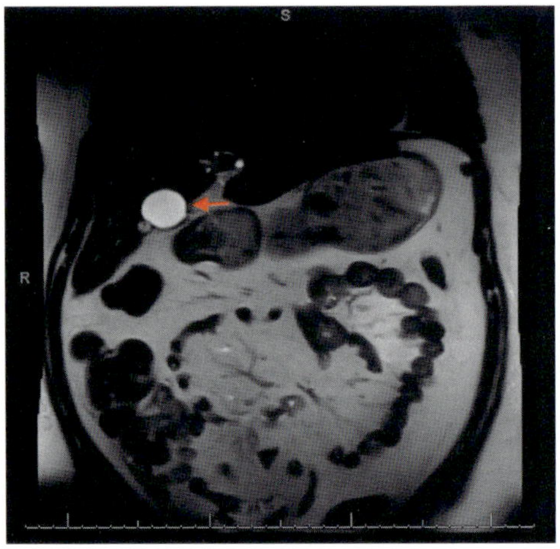

FIGURE 1: Preintervention MRCP revealing a fluid collection in continuity with the cystic duct representative of a contained bile leak (marked with arrow).

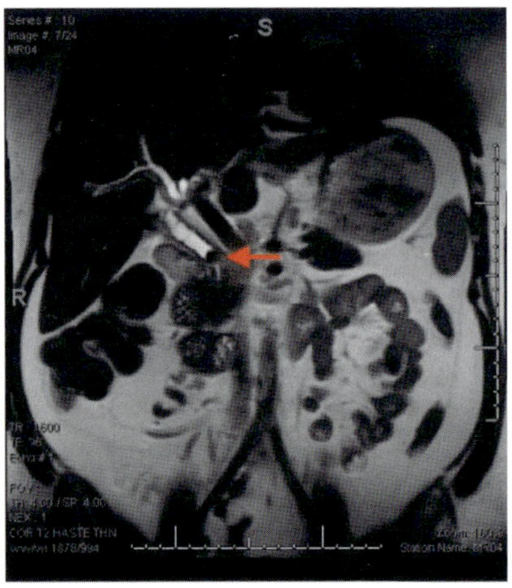

FIGURE 2: Preintervention MRCP revealing a nine-millimeter stone in the cystic duct (marked with arrow).

endoscopist who has performed >30 interventions using the SpyGlass system was the primary operator and the case was performed under general anesthesia. A Pentax ED-3490TK therapeutic duodenoscope (Pentax Medical; Tokyo, Japan) was used to facilitate passage of the SpyGlass system. The 10 Fr SpyGlass cholangioscope measuring 250 cm in length was then used to directly visualize the stone in the cystic duct (Figure 5). The visualized stone was irrigated using saline prior to EHL, which was achieved using a Nortech Autolith system (Northgate Technologies Inc.; Elgin, IL) and a 1.9 Fr EHL probe. Power was set to 90 W with a rate of 3 pulsations/second, the latter of which was escalated as needed to achieve stone fragmentation. Subsequent balloon sweeps of the cystic duct successfully cleared stone fragments (Figure 6) and repeat MRCP (Figure 7) one year after hospital discharge revealed no evidence of fluid collection or stone in the cystic duct.

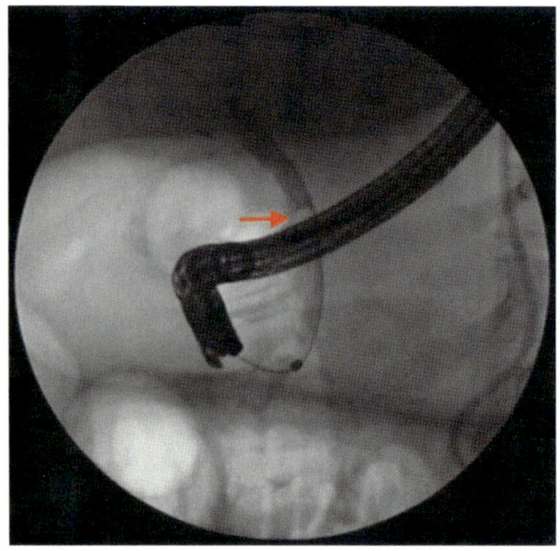

FIGURE 3: ERCP revealing a stone in the cystic duct (marked with arrow).

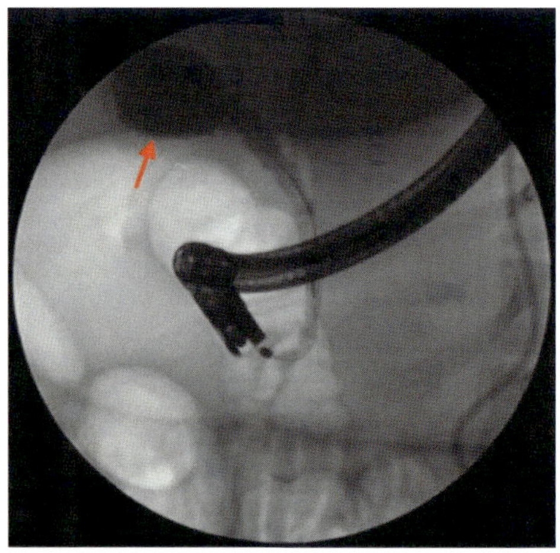

FIGURE 4: ERCP revealing proximal cystic duct dilatation and extravasation of contrast suggestive of a contained bile leak in this patient with a history of cholecystectomy. The contained bile leak is marked with an arrow.

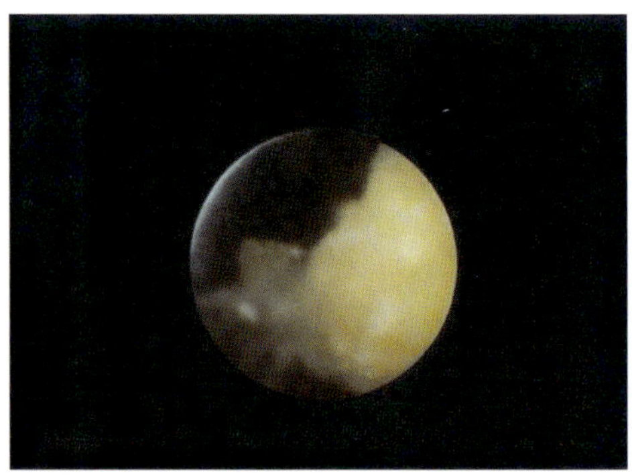

FIGURE 5: Nine-millimeter cystic duct stone visualized using peroral cholangioscopy.

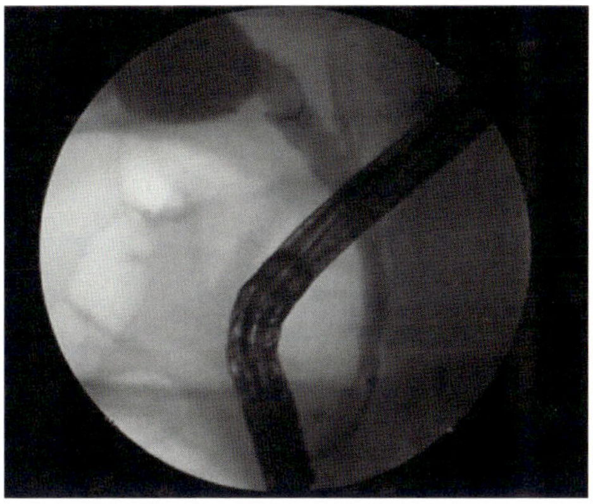

Figure 6: Occlusion cholangiogram after cystic duct stone removal.

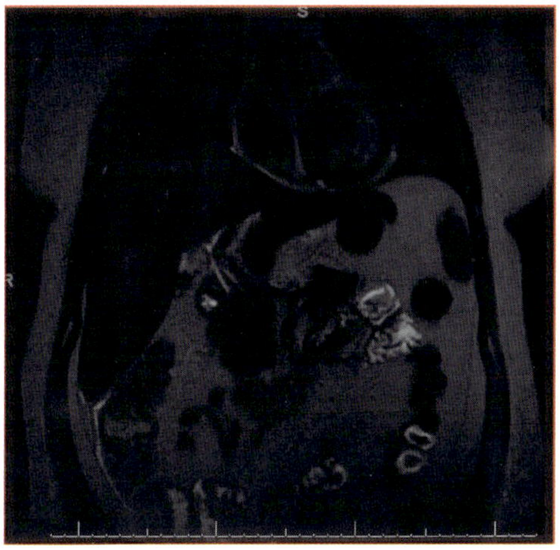

Figure 7: Postintervention MRCP revealing stone extraction and resolution of previously seen fluid collection.

3. Discussion

Mirizzi syndrome is a rare entity generally encountered in either the preoperative or intraoperative stages of cholecystectomy, with few case reports citing postcholecystectomy disease. Increased remnant cystic duct length and low insertion of the duct are hypothesized to predispose to postcholecystectomy Mirizzi syndrome. It is classified into one of four categories based on the development and severity of cholecystobiliary fistulization. Type I Mirizzi syndrome, as described in the aforementioned case, involves extrinsic compression of the common hepatic duct secondary to gallbladder neck or cystic duct stone impaction [1]. Disease pathology can also intermittently occur as a sequela of inflammation. Cholecystobiliary fistula involvement of one-third of the CBD circumference, two-thirds of the CBD circumference, and fistula development leading to complete common hepatic duct wall destruction is classified as types II, III, and IV, respectively [2].

The typical clinical presentation of Mirizzi syndrome is obstructive jaundice and a cholestatic injury pattern on laboratory analysis, sometimes with evidence of cholangitis [3]. MRCP is the imaging modality of choice to obtain a diagnosis [4]. As previously mentioned, Mirizzi syndrome is most commonly discovered in the preoperative evaluation of patients with cholelithiasis preparing to undergo cholecystectomy. Antoniou et al. found a decrease in surgical conversion, procedural complications, and need for reoperation in patients diagnosed with Mirizzi syndrome in the preoperative setting, thus emphasizing the importance of consideration of this condition [5]. Surgery is the most common treatment modality for Mirizzi syndrome, with the specific approach based on the type of disease present, technical skill of the surgeon, and the perioperative setting in which the disease is discovered. The cystic duct stones found in Mirizzi syndrome lead to a large inflammatory response which makes surgical dissection of the triangle of Calot quite difficult; thus one can expect this to be further complicated in patients who are status postcholecystectomy, in which the surgeon is faced with both surgical adhesion and severe inflammation [1, 6]. Type I Mirizzi syndrome is typically managed via open or laparoscopic cholecystectomy, either total or subtotal [1]. As expected, the presence of a cholecystobiliary fistula in types II–IV necessitates a more complicated approach to treatment. Type II Mirizzi syndrome requires subtotal cholecystectomy with bile duct reconstruction using residual gallbladder wall [1, 7]. Lastly, treatment for Mirizzi syndrome types III and IV relies on bilioenteric anastomosis [1].

Due to the need for management solutions in poor surgical candidates, as well as the inherent risk of bile duct injury associated with surgery in Mirizzi syndrome, several endoscopic and percutaneous approaches to treatment have been explored. Endoscopic therapy has been reported with the use of direct stone removal via balloon or basket as well as electrohydraulic and laser lithotripsy [3, 8, 9]. Cystic duct stump cannulation is accomplished using either fluoroscopy or direct cholangioscopy visualization. We have traditionally attempted initial cannulation using fluoroscopic guidance; however, when this is not possible a cholangioscope is introduced to localize the cystic duct stump opening and subsequently cannulate using direct visualization. Bhandari et al. recently reported a 94% success rate in single session cholangioscopy-guided laser lithotripsy in the setting of endoscopic or surgical failure [10]. Peroral cholangioscopy, while once plagued by several limitations such as restricted maneuverability, cumbersome setup, expensive maintenance, and a dual operator requirement, has become a nonsurgical, safe, and effective treatment modality with various indications in biliary pathology [11]. Boston Scientific Corporation's SpyGlass direct visualization system (Boston Scientific, Marlborough, MA) was used in this case report. SpyGlass-directed therapy has been shown to have success rates of 90–100% in the treatment of biliary stones [11]. Stone removal using the SpyGlass system is accomplished using either EHL or laser lithotripsy, with EHL shown to be superior to the more traditionally utilized extracorporeal shock wave lithotripsy [12, 13]. Complication rates of peroral cholangioscopy using the SpyGlass system are low. The most common complication reported has been acute cholangitis, with an incidence of approximately 3%, while the incidence rate of other complications such as abdominal pain, bacteremia, and pancreatitis tends to mimic those one can experience with routine ERCP [11].

Postcholecystectomy Mirizzi syndrome is an exceptionally rare phenomenon with a limited number of case reports currently available to describe the process and its complicated management. Although rare, one would expect the incidence of postcholecystectomy Mirizzi syndrome to increase as a direct result of the predominance of laparoscopic cholecystectomies in surgical practice, in which the target of surgical dissection is the junction between the cystic duct and gallbladder, thus predisposing to an increase in cystic duct stump length. Conventional balloon passage failed in our case due to large stone size in relation to duct size. No adverse events were experienced in the presented case. We therefore conclude that endoscopic management of postcholecystectomy Mirizzi syndrome can provide the patient with a safe, minimally invasive treatment modality for a problem which typically requires surgical intervention.

References

[1] M. A. Beltrán, "Mirizzi syndrome: history, current knowledge and proposal of a simplified classification," *World Journal of Gastroenterology*, vol. 18, no. 34, pp. 4639–4650, 2012.

[2] D. G. Adler and K. Eliason, "Mirizzi's syndrome presenting after laparoscopic cholecystectomy," *Gastrointestinal Endoscopy*, vol. 83, no. 3, pp. 668–669, 2016.

[3] K. F. Binmoeller, F. Thonke, and N. Soehendra, "Endoscopic treatment of Mirizzi's syndrome," *Gastrointestinal Endoscopy*, vol. 39, no. 4, pp. 532–536, 1993.

[4] N. Wani, N. Khan, A. Shah, and A. Khan, "Post-cholecystectomy Mirizzi's syndrome: magnetic resonance cholangiopancreatography demonstration," *Saudi Journal of Gastroenterology*, vol. 16, no. 4, pp. 295–298, 2010.

[5] S. A. Antoniou, G. A. Antoniou, and C. Makridis, "Laparoscopic treatment of Mirizzi syndrome: a systematic review," *Surgical Endoscopy and Other Interventional Techniques*, vol. 24, no. 1, pp. 33–39, 2010.

[6] M. Lim, J. Y. Jeon, J. W. Kwon et al., "Laparoscopic treatment for post-cholecystectomy Mirizzi syndrome," *Korean Journal of Hepato-Biliary-Pancreatic Surgery*, vol. 17, no. 2, p. 79, 2013.

[7] O. J. Shah, M. A. Dar, M. A. Wani, and N. A. Wani, "Management of Mirizzi syndrome: a new surgical approach," *ANZ Journal of Surgery*, vol. 71, no. 7, pp. 423–427, 2001.

[8] R. E. England and D. F. Martin, "Endoscopic management of Mirizzi's syndrome," *Gut*, vol. 40, no. 2, pp. 272–276, 1997.

[9] V. P. Kodali and B. T. Petersen, "Endoscopic therapy of postcholecystectomy Mirizzi syndrome," *Gastrointestinal Endoscopy*, vol. 44, no. 1, pp. 86–90, 1996.

[10] S. Bhandari, R. Bathini, A. Sharma, and A. Maydeo, "Usefulness of single-operator cholangioscopy-guided laser lithotripsy in patients with Mirizzi syndrome and cystic duct stones: experience at a tertiary care center," *Gastrointestinal Endoscopy*, vol. 84, no. 1, pp. 56–61, 2016.

[11] J. B. Williamson and P. V. Draganov, "The Usefulness of SpyGlass™ choledochoscopy in the diagnosis and treatment of biliary disorders," *Current Gastroenterology Reports*, vol. 14, no. 6, pp. 534–541, 2012.

[12] H. Issa, B. Bseiso, and A. H. Al-Salem, "Successful laser lithotripsy using peroral SpyGlass cholangioscopy in a patient with Mirizzi syndrome," *Endoscopy*, vol. 43, no. 2, pp. E166–E167, 2011.

[13] A. M. Aljebreen, O. R. Alharbi, N. Azzam, and M. A. Almadi, "Efficacy of spyglass-guided electrohydraulic lithotripsy in difficult bile duct stones," *Saudi Journal of Gastroenterology*, vol. 20, no. 6, pp. 366–370, 2014.

13

Metastatic Periampullary Tumor from Hepatocellular Carcinoma Presenting as Gastrointestinal Bleeding

Amir Kashani,[1] Nicholas N. Nissen,[2] Maha Guindi,[3] and Laith H. Jamil[1]

[1]*Department of Gastroenterology, Cedars-Sinai Medical Center, 8700 Beverly Boulevard, Los Angeles, CA 90048, USA*
[2]*Hepatobiliary and Pancreatic Surgery, Cedars-Sinai Medical Center, 8700 Beverly Boulevard, Los Angeles, CA 90048, USA*
[3]*Department of Pathology and Laboratory Medicine, Cedars-Sinai Medical Center, 8700 Beverly Boulevard, Los Angeles, CA 90048, USA*

Correspondence should be addressed to Laith H. Jamil; laith.jamil@cshs.org

Academic Editor: Naohiko Koide

Periampullary tumors constitute a number of diverse neoplastic lesions located within 2 cm of the major duodenal papilla; among these, metastatic lesions account for only a small proportion of the periampullary tumors. To our knowledge, a metastatic periampullary tumor from hepatocellular carcinoma has never been reported. A 62-year-old male reported to our institute for fatigue and low hemoglobin. His medical history was remarkable for multifocal hepatocellular carcinoma (HCC) treated with selective transcatheter arterial chemoembolization (TACE). An esophagogastroduodenoscopy (EGD) was performed which revealed a periampullary mass. Histopathology was consistent with metastatic moderately differentiated HCC. Two endoloops were deployed around the base of the mass one month apart. The mass eventually sloughed off and patient's hemoglobin level stabilized. We postulated that periampullary metastasis in this patient was the result of tumor fragments migration through the biliary tracts and that TACE which increases tumor fragments burden might have played a contributory role. Metastasis of HCC to the gastrointestinal (GI) tract should be considered as a cause of GI bleeding.

1. Introduction

Common sites of metastases from hepatocellular carcinoma (HCC) are the lung, bone, lymph nodes, and adrenal glands [1]. Gastrointestinal (GI) metastases from HCC are rare, with most cases reported in the stomach and duodenum [2]. The suggested mechanism of metastasis is mainly direct invasion of a tumor contiguous with the GI tract [2]. In this paper, we describe a patient with an isolated metastatic periampullary tumor from HCC who presented with GI bleeding. This finding is unusual for two reasons: first, HCC does not tend to metastasize to the small bowel and, second, metastatic periampullary tumors are very uncommon [2, 3]. We also will elaborate on the possible pathogenesis of periampullary metastasis in our patient.

2. Case Report

A 62-year-old male presented to our institute with fatigue. His medical history was notable for cirrhosis secondary to chronic hepatitis C, complicated by multifocal hepatocellular carcinoma (HCC), which had been lately diagnosed following an episode of obstructive jaundice. Later he underwent multiple biliary interventions including sphincterotomy, dilatation, and stent placement due to recurrent strictures. Cytopathology of the biliary materials had revealed necrotic tissue containing HCC cells. Also, a few months prior to the current presentation, he underwent selective transcatheter arterial chemoembolization (TACE) of three discrete areas of the tumor within the right hepatic lobe. His blood laboratory test upon presentation showed a hemoglobin level of 5.1 g/dL (reference value: 11.6–15.4 g/dL), so he was admitted for further evaluation. An esophagogastroduodenoscopy (EGD) was performed, which revealed columns of grade II and III esophageal varices (EVs), in addition to a 3 by 2 cm periampullary mass at the site of prior sphincterotomy with no sign of active bleeding (Figure 1(a)). This mass was not evident on any of the several previous endoscopic procedures. Histopathology confirmed this mass as a metastatic lesion

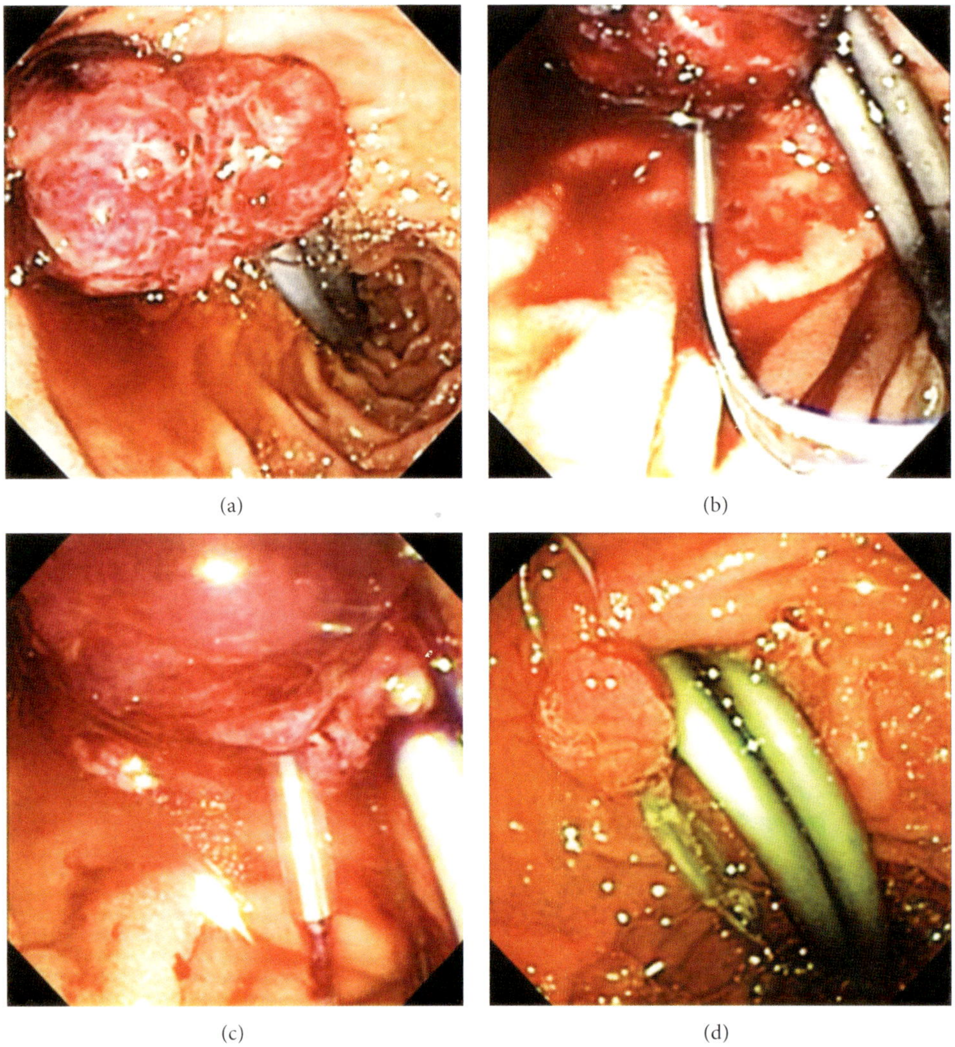

Figure 1: (a) A 3 × 2 cm ulcerated periampullary mass; previous biliary stents in place. ((b), (c)) First and second endoloops were deployed at the base of the mass one month apart. (d) Tumor remnant tissue one month after the second endoloop; two endoloops are still in place.

showing the characteristics of moderately differentiated HCC (Figure 2(a)). Immunohistochemistry studies were positive for hepatocyte paraffin-1, glypican-3, and carcinoembryonic antigen (polyclonal) (Figures 2(b), 2(c), and 2(d)). Thereafter, an extensive metastatic workup was performed which did not reveal any metastatic sites other than the periampullary mass seen on abdominal magnetic resonance imaging (Figure 3). Due to ongoing blood loss, a series of empiric endoscopic band ligations of the EVs were performed until the varices were resolved; however, the patient's hemoglobin level continued to decline. On repeat EGD, the periampullary mass was visualized with adherent blood clots. An endoloop was then deployed around the base of the mass (Figure 1(b)). However, the patient's hemoglobin gradually continued to drop. One month later, a second EGD showed evidence of only minimal necrosis; thus a second endoloop was deployed (Figure 1(c)). One month later, a follow-up endoscopy showed the mass had sloughed off with only slight remnant tissue (Figure 1(d)). Subsequently, the patient's hemoglobin level stabilized without any further blood transfusion required. However, he expired a few months later due to liver failure.

3. Discussion

Periampullary tumors constitute a number of diverse neoplastic lesions located within two cm of the major duodenal papilla [4]. Among these, metastatic lesions constitute only a small proportion of periampullary tumors [3]; melanoma, choriocarcinoma, liposarcoma, squamous carcinoma of the lung, and renal cell carcinoma are the reported origins of these metastatic tumors [3, 5]. Although duodenal metastasis from HCC is occasionally reported, to our knowledge an HCC-originating metastatic tumor, involving the periampullary region, has never been reported in the literature. In a postmortem study in patients with HCC, duodenal metastasis is reported in 4% of cases [6]. Meanwhile, premortem metastasis to the duodenum is limited only to a few

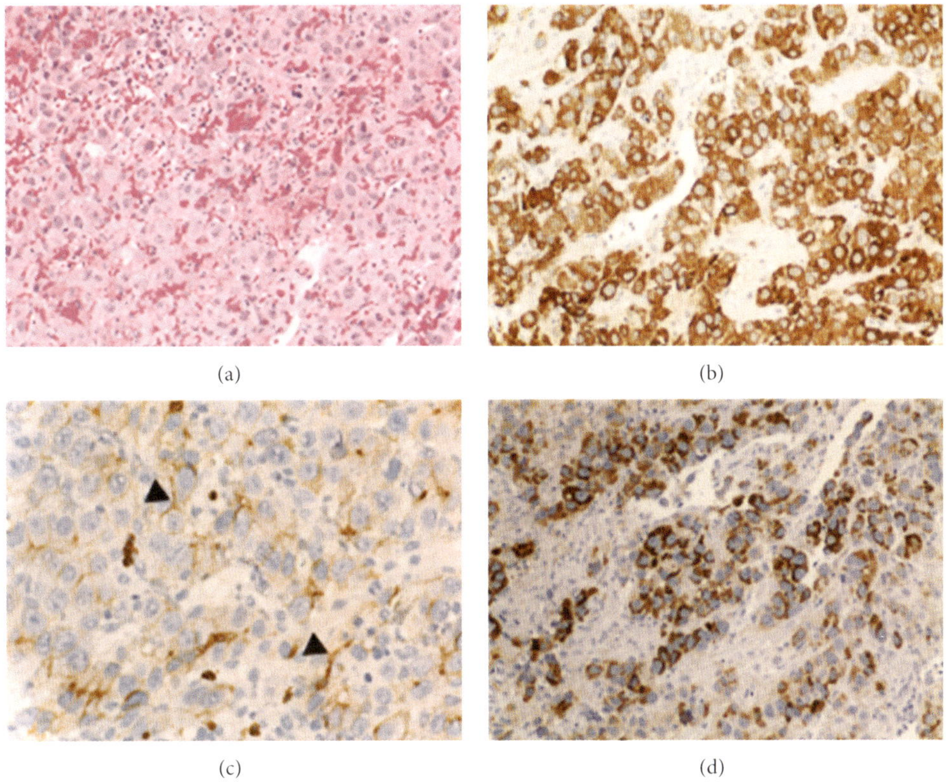

FIGURE 2: (a) (H&E, 20×) Poorly differentiated hepatocellular carcinoma composed of large epithelial cells with abundant pink cytoplasm and central atypical nuclei. (b) (H&E, 20×) Glypican-3 immunostain positive (brown chromogen). (c) (H&E, 40×) Polyclonal carcinoembryonic antigen immunostain highlights a positive canalicular pattern (arrowheads). (d) (H&E, 40×) Hepatocyte paraffin-1 immunostain (brown chromogen).

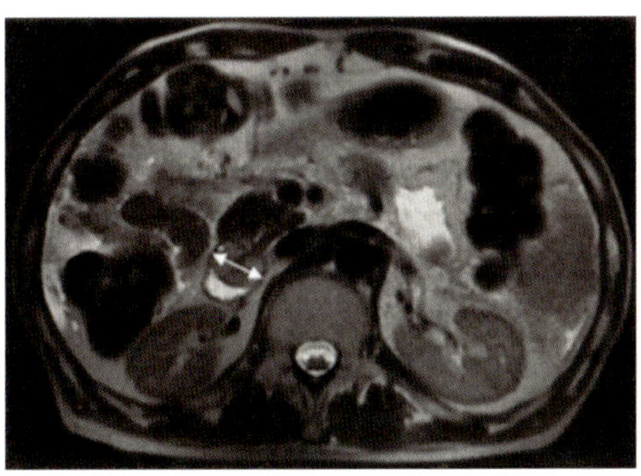

FIGURE 3: Abdominal magnetic resonance imaging shows a pedunculated mass at the level of ampulla with mild enhancement (double arrow).

case reports and series [7–9]. The main suggested route of metastasis is direct invasion of a bulky HCC tumor adjacent to the GI tract [2]. Hence, duodenal invasion is generally seen when the tumor involves the right hepatic lobe, which is in proximity to the first portion of the duodenum [7]. Anatomically, left lobe tumors tend to invade the stomach [10]. The direct invasion can be confirmed by abdominal imaging modalities such as magnetic resonance imaging or computed tomography scan [7, 11]. A less common mechanism of metastasis is hematogenous/lymphatic dissemination [8, 9, 12]. This route of metastasis is tentatively suggested when a direct invasion is excluded and remote metastases to the other organs have been revealed by imaging studies [8]. The presence of portal vein thrombosis is known as a strong indicator of presumed hematogenous spreading of HCC [2]. Due to anatomic correspondence, in which a contiguous liver tumor is invading the duodenum, the proximal duodenum is generally involved, while in hematogenous metastasis involvement of the distal duodenum is also reported [8]. In the absence of remote metastases, isolated duodenal involvement via a hematogenous route is extremely rare [2, 9]. Herein we report a novel case of isolated periampullary metastasis from HCC. In the absence of radiologic evidence of HCC direct invasion to the duodenum, the possibility of this route of metastasis is excluded. Also, imaging modalities did not reveal any evidence of remote metastases, lymphatic involvement, or portal vein thrombosis. Therefore, the possibility of hematogenous/lymphatic dissemination was not deemed high. Involvement of the biliary tracts by cancerous cells is an uncommon finding, which is reported in only 4% of patients with HCC [6]. This can lead to biliary obstruction via impacting the major duodenal papilla with tumor fragments [13]. Moreover, migration of the tumor fragments through the biliary system, although rare, is a suggested route of metastasis in primary liver malignancies [14]. In the present patient, cytology result of the biliary material aspiration on multiple interventions that had been performed due to obstruction confirmed the presence of malignant HCC cells. We postulated that metastasis in our patient was due to invasion of HCC into the biliary ducts, leading to recurrent strictures, which required multiple biliary interventions; this subsequently caused cancerous cells to spread to the periampullary region. Moreover, performing TACE is known to cause tumor necrosis, which leads to an increase in the burden of tumor fragments in the biliary system [15]. In the current patient, it is presumed that TACE might stand as another contributing factor to periampullary metastasis.

Gastrointestinal hemorrhage in patients with HCC is predominantly originating from EVs; gastrointestinal metastases account for about 5% of GI bleeding in these patients [16]. Duodenal metastatic lesions from HCC, although rare, usually manifest as upper GI bleeding, which might be obscured in the context of concurrent cirrhosis and variceal bleeding [7]. In our patient, several band ligations of EVs were performed; however these did not stop the drop in the patient's hemoglobin level. Only after endoscopic treatment of the periampullary tumor was the patient's hemoglobin stabilized. So in patients with HCC and GI bleeding where metastatic lesions to the GI tract are found, these should be considered as the possible source of hemorrhage, especially when bleeding EVs or other sources are not evident. In addition to supportive care, surgical or endoscopic interventions and transarterial embolization are the suggested therapeutic options for bleeding GI metastatic lesions from HCC [7]. Due to the unique location of the tumor in the current patient, we were able to control the bleeding with endoloops which cut off tumor blood perfusion leading to tumor necrosis.

In conclusion, we described a novel case of periampullary metastasis from HCC which presented as GI bleeding. The biliary system is a possible route of metastasis to the periampullary region in patients with liver malignancies. In HCC patients presenting with GI bleeding, metastasis to the GI tract from HCC should be considered as a possible source.

Authors' Contribution

Amir Kashani contributed to data collection, review of the literatures, and drafting the paper. Nicholas N. Nissen contributed to data collection, review of the literatures, and scientific revision of the paper. Maha Guindi contributed to data collection and scientific revision of the paper. Laith H. Jamil contributed to data collection, review of the literatures, and scientific revision of the paper.

References

[1] P. P. Anthony, "Primary carcinoma of the liver: a study of 282 cases in Ugandan Africans," *Journal of Pathology*, vol. 110, no. 1, pp. 37–48, 1973.

[2] C.-P. Lin, J.-S. Cheng, K.-H. Lai et al., "Gastrointestinal metastasis in hepatocellular carcinoma: radiological and endoscopic studies of 11 cases," *Journal of Gastroenterology and Hepatology*, vol. 15, no. 5, pp. 536–541, 2000.

[3] H. Medina-Franco, N. B. Halpern, and J. S. Aldrete, "Pancreaticoduodenectomy for metastatic tumors to the periampullary region," *Journal of Gastrointestinal Surgery*, vol. 3, no. 2, pp. 119–122, 1999.

[4] J. H. Kim, M. J. Kim, J. J. Chung, W. J. Lee, H. S. Yoo, and J. T. Lee, "Differential diagnosis of periampullary carcinomas at MR imaging," *Radiographics*, vol. 22, no. 6, pp. 1335–1352, 2002.

[5] T. A. Sohn, C. J. Yeo, J. L. Cameron, A. Nakeeb, and K. D. Lillemoe, "Renal cell carcinoma metastatic to the pancreas: results of surgical management," *Journal of Gastrointestinal Surgery*, vol. 5, no. 4, pp. 346–351, 2001.

[6] J. Kaczynski, G. Hansson, and S. Wallerstedt, "Metastases in cases with hepatocellular carcinoma in relation to clinicopathologic features of the tumour. An autopsy study from a low endemic area," *Acta Oncologica*, vol. 34, no. 1, pp. 43–48, 1995.

[7] J. D. Liang, C. H. Chen, S. J. Hsu et al., "Hepatocellular carcinoma with duodenal invasion and metastasis," *Journal of Gastroenterology and Hepatology*, vol. 27, no. 4, pp. 677–683, 2012.

[8] C. Chung, J. Al Ali, D. A. Owen, A. A. Weiss, E. M. Yoshida, and I. T. Tai, "A rare case of isolated duodenal metastases from hepatocellular carcinoma associated with p53 and ki-67 expression: a case report," *Cases Journal*, vol. 2, no. 12, article no. 9344, 2009.

[9] N. Priyathersini, S. Rajendiran, R. B. Sudagar Singh et al., "Isolated duodenal metastasis of hepatocellular. Carcinoma: a rare presentation," *Indian Journal of Clinical Practice*, vol. 22, no. 11, pp. 587–589, 2012.

[10] M. S. Park, K. W. Kim, J. S. Yu et al., "Radiologic findings of gastrointestinal tract involvement in hepatocellular carcinoma," *Journal of Computer Assisted Tomography*, vol. 26, no. 1, pp. 95–101, 2002.

[11] T.-L. Lin, A. Q. Yap, J.-H. Wang et al., "Long term survival in patients with hepatocellular carcinoma directly invading the gastrointestinal tract: case reports and literature review," *Surgical Oncology*, vol. 20, no. 4, pp. e207–e214, 2011.

[12] Y. Sone, T. Imaeda, M. Suzuki et al., "A case of hepatocellular carcinoma with a duodenal invasion from metastatic lymph node," *Gan No Rinsho*, vol. 35, no. 6, pp. 756–760, 1989 (Japanese).

[13] N. Kobayashi, H. Kirikoshi, T. Higurashi et al., "Tumor fragment impacted at the major duodenal papilla causing obstructive jaundice in a patient with hepatocellular carcinoma," *Gastrointestinal Endoscopy*, vol. 68, no. 5, pp. 999–1000, 2008.

[14] Y. Huang, G. J. Liu, M. De Lu, and B. Liao, "Gallbladder metastatic combined hepatocellular carcinoma and cholangiocarcinoma without primary intrahepatic tumor," *Digestive Diseases and Sciences*, vol. 58, no. 9, pp. 2733–2735, 2013.

[15] L. Spahr, J.-L. Frossard, C. Felley, M.-A. Brundler, P. E. Majno, and A. Hadengue, "Biliary migration of hepatocellular carcinoma fragment after transcatheter arterial chemoembolization therapy," *European Journal of Gastroenterology & Hepatology*, vol. 12, no. 2, pp. 243–244, 2000.

[16] W. Yeo, J. Y. Sung, S. C. Ward et al., "A prospective study of upper gastrointestinal hemorrhage in patients with hepatocellular carcinoma," *Digestive Diseases and Sciences*, vol. 40, no. 12, pp. 2516–2521, 1995.

14

Visceral Kaposi's Sarcoma Presenting as Upper Gastrointestinal Bleeding

Naomi Hauser, Devon McKenzie, Xavier Fonseca, and Jose Orsini

Department of Medicine, New York University School of Medicine, Woodhull Medical and Mental Health Center, Brooklyn, NY 11206, USA

Correspondence should be addressed to Naomi Hauser; naomi.hauser@gmail.com

Academic Editor: Haruhiko Sugimura

Since the advent of highly active antiretroviral therapy (HAART), the incidence of acquired immunodeficiency syndrome- (AIDS-) related Kaposi's sarcoma (KS) has decreased dramatically. While cutaneous KS is the most common and well-known manifestation, knowledge of alternative sites such as the gastrointestinal (GI) tract is important. GI-KS is particularly dangerous because of its potential for serious complications including perforation, obstruction, or bleeding. We report a rare case of GI-KS presenting as upper GI bleeding in a human immunodeficiency virus- (HIV-) infected transgendered individual. Prompt diagnosis and early initiation of therapy are the cornerstones for management of this potentially severe disease.

1. Introduction

While KS is a rare type of cancer in the United States, accounting for approximately 0.001% of all diagnosed malignancies [1], it affects HIV-infected patients at a rate of up to 1000 times greater than the general population [2]. It is the most prevalent malignancy among HIV-infected patients when HAART is not readily accessible [3, 4]. KS most commonly involves mucocutaneous sites such as the skin and oropharynx, but visceral involvement is not unusual [5, 6]. Site identification is important for prognosis and treatment. Even though HAART is seen to curb visceral involvement of KS in those with known cutaneous disease [7], the need for additional treatment, such as surgery and/or chemotherapy, may depend on the extent of visceral disease [6, 8–10]. GI tract involvement is usually asymptomatic, but when symptoms are present, they are typically nonspecific and may include abdominal pain, dyspepsia, nausea, vomiting, or diarrhea [11]. As Nagata et al. described, GI-KS can take on a variety of endoscopic appearances ranging from flat, maculopapular lesions to polypoid masses of variable sizes and consistencies [6]. Larger and more friable lesions have the potential to become severe enough to cause hemorrhage, perforation, or obstruction within the GI tract [12, 13]. We present an uncommon case of AIDS-related GI-KS with vague, nonspecific symptoms complicated by GI bleeding. Our case illustrates the need for increased awareness of the varied manifestations and complications of AIDS-related KS. A high index of suspicion along with established criteria for investigation is needed for the diagnosis and treatment of AIDS-related GI-KS, especially in cases of rapidly developing disease.

2. Case Report

A 35-year-old Hispanic transgendered female, born male, was brought to the emergency department (ED) complaining of cough, subjective fever, abdominal pain, nausea, and vomiting for a few days, as well as unintentional weight loss and "feeling unwell" for the previous 3 months. She reported being diagnosed with HIV infection 2 months earlier and having a negative HIV test 7 months before becoming seropositive. She was HAART-naive at the time of the ED visit. Her past medical history was significant for chronic constipation for which she used daily laxatives. On arrival to the ED, her vital signs were within normal limits. Physical examination was notable for laryngeal stridor, bilateral crackles, and coarse breath sounds, as well as for left lower quadrant tenderness to palpation. Remarkable laboratory findings included a platelet count of 74,000/μL (130,000–400,000), activated partial thromboplastin time of 36.3 seconds (20.4–33.4), a sodium level of 129 mmol/L (135–147), and a potassium level of 5.5 mmol/L (3.5–5.3). Complete blood count (CBC) and liver function tests (LFTs) were within normal limits. A chest X-ray (CXR) revealed no infiltrates. The patient was discharged home with prescriptions for metoclopramide and esomeprazole.

Six days later, the patient returned to the ED complaining of blood-streaked vomit and stool, odynophagia, constipation, and generalized body pain. Vital signs were within normal limits and physical examination disclosed epigastric tenderness. Fecal occult blood test was positive and laboratory findings revealed a 3 g/dL drop in hemoglobin (Hgb) (from 12.8 g/dL to 9.7 g/dL; 12.0–16.0), a 9% drop in hematocrit (Hct) (from 35.9% to 26.9%; 37.0–47.0), worsening thrombocytopenia to 43,000/μL, and a CD_4 T-cell count of 8 cells/mm^3 (544–1894). Coagulation profile was within normal limits. The patient was transfused one unit of packed red blood cells and admitted with a diagnosis of GI hemorrhage, likely secondary to gastroduodenal ulcer. Thorough physical examination was performed on the floor and revealed palpable red maculopapular, nonpainful, nonpruritic skin lesions on the back, thighs, and arms. At that time, the diagnosis of cutaneous KS was sought. Gastroenterology service was consulted and oral fluconazole 100 mg daily was initiated for possible *Candida* esophagitis causing the patient's odynophagia. During this admission, the patient had one episode of coffee-ground emesis without hematochezia or melena. A barium esophagram was unremarkable. HIV-1 viral load by PCR was 172,213 copies/mL and human herpesvirus-(HHV-) 8 was detected in the patient's plasma. Her clinical condition improved without further clinical evidence of GI bleeding. She was discharged on hospital day 5 on HAART, *Pneumocystis jirovecii* and *Mycobacterium avium* complex prophylaxis, and with instructions to return to HIV and GI outpatient clinics. Esophagogastroduodenoscopy (EGD) was scheduled to be performed as an outpatient.

The patient returned to the ED for a third time 2 weeks after discharge complaining of nausea, vomiting, and abdominal pain for 3 days. All vital signs were within normal limits, with the exception of a temperature of 102.5°F. Significant laboratory findings included Hgb of 8.7 g/dL, Hct of 25.4%, platelet count of 86,000/μL, and sodium level of 126 mmol/L. Lactic acid level was within normal limits. Her CD_4 T-cell count had risen to 20 cells/mm^3 and her HIV-1 viral load had dropped to 3,530 copies/mL. Urine toxicology screen, blood cultures, cerebrospinal fluid analysis, and CXR were all negative. Urine cultures were not completed. Empiric intravenous antimicrobial therapy was initiated consisting of cefepime 1 g every 12 hours and vancomycin 1 g every 12 hours. Abdominal computed tomography (CT) with oral and intravenous contrast showed severe thickening of the antral portion of the stomach.

EGD revealed multiple friable and possibly obstructive tumors of varying sizes in the stomach and duodenum (Figures 1 and 2). Cytopathology of the lesions showed high vascularity and spindle cells (Figure 3) and stained positively for HHV-8 (Figure 4), findings consistent with KS. The patient was discharged with instructions to continue with HAART regimen and follow up with HIV and hematology/oncology clinics. Six months after her initial ED presentation, the patient's CD_4 count had risen to 78 cells/mm^3 and repeat abdominal CT showed a decrease in the thickening of the gastric antrum. She began chemotherapy with doxorubicin one month later and completed four cycles before being lost for followup.

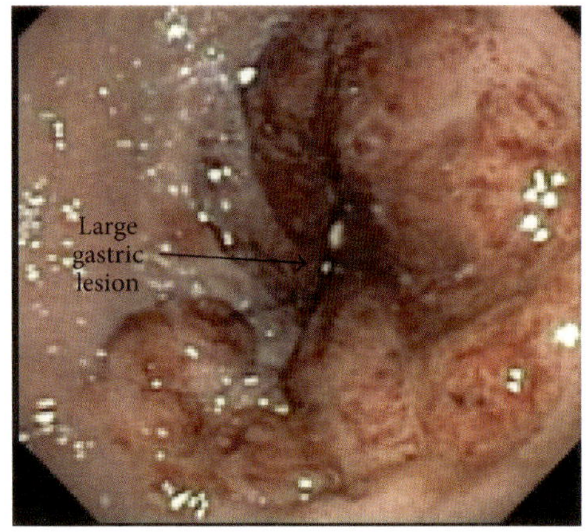

Figure 1: Large gastric lesion.

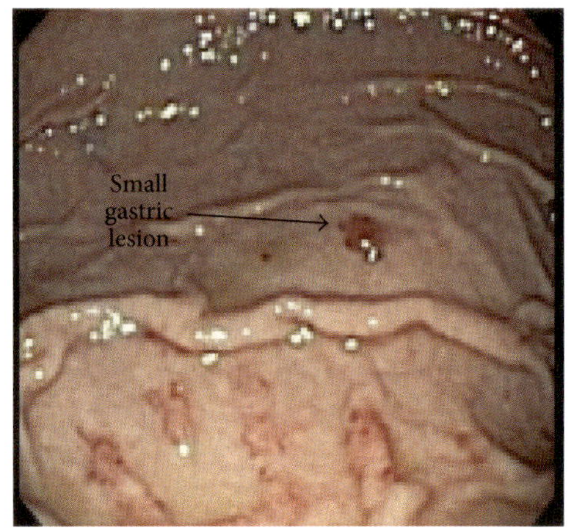

Figure 2: Small gastric lesion.

3. Discussion

Since the widespread adoption of HAART in the treatment of HIV infection, the incidence of KS has dramatically decreased among the HIV-infected population. Visceral involvement is often asymptomatic and frequently diagnosed postmortem [14]. Knowledge of visceral KS in general and GI-KS in particular remains important in light of the possible complications such as hemorrhage and obstruction as presented in our case. Acute GI bleeding due to GI-KS has been infrequently reported in the literature [14–16]. Neoplastic lesions are the most common causes of HIV-related upper GI bleeding, with GI-KS most frequently being asymptomatic, and gastrointestinal non-Hodgkin lymphoma

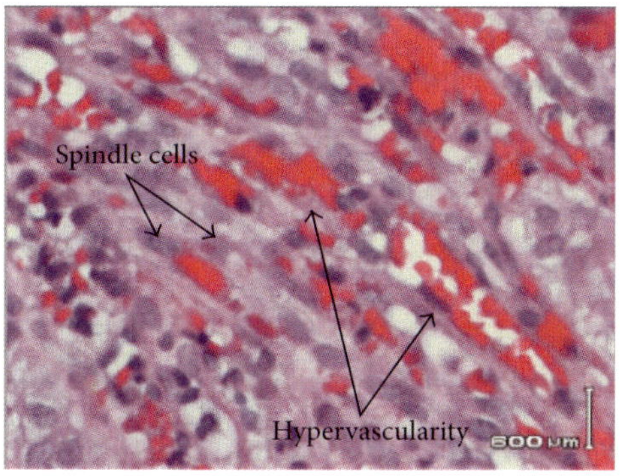

FIGURE 3: Gastric lesion biopsy displaying spindle cells and hypervascularity.

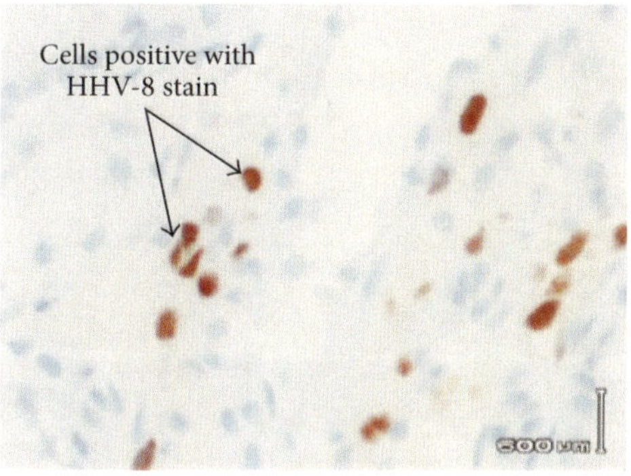

FIGURE 4: Gastric lesion biopsy showing cells positive with HHV-8 stain (brown).

often presenting with pain or gastric outlet obstruction [17]. Other GI malignancies to be considered include the much more common adenocarcinoma, which comprises nearly 95% of gastric malignancies in the general population [18]. Leiomyomas, rhabdomyosarcomas, pleomorphic sarcomas, and GI stromal tumors are additional spindle cell tumors that may be appropriate to consider as differential diagnoses [19]. Mansfield et al. analyzed 16 cases of acute upper GI bleeding associated with GI-KS reported in the literature, a handful of which were AIDS-related KS, most of the others following renal transplant and immunosuppression [14].

Nagata et al. outlined the need to determine indications for EGD in diagnosing GI-KS. They suggested that endoscopy is clearly indicated in HIV/AIDS patients with GI symptoms and cutaneous KS but that GI-KS is often present in their absence [6]. Although the mainstay of treatment is initiating/continuing HAART, early diagnosis is important in severe cases for which additional therapy is both needed and available [6, 7, 12]. Guidelines for endoscopic investigation may help prevent diagnosis of GI-KS at later stages of disease when combination therapy would no longer be tolerated [20]. Although unusual, our case illustrates the need for increased awareness of GI-KS as a potentially dangerous complication of HIV infection and as a possible etiology of upper GI bleeding. Indications for EGD in such patients should be evaluated and determined in order to prevent late diagnosis of this disease.

References

[1] N. Howlader, A. M. Noone, M. Krapcho et al., "SEER Cancer Statistics Review, 1975–2011," National Cancer Institute, Bethesda, Md, USA, based on November 2013 SEER data submission, posted to the SEER web site, April 2014, http://seer.cancer.gov/archive/csr/1975_2011/.

[2] S. Gopal, C. J. Achenbach, E. L. Yanik, D. P. Dittmer, J. J. Eron, and E. A. Engels, "Moving forward in HIV-associated cancers," *Journal of Clinical Oncology*, vol. 32, no. 9, pp. 876–880, 2014.

[3] O. Radu and L. Pantanowitz, "Kaposi sarcoma," *Archives of Pathology and Laboratory Medicine*, vol. 137, no. 2, pp. 289–294, 2013.

[4] L. A. Torre, F. Bray, R. L. Siegel, J. Ferlay, and J. Lortet-Tieulent, "Global cancer statistics, 2012," *CA: A Cancer Journal for Clinicians*, vol. 65, no. 2, pp. 87–108, 2015.

[5] L. Pantanowitz and B. J. Dezube, "Kaposi sarcoma in unusual locations," *BMC Cancer*, vol. 8, article 190, 2008.

[6] N. Nagata, T. Shimbo, H. Yazaki et al., "Predictive clinical factors in the diagnosis of gastrointestinal Kaposi's sarcoma and its endoscopic severity," *PLoS ONE*, vol. 7, no. 11, Article ID e46967, 2012.

[7] G. Nasti, F. Martellotta, M. Berretta et al., "Impact of highly active antiretroviral therapy on the presenting features and outcome of patients with acquired immunodeficiency syndrome-related Kaposi sarcoma," *Cancer*, vol. 98, no. 11, pp. 2440–2446, 2003.

[8] A. Mocroft, O. Kirk, N. Clumeck et al., "The changing pattern of Kaposi sarcoma in patients with HIV, 1994–2003: the EuroSIDA study," *Cancer*, vol. 100, no. 12, pp. 2644–2654, 2004.

[9] S. Lodi, M. Guiguet, D. Costagliola, M. Fisher, A. de Luca, and K. Porter, "Kaposi sarcoma incidence and survival among HIV-infected homosexual men after HIV seroconversion," *Journal of the National Cancer Institute*, vol. 102, no. 11, pp. 784–792, 2010.

[10] J. H. Gallafent, S. E. Buskin, P. B. de Turk, and D. M. Aboulafia, "Profile of patients with Kaposi's sarcoma in the era of highly active antiretroviral therapy," *Journal of Clinical Oncology*, vol. 23, no. 6, pp. 1253–1260, 2005.

[11] S. Attia, B. J. Dezube, J. R. Torrealba et al., "AIDS-related Kaposi's sarcoma of the gastrointestinal tract," *Journal of Clinical Oncology*, vol. 28, no. 16, pp. e250–e251, 2010.

[12] E. M. Yoshida, N. H. L. Chan, C. Chan-Yan, and R. M. Baird, "Perforation of the jejunum secondary to AIDS-related gastrointestinal Kaposi's sarcoma," *The Canadian Journal of Gastroenterology*, vol. 11, no. 1, pp. 38–40, 1997.

[13] J. Halankar, E. Martinovic, and P. Hamilton, "Kaposi's sarcoma presenting as acute small bowel obstruction diagnosed on multidetector computed tomography with histopathological correlation," *Case Reports in Radiology*, vol. 2015, Article ID 581470, 4 pages, 2015.

[14] S. A. Mansfield, S. P. A. Stawicki, R. C. Forbes, T. J. Papadimos, and D. E. Lindsey, "Acute upper gastrointestinal bleeding secondary to Kaposi sarcoma as initial presentation of HIV infection," *Journal of Gastrointestinal and Liver Diseases*, vol. 22, no. 4, pp. 441–445, 2013.

[15] C. H. Lin, C. W. Hsu, Y. J. Chiang, K. F. Ng, and C. T. Chiu, "Esophageal and gastric Kaposi's sarcomas presenting as upper gastrointestinal bleeding.," *Chang Gung medical journal*, vol. 25, no. 5, pp. 329–333, 2002.

[16] F. Parente, M. Cernuschi, L. Valsecchi et al., "Acute upper gastrointestinal bleeding in patients with AIDS: a relatively uncommon condition associated with reduced survival," *Gut*, vol. 32, no. 9, pp. 987–990, 1991.

[17] F. Bhaijee, C. Subramony, S. Tang, and D. J. Pepper, "Human Immunodeficiency Virus-associated gastrointestinal disease: common endoscopic biopsy diagnoses," *Pathology Research International*, vol. 2011, Article ID 247923, 8 pages, 2011.

[18] V. Virmani, A. Khandelwal, V. Sethi, M. Fraser-Hill, N. Fasih, and A. Kielar, "Neoplastic stomach lesions and their mimickers: spectrum of imaging manifestations," *Cancer Imaging*, vol. 12, no. 1, pp. 269–278, 2012.

[19] M. Arora and E. M. Goldberg, "Kaposi sarcoma involving the gastrointestinal tract," *Gastroenterology and Hepatology*, vol. 6, no. 7, pp. 459–462, 2010.

[20] C.-Y. Chung, S.-W. Park, E. Myung et al., "AIDS-related gastrointestinal kaposi sarcoma in Korea: a case report and review of the literature," *The Korean Journal of Gastroenterology*, vol. 60, no. 3, pp. 166–171, 2012.

15

Primary Hepatic Lymphoma Is Difficult to Discriminate from a Liver Abscess

Nobuhiro Takeuchi[1] and Kazuyoshi Naba[2]

[1] *Department of Gastroenterology, Kawasaki Hospital, Kobe, Hyogo 652-0042, Japan*
[2] *Department of Laboratory Medicine, Kawasaki Hospital, Kobe, Hyogo 652-0042, Japan*

Correspondence should be addressed to Nobuhiro Takeuchi; takeuchi_nobuhiro@kawasaki-hospital-kobe.or.jp

Academic Editors: H. Akiho, I. C. Lawrance, I. M. Leitman, A. J. Lembo, and I. Siddique

An 82-year-old woman presented with a high-grade fever of 40°C and was admitted to our institution for intensive examination and treatment. Noncontrast abdominal computed tomography (CT) revealed low-density masses at segments 5 and 8, suggestive of a liver abscess. On further examination, a contrast-enhanced abdominal CT showed a 30 × 30 mm mass with an enhanced margin at segment 8 in the arterial phase; the contrast agents were washed out in the venous phase. In addition, a 63 × 52 mm mass with a density lower than that of liver parenchyma was observed at segment 8 in the portal phase. On the basis of these findings, either a liver abscess or hepatocellular carcinoma was suspected. To confirm the diagnosis, a fine needle biopsy was scheduled. Histopathological analysis of the biopsied specimens confirmed the diagnosis of diffuse large B-cell lymphoma. Chemotherapy was not indicated owing to the patient's age and poor performance status; thus, best supportive care was planned. On day 22 after admission, the patient died of pneumonia. We experienced a case of PHL that was difficult to discriminate from a liver abscess. Imaging alone is insufficient to diagnose PHL; therefore, fine needle biopsy is recommended for a definitive diagnosis.

1. Introduction

Primary hepatic lymphoma (PHL) is a rare entity comprising only 0.48% of all malignant lymphoma. PHL is sometimes difficult to diagnose accurately as there are no specific imaging characteristics associated with this disease and confirmation requires a fine needle biopsy. Here we present a case of PHL that was difficult to discriminate from a liver abscess; fine needle biopsy facilitated diagnosis confirmation.

2. Case Presentation

An 82-year-old woman presented with a high-grade fever of 40°C and was admitted to our institution for intensive examination and treatment. The patient's medical history included type 2 diabetes mellitus diagnosed at 52 years, and oral hypoglycaemic agents were administered thereafter. She had no history of alcohol consumption or smoking. On admission, her consciousness level was alert; height, 145.6 cm; weight, 49.7 kg; body mass index, 23.4 kg/m^2; blood pressure, 120/67 mmHg; heart rate, 81/min; respiratory rate, 14/min; body temperature, 38.0°C; saturated oxygen in arterial blood, 96% (room air). Mild anaemia was evident in her palpebral conjunctiva. Chest auscultation revealed no abnormal findings. The abdomen was soft and flat, with normal bowel sounds; slight tenderness was observed over the upper abdomen. Leg oedema was not evident. Chest radiography revealed a cardiothoracic ratio of 50.0%, without evidence of pulmonary congestion or pleural effusion. Abdominal radiography revealed no abnormal gas distribution. Noncontrast abdominal computed tomography (CT) revealed low-density masses at segments 5 and 8, suggestive of a liver abscess (Figures 1(a) and 1(b)). For further examinations, including contrast-enhanced abdominal CT, magnetic resonance imaging (MRI) and ultrasonography were scheduled. Contrast-enhanced abdominal CT showed a 30 × 30 mm mass with an enhanced margin at segment 8 in the arterial phase (Figures 2(a) and 2(b)). The contrast agents were washed out in the venous phase. In addition, a 63 × 52 mm mass with a density lower than that of liver

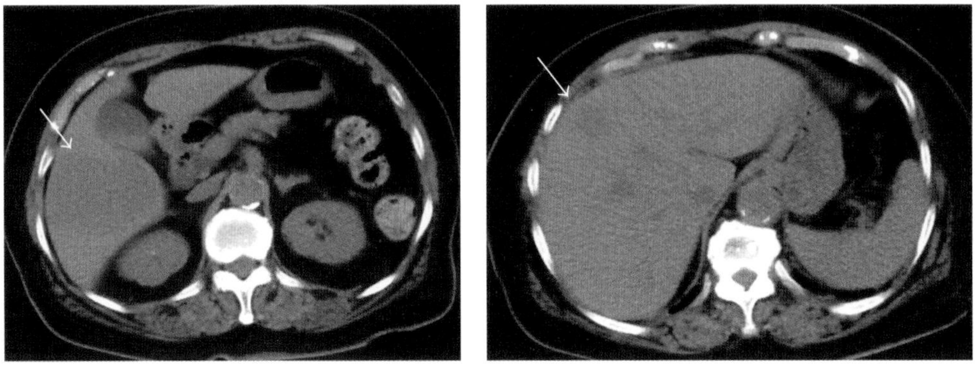

(a) (b)

Figure 1: Noncontrast abdominal computed tomography. Low-density masses were revealed at segments 5 and 8, suggestive of a liver abscess ((a) and (b)).

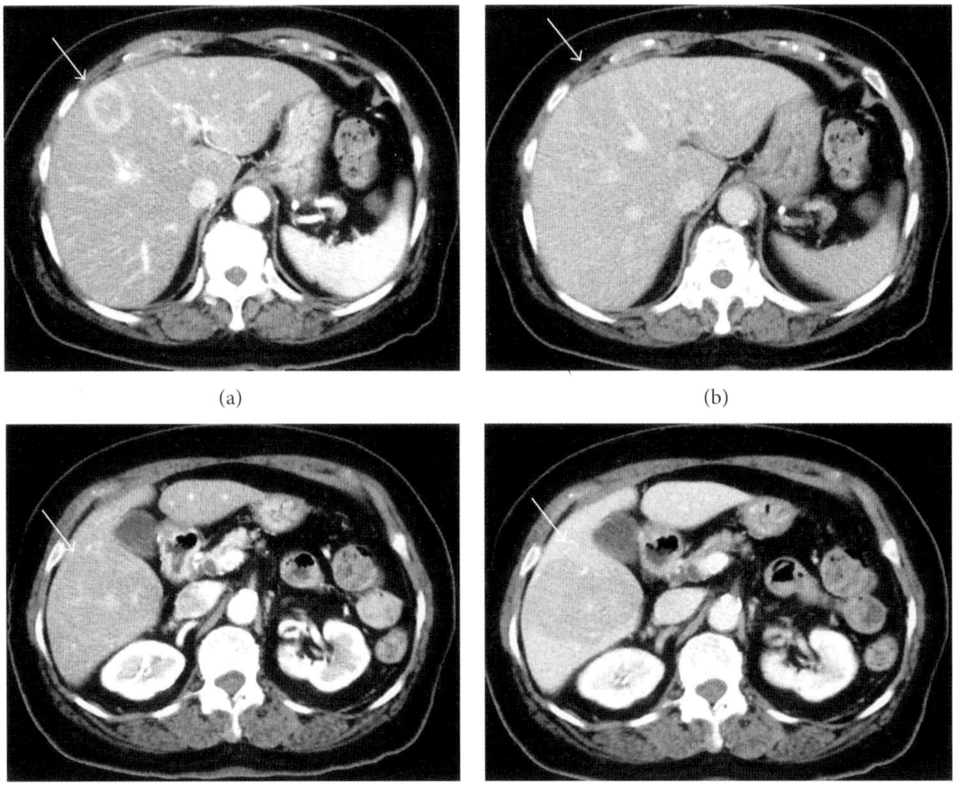

(a) (b) (c) (d)

Figure 2: Contrast-enhanced abdominal computed tomography. A 30 × 30 mm mass with an enhanced margin was revealed at segment 8 in the arterial phase (a). The contrast agents were washed out in the venous phase (b). A 63 × 52 mm mass with a density lower than that of liver parenchyma was revealed at segment 8 in the portal phase (c). On the basis of these findings, either a liver abscess or hepatocellular carcinoma was suspected.

parenchyma was observed at segment 8 in the portal phase (Figures 2(c) and 2(d)). On the basis of these findings, either a liver abscess or hepatocellular carcinoma was suspected. Noncontrast abdominal MRI revealed masses, 3.2 cm, 7 cm, and 2.2 cm in size, at segments 5, 6, and 8, respectively (Figures 3(a)–3(f)), which exhibited high signal intensity on T2- and diffusion-weighted imaging. Penetrating vessels were evident among these masses, suggestive of hepatic lymphoma (Figure 2(b)). Ultrasonography revealed low-echo masses, 3 cm, 6 cm, and 3 cm in size, at segments 5, 6, and 8, respectively (Figures 4(a)–4(d)). To confirm the diagnosis, a fine needle biopsy was scheduled. Histopathological analysis of the biopsied specimens showed diffuse and atypical large cells by hematoxylin and eosin staining (Figures 5(a) and 5(b)).

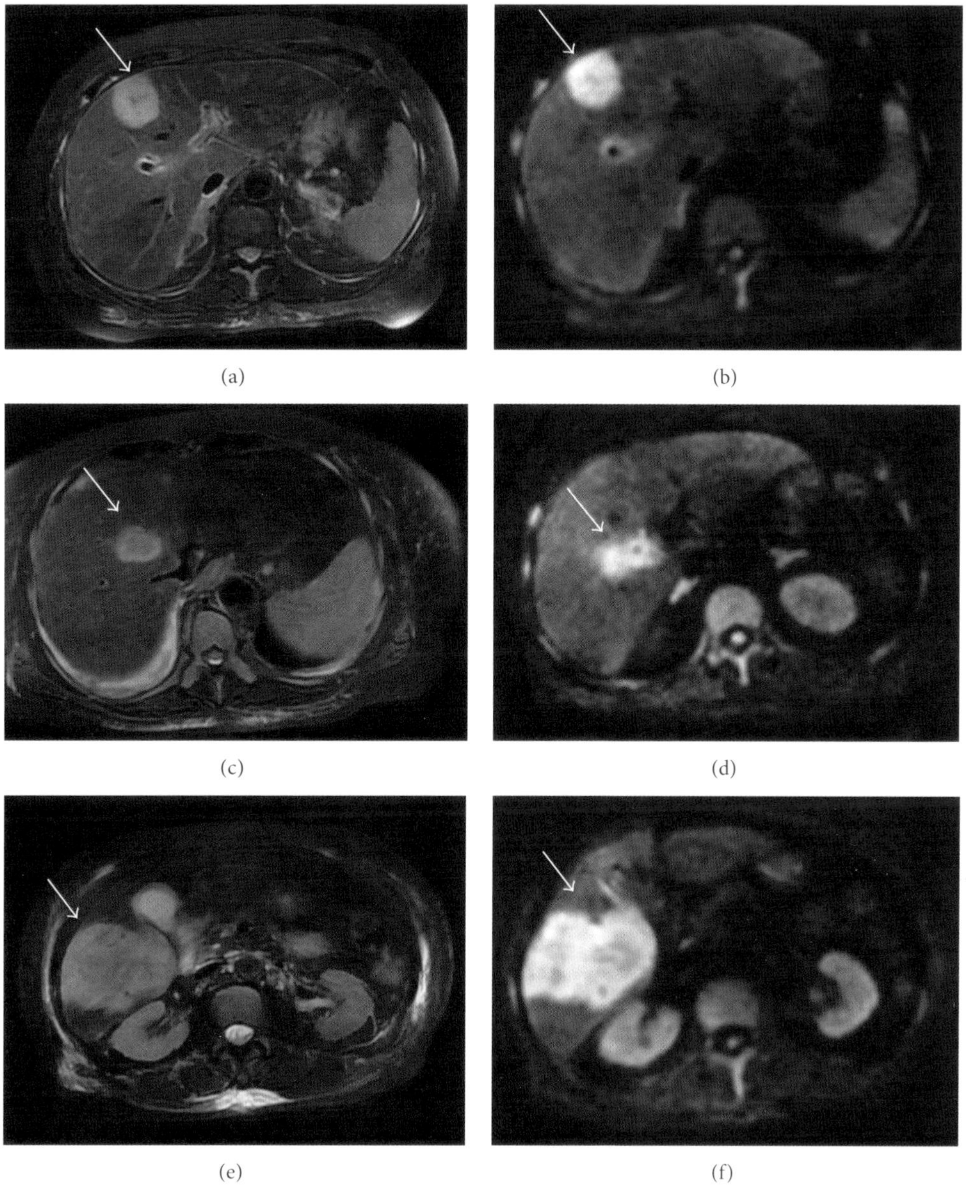

FIGURE 3: Noncontrast abdominal magnetic resonance imaging. Masses, 3.2 cm, 7 cm, and 2.2 cm in size, were revealed at segments 5, 6, and 8, respectively ((a)–(f)). These masses exhibited high signal intensity on T2- and diffusion-weighted imaging. Penetrating vessels were evident among the masses, suggesting hepatic lymphoma.

Immunohistochemical staining was positive for anti-LCA (CD45) and anti-L26 antibodies and negative for anti-CD3, anti-CD30, and anti-cytokeratin AE1/AE3 antibodies; Ki-67 staining was positive in 53% of cells (Figures 5(c)–5(h)). On the basis of the imaging and liver biopsy results, a diagnosis of PHL, diffuse large B-cell lymphoma, was confirmed. Bone marrow biopsies revealed no evidence of tumour cells invasion. Serum soluble interleukin-2 receptor levels were markedly high (23,200 U/mL). Gallium-67 scintigraphy revealed 2 prominent hot spots in the liver (Figure 6). Chemotherapy was not indicated owing to the patient's age and poor performance status; thus, best supportive care was planned. On day 22 after admission, the patient died of pneumonia.

3. Discussion

PHL has been diagnosed in patients with an age of 8–78 years (average, 48 years) and predominantly occurs in men [1]. Its clinical symptoms include right upper abdominal pain (43%), weight loss (35%), and fever (22%) [1], and it has been associated with hepatitis B [2], hepatitis C [3], and human immunodeficiency viruses [4]. PHL patient positivity for the hepatitis B surface antigen and hepatitis C antibody is

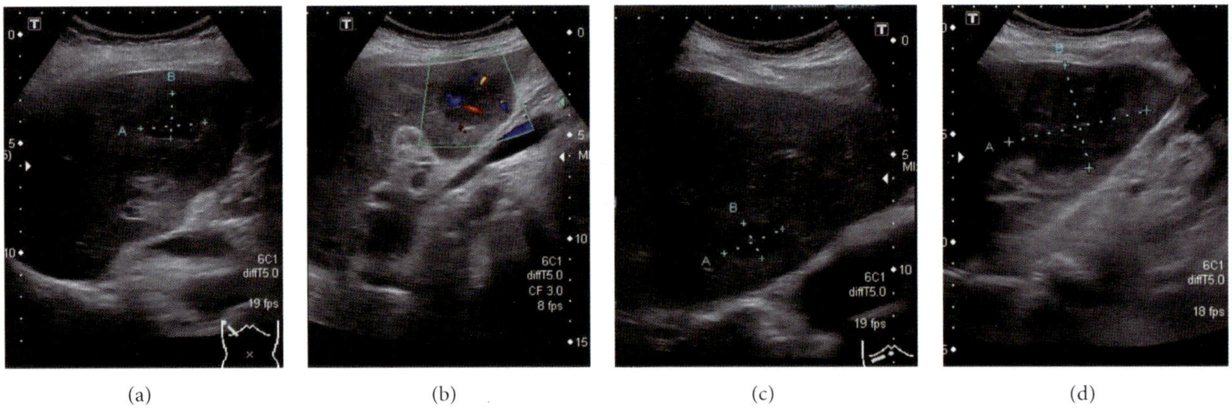

FIGURE 4: Ultrasonography. Low-echo masses, 3 cm, 6 cm, and 3 cm in size, were revealed at segments 5, 6, and 8, respectively ((a)–(d)). Penetrating vessels were evident among the masses (b).

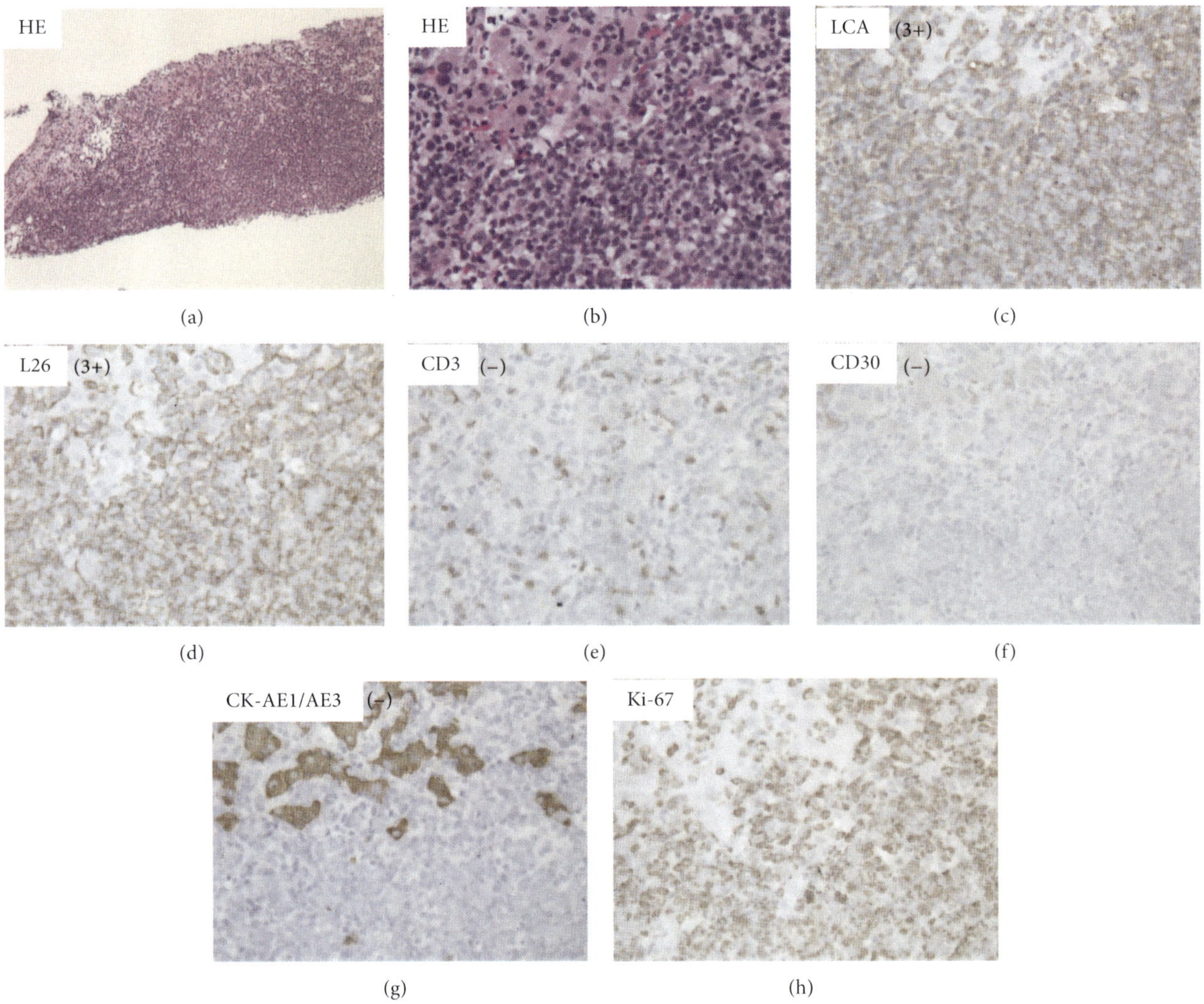

FIGURE 5: Histopathological findings. Histopathological findings from the biopsy specimens revealed the following. Diffuse and atypical large cells were revealed by hematoxylin and eosin staining ((a) and (b)). Immunohistochemical staining was positive for anti-LCA (CD45) and anti-L26 antibodies and negative for anti-CD3, anti-CD30, and anti-cytokeratin AE1/AE3 antibodies; Ki-67 staining was positive in 53% of cells ((c)–(h)).

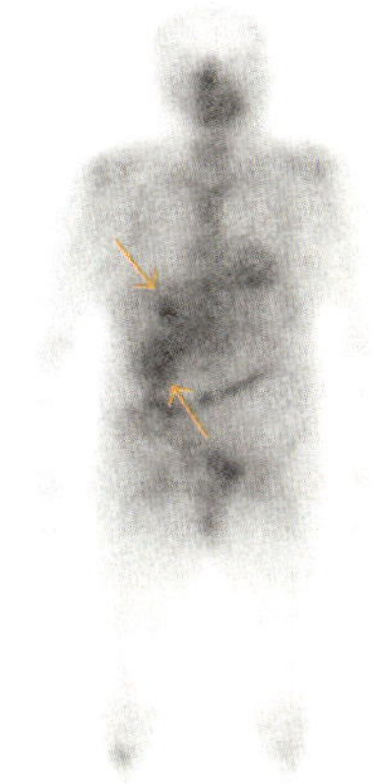

FIGURE 6: Gallium-67 scintigraphy. Two prominent hot spots were revealed in the liver.

reportedly 22% and 58% of cases, respectively [5]. PHL affects the right lobe and bilateral lobes in 34.6% and 62.0% of cases, respectively [1]. The disease exhibits several morphologies: mononodular (71.2%), multinodular (25.0%), and diffuse (3.8%). Most PHL is derived from B-cell lymphoma (88.6%) and histologically diffuse large B-cell lymphoma (52.5%) [1].

The imaging findings for PHL comprise a low-density mass on noncontrast CT, a marginally or internally enhanced mass on contrast-enhanced CT, and a homogeneously low-echo mass on ultrasonography. It is impossible to confirm a PHL diagnosis by imaging alone as there are no characteristic imaging findings associated with this disease. While images of vessels penetrating tumours are suggestive of PHL, these vessels have a relatively low impact on the vascular structure of the liver. For a definite PHL diagnosis, histopathological examination of a fine needle biopsy is mandatory and has a reported accuracy of 85% [6]. The risk of tumour seeding by fine needle biopsy is low, at 0.005% [7], and, therefore, is recommended in cases where imaging results are suggestive of PHL.

PHL treatment options include resection of the affected lesion, a combination of chemotherapy and radiotherapy, and a combination of resection and chemotherapy, although no established treatment regimen exists. Niimi et al. [8] reported a case where histological examination of resected tumours after chemotherapy revealed no evidence of tumour cells. In general, PHL has a poor prognosis and the mean survival time following chemotherapy is 14 months. In contrast, the mean survival time following surgical treatment is 32.1 months [9], and localized PHL that can be completely resected has a relatively good prognosis. In patients with localized PHL, surgery is recommended as the first-line treatment.

4. Conclusion

We reported a case of PHL that was difficult to discriminate from a liver abscess. Imaging alone is insufficient to diagnose PHL; therefore, fine needle biopsy is recommended for a definitive diagnosis.

References

[1] L. Memeo, I. Pecorello, A. Ciardi, E. Aiello, A. De Quarto, and U. Di Tondo, "Primary non-Hodgkin's lymphoma of the liver," *Acta Oncologica*, vol. 38, no. 5, pp. 655–658, 1999.

[2] T. S. Talamo, A. Dekker, J. Gurecki, and G. Singh, "Primary hepatic malignant lymphoma. Its occurrence in a patient with chronic active hepatitis, cirrhosis, and hepatocellular carcinoma associated with hepatitis B viral infection," *Cancer*, vol. 46, no. 2, pp. 336–339, 1980.

[3] C. Ferri, F. Caracciolo, A. L. Zignego et al., "Hepatitis C virus infection in patients with non-Hodgkin's lymphoma," *British Journal of Haematology*, vol. 88, no. 2, pp. 392–394, 1994.

[4] C. M. Reichert, T. J. O'Leary, and D. L. Levens, "Autopsy pathology in the acquired immune deficiency syndrome," *American Journal of Pathology*, vol. 112, no. 3, pp. 357–382, 1983.

[5] K. Kai, T. Beppu, Y. Imamura et al., "A resected case of primary lymphoma of the liver: review of twenty-seven resected cases in Japan," *Japanese Journal of Gastroenterological Surgery*, vol. 38, no. 6, pp. 644–649, 2005.

[6] S. F. Quinn, R. C. Sheley, H. A. Nelson, T. A. Demlow, R. E. Wienstein, and B. L. Dunkley, "The role of percutaneous needle biopsies in the original diagnosis of lymphoma: a prospective evaluation," *Journal of Vascular and Interventional Radiology*, vol. 6, no. 6, pp. 947–952, 1995.

[7] E. H. Smith, "The hazards of fine-needle aspiration biopsy," *Ultrasound in Medicine and Biology*, vol. 10, no. 5, pp. 629–634, 1984.

[8] Y. Niimi, A. Watanabe, H. Ishikawa et al., "A resected case of primary lymphoma of the liver after chemotherapy," *Journal of Japanese College of Surgeons*, vol. 31, pp. 724–727, 2006.

[9] V. S. Avlonitis and D. Linos, "Primary hepatic lymphoma: a review," *European Journal of Surgery*, vol. 165, no. 8, pp. 725–729, 1999.

16

Littoral Cell Angioma in a Patient with Crohn's Disease

Joel Johansson,[1] Bergthor Björnsson,[2,3] Simone Ignatova,[4] Per Sandström,[2,3] and Mattias Ekstedt[1]

[1] *Department of Gastroenterology and Department of Clinical and Experimental Medicine, Linköping University, 58185 Linköping, Sweden*
[2] *Department of Surgery, County Council of Östergötland, 58185 Linköping, Sweden*
[3] *Division of Surgery, Department of Clinical and Experimental Medicine, Faculty of Health Sciences, Linköping University, 581 85 Linköping, Sweden*
[4] *Department of Pathology, Linköping University Hospital, 581 85 Linköping, Sweden*

Correspondence should be addressed to Joel Johansson; joejo597@student.liu.se

Academic Editor: Haruhiko Sugimura

Littoral cell angioma is a rare vascular tumor of the spleen. The pathogenesis is unknown but the lesion is associated with several malignancies and immunological disorders. The diagnosis requires histopathological examination. The malignant potential of this lesion is unknown, which is why splenectomy is recommend for all cases. Symptomatic cases generally suffer from hypersplenism and pyrexia. A previously healthy 20-year-old female was diagnosed with colonic Crohn's disease; as part of the work-up a magnetic resonance enterography was performed which showed multiple signal changes of the spleen. The patient reported chronic abdominal pain in the left upper quadrant, malaise, and fever. The unknown splenic lesions prompted a laparoscopic splenectomy; pathology revealed a littoral cell angioma. The abdominal pain and malaise remitted but the fever persisted one year despite adequate treatment of the patient's Crohn's disease. Littoral cell angioma is associated with immune-dysregulation including Crohn's disease with several reported cases. Signs and symptoms of hypersplenism and splenic lesions on imaging should raise suspicion of littoral cell angioma in patients with Crohn's disease. Magnetic resonance enterography to assess disease severity in Crohn's disease may provide an opportunity to study the prevalence and natural history of this rare splenic tumor.

1. Introduction

Littoral cell angioma, LCA, is a primary vascular tumor of the spleen, first described by Falk et al. in 1991 [1]. It is a rare neoplasm which is thought to arise from the splenic cords showing both endothelial and histiocytic phenotype [1]. It has been associated with both malignancies [2] and immune-dysregulation [3]. Around 150 cases have been reported and although radiological features have been described for US, MRI, and CT, findings are unspecific and diagnosis usually requires histopathology [4] on image guided biopsy specimen [5] or splenectomy specimen. The LCA is frequently an incidental finding on imaging but some cases are symptomatic. Symptomatic cases typically develop signs and symptoms of hypersplenism including anemia, splenomegaly, and thrombocytopenia as well as constitutional symptoms including fever [3]. Treatment is splenectomy as it cures symptoms and malignant lesions cannot be excluded with imaging [6]. We report a case of LCA in a patient with new onset of Crohn's disease, naive to biologics, and with little exposure to immunosuppressive agents before the incidental finding of LCA on magnetic resonance enterography, MRE.

2. Case Presentation

A 20-year-old, previously healthy female with a two-month history of abdominal pain, bloody diarrhoea, and tenesmus was referred to the Gastroenterology Clinic at the Linköping University Hospital by her primary care physician. She underwent colonoscopy that revealed a friable erythematous area with contact bleeding that spanned from the splenic flexure and 15 cm down the descending colon; biopsies were taken throughout the procedure. These findings were interpreted as Crohn's disease because of the distribution of inflammation

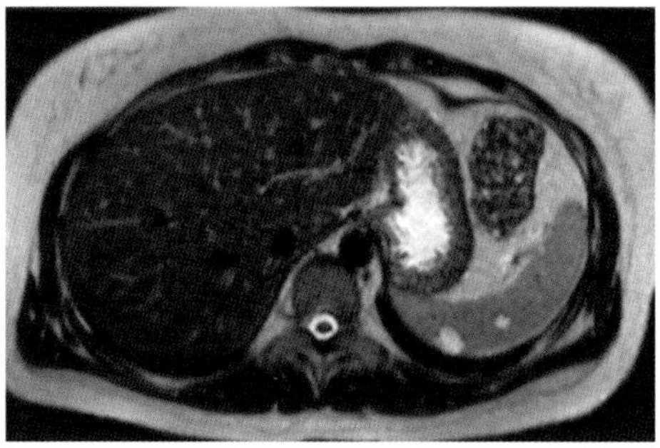

(a)

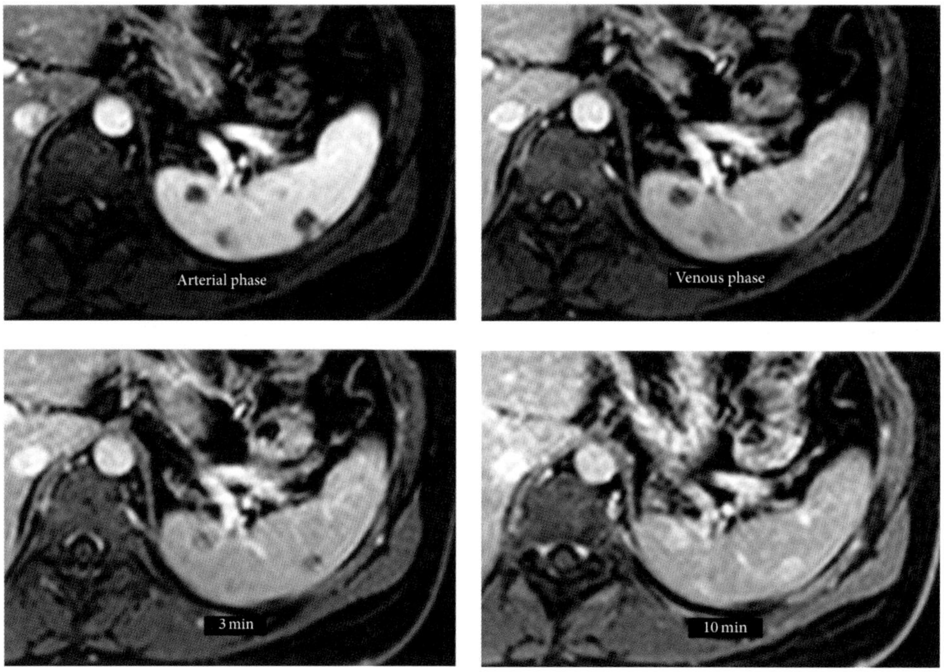

(b)

FIGURE 1: (a) Multiple lesions throughout the spleen up to 15 mm in size. They have a high signal on T2 and SPIR. (b) Signal intensity was low on T1 sequences. After gadolinium contrast, no attenuation was seen in the arterial phase, heterogeneous contrast enhancement in the portal venous phase, and after 3 minutes the enhancement is stronger in the periphery than central in the lesions. After 10 minutes the signal is stronger in the lesions than the surrounding splenic tissue. The signal pattern is in keeping with hemangiomas. On histopathological examination the diagnosis of LCA was confirmed.

although histology-pathology showed unspecific inflammation more closely related to ulcerative colitis. The patient was started on prednisolone which was tapered as planned over 8 weeks. Follow-up with fecal calprotectin showed no response and the patient was started on balsalazide.

When the patient came for follow-up at 9 months she suffered from fever and bloody diarrhoea once daily. This was regarded as colonic Crohn's disease and budesonide was added to balsalazide, An MRE was made one month after the follow-up and it revealed no small bowel engagement; however it showed multiple signal changes in the spleen, benign cysts where suspected. A contrast enhanced ultrasound was made that showed indentations in the superior portion of the spleen as well as multiple minor cystic lesions and a central 1 cm lesion with late contrast loading, possibly a hemangioma. After two months the effect of budesonide wore off and the patient again suffered from bloody diarrhoea. Sigmoidoscopy showed proctitis with diminished vascularity and contact bleeding. Budesonide was switched to mesalamine which had no effect; therefore azathioprine was tried but a colonoscopy one month later showed inflammation from the sigmoid colon till the splenic flexure. The MRE images were once again examined and it was decided that an MRI was necessary to establish the nature of the splenic lesions. The MRI showed multiple lesions with a contrast pattern of hemangiomas (Figures 1(a) and 1(b)). Two months after the MRI she presented acutely to the gastroenterology outpatient clinic with sudden worsening of abdominal pain that had been present for one month. There were no associated GI or micturition symptoms, body temperature of 38, 3°C with abdominal tenderness in the upper left quadrant, no guarding, rigidity, or mass.

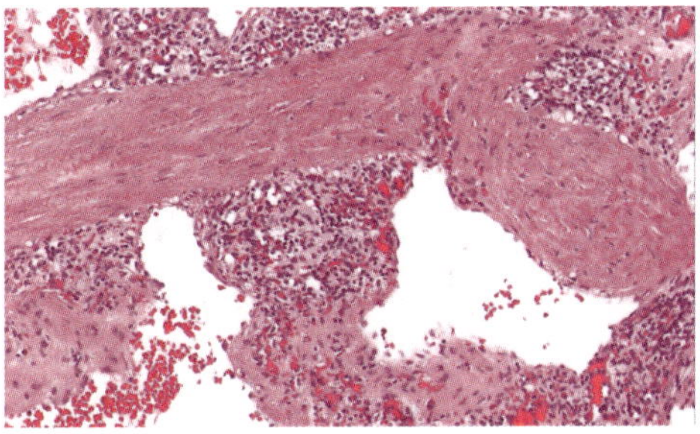

FIGURE 2: Photomicrograph ×20 magnification. Littoral cell angioma of the spleen composed of small anastomosing and irregular channels reminiscent of splenic sinuses and covered of neoplastic plump "littoral" cells with low mitotic activity.

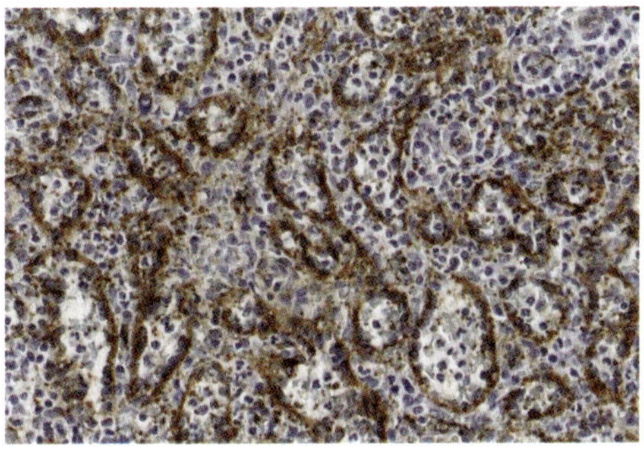

FIGURE 3: Photomicrograph ×20 magnification. The neoplastic cells express FVIII.

The patient was discussed at the upper gastrointestinal interdisciplinary round 2 months later. LCA or similar benign tumor was suspected and splenectomy was favoured due to the patient's symptoms. A laparoscopic splenectomy was performed, after adequate immunisation, without complications 3 months later. The patient got better and could eventually resume working. Repeated fecal calprotectin was negative. The pathology report confirmed LCA of the spleen (Figures 2, 3, and 4). The episodic fever persisted for one year and has been extensively investigated. A rheumatology consult (the patient reported joint pain and stiffness of the hand and has a first-degree relative with rheumatoid arthritis), capsule endoscopy and laboratory tests for VIP, pancreatic polypeptide, and gastrin all came back negative. After one year the fever gradually disappeared.

3. Discussion

Several cases link Crohn's disease to LCA [1, 7, 8]. LCA should be suspected in patients with Crohn's disease who develop signs and symptoms of hypersplenism or where imaging shows lesions of the spleen. Azathioprine, corticosteroids, and other immunosuppressive drugs have also been implicated [3]. In our patient the LCA was found on MRE before azathioprine treatment was initiated. The courses of prednisolone, budesonide, and balsalazide prior to MRE were all relatively short. In the cases where LCA has been tied

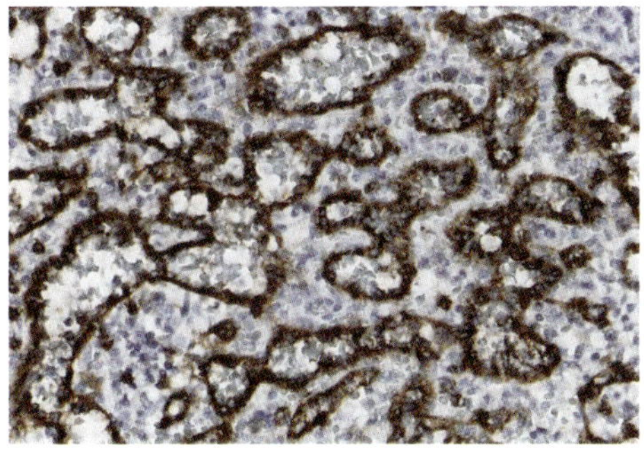

FIGURE 4: Photomicrograph ×20 magnification. The neoplastic cells express histiocytic antibody CD 68 as well as VIII whereas usual endothelial splenic cells only express VIII.

to immunosuppression, patients have been treated for years [9–11].

TNF-α has been suggested to play a role in the pathogenesis of LCA, both in itself in the presence of immune-dysregulation [12] and in immunosuppression with anti-TNF-α agents [10]. Since our patient has not been exposed to biologics it further strengthens the hypothesis that LCAs are associated with immune-dysregulation. It is also to our knowledge the first case where systemic symptoms persisted despite splenectomy. The episodic pyrexia points towards an immunologic component of the disease. Why only some patients develop systemic symptoms remains elusive. The pyrexia has been attributed to the patients LCA since a comprehensive work-up failed to find a cause and her Crohn's disease was in remission, repeated fecal calprotectin negative.

The LCA in our patient was discovered on MRE before the onset of symptoms. Imaging is an important part of the assessment of disease severity in Crohn's disease; this generates a lot of data. These images may provide an opportunity to study the natural history and prevalence of LCA. Since Crohn's disease seems to be a risk factor for LCA, patient cohorts may be sought through reexamination of imaging studies from patients with Crohn's disease.

4. Conclusion

LCA is a rare neoplasm associated with immune-dysregulation. Several cases link LCA with Crohn's disease. Our case is the first where pyrexia, not explained otherwise, persisted for a year after splenectomy further suggesting an immunologic association. Splenic nodules on imaging and hypersplenism should always raise suspicion of LCA in patients with Crohn's disease. The MRE studies of patients with Crohn's disease may provide an opportunity to study the natural history and prevalence of LCAs in patients with Crohn's disease.

Consent

Written informed consent was obtained from the patient for publication of this case report and accompanying images. A copy of the written consent is available for review.

References

[1] S. Falk, H. J. Stutte, and G. Frizzera, "Littoral cell angioma: a novel splenic vascular lesion demonstrating histiocytic differentiation," *The American Journal of Surgical Pathology*, vol. 15, no. 11, pp. 1023–1033, 1991.

[2] M. Bisceglia, J. Z. Sickel, F. Giangaspero, V. Gomes, M. Amini, and M. Michal, "Littoral cell angioma of the spleen: an additional report of four cases with emphasis on the association with visceral organ cancers," *Tumori*, vol. 84, no. 5, pp. 595–599, 1998.

[3] R. L. Harmon, C. A. Cerruto, and A. Scheckner, "Littoral cell angioma: a case report and review," *Current Surgery*, vol. 63, no. 5, pp. 345–350, 2006.

[4] M. Grantham, D. Einstein, K. McCarron, A. Lichtin, and D. Vogt, "Littoral cell angioma of the spleen," *Abdominal Imaging*, vol. 23, no. 6, pp. 633–635, 1998.

[5] S. Shah, A. Wasnik, A. Pandya, and R. O. Bude, "Multimodality imaging findings in image-guided biopsy proven splenic littoral cell angioma: series of three cases," *Abdominal Imaging*, vol. 36, no. 6, pp. 735–738, 2011.

[6] R. M. Abbott, A. D. Levy, N. S. Aguilera, L. Gorospe, and W. M. Thompson, "Primary vascular neoplasms of the spleen: radiologic-pathologic correlation," *Radiographics*, vol. 24, no. 4, pp. 1137–1163, 2004.

[7] J. A. Blansfield, R. T. Goldhahn Jr., and R. K. Josloff, "Littoral cell angioma of the spleen treated by laparoscopic splenectomy," *Journal of the Society of Laparoendoscopic Surgeons*, vol. 9, no. 2, pp. 222–224, 2005.

[8] J. J. Sarandria, M. Escano, F. Kamangar, S. O. Farooqui, E. Montgomery, and S. C. Cunningham, "Littoral cell angioma: gastrointestinal associations," *Gastrointestinal Cancer Research*, vol. 7, no. 2, pp. 63–64, 2014.

[9] Y. M. Tan, K. L. Chuah, and W. K. Wong, "Littoral cell angioma of the spleen," *Annals of the Academy of Medicine Singapore*, vol. 33, no. 4, pp. 524–526, 2004.

[10] M. Cappello, I. Bravatà, G. Cocorullo, M. Cacciatore, and A. M. Florena, "Splenic littoral cell hemangioendothelioma in a patient with crohn's disease previously treated with immunomodulators and anti-TNF agents: a rare tumor linked to deep immunosuppression," *American Journal of Gastroenterology*, vol. 106, no. 10, pp. 1863–1865, 2011.

[11] E. Tholouli, J.-A. Roulson, R. Byers, I. Burton, and J. A. Liu Yin, "Littoral cell angioma of the spleen in a patient with severe aplastic anaemia," *Haematologica*, vol. 88, no. 11, Article ID ECR33, 2003.

[12] S. Cordesmeyer, M. Pützler, U. Titze, H. Paulus, and M. W. Hoffmann, "Littoral cell angioma of the spleen in a patient with previous pulmonary sarcoidosis: a TNF-α related pathogenesis?" *World Journal of Surgical Oncology*, vol. 9, article 106, 2011.

17

Metastatic Melanoma of the Gallbladder in an Asymptomatic Patient

Asad Khan,[1] Sejal Patel,[2] Daniel J. Zaccarini,[3] and Mary McGrath[4]

[1]SUNY Upstate Medical University, Syracuse, NY 13210, USA
[2]Department of Radiology, SUNY Upstate Medical University, Syracuse, NY 13210, USA
[3]Department of Pathology, SUNY Upstate Medical University, Syracuse, NY 13210, USA
[4]Department of Nuclear Medicine, SUNY Upstate Medical University, Syracuse, NY 13210, USA

Correspondence should be addressed to Asad Khan; khanasa@upstate.edu

Academic Editor: Gregory Kouraklis

Malignant Melanoma (MM) is among the most dangerous malignancies with some of the least known survival rates. Melanoma most commonly metastasizes to regional lymph nodes, the lungs, and brain. Metastatic disease of the gallbladder (GB) is exceptionally rare making it difficult to diagnose. The fact that typically patients do not present until they are symptomatic—only after widespread metastatic disease has already occurred—is further complicating the diagnosis of MM of the GB. For this reason, MM of the GB is rarely discovered in living patients. In fact, review of the literature showed only 40 instances in which metastatic disease of the GB was reported in living patients. We describe the presentation and management of a patient who had metastatic disease of the GB. However, our case is unique because his malignancy was discovered incidentally while he was asymptomatic. He was successfully treated with an open cholecystectomy. We have presented this case in order to make the necessity of meticulous investigation of potential metastasis in patients with a known history of cutaneous melanoma clear.

1. Introduction

Metastatic melanoma is among the most aggressive malignancies with some of the least known survival rates with a median survival of 6–10 months after surgery and 18% survival at five years [1]. Melanoma most commonly metastasizes to regional lymph nodes, the lungs, and brain [2, 3]. Metastatic disease of the gastrointestinal (GI) system is unusual and only occurs in 2–4% of patients [4]. Within the GI system metastatic disease most commonly occurs in the intestines, colon, and the stomach [4].

Metastatic disease of the gallbladder is rare and associated with a poor prognosis with a mean survival rate of 8.4 months [5]. Furthermore, patients typically do not report symptoms during their lifetime because involvement of the gallbladder seldom produces symptoms [6]. For this reason, melanoma of the gallbladder is rarely discovered in living patients [6]. A review of the literature shows only 40 instances in which metastatic disease of the gallbladder was reported in living patients [7].

We herein report a case of a 57-year-old gentleman with a history of cutaneous melanoma of the shoulder that was incidentally discovered to have metastatic melanoma of the gallbladder, which was successfully treated with open cholecystectomy. Our patient's case is particularly unique due to discovery of the mass while being alive and asymptomatic.

2. Case Presentation

A 57-year-old gentleman was diagnosed with depth of 2.71 mm, Clark level IV, ulcerated cutaneous melanoma of the left shoulder and back, which showed perivascular invasion and superficial spreading. Preoperative lymphoscintigraphy showed a focus of increased activity in the left axilla, which was removed and negative on final pathology for metastatic melanoma.

The patient was treated with wide local excision and a total of four sentinel lymph nodes were removed, which were negative for malignancy. He also underwent metastatic workup including CT of the chest, abdomen, and pelvis that

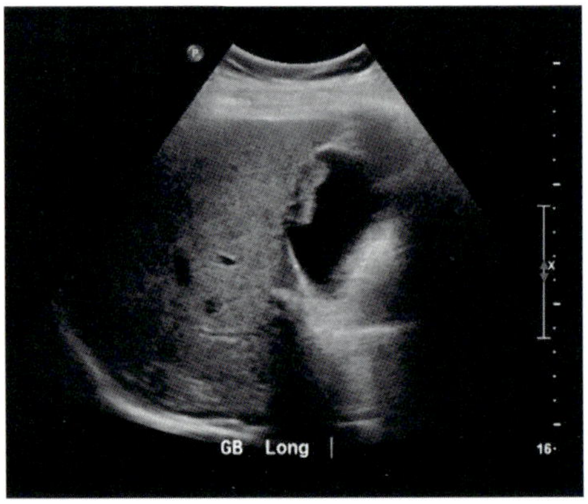

Figure 1: Ultrasound of the gallbladder demonstrating an irregular lesion along the gallbladder wall measuring 2.9 × 1.0 cm.

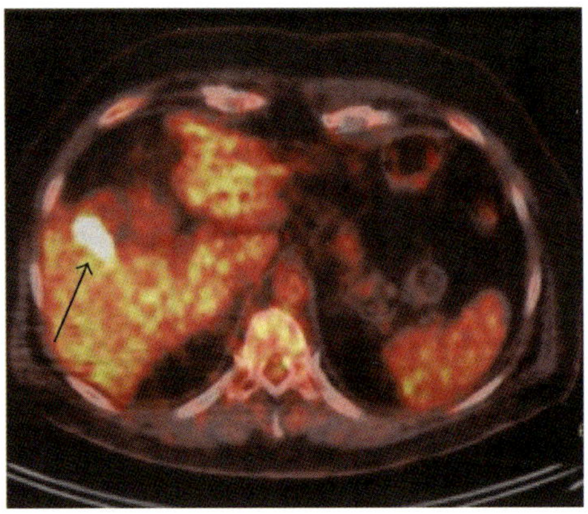

Figure 2: Fused PET/CT axial image demonstrating intense increased activity in the gallbladder (black arrow).

was negative for any distant metastasis; however, it did show some hepatic cysts that warranted follow-up imaging.

A sonographic exam of the right upper quadrant of the abdomen was performed for evaluation of liver cysts and incidentally noted an irregular lesion along the gallbladder wall (Figure 1). A follow-up MRI was recommended, which showed multiple hepatic cysts and a nonspecific gallbladder mass measuring 2.8 cm in transverse diameter. The decision was then made to proceed with PET scan and MRI of the brain for staging given the history of high-risk melanoma. The PET scan showed a focus of increased metabolic activity with maximum SUV of 22.1 within the gallbladder in the region of abnormality visualized on the ultrasound and MRI (Figures 2 and 3). The patient underwent cholecystectomy with final pathology remarkable for metastatic melanoma (Figure 4).

3. Discussion

Melanoma is a cancer of melanocytes, which are dendritic cells responsible for producing melanin, and represents approximately <5% of all skin cancers [8]. It is associated with high mortality due to the potential for wide spread metastatic

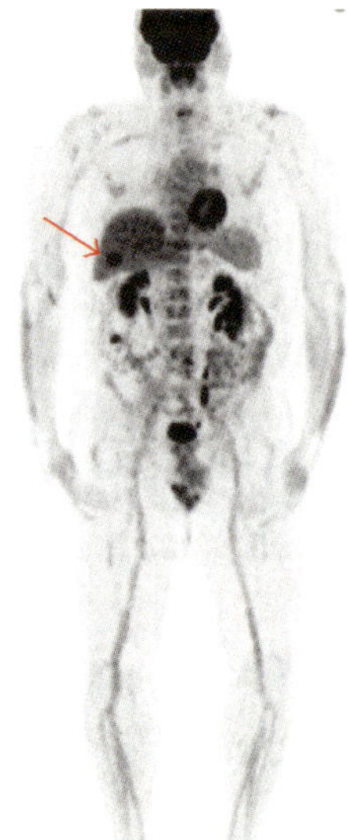

Figure 3: Whole body MIP image showing abnormal focal activity in the region of the gallbladder (red arrow).

disease. Once metastatic disease has occurred, prognosis is very poor with a mean survival rate of approximately 8.4 months [5].

Autopsy reports show the prevalence of metastatic disease of the gallbladder is between 15 and 20% [6]. Melanoma is the most common metastatic malignancy of the gallbladder, accounting for about 50–67% [9]. Despite these statistic data, most patients are asymptomatic and do not present until widespread disease has occurred [10–12]. Thus accurate diagnosis requires a strong degree of suspicion. Among the symptomatic patients, acute cholecystitis is the most common presentation, followed by jaundice and obstruction of the common bile duct [13]. Incidences of hemobilia and biliary fistula have also been reported [14].

Ultrasound is the preferred imaging modality for evaluation of the gallbladder in symptomatic patients or in patients in whom metastatic disease of the gallbladder is suspected [15]. Typical ultrasound findings include a sole or multiple infiltrative polypoid lesions not showing acoustic shadow, larger than 1 cm, and attached to the GB wall [4]. Doppler ultrasound has been shown to be useful in detecting the presence of remarkably increased blood flow within the lesions [16].

While the examination of choice in detecting metastatic melanoma of the gallbladder is straightforward, the treatment is much less definitive. There is limited experience in the management of metastatic melanoma of the gallbladder due to its rarity. In general, patients with disease limited to the GB should be aggressively treated with surgery with a goal of avoiding symptoms or tumor complications and significant improvement in survival and prognosis [1]. One study done by Dong et al. found that patients who had surgery for isolated gallbladder metastases had a 100% survival at 1 year compared with 0% for those with unresectable tumors with multiple metastases [10]. When considering surgical approach, open

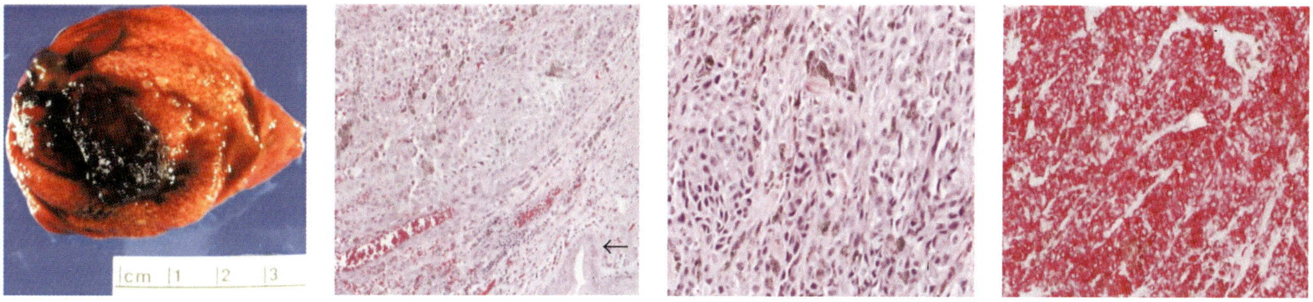

(a) (b) (c) (d)

FIGURE 4: (a) Gallbladder mucosa with dark brown pigmented polypoid lesion measuring 2.7 × 1.5 × 1.3 cm. (b) Sheets of malignant epithelioid cells are seen with eosinophilic cytoplasm and prominent nucleoli. Gallbladder epithelium can be seen (arrow). (c) Higher power showing malignant cells with hyperchromatic large atypical nuclei with eosinophilic cytoplasm and scattered brown pigment. (d) Immunohistochemistry for melanocytic marker HMB-45 showing diffuse and strong staining.

cholecystectomy is preferred over laparoscopic technique, which has been associated with port site recurrence [1, 17].

One promising avenue for the future in the treatment of metastatic melanoma is chemoimmunotherapy. One study documented the use of high-dose interleukin-2 in tumor remission in approximately 15% of patients [18]. However, the use of interleukin-2 is limited on a large scale due to toxicity and difficulties with its administration. The BRAF inhibitor, vemurafenib, has demonstrated improved progression-free and overall survival compared with chemotherapy in a randomized trial [19]. The use of vemurafenib in patients who are BRAF V600E positive has become the standard of care [19]. Other studies have shown that combining the use of BRAF inhibitors with the use of MEK inhibitors lowers the incidence of adverse reactions, prolongs disease-free survival, and delays the resistance that has been seen in BRAF inhibitor use alone [20].

4. Conclusion

Metastatic melanoma is among the most ominous malignancies due to its aggressive course and poor prognosis. We have presented this case in order to make the necessity of meticulous investigation of potential metastases in patients with a known history of cutaneous melanoma clear. Metastatic melanoma of the gallbladder is considered an especially rare event and diagnosis is difficult because most cases of gallbladder metastasis are asymptomatic. Various studies indicate that the key to prolonging survival is aggressive treatment once metastatic disease is discovered. Acceptable treatment options include cholecystectomy and chemoimmunotherapy.

Disclosure

There were no sources of financial or material support for this case report. The SUNY Upstate IRB does not require review of case reports that do not meet the definition of human subject research.

References

[1] U. Marone, C. Caracò, S. Losito et al., "Laparoscopic cholecystectomy for melanoma metastatic to the gallbladder: Is it an adequate surgical procedure? Report of a case and review of the literature," *World Journal of Surgical Oncology*, vol. 5, article no. 141, 2007.

[2] M. O. Meyers, D. J. Frey, and E. A. Levine, "Pancreaticoduodenectomy for melanoma metastatic to the duodenum: A case report and review of the literature," *American Surgeon*, vol. 64, no. 12, pp. 1174–1176, 1998.

[3] J. Gogas, D. Mantas, H. Gogas, E. Kouskos, C. Markopoulos, and S. Vgenopoulou, "Metastatic melanoma in the gallbladder: report of a case," *Surgery Today*, vol. 33, no. 2, pp. 135–137, 2003.

[4] M. F. Haskaraca, M. Ozsoy, İ. Özsan, and K. Kurt, "Primary malignant melanoma of the gallbladder: a case report and review of the literature," *Case Reports in Surgery*, vol. 2012, Article ID 693547, 4 pages, 2012.

[5] M. Guida, A. Cramarossa, A. Gentile et al., "Metastatic malignant melanoma of the gallbladder: a case report and review of the literature," *Melanoma Research*, vol. 12, no. 6, pp. 619–625, 2002.

[6] T. Das Gupta and R. Brasfield, "Metastatic melanoma. A clinicopathological study," *Cancer*, vol. 17, pp. 1323–1339, 1964.

[7] J.-P. A. Martel, C. A. McLean, and R. N. Rankin, "Best cases from the AFIP: melanoma of the gallbladder," *Radiographics*, vol. 29, no. 1, pp. 291–296, 2009.

[8] M. K. Samplaski, E. L. Rosato, A. K. Witkiewicz, M. J. Mastrangelo, and A. C. Berger, "Malignant melanoma of the gallbladder: a report of two cases and review of the literature," *Journal of Gastrointestinal Surgery*, vol. 12, no. 6, pp. 1123–1126, 2008.

[9] R. S. Nelson and F. Lanza, "Malignant melanoma metastatic to the upper gastrointestinal tract," *Gastrointestinal Endoscopy*, vol. 24, no. 4, pp. 156–158, 1978.

[10] X. D. Dong, P. DeMatos, V. G. Prieto, and H. F. Seigier, "Melanoma of the gallbladder: a review of cases seen at Duke University Medical Center," *Cancer*, vol. 85, no. 1, pp. 32–39, 1999.

[11] R. G. B. Langley, E. M. Bailey, and A. J. Sober, "Acute cholecystitis from metastatic melanoma to the gall-bladder in a patient with a low-risk melanoma," *British Journal of Dermatology*, vol. 136, no. 2, pp. 279–282, 1997.

[12] P. Cellerino, F. Corsi, E. Morandi, D. Foschi, and E. Trabucchi, "Metastatic melanoma of the gallbladder," *European Journal of Surgical Oncology*, vol. 26, no. 8, pp. 815-816, 2000.

[13] S. Vernadakis, G. Rallis, N. Danias et al., "Metastatic melanoma of the gallbladder: an unusual clinical presentation of acute cholecystitis," *World Journal of Gastroenterology*, vol. 15, no. 27, pp. 3434–3436, 2009.

[14] N. Daunt and D. M. King, "Metastatic melanoma in the biliary tree," *British Journal of Radiology*, vol. 55, no. 659, pp. 873-874, 1982.

[15] S. T. Hahn, S. H. Park, H. S. Choi, C. Kim, K. S. Shinn, and C. S. Kim, "Ultrasonographic features of metastatic melanoma of the gallbladder," *Journal of Clinical Ultrasound*, vol. 21, no. 8, pp. 542–546, 1993.

[16] N. A. Avila, T. H. Shawker, and D. Fraker, "Color-flow Doppler ultrasonography in metastatic melanoma of the gallbladder," *Journal of Clinical Ultrasound*, vol. 22, no. 5, pp. 342–347, 1994.

[17] S. C. Katz, W. B. Bowne, J. D. Wolchok, K. J. Busam, D. P. Jaques, and D. G. Coit, "Surgical management of melanoma of the gallbladder: a report of 13 cases and review of the literature," *American Journal of Surgery*, vol. 193, no. 4, pp. 493–497, 2007.

[18] D. Christou, N. Katodritis, M. P. Decatris et al., "Melanoma of the gallbladder: appropriate surgical management and review of the literature," *Clinical Case Reports*, vol. 2, no. 6, pp. 313–318, 2014.

[19] A. A. Tarhini, J. M. Kirkwood, W. E. Gooding, C. Cai, and S. S. Agarwala, "Durable complete responses with high-dose bolus interleukin-2 in patients with metastatic melanoma who have experienced progression after biochemotherapy," *Journal of Clinical Oncology*, vol. 25, no. 25, pp. 3802–3807, 2007.

[20] R. Fisher and J. Larkin, "Vemurafenib: A new treatment for BRAF-V600 mutated advanced melanoma," *Cancer Management and Research*, vol. 4, no. 1, pp. 243–252, 2012.

18

Surgery to Treat Symptomatic Mobile Cecum Syndrome Is Safe and Associated with Good Recovery Outcomes

Manuela Cesaretti,[1] Manuela Trotta,[1] Irene Leale,[1] Giuseppe Antonio Minetti,[2] Giuseppe Cittadini,[2] Fabrizio Montecucco,[3,4,5] Giovanni Bruno Camerini,[1,3] and Giacomo Borgonovo[1,3]

[1] *Dipartimento di Scienze Chirurgiche e Diagnostiche Integrate (DISC), Università degli Studi di Genova, 8 Largo Benzi, 16132 Genoa, Italy*
[2] *Department of Radiology, Ospedale Policlinico San Martino, 10 Largo Benzi, 16132 Genoa, Italy*
[3] *Ospedale Policlinico San Martino, 10 Largo Benzi, 16132 Genoa, Italy*
[4] *First Clinic of Internal Medicine, Department of Internal Medicine, University of Genoa, 6 Viale Benedetto XV, 16132 Genoa, Italy*
[5] *Centre of Excellence for Biomedical Research (CEBR), University of Genoa, 9 Viale Benedetto XV, 16132 Genoa, Italy*

Correspondence should be addressed to Fabrizio Montecucco; fabrizio.montecucco@unige.it

Academic Editor: Yucel Ustundag

The mobile cecum syndrome includes a spectrum of conditions. The cecal volvulus represents the acute form, with typical feature of a bowel obstruction that needs immediate operative treatment. On the other hand, a chronic form of mobile cecum syndrome which is the most common form reported a history of intermittent crampy abdominal pain, distension, and constipation. In this study, five patients came to our attention during the last ten years, presenting different symptoms due to a mobile cecum. All patients were investigated by several diagnostic techniques according to the specific clinical setting. All patients were found to have the cecum and ascending colon unattached to the posterior peritoneum. Surgery was the treatment of choice. In our experience, the best diagnostic technique was computed tomography scan, especially if performed in the Trendelenburg position. We also propose virtual colonoscopy as a good option for diagnosis (in patients with chronic syndrome) and follow-up after surgery. In conclusion, laparoscopic approach guaranteed a good result, with no symptoms of recurrence, in both acute and elective treatments. The diagnosis of mobile cecum needs a high index of suspicion and a targeted radiological investigation. Surgery, especially laparoscopic cecopexy and appendectomy, is the recommended treatment.

1. Introduction

Mobile cecum is anatomically defined as an anomalous position of the right colon, cecum, and terminal ileum due to the failure of the right colon mesentery to fuse with the posterior parietal peritoneum. Embryogenesis of bowel is a complex process that begins during the 5th gestational week and involves three phases: herniation, return to the abdomen, and fixation [1, 2]. Anomalies of rotation and fixation of the gastrointestinal tract are frequently associated with other embryological defects, but per se the suspension on a mesentery of the cecum and ascending colon may allow them to freely rotate and cause a wide spectrum of symptoms included in the "mobile cecum syndrome." This condition can be asymptomatic, as it has been found in 11.2% of autopsies [3, 4]. On the other hand, it can also clinically manifest as a chronic syndrome including constipation, abdominal distension, and recurrent abdominal pain or, more rarely, as an acute bowel obstruction due to cecal volvulus (1–1.5% of all adult intestinal obstruction) [5]. This study reports a series of five patients presenting for a symptomatic mobile cecum that required surgical treatment (mostly by laparoscopy).

2. Methods

In the last ten years, five patients were admitted at the Surgery Unit of San Martino Hospital (Genoa, Italy), since they

Table 1: Summary of clinical cases' characteristics.

Clinical case	Patient age (years)/sex (F/M)	Laboratory test alteration	CT scan/virtual colonoscopy positivity	Grade of lack of peritoneal attachment of the right colon (I-II-III)	Surgical treatment	Postoperative day of discharge
			Acute form			
Case 1	20/M	Yes	Yes	II	Laparoscopy	5th day
Case 2	82/M	Yes	Yes	II	Laparotomy	7th day
Case 3	40/F	Yes	Yes	II	Laparotomy	15th day
			Chronic form			
Case 4	57/F	No	Yes	II	Laparoscopy	3rd day
Case 5	54/F	No	Yes	II	Laparoscopy	3rd day

presented different symptoms due to an anomalous position of the cecum. Two patients came after a history of recurrent lower quadrant pain and abdominal distension (chronic form of the disease); the other three patients arrived with an acute form of cecal volvulus (acute form for the disease). Patients gave written informed consent prior to entering the study. The protocol adheres to the principles of the Declaration of Helsinki. The cases of acute and chronic forms of the diseases are summarized in Table 1. The grade of lack of peritoneal attachment of the right colon was graded as follows: I (cecum retroperitoneal or with little mobility), II (wide mobility, crossing the midline), and III (maximum mobility, reaching the left abdomen) [6].

Diagnosis was obtained by several diagnostic techniques (ultrasound, abdominal radiography, computed tomography, and virtual colonoscopy), according to the specific clinical setting.

All patients were examined using a computed tomography (CT) scanner (GE LightSpeed 16) with the following scan parameters: slice thickness of 1.2 mm, tube rotation time of 0.8 s, and KV/mAs of 120/Mod. The scan was performed with the patient supine from the diaphragmatic domes to the pubic symphysis before and after injection of intravenous nonionic, uroangiographic contrast material (Ultravist 370®; Bracco, Milan, Italy) into the cubital vein with an 18-gauge needle connected to an automatic injector. The parameters were as follows: volume of 1,5 ml/kb of body weight (maximum value: 120 mL) and an injection rate of 3 ml/s. Images were obtained during the arterial and portal phase, and the scan delay was determined automatically using the Smart-Prep tracking technique. 3% diatrizoate meglumine (Gastrografin®; Bracco, Milan, Italy) was administered as positive rectal contrast material. To stress the spontaneous colic malposition, CT scans performed in Trendelenburg position were also acquired. The majority of patients were operated by laparoscopic surgery. In case of massive overdistended bowel loops, a laparotomy was chosen. Several surgical procedures were carried out according to the ischemic state of the bowel: in case of ischemic colon, a right colectomy was performed; otherwise, a cecopexy and appendectomy were performed. Laparoscopic cecopexy procedure is briefly summarized below. After the induction of general anesthesia, the patient was placed in the supine position. A 15 mm skin incision was made just below the umbilicus, a 12 mm trocar was inserted, and pneumoperitoneum was established by insufflation with carbon dioxide to 12 mmHg abdominal pressure. Two 5 mm trocars were inserted under laparoscopic guidance: one in the middle lower abdominal region and the other in the left lateral region. First step was the careful examination of the abdominal cavity, looking for evident intraperitoneal adhesions, macroscopic gastroenteric diseases, and the right colon position. Cecopexy was done by suturing the cecum and the ascending colon under a flap of parietal peritoneum expressly created with interrupted absorbable sutures.

3. Report of Cases

3.1. Acute Form of the Disease

Case 1. A 20-year-old man was admitted to the Emergency Department with a six-hour-long diffuse abdominal pain, vomiting, and constipation. His medical history did not present remarkable episodes, except for a chronic recurrence of intermittent lower right quadrant pain. No previous surgery was reported. At physical examination, he presented diffuse abdominal tenderness, more evident in upper left quadrant, with asymmetric meteorism and rebound tenderness. Digital rectal examination revealed no stools in rectal ampulla. Laboratory tests showed a white blood cell count of 13800 cells/mm^3 and elevated C-Reactive Protein (CRP) (130 mg/L).

Diagnosis of bowel obstruction was confirmed by an abdominal plain radiograph that revealed a grossly dilated bowel segment with haustra in the right abdomen. No free gas was detected. A CT scan demonstrated a dilated and twisted cecum with tip pointing to left upper quadrant, twisted mesentery, and small bowel vessels. Distal colon was collapsed. All these findings were suggestive of cecal volvulus (Figure 1).

Exploratory laparoscopy revealed a notable distension of the cecum, ileum, and jejunal loops. The cecum was rotated around its axis and located in the left abdominal quadrant. Distal colon beyond the rotation was collapsed. Free fluid was

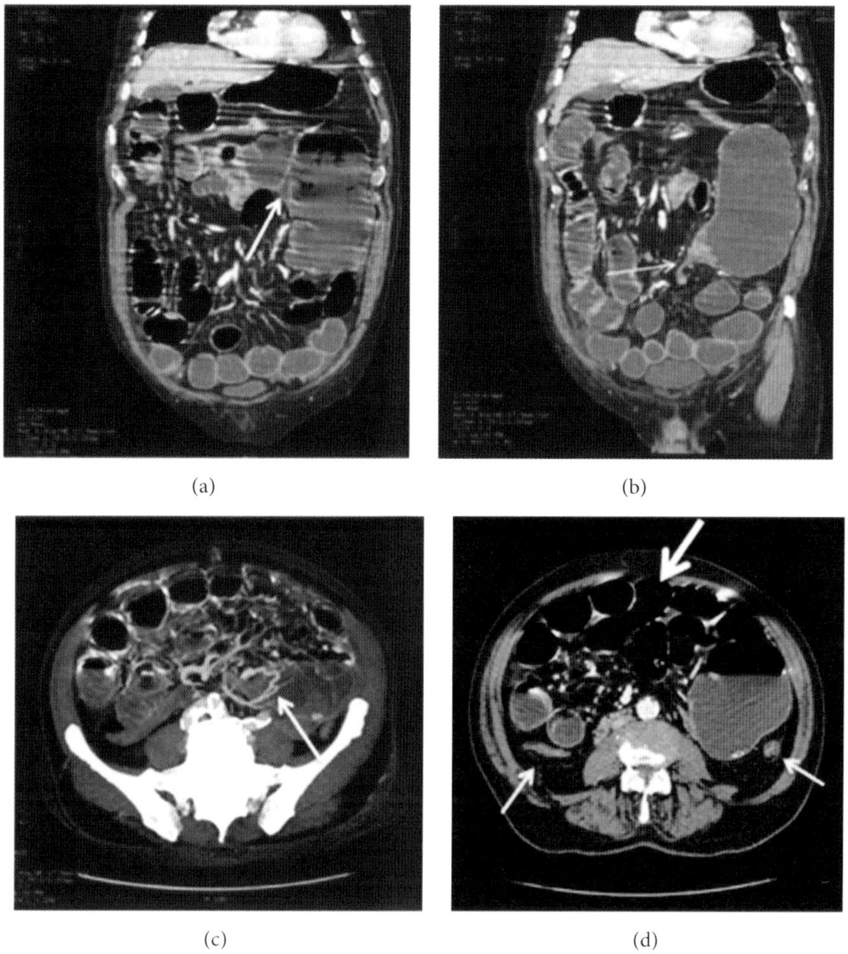

FIGURE 1: (a) Medially placed ileocecal valve (arrow). (b) Dilated, twisted cecum with tip pointing to left upper quadrant (arrow). (c) "Whirlpool" sign: tightly twisted mesentery and bowel vessels. (d) Dilated small bowel loops with air fluid levels (thick arrow) and distended gas or fluid-filled small bowel (white arrows).

found in the abdomen and it was collected for microbiological culture, which resulted to be negative. After derotation of the right colon, the intestine recovered completely, so an appendectomy and cecopexy using a right gutter peritoneal flap were performed. Postoperative course was uneventful and the patient was discharged on the 5th postoperative day. After five years, he does not suffer from abdominal pain anymore.

Case 2. An 82-year-old man presented with a two-day history of fever, acute diffuse abdominal pain, diarrhea, and then constipation. Neither vomiting nor fever was reported. Past medical history included acute prostatitis and arterial hypertension treated with amiloride chlorhydrate and hydrochlorothiazide. The patient also had a history of chronic abdominal pain and distension that was relieved by passing flatus. Physical examination revealed tenderness in the right lower quadrant. Rectal examination showed residual normal stool in rectal ampulla. Laboratories' studies showed no abnormalities except for leukocytosis (15000/mm^3). Abdominal radiography showed air fluid levels of the small bowel. CT scan demonstrated ileal peritoneal adhesion with markedly dilated small bowel loops (>2.5 cm) and collapsed colon. A nasogastric tube was placed to decompress the bowel but did not result in improvement of patient's situation. Consequently, he underwent urgent laparotomy that revealed a volvulus of the cecum. The cecum had an elongation of the ileocolic pedicle without lateral peritoneal attachments and it was situated in the upper left abdominal quadrant (Figure 2). The bowel was ischemic but not perforated; nevertheless a right colectomy was performed. Histological exam of the resected specimen showed a thin and necrotic bowel. Postoperative course was uneventful and he was discharged on the 7th postoperative day. The patient is currently asymptomatic after two years of follow-up.

Case 3. A 40-year old woman presented with a three-day history of persistent diffuse acute abdominal pain and vomiting. Her medical problems included intermittent abdominal distension and constipation for several years. An appendectomy was performed twenty years previously. No medication was reported. The abdomen was symmetrically distended with tenderness, but there was neither muscle rigidity nor Blumberg's sign. Laboratory studies revealed leukocytosis

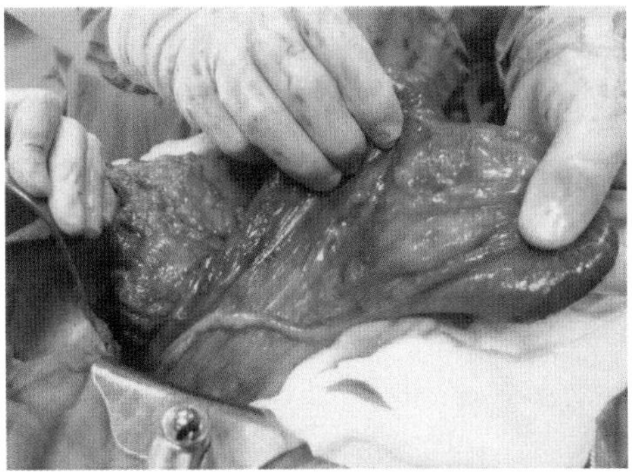

FIGURE 2: Elongation of the ileocolic pedicle without lateral peritoneal attachments and with hypermobile cecal apex, which could be directed toward the upper quadrant. A retrocecal, ascending appendix can also be noticed.

(12000/mm^3). Plain abdominal X-ray showed markedly dilated loops with air fluid levels. Transverse colon appeared collapsed. These findings suggested the presence of a bowel obstruction in the ascending colon. A CT scan confirmed it and aroused the suspicion of a volvulus of the right colon. The patient underwent urgent laparotomy that revealed dilated small bowel loops and a volvulus of the cecum located in the central abdominal quadrant. The cecum was derotated and a fixation of the right colon to the right parietocolic peritoneal space using a peritoneal flap was performed. On the 3rd day after surgery, the patient had fever due to a pneumonia treated with quinolone. She was discharged on the 15th postoperative day. She remains asymptomatic ten years after the cecopexy.

3.2. Chronic Form of the Disease

Case 4. A 57-year-old woman arrived with a five-month history of intermittent colicky periumbilical pain, constipation, and abdominal distention. Past medical history included colpohysterectomy for uterine fibroids, hiatal hernia treated conservatively, and arterial hypertension treated by atenolol. At physical examination, the patient's abdomen was distended with diffuse tenderness, without muscle guarding. The bowel sounds were normal. Laboratory blood tests were normal. During a previous emergency admission for a severe attack of abdominal pain, ultrasound and plain abdominal radiographs were performed. They showed dilated bowel and a medial position of the appendix. After one month, a virtual colonoscopy was performed and demonstrated a large right colon in the left abdominal quadrant (Figure 3(a)), so a mobile cecum syndrome was diagnosed.

The patient underwent a laparoscopy that revealed a long and mobile right colon, without attachments to the posterior abdominal wall. No other abnormalities were found. A cecopexy using a lateral peritoneal flap was performed. A complementary appendectomy was carried out as well. Postoperative course was uneventful and the patient was discharged on the 3rd postoperative day. She has not had pain for one year and another virtual colonoscopy demonstrated the physiological position of the cecum (Figure 3(b)).

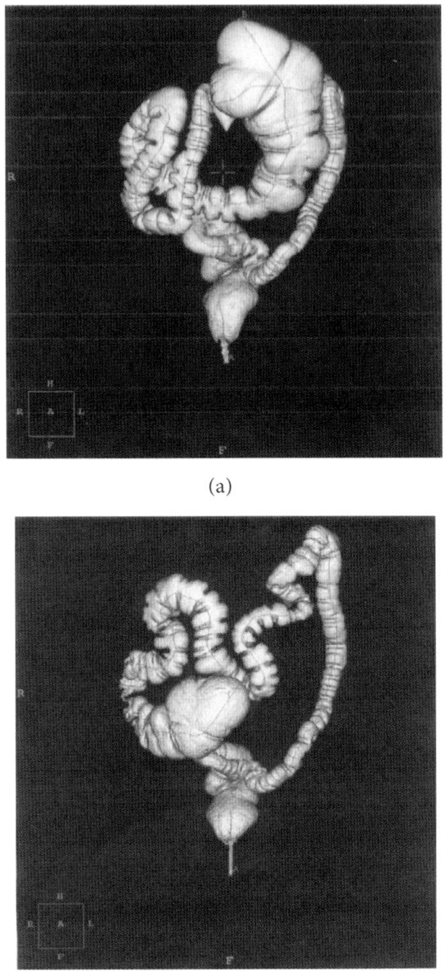

(a)

(b)

FIGURE 3: (a) Virtual colonoscopy. Three-dimensional volume-rendered CT colonography (anteroposterior view) showed an elongated right colon with the cecum dislocated in the upper left quadrant. (b) Virtual colonoscopy one year after surgery. Three-dimensional volume-rendered CT colonography (anteroposterior view) demonstrated the cecum and the ascending colon in the physiological position.

Case 5. A 54-year-old woman was admitted to our hospital with a six-month history of crampy diffuse abdominal pain and constipation. Ten years previously, she underwent a laparoscopic ovariectomy for endometriosis. At physical examination, the patient's abdomen appeared diffusely tender, without signs of peritonitis. Laboratory tests were negative. Ultrasound and plain abdominal radiographs taken at another hospital showed dilated bowel loops throughout the abdomen. Rectal contrast CT examination performed a week before surgery showed an enlarged right colon in the left abdominal quadrant. A mobile cecum syndrome was diagnosed. The patient underwent laparoscopic surgery that revealed a malposition of a mobile right colon, unattached to the posterior peritoneal abdominal wall, without signs of ischemia. Appendectomy and cecopexy were performed. The patient recovered after the operation and was discharged on the 3rd postoperative day. Four years after the surgery, no further recurrence of abdominal pain was reported.

4. Discussion

Symptomatic presentation of an anomalous cecum fixation includes recurrent abdominal pain and constipation due to the intermittent distension and sufferance of the cecum or acute bowel obstruction due to cecal volvulus. The presence of the recurrent pattern, known as mobile cecum syndrome, is reported in about 50% of the patients before the onset of acute volvulus [4]. Symptoms of the chronic syndrome are relieved after passing flatus or using laxative therapy. During symptomatic episodes, physical examination reveals abdominal tenderness and high pitched bowel sounds. Laboratory tests are negative. When there are two concomitant requisites, such as hypermobile cecum and a point of fixation with torsion, a cecal volvulus may occur. Clinically, it is an acute bowel obstruction, which has various features depending on the severity and the duration of the intestinal obstruction, ranging from the subacute obstruction to the acute fulminant pattern [5]. Symptoms are not specific, with different intensity, but the most common presentations are acute abdominal pain (80%), distension (80%), constipation (60%), and vomiting (28%) [7].

While mobile cecum syndrome could be suitable to elective surgery, cecal volvulus, if not rapidly treated, may evolve to intestinal strangulation with bowel ischemia, gangrene, and perforation. Because of this serious clinical condition, it is very important to make a prompt diagnosis. Since clinical and laboratory tests are often not specific, for both mobile cecum syndrome and acute presentation, radiological investigations play a central role in diagnosis. Patients with mobile cecum syndrome often have extensive work-ups before a correct diagnosis. Ultrasonography is always the first examination to be carried out because of its cost-effectiveness. It allows excluding appendicitis or macroscopic lesions of the intestine. Sometimes it can detect anomalies of right colon position but its findings are generally nonspecific [8]. CT scan (with endoluminal contrast in nonacute patients) can reveal medialization of appendix and a suspicion of cecum malposition. Scan performed in Trendelenburg position can show a hypermobile cecum with cecal apex directed toward the left upper quadrant. This sign is highly specific for mobile cecum. Virtual colonoscopy can be also a valid technique for both diagnosis (in patients affected by mobile cecum syndrome) and follow-up after the cecopexy. When acute bowel obstruction is suspected, radiological investigations become crucial to demonstrate the level and the cause of obstruction.

Cecal volvulus is mostly diagnosed on abdominal plain radiographs and CT images. In a large series, however, abdominal X-ray is rarely diagnostic, and therefore CT scan is usually performed [9]. Barium enema can also be used, with an accuracy of 88% [4, 9]. This technique can show a collapsed colon downstream the pivot point and if the obstruction is incomplete, barium may trickle past the site of obstruction and the twist could be visualized in detail. Because of the risk of overdistension and perforation of the cecum during this exam, it is not indicated in emergency. Additional drawbacks are signs of peritonitis, rectal bleeding, radiographic sign of gas in the bowel wall, and pneumoperitoneum [10]. Literature reports cases of occasional successful cecal volvulus reduction after barium enema administration [11]. Severe cecal distension, cecal apex in left upper quadrant, collapsed distal colon, small bowel distension, whirlpool sign (the superior mesenteric artery wrapped by coils of superior mesentery vein and bowel), ileocecal twist, and transition points are the most common CT findings [12]. Differential diagnosis includes gastric dilation, sigmoid volvulus, small bowel volvulus, and colon obstruction with a competent ileocecal valve [7]. After the achievement of a correct diagnosis, a tailored treatment should be performed. Mobile cecum syndrome should be treated surgically, due to the recurrence of abdominal pain and the risk of cecal volvulus.

Authors suggest associating appendectomy with cecopexy in order to increase the fixation to parietal peritoneum due to postappendectomy adhesions [13]. Literature reports recurrence of syndrome after simple cecopexy, but most of these procedures use only simply suturing the cecum to lateral peritoneum [3, 4]. Rabinovici and coworkers [9] reported that cecopexy has a recurrence rate of 13%. In case of cecal volvulus, endoscopy has been proposed as initial treatment. However, it is usually associated with unsuccessful reduction and high risk of perforation, and therefore it is considered as a treatment of limited interest [14, 15]. Surgery offers different options of surgical treatment, including detorsion, cecopexy (with or without appendectomy), colectomy, or cecostomy. Treatment should be tailored and based on patient's performance status, viability of the bowel, risk of recurrence, and surgeon's skill in laparoscopic procedure. There is generally an agreement on the fact that, in case of gangrene and perforation of the bowel, it should be resected. Colectomy of course eliminates the possibility of volvulus recurrence, but it is associated with higher morbidity and mortality [16]. Improvements in surgical technique and perioperative cares had led to reduction of the mortality and morbidity rate. Cecostomy should be avoided because it results in a high rate of complications. In case of early diagnosis of cecal volvulus and in the absence of a massive loops distension (>2.5 cm), a laparoscopic approach should be attempted.

Literature reports only eight cases of mobile cecum syndrome or cecal volvulus treated by laparoscopic surgery [3, 6, 17–21]. In our experience, laparoscopic cecopexy using a peritoneal flap is a valid therapeutic approach that could be adopted in both chronic and acute manifestations of anomalous cecum position with excellent results and no recurrence of symptoms in a medium term follow-up.

5. Conclusion

Anomalous position of the right colon is quite common, but it is rarely symptomatic. Indeed diagnosis of a clinically evident mobile cecum needs a high index of suspicion. CT scan is the best imaging technique available for a correct diagnosis, especially in Trendelenburg position. Surgery is the treatment of choice in order to prevent or solve volvulus of the cecum and recurrence of disease. In this report, the most performed procedure is laparoscopic cecopexy with peritoneal flap associated with appendectomy. Only one patient presented signs of bowel ischemia and a right colectomy became necessary. Laparoscopic suturing of the cecum can be performed in the same way as in open surgery but with better functional results. In our experience, recurrences were absent in a medium term follow-up.

References

[1] W. E. Ladd, "Surgical Diseases of the Alimentary Tract in Infants," *The New England Journal of Medicine*, vol. 215, no. 16, pp. 705–708, 1936.

[2] F. T. Mall, *Development of the human intestine and its position in the adult*, vol. 9, Bull Johns Hopkins Hosp, 1898.

[3] T. Tsushimi, H. Kurazumi, Y. Takemoto et al., "Laparoscopic cecopexy for mobile cecum syndrome manifesting as cecal volvulus: Report of a case," *Surgery Today*, vol. 38, no. 4, pp. 359–362, 2008.

[4] R. L. Rogers and F. J. Harford, "Mobile cecum syndrome," *Diseases of the Colon & Rectum*, vol. 27, no. 6, pp. 399–402, 1984.

[5] E. T. Consorti and T. H. Liu, "Diagnosis and treatment of caecal volvulus," *Postgraduate Medical Journal*, vol. 81, no. 962, pp. 772–776, 2005.

[6] C. A. Gomes, C. Soares, F. Catena et al., "Laparoscopic management of mobile cecum," *Journal of the Society of Laparoendoscopic Surgeons*, vol. 20, no. 4, Article ID e2016.00076, 2016.

[7] T. E. Madiba and S. R. Thomson, "The management of cecal volvulus," *Diseases of the Colon & Rectum*, vol. 45, no. 2, pp. 264–267, 2002.

[8] W.-C. Yeh, H.-P. Wang, C. Chen, H.-H. Wang, M.-S. Wu, and J.-T. Lin, "Preoperative sonographic diagnosis of midgut malrotation with volvulus in adults: The 'whirlpool' sign," *Journal of Clinical Ultrasound*, vol. 27, no. 5, pp. 279–283, 1999.

[9] R. Rabinovici, D. A. Simansky, O. Kaplan, E. Mavor, and J. Manny, "Cecal volvulus," *Diseases of the Colon & Rectum*, vol. 33, no. 9, pp. 765–769, 1990.

[10] B. Lampl, T. L. Levin, W. E. Berdon, and R. A. Cowles, "Malrotation and midgut volvulus: A historical review and current controversies in diagnosis and management," *Pediatric Radiology*, vol. 39, no. 4, pp. 359–366, 2009.

[11] C. S. O'Mara, T. H. Wilson, G. L. Stonesifer, and J. L. Cameron, "Cecal volvulus. Analysis of 50 patients with long term follow up," *Annals of Surgery*, vol. 189, no. 6, pp. 724–731, 1979.

[12] J. M. Rosenblat, A. M. Rozenblit, E. L. Wolf, R. A. DuBrow, E. I. Den, and J. M. Levsky, "Findings of cecal volvulus at CT," *Radiology*, vol. 256, no. 1, pp. 169–175, 2010.

[13] Y. El-Katib, "Volvulus of the caecum: Caecopexy polyvinyl alcohol sponge," *British Journal of Surgery*, vol. 60, no. 6, pp. 475–478, 1973.

[14] C. Theuer and W. G. Cheadle, "Volvulus of the colon," *The American Surgeon*, vol. 57, no. 3, pp. 145–150, 1991.

[15] P. Renzulli, C. A. Maurer, P. Netzer, and M. W. Büchler, "Preoperative colonoscopic derotation is beneficial in acute colonic volvulus," *Digestive Surgery*, vol. 19, no. 3, pp. 223–229, 2002.

[16] K. Hiltumen, H. Syrja, and M. Matikainen, "Colonic volvulus. Diagnosis and results of treatment in 82 patients," *European Journal of Surgery*, pp. 158-11, 1992.

[17] S. Kakizoe, Y. Kakizoe, H. Kakizoe, T. Kakizoe, and K. Kakizoe, "Experience of laparoscopic cecoplication for mobile cecum," *Endoscopy*, vol. 32, no. 1, pp. S4–S5, 2000.

[18] Y. Fukuda, Y. Higuchi, K. Shinozaki et al., "Mobile Cecum in a Young Woman with Ehlers-Danlos Syndrome Hypermobility type: A Case Report and Review of the Literature," *Internal Medicine*, vol. 56, no. 20, pp. 2791–2796, 2017.

[19] C. D. Carli, J. Bass, and B. Sweeney, "A mobile cecum predisposing to a major complication of laparoscopic assisted ileostomy," *Journal of Laparoendoscopic & Advanced Surgical Techniques*, vol. 19, no. 1, pp. S153–S154, 2009.

[20] M. Baldarelu, A. De Sanctis, J. Sarnari, M. Nisi, M. Rimini, and M. Guerrieri, "Laparoscopic cecopexy for cecal volvulus after laparoscopy case report and a review of the literature," *Minerva Chirurgica*, vol. 62, no. 3, pp. 201–204, 2007.

[21] K. Garude and S. Rao, "Mobile Cecum: An Incidental Finding," *Indian Journal of Surgery*, vol. 75, no. 4, pp. 265–267, 2013.

19

Acute Gastric Volvulus Causing Splenic Avulsion and Hemoperitoneum

Yana Cavanagh,[1] Neal Carlin,[1] Ruhin Yuridullah,[2] and Sohail Shaikh[1]

[1]*Department of Gastroenterology, New York Medical College at St. Joseph's Regional Medical Center, Paterson, NJ, USA*
[2]*Department of Medicine, New York Medical College at St. Joseph's Regional Medical Center, Paterson, NJ, USA*

Correspondence should be addressed to Yana Cavanagh; r_cavanaghy@sjhmc.org

Academic Editor: Shiro Kikuchi

Gastric volvulus is an abnormal, potentially life-threatening, torsion of the stomach. The presence of complications such as hemoperitoneum increases the diagnostic urgency; however it can also mask the presentation of gastric volvulus. We encountered a 66-year-old female who presented with symptomatic gastric outlet obstruction and was found to have hemoperitoneum and splenic avulsion on imaging. In our case, hemoperitoneum was a clinical red herring as initial imaging concentrated on the presence of hemoperitoneum and was nondiagnostic of gastric volvulus. Interestingly, our patient experienced complete resolution of her presenting symptomatology following placement of a nasogastric tube. Furthermore, endoscopic evaluation revealed no overt pathology to explain outlet obstruction. In light of these findings, gastric torsion was strongly suspected. A repeat CT scan was confirmatory, elucidated reduction of the stomach to its anatomic position, retroactively diagnosing a gastric volvulus. This case is unusual in its presentation and setting. The patient presented with two rare complications of gastric volvulus, hemoperitoneum and splenic avulsion. Additionally, ten years prior to this presentation the patient had a temporary gastrostomy tube. Gastropexy with a gastrostomy is the treatment for gastric volvulus and should have been preventative of her presentation with torsion. Furthermore, the gastric volvulus was not initially recognized radiographically due to the presence of masking radiographic findings. This case serves to highlight the utility of clinical acumen and maintain a high index of suspicion for gastric volvulus in all cases presenting with Borchardt's triad.

1. Introduction

Gastric volvulus is an abnormal rotation of the stomach that is well documented in small animals [1–4]. However, gastric volvulus is a rare entity in humans [5–7]. The peak incidence of gastric volvulus is in the fifth decade. No association with race or sex has been established; however gastric volvulus is associated with significant mortality [7, 8]. Therefore, prompt diagnosis and treatment are imperative [9, 10].

Acute gastric volvulus typically presents with pain in the upper abdomen or lower chest and is associated with vomiting. These symptoms accompanied by an inability to pass a nasogastric tube are known as Borchardt's triad, which is characteristic of gastric volvulus [7, 11]. The main consequence of the gastric volvulus is acute, intermittent, or chronic foregut obstruction [8, 12, 13]. Associated complications can include ulceration, perforation, hemorrhage, pancreatic necrosis, and omental avulsion [14–16]. On rare occasions, rotation of the stomach causing disruption of the splenic vessels or splenic rupture has been reported [9, 17].

The most frequently implemented classification of gastric volvulus is based on the axis around which the stomach rotates [18, 19]. Organoaxial gastric volvulus (Figure 1) is rotation of the stomach around its long axis. Organoaxial volvulus is the most common type, occurring in sixty percent of cases [7, 19]. It is associated with secondary etiologies such as a laxity of gastric ligaments or diaphragmatic defects [8, 19–21]. Strangulation and necrosis can occur with this type of volvulus [7].

Rotation of the stomach along its short axis or mesenteroaxial volvulus causes the antrum to become displaced above the gastroesophageal junction (Figure 2). This form of volvulus is usually partial (<180°), not generally associated with a secondary anatomic defect, and vascular compromise

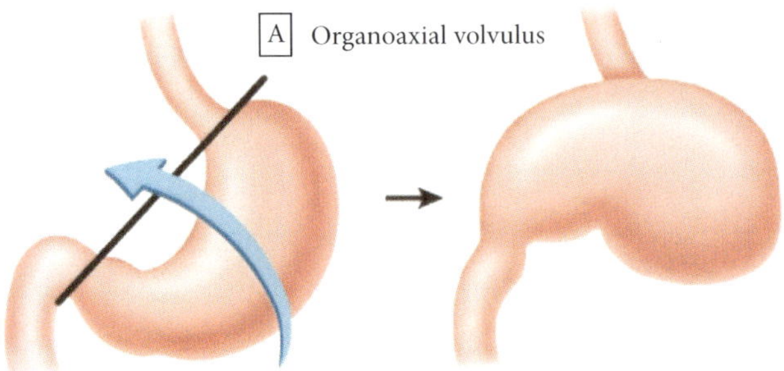

Figure 1: *Organoaxial gastric volvulus.* Rotation of the stomach along its long axis through a line that connects the gastroesophageal junction and the pylorus. The antrum rotates anterosuperiorly and the fundus rotates posteroinferiorly. The greater curvature of the stomach comes to rest superior to the lesser curvature of the stomach in an inverted position.

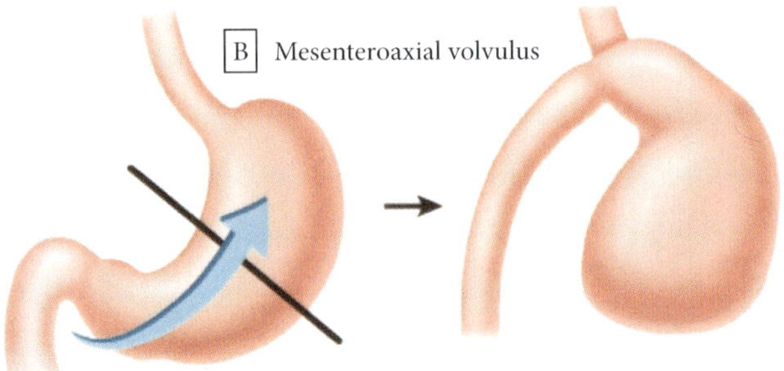

Figure 2: *Mesenteroaxial gastric volvulus.* The stomach rotates around its short axis through a perpendicular line connecting the greater and lesser curvatures of the stomach. The antrum becomes displaced above the gastroesophageal junction.

is uncommon [19]. A combined gastric volvulus, in which the stomach twists mesentericoaxially and organoaxially, is rare but can be seen in patients with chronic volvulus [18, 22]. Gastric volvulus can also be described as idiopathic (type I) or acquired (type II) [7, 23].

2. Case Report

We encountered an unusual case of organoaxial gastric volvulus resulting in splenic laceration and hemoperitoneum in a patient with a distant history of gastrostomy tube. A 66-year-old Hispanic female with a history of stroke and residual expressive aphasia as well as right sided hemiparesis presented with acute onset abdominal pain of one-day duration. The pain was described as 7/10, achy, and diffuse. It was associated with multiple episodes of nonbloody emesis of food contents and white frothy fluid. There were no alleviating or aggravating factors noted and she had never experienced similar symptoms in the past. She denied preceding trauma, chest pain, change in bowel habits, consumption of new/unusual foods, or sick contacts.

On physical examination, the patient appeared uncomfortable and had a well-healed cicatrix from previous gastrostomy tube in the left upper quadrant. Her examination

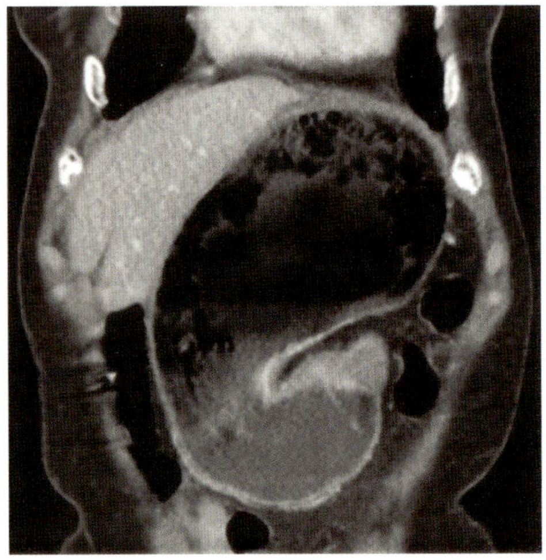

Figure 3: CT of abdomen and pelvis with contrast showing a markedly distended abdomen without focal wall thickening. The J-shaped stomach is rotated along its long axis, displaying a gastric volvulus. Fluid, consistent with blood, is seen tracking along the paracolic gutters and the pelvis.

revealed abdominal distention as well as moderate tenderness to light palpation, diffusely. Pertinent negatives included the absence of guarding, rigidity, or rebound tenderness. Her laboratory evaluation revealed an acute normocytic anemia with a hemoglobin of 11.9 and hematocrit of 36.9. A complete metabolic panel was unremarkable and her lactic acid was 1.1. An emergent CT scan of the abdomen and pelvis reported a grossly distended stomach with gastric outlet obstruction, as well as a moderate amount of hyperdense intraperitoneal fluid, highly concerning for hemoperitoneum (Figure 3).

While awaiting abdominal CT findings, a nasogastric tube (NGT) was placed for symptomatic care. One and a half liters of nonbloody, nonbilious gastric fluid was aspirated with concomitant resolution of her presenting complaints upon decompression of her stomach. Gastroscopy was performed to further elucidate the etiology of the patient's gastric outlet obstruction. Endoscopy revealed distal Los Angeles Grade C esophagitis, a deeply J-shaped stomach, a 10 mm gastric body ulcer with pigmented spots, and nonbleeding erosive gastropathy in the antrum. The duodenum was easily accessible and unremarkable (Figure 4). Following gastroscopy and further review of the initial imaging, a reduced gastric volvulus was strongly suspected and a repeat CT scan was pursued. It revealed the stomach in an anatomically differing position from initial imaging, confirming the presumptive diagnosis, as well as persistent stable hemoperitoneum and a 0.9 cm linear defect involving the posteroinferior margin of the spleen (Figure 5).

As the volvulus resolved with medical management, no surgical interventions were pursued. The potential for recurrence of the volvulus was discussed with the patient and her family and symptomatic care was preferred. The NGT remained in place for one day while the patient's diet was advanced to clear liquids and then to regular diet. The patient tolerated diet and was discharged home in stable condition.

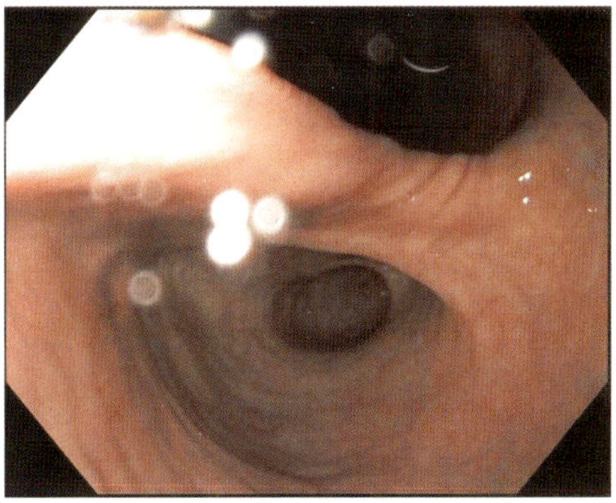

FIGURE 4: Retroflexed endoscopic view of the lesser curvature of the body of the stomach, antrum, and fundus, depicting the deeply J-shape anatomy of the stomach.

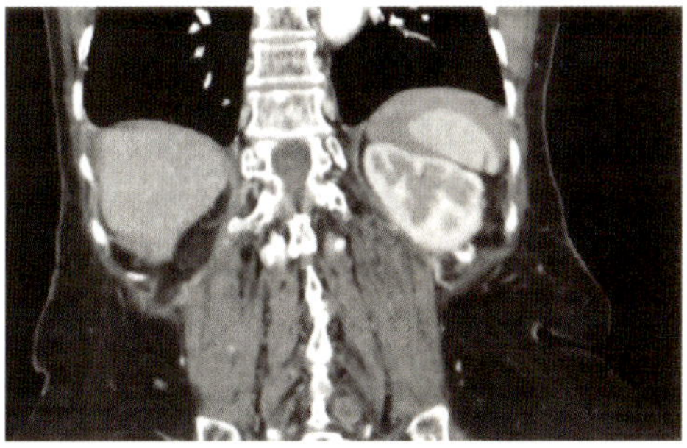

FIGURE 5: Repeat CT of abdomen and pelvis with contrast revealing an apparent linear defect measuring 0.9 cm involving the posteroinferior margin of the spleen. Again seen, consistent with prior study is the presence of a moderate amount of hyperdense free intraperitoneal fluid, indicative of hemoperitoneum.

3. Discussion

Gastric volvulus is an abnormal rotation of the stomach along its either long or short axis. Prompt diagnosis and treatment are imperative in order to avoid potential complications such as ulceration, perforation, hemorrhage, pancreatic necrosis, and omental avulsion. In our case, the patient presented with acute onset abdominal pain associated with multiple episodes of emesis. CT scan revealed a distended, deeply J-shaped stomach, gastric outlet obstruction, and moderate hemoperitoneum. Although no torsion was reported on initial imaging, a high level of suspicion was maintained for gastric volvulus due to the congruency between the patient's presentation and Borchardt's triad. Gastroscopy displayed no overt etiology for gastric outlet obstruction, which was further supportive of a reduced volvulus, as placement of the NGT likely reduced the stomach to its anatomic position and therefore resulted in resolution of the patient's symptomatology.

Repeat CT scan performed after endoscopy confirmed our supposition and showed the stomach was reduced to its normal anatomical position. Additionally, it revealed a 0.9 cm linear defect of the spleen, consistent with gastric volvulus causing splenic avulsion by placing traction on the splenogastric ligaments and resulting in hemoperitoneum. These radiographic findings and the patient's clinical course pointed to an initially overlooked radiographic finding of gastric volvulus due to the presence of red herring findings such as hemoperitoneum (Figure 6).

Our patient's unique presentation makes this case noteworthy. Gastric volvulus, particularly when accompanied by other complications, is rare. The treatment of gastric volvulus generally involves reduction of the stomach to its anatomic position and gastropexy by gastrostomy tube. This fixates the stomach to the abdominal wall, to prevent repeat torsion. Exceedingly interestingly, our patient previously had a gastrostomy tube following her cerebrovascular accident, which should have been preventative of future torsion. However, the deeply J-shaped anatomy of our patient's stomach nullified this additional point of fixation. The location of her previous PEG was the distal antrum, allowing ample unfixed proximal stomach to result in organoaxial rotation. As a result of this case, we urge maintaining a keen clinical eye and high level of suspicion for all cases presenting with Borchardt's triad, despite other potentially distracting radiographic and physical findings.

Disclosure

The manuscript was presented as a poster at the World Congress of Gastroenterology at American College of Gastroenterology 2017 abstract presentation.

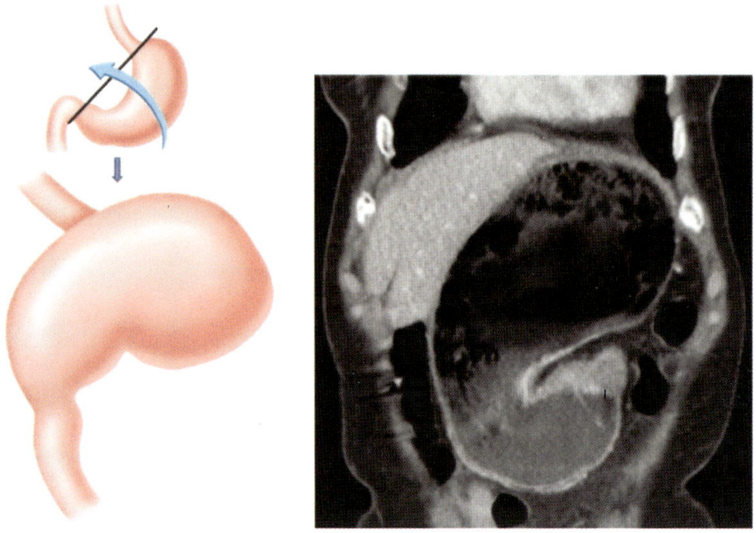

Figure 6: *Organoaxial gastric volvulus.* Rotation of the stomach along its long axis through a line that connects the gastroesophageal junction and the pylorus.

References

[1] T. W. Fossum, *Small Animal Surgery*, Mosby, St. Louis, Missouri, USA, 2002, pp. 542–544.

[2] D. L. Millis, J. Nemzek, C. Riggs, and R. Walshaw, "Gastric dilatation-volvulus after splenic torsion in two dogs.," *Journal of the American Veterinary Medical Association*, vol. 207, no. 3, pp. 314-315, 1995.

[3] D. Slatter, *Textbook of Small Animal Surgery*, WB Saunders, Philadelphia, Pennsylvania, USA, 2003.

[4] F. Rashid, T. Thangarajah, D. Mulvey, M. Larvin, and S. Y. Iftikhar, "A review article on gastric volvulus: A challenge to diagnosis and management," *International Journal of Surgery*, vol. 8, no. 1, pp. 18–24, 2010.

[5] E. S. Dudley and G. P. Boivin, "Gastric Volvulus in Guinea Pigs: Comparison with other species," *Journal of the American Association for Laboratory Animal Science*, vol. 50, no. 4, pp. 526–530, 2011.

[6] M.-H. Wu, Y.-C. Chang, C.-H. Wu, S.-C. Kang, and J.-T. Kuan, "Acute gastric volvulus: a rare but real surgical emergency," *The American Journal of Emergency Medicine*, vol. 28, no. 1, pp. 118.e5–118.e7, 2010.

[7] B. Chau and S. Dufel, "Gastric volvulus," *Emergency Medicine Journal*, vol. 24, no. 6, pp. 446-447, 2007.

[8] D. P. McElreath, K. W. Olden, and F. Aduli, "Hiccups: A subtle sign in the clinical diagnosis of gastric volvulus and a review of the literature," *Digestive Diseases and Sciences*, vol. 53, no. 11, pp. 3033–3036, 2008.

[9] A. S. Hudspeth and J. M. Mcwhorter, "Gastric Volvulus Causing Rupture of the Spleen," *JAMA Surgery*, vol. 102, no. 3, pp. 232-233, 1971.

[10] A. Berti, "Singolare attortigliamento dell'esofago col duodeno sequito da rapida morte," *Gazzetta Medica Italiana*, vol. 9, pp. 139–141, 1866.

[11] M. Borchardt, "Kur Pathologie and Therapie des magen volvulus," *Archiv Fur Klinische Chirurgie*, vol. 74, pp. 243–260, 1904.

[12] R. K. Cribbs, K. W. Gow, and M. L. Wulkan, "Gastric volvulus in infants and children," *Pediatrics*, vol. 122, no. 3, pp. e752–e762, 2008.

[13] D. Godshall, U. Mossallam, and R. Rosenbaum, "Gastric volvulus: Case report and review of the literature," *The Journal of Emergency Medicine*, vol. 17, no. 5, pp. 837–840, 1999.

[14] G. Shivanand, S. Seema, D. N. Srivastava et al., "Gastric volvulus: Acute and chronic presentation," *Clinical Imaging*, vol. 27, no. 4, pp. 265–268, 2003.

[15] S. K. Oh, B. K. Han, T. L. Levin, R. Murphy, N. M. Blitman, and C. Ramos, "Gastric volvulus in children: The twists and turns of an unusual entity," *Pediatric Radiology*, vol. 38, no. 3, pp. 297–304, 2008.

[16] J. Estevão-Costa, M. Soares-Oliveira, J. Correia-Pinto, C. Mariz, J. L. Carvalho, and J. E. da Costa, "Acute gastric volvulus secondary to a Morgagni hernia," *Pediatric Surgery International*, vol. 16, no. 1-2, pp. 107-108, 2000.

[17] H. Kotobi, F. Auber, E. Otta, N. Meyer, G. Audry, and P. G. Hélardot, "Acute mesenteroaxial gastric volvulus and congenital diaphragmatic hernia," *Pediatric Surgery International*, vol. 21, no. 8, pp. 674–676, 2005.

[18] A. C. Singleton, "Chronic Gastric Volvulus," *Radiology*, vol. 34, no. 1, pp. 53–61, 1940.

[19] C. M. Peterson, J. S. Anderson, A. K. Hara, J. W. Carenza, and C. O. Menias, "Volvulus of the gastrointestinal tract: Appearances at multimodality imaging," *RadioGraphics*, vol. 29, no. 5, pp. 1281–1293, 2009.

[20] W. J. Teague, R. Ackroyd, D. I. Watson, and P. G. Devitt, "Changing patterns in the management of gastric volvulus over 14 years," *British Journal of Surgery*, vol. 87, no. 3, pp. 358–361, 2000.

[21] J. A. Wasselle and J. Norman, "Acute gastric volvulus: Pathogenesis, diagnosis, and treatment," *American Journal of Gastroenterology*, vol. 88, no. 10, pp. 1780–1784, 1993.

[22] B. S. Hurst, S. C. Gardner, K. E. Tucker, C. A. Awoniyi, and W. D. Schlaff, "Delayed oral estradiol combined with leuprolide increases endometriosis-related pain," *Journal of the Society of Laparoendoscopic Surgeons*, vol. 4, no. 2, pp. 97–101, 2000.

[23] D. L. Miller, M. D. Pasquale, R. P. Seneca, and E. Hodin, "Gastric Volvulus in the Pediatric Population," *JAMA Surgery*, vol. 126, no. 9, pp. 1146–1149, 1991.

20

CMV Colitis in Immunocompetent Patients: 2 Cases of a Diagnostic Challenge

Maria Paparoupa,[1] Viola Schmidt,[1] Helgard Weckauf,[2] Huy Ho,[1] and Frank Schuppert[1]

[1] *Department of Gastroenterology, Endocrinology, Diabetology and General Medicine, Klinikum Kassel, Mönchebergstraße 41-43, 34125 Kassel, Germany*
[2] *Institute of Pathology, Klinikum Kassel, Mönchebergstraße 41-43, 34125 Kassel, Germany*

Correspondence should be addressed to Maria Paparoupa; maria.paparoupa@yahoo.com

Academic Editor: Olga I. Giouleme

CMV infections are generally thought to be opportunistic by immunosuppression. Many literature cases though indicate that CMV infections can be also observed in immunocompetent patients. We present an unusual case of an extensive concentric benign stenosis due to CMV colitis and a case of coexistence with Crohn's Disease, both observed in nonimmunosuppressed individuals. The right diagnosis was set after implementation of multiple unsuccessful treatment strategies. Our purpose is therefore to familiarize clinicians involved with the diagnosis and treatment of gastroenterological diseases with this entity.

1. Introduction

CMV infections are generally thought to be opportunistic in patients with immunosuppressive diseases like HIV/AIDS, underlying malignancies, and organ- or bone marrow-transplantation and patients under treatment with chemotherapeutics or steroids [1–4]. However a rapidly rising number of literature cases worldwide indicate that CMV infections can be also observed in immunocompetent individuals, causing primarily gastrointestinal manifestations, like ulcerative colitis, pseudopolyps, or tumors, and ischemic and hemorrhagic enterocolitis [5–9]. The first case reporting verification of CMV colitis in an immunocompetent patient was published in 1992 [10]. Since then, particular underlying conditions are linked with a high risk of CMV colitis in apparently nonimmunocompromised patients, like chronic renal insufficiency and hemodialysis, aging, coinfection with bacterial gastrointestinal infections, and food allergy [11–19]. A notable connection between CMV colitis and colitis ulcerosa stands out in the literature [20–25], while only a single reported case correlates the first one with Crohn's Disease [26]. We present an unusual case of a persistent benign colon stenosis due to CMV colitis and a case of coexistence with Crohn's Disease, both observed in nonimmunosuppressed individuals. The right diagnosis was set after rigorous diagnostic procedures and implementation of multiple unsuccessful treatment strategies.

2. Cases Description

A 77-year-old man presented to our Department of Gastroenterology with subileus symptoms and blood spots on his stool. COPD and laparoscopic cholecystectomy several years ago were reported as his medical history. A partial colonoscopy revealed multiple sigma diverticula with signs of inflammation and the patient was treated with oral mesalazine (Salofalk Granu-Stix 2000 mg/day) and antibiotics (ceftriaxone and metronidazole) for 2 weeks, leading to discrete relief of his symptoms. Two months later a control colonoscopy was performed; edema and erythema of mucosa were not present any more, but a persisting stenosis 40 cm from anus was almost occluding colon lumen (Figure 1). The colonoscope could not be advanced beyond the mass. All sigma diverticula presented unobtrusively and new biopsies were taken from the stenosis site. Histologic analysis confirmed a chronic inflammatory mucosal alteration and

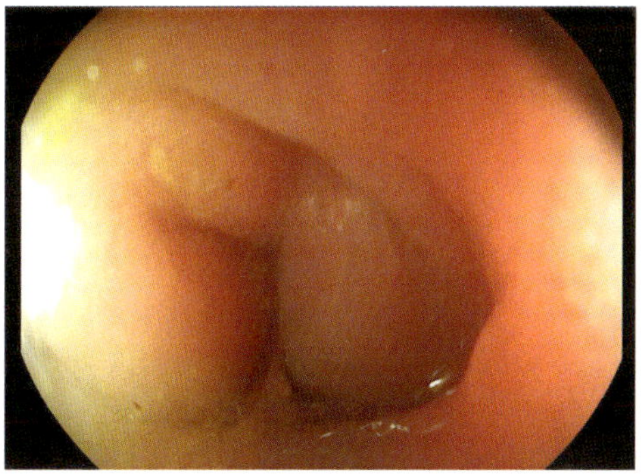

Figure 1: Persisting stenosis 40 cm from anus almost occluding colon lumen. The colonoscope could not be advanced beyond the mass.

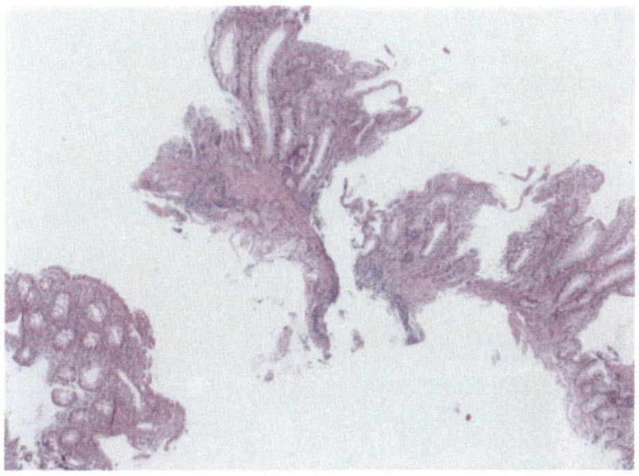

Figure 2: Light microscopy presenting biopsies of colonic mucosa with chronic inflammation and disorders of mucosal architecture (H & E, 100x).

lymphofollicular hyperplasia of submucosa compatible with diverticula-associated colitis (Figures 2 and 3). By unclear distinctive stenosis of colon lumen and histological signs of chronic inflammation, atypical manifestation of IBD (inflammatory bowel disease) was hypothesized and immunosuppressive therapy with steroids was initiated, without clinical response. As last step of our diagnostic strategy, we performed serological and microbiological tests, in order to exclude gastrointestinal pathogens. Surprisingly, CMV-IgM Titer was positive and CMV-IgG Titer found greater than 200 RE/mL. After receiving this result, antiviral treatment with ganciclovir (Cymevene 600 mg/day) was initiated. A month later colon stenosis was slightly detectable and patient's subileus symptoms were no more present (Figure 4).

In the second case, a 66-year-old man with Crohn's Disease in remission complained about diffuse abdominal pain, diarrhea, and weight loss starting 2 weeks ago. A high colonoscopy revealed multiple ulcerative lesions and hemorrhagic colitis leading to the diagnosis of acute Crohn's Disease exacerbation (Figure 5). We initiated immunosuppression with corticosteroids, with no clinical response, and then escalated to azathioprine. In the control colonoscopy, several days under immunosuppressive treatment, endoscopic findings remained unchanged (Figure 6).

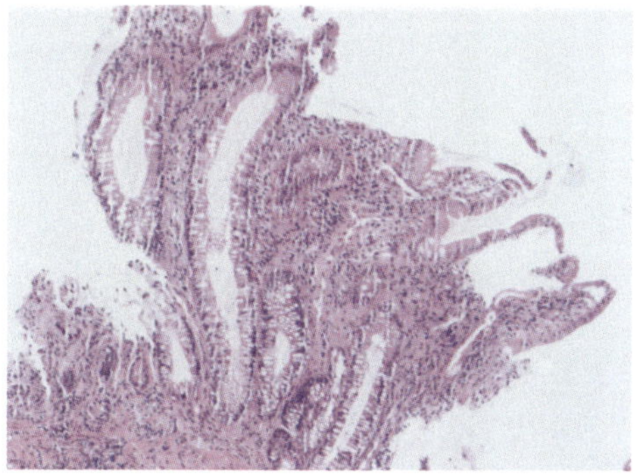

Figure 3: Histologic picture 2 in higher analysis (H & E, 200x).

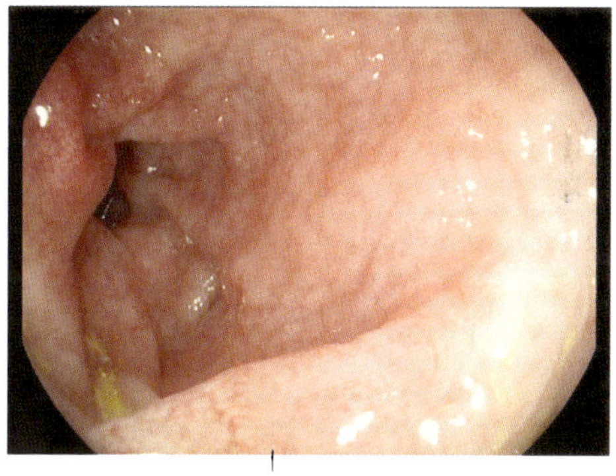

Figure 4: Colon stenosis slightly detectable in control colposcopy one month later.

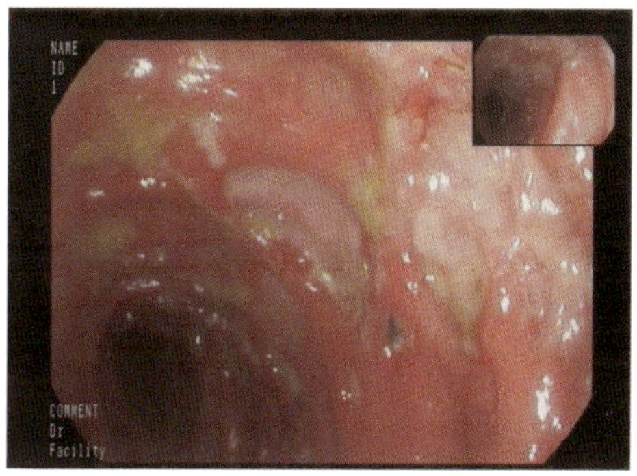

Figure 5: Multiple ulcerative lesions and hemorrhagic colitis.

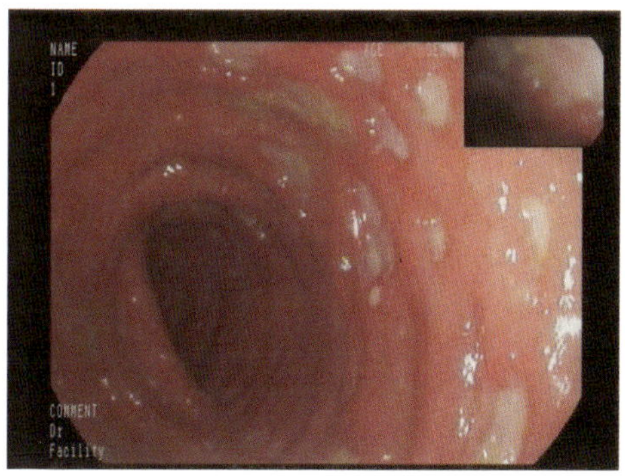

Figure 6: Endoscopic findings remained unchanged despite immunosuppressive therapy.

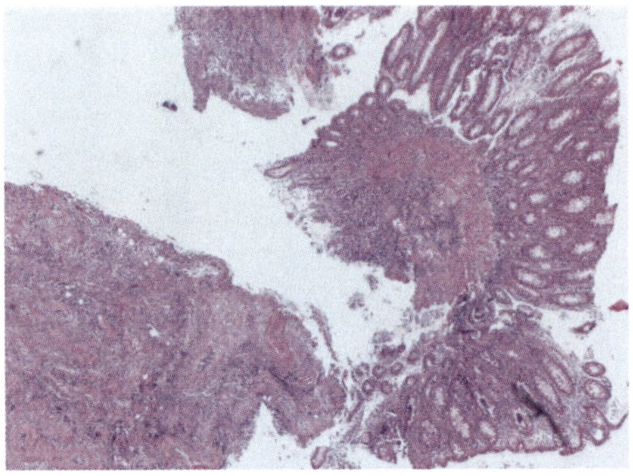

FIGURE 7: Highly active inflammation of colonic mucosa with an ulcerative lesion on the bottom of the picture (H & E, 100x).

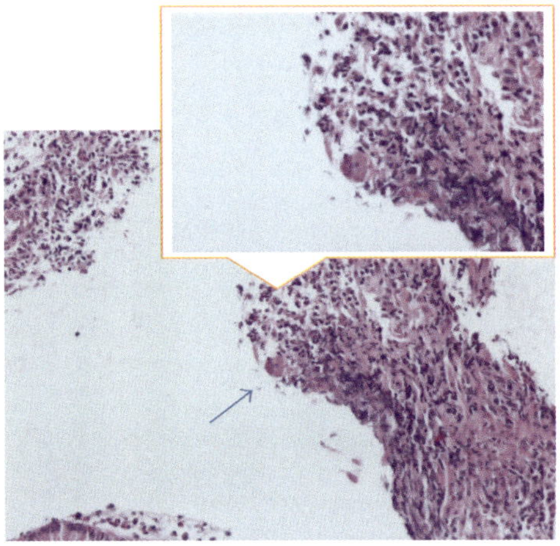

FIGURE 8: Virus infected cell at the edge of an ulcerous defect, known as "owl eye" cell, marked with an arrow and detailedly shown in the window (H & E, 400x).

A new course of multiple step colon biopsies was conducted; multiple deeply reaching ulcers and lymphoid aggregates in the submucosa were detected (Figure 7). After a rigorous microscopic examination of histological samples, a typical intracellular inclusion of CMV virus known as "owl eye" was surprisingly detected on the border line of an ulcerative lesion (Figure 8). Elevation of CMV-IgM and IgG Titer in serum confirmed the diagnosis of CMV colitis and our patient was treated with intravenous ganciclovir (10 mg/kg/day), leading to complete clinical remission.

3. Discussion

These are two unusual cases of CMV colitis, manifested in immunocompetent patients, who presented to our Department for Internal Medicine and Gastroenterology over the last year. In both cases, patient symptoms and endoscopic findings imitated other more common conditions, like sigma diverticulitis and acute exacerbation of Crohn's Disease. This was the main reason for the delayed diagnosis. The implementation of multiple unsuccessful therapeutic strategies forced us to search further, without actually having CMV colitis in mind. In both cases the right diagnosis was set incidentally after positive CMV serology or typical histologic finding of "owl eye" cell. Our purpose is therefore to awaken clinicians involved with the treatment of gastroenterological diseases on the entity of CMV colitis in nonimmunocompromised patients.

In the first case, CMV colon infection presented as a persisting stenosis, which was initially almost occluding colon lumen. A similar case of an extensive colonic stenosis due to CMV colitis has been already described from Novakova et al. [27] in a 2-month-old immunocompetent male, infected via breast milk. In this case, stenosis was persisting after antiviral therapy and corticosteroids were initiated. Our patient showed no clinical response under steroids, but healed after antiviral therapy. According to literature reports, colonic occlusion due to CMV infection can be so severe and persistent that surgical removal is the ultimate therapeutic option [28]. However, inflammatory hyperplastic tissue forms more frequently pseudopolyps or tumor masses and not an extensive concentric benign stenosis like in our case and is mostly observed in immunocompromised compared to in immunocompetent patients [5, 6, 29–31].

The second case presented with multiple ulcerative lesions and hemorrhagic mucosa in a patient with known Crohn's Disease in remission. Clinical manifestations and endoscopic findings were compatible with acute Crohn's Disease exacerbation, but immunosuppressive treatment was unsuccessful. Shahani reported a case where diagnosis of Crohn's Disease followed the diagnosis of CMV colitis, as extraintestinal manifestations of IBD complicated the clinical course and antiviral therapy failed to improve the gastrointestinal symptoms of the patient [26]. According to scientific literature, CMV colitis can induce an acute exacerbation of IBD in remission [24] or complicate preexisting active and more often steroids refractory colitis flare [28]. In conclusion, CMV infection should be ruled out in patients with IBD exacerbation before starting immunosuppression and, on the contrary, IBD should be suspected in immunocompetent patients with CMV colitis.

Consent

Patients' informed consent is available.

References

[1] B. Salzberger, G. Fätkenheuer, A. Schwenk et al., "Foscarnet and ganciclovir combination therapy for CMV disease in HIV-infected patients," *Infection*, vol. 22, no. 3, pp. 197–200, 1994.

[2] D. J. C. Ramsey and S. A. Schey, "Cytomegalovirus colitis after autologous transplantation for multiple myeloma," *British Journal of Haematology*, vol. 110, no. 4, pp. 894–896, 2000.

[3] T. L. Lemonovich and R. R. Watkins, "Update on cytomegalovirus infections of the gastrointestinal system in solid organ transplant recipients," *Current Infectious Disease Reports*, vol. 14, no. 1, pp. 33–40, 2012.

[4] C. Polprasert, C. Wongjitrat, and N. Wisedopas, "Case report: severe CMV colitis in a patient with follicular lymphoma after chemotherapy," *Journal of the Medical Association of Thailand*, vol. 94, no. 4, pp. 498–500, 2011.

[5] A. S. Vegunta, S. K. Dasar, S. K. Joshi, and R. V. Rao, "Spontaneous partial vanishing cytomegalovirus pseudotumour of colon in an immunocompetent patient," *Journal of Clinical and Diagnostic Research*, vol. 9, no. 8, pp. TD07–TD09, 2015.

[6] A. Agaimy, J. Mudter, B. Märkl, and R. Chetty, "Cytomegalovirus infection presenting as isolated inflammatory polyps of the gastrointestinal tract," *Pathology*, vol. 43, no. 5, pp. 440–446, 2011.

[7] Z. Naseem, R. Hendahewa, M. Mustaev, and G. Premaratne, "Cytomegalovirus enteritis with ischemia in an immunocompetent patient: a rare case report," *International Journal of Surgery Case Reports*, vol. 15, pp. 146–148, 2015.

[8] T. Hasegawa, K. Aomatsu, M. Nakamura, N. Aomatsu, and K. Aomatsu, "Cytomegalovirus colitis followed by ischemic colitis in a non-immunocompromised adult: a case report," *World Journal of Gastroenterology*, vol. 21, no. 12, pp. 3750–3754, 2015.

[9] A. Rankin, K. Cuthill, M. Subesinghe, and D. Goldsmith, "Life-threatening rectal bleeding due to cytomegalovirus colitis in a haemodialysis patient," *NDT Plus*, vol. 2, no. 3, pp. 239–241, 2009.

[10] S. D. Blair, A. Forbes, and R. A. Parkins, "CMV colitis in an immunocompetent adult," *Journal of the Royal Society of Medicine*, vol. 85, no. 4, pp. 238–239, 1992.

[11] S.-H. Kim, W. S. Kim, H. W. Kim et al., "A case of cytomegalovirus colitis in an immunocompetent hemodialysis patient," *Hemodialysis International*, vol. 15, no. 2, pp. 297–300, 2011.

[12] A. R. Farah Musa, T. Fülöp, K. Kokko, B. Kanyicska, J. R. Lewin, and É. Csongrádi, "Cytomegalovirus colitis in a critically ill, dialysis-dependent, acute kidney injury patient without immunosuppressive therapy," *Clinical Nephrology*, vol. 84, no. 1, pp. 44–49, 2015.

[13] M. R. Lockwood, J. Liddle, and P. Kitsanta, "Cytomegalovirus colitis—an unusual cause for diarrhoea in an elderly woman," *Age and Ageing*, vol. 35, no. 2, pp. 198–200, 2006.

[14] B. Fleischer, J. Morgenthaler, G. Tippel, A. Kuhfus, U. Gieseler, and M. Stolte, "Cytomegalovirus-induced colitis in an immunocompetent old patient," *Medizinische Klinik*, vol. 101, no. 10, pp. 835–838, 2006.

[15] T.-N. Chau, L.-K. Lau, K.-C. Lee, M.-L. Kwok, S.-T. Lai, and H. Yuen, "Association of self-limited cytomegalovirus colitis and shigellosis in an immunocompetent patient," *European Journal of Gastroenterology and Hepatology*, vol. 8, no. 8, pp. 819–822, 1996.

[16] M. Kurtz and M. Morgan, "Concomitant Clostridium difficile colitis and cytomegalovirus colitis in an immunocompetent elderly female," *BMJ Case Reports*, Article ID bcr2012007273, 2012.

[17] I. M. Dumitru, E. Dumitru, G. Resul, L. Curtali, S. Paris, and S. Rugina, "Concomitant CMV and *Clostridium difficile* colitis in an immunocompetent patient treated with Ganciclovir and fecal transplantation," *Journal of Gastrointestinal and Liver Diseases*, vol. 23, no. 2, pp. 221–222, 2014.

[18] T. W. Jonkhoff-Slok, R. H. Veenhoven, E. R. de Graeff-Meeder, and H. A. Büller, "An immunocompetent infant with cow's milk allergy and cytomegalovirus colitis," *European Journal of Pediatrics*, vol. 156, no. 7, pp. 528–529, 1997.

[19] J.-H. Ko, K. R. Peck, W. J. Lee et al., "Clinical presentation and risk factors for cytomegalovirus colitis in immunocompetent adult patients," *Clinical Infectious Diseases*, vol. 60, no. 6, pp. e20–e26, 2015.

[20] M. Maté del Tío, J. M. Peña Sánchez de Rivera, J. Larrauri Martínez, M. C. Garcés Jiménez, and F. J. Barbado Hernández, "Association of cytomegalovirus colitis and the 1st episode of ulcerative colitis in an immunocompetent patient," *Gastroenterología y Hepatología*, vol. 19, no. 4, pp. 206–207, 1996.

[21] C. Rachima, E. Maoz, S. Apter, M. Thaler, E. Grossman, and T. Rosenthal, "Cytomegalovirus infection associated with ulcerative colitis in immunocompetent individuals," *Postgraduate Medical Journal*, vol. 74, no. 874, pp. 486–489, 1998.

[22] M. Kraus, C. Meyenberger, and W. Suter, "Generalised intestinal CMV infection with protein losing syndrome in ulcerative colitis," *Schweizerische Medizinische Wochenschrift*, vol. 130, no. 43, pp. 1600–1605, 2000.

[23] K. L. Streetz, T. Buhr, H. Wedemeyer et al., "Acute CMV-colitis in a patient with a history of ulcerative colitis," *Scandinavian Journal of Gastroenterology*, vol. 38, no. 1, pp. 119–122, 2003.

[24] N. S. Malhi, D. K. Bhasin, N. M. Gupta, K. Vaiphei, and K. Singh, "Exacerbation of ulcerative colitis by cytomegalovirus infection in an immunocompetent Indian patient," *Tropical Gastroenterology*, vol. 23, no. 2, pp. 88–90, 2002.

[25] S. Yangzhen, K. Liu, T. Xu, Y. Yang, and Y. Zhang, "Synchronous onset of CMV colitis and ulcerative colitis in an immunocompetent patient: a case report," *West Indian Medical Journal*, 2015.

[26] L. Shahani, "CMV infection complicating the diagnosis of Crohn's disease in an immunocompetent patient," *BMJ Case Reports*, 2012.

[27] V. Novakova, K. Hamprecht, A. M. Müller, J. Arellano-Galindo, M. Ehlen, and G. Horneff, "Severe postnatal CMV colitis with an extensive colonic stenosis in a 2-month-old male immunocompetent term infant infected via breast milk," *Journal of Clinical Virology*, vol. 59, no. 4, pp. 259–263, 2014.

[28] T. Nakamura, R. Nakamura, K. Maruyama et al., "Refractory ulcerative colitis complicated by a cytomegaloviral infection requiring surgery: report of a case," *Surgery Today*, vol. 34, no. 1, pp. 68–71, 2004.

[29] S. Kawasaki, S. Osawa, K. Sugimoto et al., "Cecal vanishing tumor associated with cytomegalovirus infection in an immunocompetent elderly adult," *World Journal of Gastrointestinal Oncology*, vol. 2, no. 11, pp. 417–420, 2010.

[30] A. Maiorana, P. Torricelli, F. Giusti, and N. Bellini, "Pseudoneoplastic appearance of cytomegalovirus-associated colitis in nonimmunocompromised patients: report of 2 cases," *Clinical Infectious Diseases*, vol. 37, no. 5, pp. e68–e71, 2003.

[31] A. De Jesus, S. A. Grossman, and O. Paun, "Cytomegalovirus associated colonic pseudotumor: a consequence of iatrogenic immunosuppression in a patient with primary brain tumor receiving radiation and temozolomide," *Journal of Neuro-Oncology*, vol. 94, no. 3, pp. 445–448, 2009.

21

Marked Direct Hyperbilirubinemia due to Ceftriaxone in an Adult with Sickle Cell Disease

Daniyeh Khurram, Leonid Shamban, Robert Kornas, and Maryann Paul

Department of Internal Medicine, Providence Hospital and Medical Center, 16001 W. Nile Mile Road, Southfield, MI 48075, USA

Correspondence should be addressed to Daniyeh Khurram; daniyeh_k@yahoo.com

Academic Editor: Yoshihiro Moriwaki

Drugs are a significant cause of liver injury. Drug-induced liver injury (DILI) can cause acute hepatitis, cholestasis, or a mixed pattern. Ceftriaxone is a commonly used antibiotic and has been associated with reversible biliary sludge, pseudolithiasis, and cholestasis. A 32-year-old male with sickle cell disease was admitted to the hospital for acute sickle cell crisis. On the second day of hospitalization, he developed cough and rhonchi with chest X-ray revealing right middle lobe infiltrates. Ceftriaxone and azithromycin were initiated. Subsequently, he developed conjugated hyperbilirubinemia and mild transaminitis. His total bilirubin trended upwards from 3.3 mg/dL on admission to 17 mg/dL. It was predominantly conjugated bilirubin, with preadmission bilirubin levels of 3-4 mg/dL. His transaminases were mildly elevated as well compared to previous levels. Extensive workup for bilirubin elevation was unremarkable. Ceftriaxone was switched to levofloxacin and the hyperbilirubinemia improved. On ambulatory follow-up, his bilirubin remained below 4 mg/dL. Ceftriaxone may be associated with marked direct hyperbilirubinemia particularly in sickle cell patients with chronic liver chemistry abnormalities. In the case of elevated bilirubin with concomitant ceftriaxone use, elimination of the offending agent should be considered.

1. Introduction

Medications account for approximately half of all cases of acute liver failure [1]. Drug-induced liver injury (DILI) can present with a wide range of acute and chronic liver diseases, including acute hepatitis, cholestasis, or a mixed pattern [2]. Many drugs have been associated with relatively high to very low rates of DILI; some of most common classes are acetaminophen products, statins, NSAIDs, and antibiotics [3]. Ceftriaxone, a third generation cephalosporin, is in widespread use due to its long half-life, broad-spectrum coverage, high tissue penetration rate, and favorable safety profile [4]. Ceftriaxone is known to cause cholestasis in neonates [5] and caution is urged for use in children due to reported cases of intrahepatic cholestasis [6]. Most of the documented cases of ceftriaxone associated hepatobiliary pathology are in neonates and children; few cases have been documented in adults [7]. Cases of ceftriaxone-induced liver injury in adults consist of reversible biliary sludge and pseudolithiasis [8]. We report a case of an adult male with an acute sickle cell crisis who developed significant conjugated hyperbilirubinemia, secondary to ceftriaxone administration.

2. Case

A 32-year-old obese African American male, with a history of sickle cell disease, presented to the hospital with severe pain in his legs and back that had become progressively worse for three days prior to presentation. For his sickle cell crisis, he has had multiple blood transfusions, but none within recent years. His medications consisted of hydroxyurea and morphine sulfate. His initial vital signs were heart rate of 72 beats per minute, blood pressure of 118/60 mmHg, respiratory rate of 18 breaths per minute, and temperature of 98.9 Fahrenheit. On examination, the patient was in distress and writhing in pain but otherwise no additional abnormalities were noted. According to the patient, these symptoms were typical of his sickle cell crisis.

Initial laboratory studies revealed a hemoglobin of 10 g/dL, reticulocyte count of 22%, haptoglobin of <10 mg/dL,

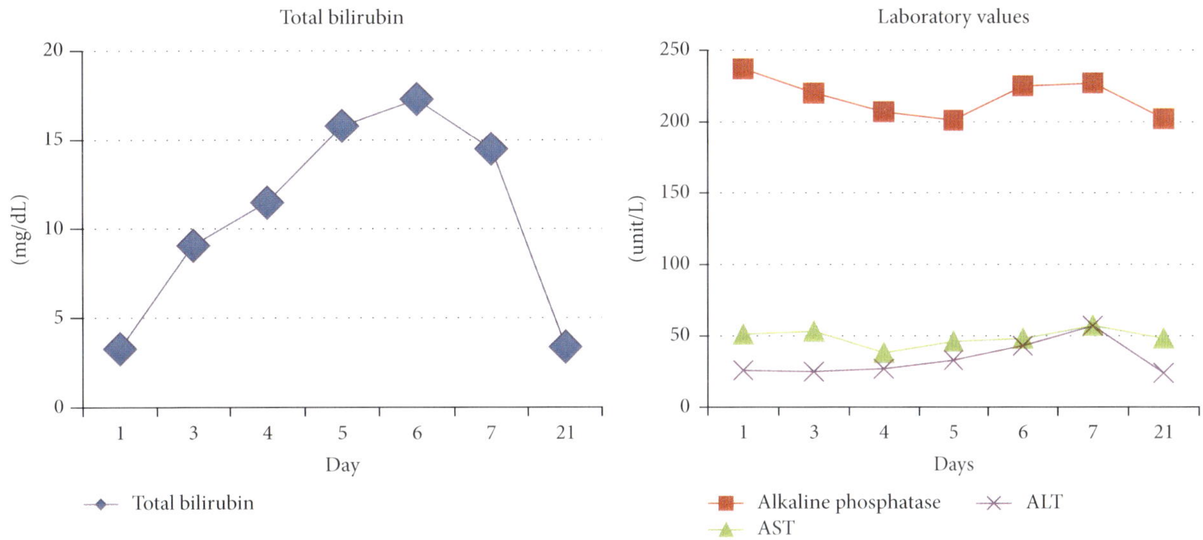

FIGURE 1: Trend of total bilirubin, alkaline phosphatase, AST, and ALT values from admission till outpatient follow-up.

and LDH of 462 units/L, and no electrolyte or kidney function abnormalities were noted. His total bilirubin on admission was 3.3 mg/dL (1.0 mg/dL upper limit of normal (UPLN)), AST was 51 unit/L (35 unit/L UPLN), ALT was 26 unit/L, ALP was 237 unit/L (129 unit/L UPLN), and GGT was 157 unit/L (60 unit/L UPLN) with albumin 4.1 gm/dL. His platelets and coagulation panel were within normal limits. Upon review of his prior records, it was determined that his liver chemistry panel was at baseline. Thus, based on the physical examination and laboratory findings, the patient was diagnosed with acute sickle cell crisis and was admitted to the hospital. He was started on a morphine (patient controlled analgesia) pump, hydroxyurea, intravenous fluids, and oxygen supplementation.

Initial chest X-ray done in the emergency room did not show any infiltrates or consolidations. However, on the second day, he developed cough and rhonchi in the right lung field on auscultation. Repeat chest X-ray revealed right middle lobe infiltrate and the patient was started on ceftriaxone and azithromycin for community acquired pneumonia.

Throughout the course of his hospitalization, the patient developed pronounced scleral icterus with acutely increased total bilirubin. There was minimal change in the other liver chemistries (Figure 1). A medication review was completed to investigate the cause of the direct hyperbilirubinemia. Ceftriaxone was continued since the most common adverse drug reaction with this medication reported is transaminitis. A complete additional workup was then pursued, as seen in Table 1. Ultrasonography of the liver and gallbladder did not demonstrate any abnormality. Furthermore, a subsequent ultrasound with additive arterial and venous evaluation did not reveal evidence of thrombosis.

After several days with intravenous hydration and appropriate pain control, the patient's pain symptoms returned to baseline. His laboratory values also improved, except for persistent hyperbilirubinemia that peaked at 17 mg/dL. His respiratory status improved as well. At this time, the ceftriaxone and azithromycin were changed to levofloxacin. Two days after changing the antibiotics, the total bilirubin started trending downwards to 15 mg/dL, and the patient was discharged with oral antibiotics. Repeat outpatient liver chemistries depicted total bilirubin levels returning to baseline values.

3. Discussion

Persistent liver chemistry elevations are consistent abnormalities seen in sickle cell patients [9]. Sickle cell disease has many effects on the hepatobiliary system [10] and can result in conjugated and unconjugated hyperbilirubinemia, with the most concerning condition being sickle cell intrahepatic cholestasis [11]. However, this is often a fatal condition associated with acute liver failure [12], requiring exchange transfusion.

Our patient developed marked elevation of his total and direct bilirubin in the hospital. This correlated with the administration of ceftriaxone. Extensive workup was done to exclude other etiologies. Review of his hematologist's records showed a chronic elevation of his total bilirubin with his highest documented reading at 4-5 mg/dL along with chronically mildly elevated ALT/AST levels in the range of 40–50 unit/L. He did not meet criteria for sickle cell intrahepatic cholestasis [11] because he did not have any significant elevation of his transaminases nor was there evidence of abnormal synthetic liver function. Furthermore, the rise in his bilirubin level did not correlate with an elevated LDH.

Ten percent of patients with sickle cell crisis can present with an acute sickle hepatic crisis [13]. These patients will have mildly elevated transaminase levels and a markedly increased serum bilirubin level [14]. These patients will also have significant right upper quadrant pain and generalized abdominal discomfort [11]. Our patient did not have these presenting symptoms; therefore, an alternative diagnosis was considered and pursued. The workup was negative, except for

TABLE 1: Serologic evaluation of elevated direct hyperbilirubinemia.

Serological evaluation of direct hyperbilirubinemia	Patient's value	Normal value
Serum copper level	243	72–166 mcg/dL
Ceruloplasmin	59	15–30 mg/dL
Ferritin	1,850	30–400 ng/mL
Iron	81	59–159 mcg/dL
Total Iron Binding Capacity (TIBC)	207	228–428 mcg/dL
Unsaturated Iron Binding Capacity (UIBC)	126	112–346 mcg/dL
Iron saturation	39	20–55%
Folate	9.6	3.1–17.5 ng/mL
Vitamin B12	697	211–946 pg/mL
Serum zinc	130	60–130 mcg/dL
Hepatitis A total	Negative	Negative
Hepatitis B core antibody IgM	Negative	Negative
Hepatitis B surface antibody	Negative	0.0–9.9 Iunits/mL
Hepatitis B surface antigen	Negative	Negative
Hepatitis C antibody	Negative	Negative
Total IgG	1480	700–1600 mg/dL
Total IgA	376	70–400 mg/dL
Total IgM	19	40–230 mg/dL
Antinuclear Antibody (ANA)	Negative	Negative
Mitochondrial antibody	Nondetected	Nondetected
Smooth muscle antibody	Nondetected	Nondetected

elevated ferritin and copper levels. A concern for secondary hemochromatosis was raised. Yet, the remainder of his iron studies and his blood transfusion history was not significant. The elevated ferritin and copper levels were attributed to an ongoing inflammatory process that has been described in numerous conditions [15]. Of note, there was no clinical evidence of Wilson's disease.

Although a definitive diagnosis of DILI due to ceftriaxone requires a tissue sample for analysis, a liver biopsy was not pursued. Percutaneous liver biopsy in sickle cell crisis has been associated with increased mortality, and studies recommend delaying the biopsy until the acute crisis has resolved if etiology is still in question [16]. Additionally, it is important to distinguish two similar conditions in sickle cell patients, benign hyperbilirubinemia and chronic intrahepatic cholestasis. Both these conditions appear with a significantly elevated direct bilirubin and mild elevated transaminases that can mimic ceftriaxone associated cholestasis [11]. Benign hyperbilirubinemia has been described in several pediatric patients on routine laboratory studies, while chronic intrahepatic cholestasis requires exchange transfusion for the bilirubin levels to decrease [11]. Our patient did not require exchange transfusion and his bilirubin began to improve within 48 hours of discontinuing ceftriaxone.

Of note, azithromycin has been associated with cholestasis-induced hepatitis [17]. Liver injury caused by azithromycin is typically cholestatic, arising within 1 to 3 weeks of starting treatment. It occasionally arises after azithromycin is stopped and can occur even after a short, 2- or 3-day course [18]. Recovery typically occurs within 4 to 8 weeks of stopping the medication [18].

The Naranjo Adverse Drug Reaction Probability Score was used to determine the probability of a drug interaction. Both azithromycin and ceftriaxone suggest the possibility of reaction [19]. However, his clinical course fits more with ceftriaxone. Ceftriaxone can cause biliary sludge and disease can arise within a few days of starting therapy [20]. Resolution of symptoms is typically rapid once ceftriaxone is stopped, although sludge and gallstones may be detectable by ultrasound for several months [20]. The time to resolution in our patient matches that of ceftriaxone, rather than azithromycin. Furthermore, the patient denied having been treated with ceftriaxone in the past. He did admit to using azithromycin for upper respiratory tract infection, supporting the possibility that ceftriaxone was the major drug involved.

4. Conclusion

This case highlights the possibility of ceftriaxone associated marked direct hyperbilirubinemia in young adults, especially in sickle cell patients with chronic liver chemistry abnormalities due to chronic hemolysis. In cases of elevated bilirubin in the presence of ceftriaxone, discontinuation of antibiotic should be considered and bilirubin levels should be trended until levels reach baseline. If levels do not return to baseline, other etiologies should be pursued. Furthermore, ceftriaxone should be used with caution in individuals predisposed to developing hyperbilirubinemia.

References

[1] I. Kaur and J. Singh, "Cholestatic hepatitis with intravenous ceftriaxone," *Indian Journal of Pharmacology*, vol. 43, no. 4, pp. 474–475, 2011.

[2] N. Kaplowitz, "Drug-induced Liver Injury," *Clinical Infectious Diseases*, vol. 38, supplement 2, pp. S44–S48, 2004.

[3] N. M. Bass, "Drug-induced liver disease," in *Current Diagnosis and Treatment in Gastroenterology*, S. Friedman, K. McQuaid, and J. Grendell, Eds., pp. 664–679, McGraw-Hill, New York, NY, USA, 2nd edition, 2003.

[4] B. Katzung, *Basic and Clinical Pharmacology*, McGraw-Hill, New York, NY, USA, 11th edition, 2009.

[5] M. S. Ravisha and S. V. Godambe, "Ceftriaxone induced cholestasis in a neonate: a case report," *Indian Journal of Medical Sciences*, vol. 58, no. 2, pp. 73–74, 2004.

[6] M. Riccabona, R. Kerbl, W. Schwinger, D. Spork, M. Millner, and H. M. Grubbauer, "Ceftriaxone-induced cholelithiasis—a harmless side-effect?" *Klinische Padiatrie*, vol. 205, no. 6, pp. 421–423, 1993.

[7] M. J. Bell, D. C. Stockwell, N. L. C. Luban et al., "Ceftriaxone-induced hemolytic anemia and hepatitis in an adolescent with hemoglobin SC disease," *Pediatric Critical Care Medicine*, vol. 6, no. 3, pp. 363–366, 2005.

[8] N. Araz, V. Okan, M. Demirci, and M. Araz, "Pseudolithiasis due to ceftriaxone treatment for meningitis in children: report of 8 cases," *Tohoku Journal of Experimental Medicine*, vol. 211, no. 3, pp. 285–290, 2007.

[9] F. Traina, S. G. Jorge, A. Yamanaka, L. R. De Meirelles, F. F. Costa, and S. T. O. Saad, "Chronic liver abnormalities in sickle cell disease: a clinicopathological study in 70 living patients," *Acta Haematologica*, vol. 118, no. 3, pp. 129–135, 2007.

[10] H. Issa and A. H. Al-Salem, "Hepatobilary manifestations of sickle cell anemia," *Gastroenterology Research*, vol. 3, no. 10, pp. 1–8, 2010.

[11] I. Khurshid, L. Anderson, G. H. Downie, and G. S. Pape, "Sickle cell disease, extreme hyperbilirubinemia, and pericardial tamponade: case report and review of the literature," *Critical Care Medicine*, vol. 30, no. 10, pp. 2363–2367, 2002.

[12] S. Banerjee, C. Owen, and S. Chopra, "Sickle cell hepatopathy," *Hepatology*, vol. 33, no. 5, pp. 1021–1028, 2001.

[13] T. T. Schubert, "Hepatobiliary system in sickle cell disease," *Gastroenterology*, vol. 90, no. 6, pp. 2013–2021, 1986.

[14] H. J. Rosenblate, R. Eisenstein, and A. W. Holmes, "The liver in sickle cell anemia. A clinical-pathologic study," *Archives of Pathology*, vol. 90, no. 3, pp. 235–245, 1970.

[15] C. Moore, M. Ormseth, and H. Fuchs, "Causes and significance of markedly elevated serum ferritin levels in an academic medical center," *Journal of Clinical Rheumatology*, vol. 19, no. 6, pp. 324–328, 2013.

[16] N. Zakaria, A. Knisely, B. Portmann et al., "Acute sickle cell hepatopathy represents a potential contraindication for percutaneous liver biopsy," *Blood*, vol. 101, no. 1, pp. 101–103, 2003.

[17] C. Maggioli, L. Santi, G. Zaccherini, V. Bevilacqua, F. Giunchi, and P. Caraceni, "A case of prolonged cholestatic hepatitis induced by azithromycin in a young woman," *Case Reports in Hepatology*, vol. 2011, Article ID 314231, 4 pages, 2011.

[18] US National Library of Medicine and LiverTox, "Clinical and research information on Drug-Induced Liver Injury. Azithromycin," 2015, http://livertox.nlm.nih.gov/Azithromycin.htm.

[19] U.S. National Library of Medicine. LiverTox, Clinical and research information on Drug-Induced Liver Injury. Adverse Drug Reaction Probability Scale (Naranjo) in Drug Induced Liver Injury, 2015, http://livertox.nih.gov/Narajo.html.

[20] U.S National Library of Medicine, LiverTox. Clinical and research information on Drug-Induced Liver Injury. Ceftriaxone, 2015, http://livertox.nlm.nih.gov/Ceftriaxone.htm.

22

A Timely Intervention: Endoscopic Retrieval of a Swallowed Magnetized Activity Watch

Jason S. Radowsky, Joseph S. Lee, and Andrew T. Schlussel

Department of General Surgery, Brian Allgood Army Community Hospital, Yongsan 96205, Republic of Korea

Correspondence should be addressed to Andrew T. Schlussel; andrew.t.schlussel@gmail.com

Academic Editor: Yoshihiro Moriwaki

The accidental ingestion of a foreign object often presents a difficult scenario for the clinician. This includes not only the decision to retrieve the material but also the appropriate technique to use. We present the case of a young asymptomatic girl who swallowed a magnetic activity watch, which was then successfully retrieved with an endoscopic snare. To our knowledge, this is the first documented case of salvaging an operational watch from the stomach using an endoscopic technique.

1. Introduction

Foreign body ingestion is a challenging medical dilemma for both surgeons and gastroenterologists, with the greatest incidence seen in the psychiatric, elderly, and pediatric populations. The mechanism of ingestion varies based on the cohort studied. The psychiatric population may have an altered decision-making capability or will swallow objects for a secondary gain [1]. The elderly often have altered mental status, decreased oropharyngeal sensation and control, and ill-fitting dental appliances. The vast majority of cases, > 80%, occur in children. However, only 10–20% require endoscopic removal, with < 1% mandating an operation to remove the foreign body [2, 3]. Younger children demonstrate the greatest risk as their senses are developing and begin to explore their own environment, frequently placing objects in their mouth [4]. The object ingested, anatomical location, and age of the patient are important factors when making the clinical decision to pursue extraction through an invasive technique or to manage the patient expectantly in hopes of transit through the gastrointestinal tract [5]. An endoscopic or operative approach to extract dentures, batteries, or magnets is strongly recommended, as these objects portend a greater risk of intestinal laceration, perforation, obstruction, or luminal necrosis [4, 6, 7].

As one may expect, there is a paucity of data in the literature regarding the extraction of an ingested watch or object with similar dimensions. One case report has discussed the extraction of a watch through an open gastrostomy, three cases have utilized an endoscopic approach for retrieval of an impacted watch in the proximal esophagus, and one report discussed successive esophageal balloon dilation, to dislodge the timepiece, pushing it distally into the stomach to allow for passage [8–11]. To our knowledge this is the first documented case of a watch extraction from the stomach using a flexible endoscope.

2. Case Report

This is a case of a healthy, well-developed, 13-year-old girl who was reported to have accidentally swallowed a Shine Misfit fitness tracking watch (Misfit Wearables, Burlingame, CA, USA). While swimming, she removed the magnetized functional portion of the watch from its band and placed this in her mouth at which time it was swallowed by mistake. At the time of presentation, the object was identified in the stomach on an emergency department X-ray at our community-sized hospital. The patient was initially managed conservatively and was informed to return the following day for serial imaging (Figure 1). After approximately 30 hours, the watch was still retained in the stomach. Due to the failure of distal progression through the pylorus and concern for obstruction at the ileocecal valve, the decision was made to proceed with an endoscopic intervention in the operating

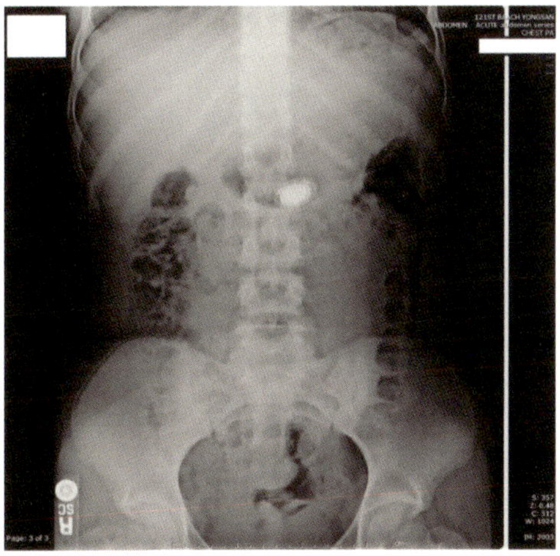

Figure 1: Supine abdominal X-ray showing watch in the stomach.

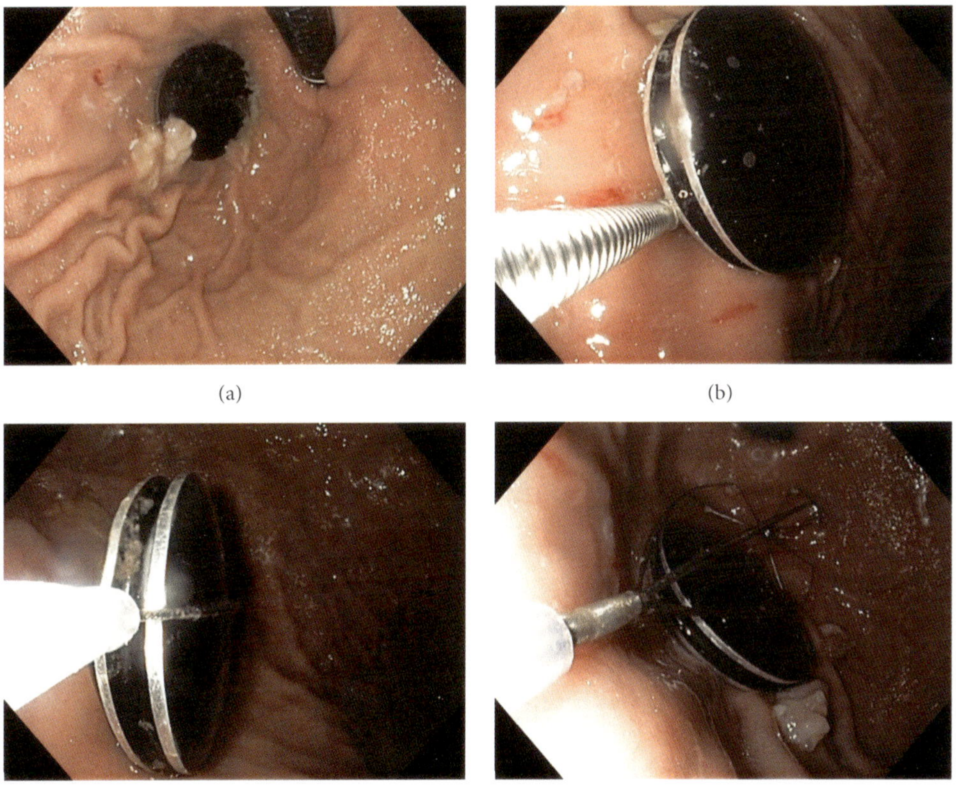

(a) (b)

(c) (d)

Figure 2: Watch shown in gastric fundus on retroflexion (a) and failed attempts at retrieval using biopsy forceps (b), transverse capture with a snare (c), and wire basket (d).

room. The watch was magnetized, measuring 28.5 × 8.0 × 28.5 mm (width × depth × height), which precluded grasping the device [12]. The size and smooth oval shape of the watch made capturing it with a wire basket or endoscopic snare difficult (Figure 2). Finally, with no additional interventional equipment available, a snare was used to manipulate the device into the esophagus, where it was then secured utilizing an end-on lassoing technique around the groove of the watch. Once the device was fully encircled, it could then be safely removed through the oropharynx (Figure 3). Following this 72 min procedure, the patient recovered well and was discharged home the following day with no apparent sequela from the event. The watch retained normal function despite the low pH of the stomach and manipulation upon retrieval. When synchronized to her mobile device, the Shine Misfit watch accurately recorded all advertised data points to include steps taken, calories burned, sleep cycles, and maintained accurate time. The patient's father provided

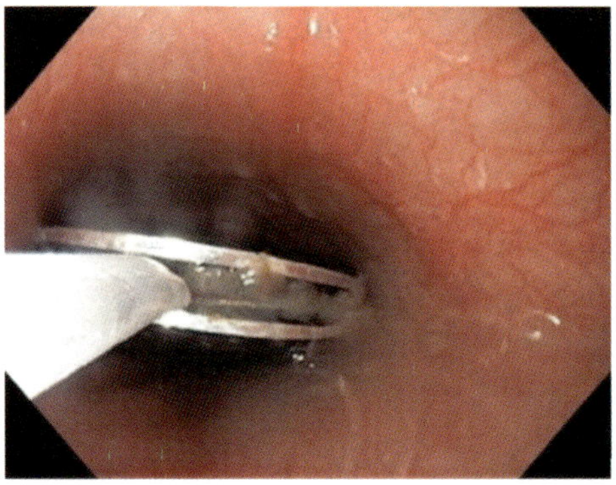

Figure 3: Successful end-on lassoing in the groove of the watch with the snare.

consent for the use of the images and information in this case report.

3. Discussion

The accidental ingestion of a foreign object is far more common in pediatric, elderly, psychiatric, and incarcerated patients when compared to the adolescent or healthy adult population. Once in the stomach, 80% of these objects will eventually pass out of the body; therefore, intervention remains uncommon as long as the patient is asymptomatic [13]. The decision to proceed with endoscopic retrieval, in this case, was prompted by a failure in the progression of the watch for greater than 24 hours. In addition, there was an uncertainty to the maintenance of the watch's structural integrity when exposed to a low pH for an extended period of time. The device is advertised as being waterproof to 50 meters; however, this did not allay the surgeon or patients' concern for battery exposure and the risk of a caustic perforation [12]. Several studies have shown that sharp foreign bodies, severe symptoms, long duration from ingestion to endoscopy, and existence of mucosal injury are significant risk factors predictive of complications related to removal of foreign bodies [14, 15]. We believe that early detection and a timely endoscopic removal were two factors that contributed to successful retrieval for this case.

As this retrieval occurred at a small community hospital, a limited variety of endoscopic tools were available. While there are no published guidelines for which endoscopic snare or grasper to utilize during foreign body recovery, the American Society for Gastrointestinal Endoscopy (ASGE) provides recommendations regarding the dimensions, configurations, and indications for many commercially available devices [16]. In addition, the ASGE has published intervention timing guidelines based on patient symptoms, object type and size, and anatomic location. Although a magnetized digital watch is not included in these published categories, disk batteries and coins larger than 2 cm are recommended to be extracted 1-2 days following ingestion [17].

In conclusion, the retrieval of a magnetized watch from the stomach with a flexible endoscope is a safe and efficacious procedure. It is critical that the physician must consider patient size, as well as the device size and design, to formulate an appropriate management plan. The patient should understand the endoscopic and operative risks and should be counseled on the need for a timely intervention when observation has failed.

Copyright Protection

Our team is comprised of military service members and employees of the US Government. This work was prepared as part of our official duties. Title 17 U.S.C. 105 provides that "Copyright protection under this title is not available for any work of the United States Government." Title 17 U.S.C. 101 defines a US Government work as a work prepared by a military service member or employee of the US Government as part of that person's official duties.

Disclaimer

This is an original work by the authors. The opinions expressed are the authors' and the authors' alone. They do not necessarily reflect the opinion of the United States Government, the United States Department of Defense, or Brian Allgood Army Community Hospital.

Authors' Contribution

Conception and design were carried out by Jason S. Radowsky. Creation of media was done by Andrew T. Schlussel. Drafting of the paper was carried out by Jason S. Radowsky. Critical revision was done by Joseph S. Lee and Andrew T. Schlussel. Supervision was done by Andrew T. Schlussel.

Acknowledgment

The authors would like to gratefully thank SGT Sky S. Park, LPN, who acted as their endoscopic technician and who contributed his experience and assistance to safely and efficiently complete this intervention.

References

[1] I. C. Grimes, B. J. Spier, L. R. Swize, M. J. Lindstrom, and P. R. Pfau, "Predictors of recurrent ingestion of gastrointestinal foreign bodies," *Canadian Journal of Gastroenterology*, vol. 27, no. 1, pp. e1–e4, 2013.

[2] D. C. Little, S. R. Shah, S. D. St Peter et al., "Esophageal foreign bodies in the pediatric population: our first 500 cases," *Journal of Pediatric Surgery*, vol. 41, no. 5, pp. 914–918, 2006.

[3] W. Cheng and P. K. H. Tam, "Foreign body ingestion in children: experience with 1,265 cases," *Journal of Pediatric Surgery*, vol. 34, no. 10, pp. 1472–1476, 1999.

[4] S. J. Sharpe, L. M. Rochette, and G. A. Smith, "Pediatric battery-related emergency department visits in the United States, 1990–2009," *Pediatrics*, vol. 129, no. 6, pp. 1111–1117, 2012.

[5] I. Rahman, P. Patel, P. Boger et al., "Therapeutic upper gastrointestinal tract endoscopy in Pediatric Gastroenterology," *The World Journal of Gastrointestinal Endoscopy*, vol. 7, no. 3, pp. 169–182, 2015.

[6] S. N. Bandyopadhyay, S. Das, S. K. Das, and A. Mandal, "Impacted dentures in the oesophagus," *Journal of Laryngology and Otology*, vol. 128, no. 5, pp. 468–474, 2014.

[7] M. Strickland, D. Rosenfield, and A. Fecteau, "Magnetic foreign body injuries: a large pediatric hospital experience," *Journal of Pediatrics*, vol. 165, no. 2, pp. 332–335, 2014.

[8] E. B. Duboys, "Watch in the stomach," *Journal of the American Medical Association*, vol. 245, no. 17, p. 1731, 1981.

[9] A. Almaç and M. Gönüllü, "Wrist watch in the esophagus," *Journal of Otolaryngology*, vol. 17, no. 4, p. 200, 1988.

[10] N. Aggarwal and D. Sinha, "An amazing case of working wrist watch in the esophagus," *Indian Journal of Otolaryngology and Head and Neck Surgery*, vol. 58, no. 1, pp. 105–106, 2006.

[11] Y. T. Jeen, J. Chun, C. W. Song et al., "Endoscopic removal of sharp foreign bodies impacted in the esophagus," *Endoscopy*, vol. 33, no. 6, pp. 518–522, 2001.

[12] Misfit Wearables, Misfit Shine, March 2015, http://misfit.com/products/shine.

[13] V. Selivanov, G. F. Sheldon, J. P. Cello, and R. A. Crass, "Management of foreign body ingestion," *Annals of Surgery*, vol. 199, no. 2, pp. 187–191, 1984.

[14] Y.-K. Park, K.-O. Kim, J.-H. Yang, S.-H. Lee, and B.-I. Jang, "Factors associated with development of complications after endoscopic foreign body removal," *Saudi Journal of Gastroenterology*, vol. 19, no. 5, pp. 230–234, 2013.

[15] J. H. Park, C. H. Park, J. H. Park et al., "Review of 209 cases of foreign bodies in the upper gastrointestinal tract and clinical factors of successful endoscopic removal," *The Korean Journal of Gastroenterology*, vol. 43, no. 4, pp. 226–233, 2004.

[16] D. L. Diehl, D. G. Adler, J. D. Conway et al., "Endoscopic retrieval devices," *Gastrointestinal Endoscopy*, vol. 69, no. 6, pp. 997–1003, 2009.

[17] S. O. Ikenberry, T. L. Jue, M. A. Anderson et al., "Management of ingested foreign bodies and food impactions," *Gastrointestinal Endoscopy*, vol. 73, no. 6, pp. 1085–1091, 2011.

Small Intestinal and Mesenteric Multiple Gastrointestinal Stromal Tumors Causing Occult Bleeding

Tolga Dinc, Selami Ilgaz Kayilioglu, Ahmet Erdogan, Erdinc Cetinkaya, Ozgur Akgul, and Faruk Coskun

Ankara Numune Training and Research Hospital, Department of General Surgery, 06100 Ankara, Turkey

Correspondence should be addressed to Tolga Dinc; tolga¯dr@hotmail.com

Academic Editor: Shiro Kikuchi

Gastrointestinal stromal tumors are the meseancymal neoplasms which may involve any part of gastrointestinal tract. C-Kit and platelet derived factor receptor alpha polypeptide are believed to be responsible for the genetic basis. This case presentation aimed to discuss the diagnostic and therapeutic modality of multiple small intestinal, omental, and mesenteric GISTs with different sizes which caused occult bleeding in a 43-year-old male patient.

1. Introduction

Gastrointestinal stromal tumor (GIST) was first described by Mazur and Clark in 1983. It is a rare tumor that may involve all parts of gastrointestinal tract [1]. It is believed that mutations of c-Kit protooncogene and platelet derived growth factor receptor alpha polypeptide underlie the genetic basis of the disease. These mutations cause uncontrolled proliferation of Cajal cells by increasing tyrosine kinase activity [2]. GISTs constitute 0.2% of all gastrointestinal tumors and they are mostly located in stomach. Some rare forms may be located in small intestine, omentum, and peritoneum. Only 10–30% of them show malignant transformation [3, 4]. This case presentation aimed to discuss, in the light of the literature, the diagnostic and therapeutic modality of multiple small intestinal, omental, and mesenteric GISTs with different sizes which caused occult bleeding in a young male patient.

2. Case Presentation

A 43-year-old male patient who was admitted to emergency department with abdominal pain, nausea, palpitation, and fatigue was describing a vague pain in the right lower quadrant of abdomen. He had no concomitant disease other than a previous diagnosis of iron deficiency anemia. He had been receiving oral iron preparations. His family history revealed nothing abnormal. On physical examination, conjunctiva was found to be pale. Blood pressure was measured as 100/70 mmHg, heart rate was 110/min., and measured body temperature was within normal limits. On abdominal examination, a 5 cm sized mobile mass was palpated in the right lower quadrant. Complete blood count showed hemoglobin level of 9.2 g/dL and hematocrit of 27.5%, while white blood cell and platelet counts were normal. Since abdominal ultrasonographic (USG) examination demonstrated a hypoechoic right lower quadrant lesion with a size of about 6 cm which had vascularisation on color Doppler ultrasonographic examination, the patient was referred to hematology outpatient clinic for the investigation of the etiology of intraabdominal lymphadenopathy and anemia. The patient in whom performed endoscopic interventions detected nothing pathological underwent computed tomography (CT) which demonstrated semisolid mass lesions with lobulated margins and necrotic centers, which were 3 cm in the middle of the abdomen, 5 cm in the left upper quadrant, 5 cm in mesentery adjacent to superior mesenteric artery, and 6 cm in the right lower quadrant (Figure 1). Tumor markers were found to be normal. The patient was referred to the department of general surgery with the diagnosis of intraabdominal mass.

The patient was taken to operation after necessary preoperative arrangements were made. Laparotomy with midline

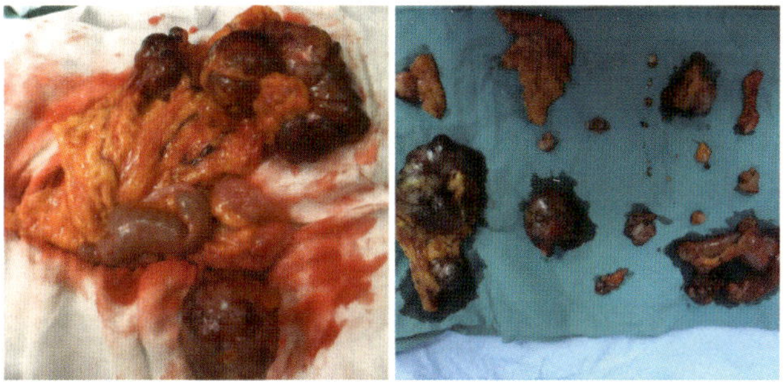

FIGURE 1: Peroperative and postresection images of the lesions.

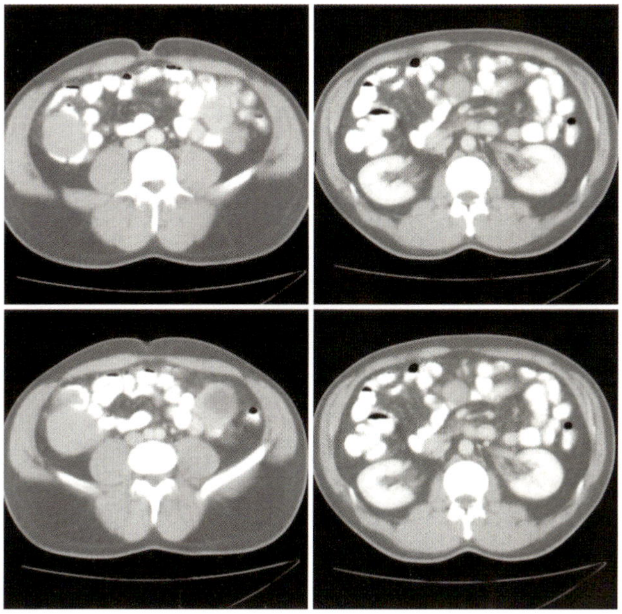

FIGURE 2: Computed tomography images of the lesions.

incision was performed. Abdominal exploration revealed semisolid mass lesions which were related to intestines, had lobulated margins, and were measured as 4, 5, and 6 cm, being 80, 100, and 180 cm away from treitz ligament, respectively (Figure 2). In addition, there were multiple lesions with different sizes on omentum and mesentery. Peritoneum, liver, and other organs were intact. Three masses adjacent to the intestines were excised. Tumors in the other locations were resected with safe surgical margins. In addition, diverticulectomy was performed in the patient with Meckel diverticulum 4 cm in size; prophylactic appendectomy was also carried out. A drain was placed in the abdomen following bleeding control and anatomic layers were then closed and the operation was terminated.

No problems were confronted during postoperative period. Bowel movements started on the 3rd postoperative day and oral feeding was started and drain was removed. The patient was discharged from the hospital with normal vital signs on the 5th postoperative day. His medical treatment was arranged to include iron preparations, proton pump inhibitor, and oral antibiotic.

Histopathological analysis of the lesions was reported as gastrointestinal stromal tumor. CD117 (c-Kit) was highly positive in more than 75% of the cells. S100 and Vimentin staining were found positive in immunohistochemical analysis, whereas CD34, SMA, Desmin, and Pancreatin were found negative. The patient was referred to relevant clinic for imatinib treatment.

3. Discussion

Gastrointestinal stromal tumor is a very rare neoplasm of digestive system with an annual incidence of 1.5/100000 [5]. GIST is a mesenchymal tumor of digestive system and may involve any region from mouth to anus. 90% of the patients are over the age of 40 and the peak incidence occurs between the ages 60 and 65. Its prevalence is slightly higher in males, while it is not affected by geographic region and ethnicity [2]. Common locations of the disease are stomach in 60–70%, small intestine in 20–30%, and esophagus, colon, and rectum in 5–15%; omentum, peritoneum, and mesentery are rarely involved [4]. The most common sites for metastasis are liver and peritoneum, while lymph node involvement is a quite rare condition [4].

It is quite difficult to make preoperative diagnosis of GISTs other than gastric and colorectal forms. Most of the patients are asymptomatic and present with nonspecific symptoms. Failure to visualize small intestine by endoscopic procedures, tendency of the lesion to demonstrate exophytic extension, and limitations in the evaluation of small intestine by CT under emergency conditions have an impact on the difficulty of the diagnosis [6, 7]. GISTs causing bleeding have been described in the literature [8, 9]. Our case also had occult bleeding; he had been referred to hospitals for many times with the symptoms of anemia; he had been repeatedly examined and tested but no diagnosis could be achieved. He had received medical treatment for iron deficiency anemia. Patients with GIST may have bleeding. Bleeding is more common in small intestinal GISTs when compared to gastric, colonic, and rectal GISTs [7]. The origin of bleeding in small intestinal GISTs has been thought to be ulcerated tumoral mucosa, even if it is extraintestinal [7, 10]. Moreover, since stromal collagen is less in amount in the patients with GIST, it is suggested that these patients have thin-walled vessels which are prone to bleeding [11]. Although it is rare, GIST should be considered in the patients presenting with anemia in which the etiology cannot be explained by colonoscopy and endoscopy.

Radiological examination, especially careful evaluation of abdominal CT, is very important in making the diagnosis of the disease. CT gives information on the localization and size of tumor, extension to liver, and peritoneal involvement. It is the most effective imaging modality in the diagnosis of GIST [12]. However, necrotic areas in the center of tumor may not be differentiated from cystic degeneration and abscess, which may lead to misdiagnosis [13]. CT appearance of most GISTs is an exophytic lesion >5 cm in size which is well demarcated and has lobulated margins, necrosis, or hemorrhage at the center but no calcification [10, 14, 15]. CT examination of our case revealed 3 separate mass lesions which were 3–6 cm in size and originating from small intestine and a mesenteric lesion 5 cm in size. All lesions had necrotic areas in the center and lobulated margins. CT images of our patient were consistent with CT images of other patients with GIST reported in the literature.

The main point of the treatment is surgical removal of the tumor, which is best to achieve cure. It is important to preserve pseudocapsule of tumor, while extensive intestinal resection is not necessary [16]. Preservation of capsule is important in that it prevents intraabdominal seeding during surgery [17]. Rupture of tumor negatively affects the prognosis [15, 18]. In our patient, tumor was removed leaving negative surgical margins and the integrity of pseudocapsule was not disrupted.

Mesenteric GISTs are quite rarely seen. c-Kit and platelet derived growth factor receptor alpha mutations can be detected in most of the cases. Presence of any of these mutations is important for diagnosis [19].

Since GIST generally does not spread to lymph nodes, lymphadenectomy is usually not required in surgical treatment of GIST [16, 17]. In our case, no lymphadenopathy was detected peroperatively and lymph node dissection was not performed.

Literature data suggest that tumors smaller than 10 cm are less likely to metastasize, have lower mitotic index and no intraperitoneal spread, and may be treated by R0 surgery [20, 21]. Our case also had tumors less than 10 cm in size, which were excised according to the above criteria.

4. Conclusion

Small intestinal GIST should be considered in the patients presenting with nonspecific abdominal pain and the symptoms of anemia. This disease should be remembered in the patients with normal endoscopic examinations, in whom large mesenteric lymph nodes which are conglomerated, have lobulated margins and necrotic centers, and are located adjacent to intestine are present. In addition, it should be kept in mind that it may have multiple origins and various sizes and may involve multiple organs.

References

[1] K. Kramer, M. Siech, J. Sträter, A. Aschoff, and D. Henne-Bruns, "GI hemorrhage with fulminant shock induced by jejunal gastrointestinal stromal tumor (GIST) coincident with duodenal neuroendocrine carcinoma (NET) + neurofibromatosis (NF)—case report and review of the literature," *Zeitschrift für Gastroenterologie*, vol. 43, no. 3, pp. 281–288, 2005.

[2] P. Sornmayura, "Gastrointestinal stromal tumors: a pathology view point," *Journal of the Medical Association of Thailand*, vol. 92, no. 1, pp. 124–135, 2009.

[3] H. Choi, "Response evaluation of gastrointestinal stromal tumors," *Oncologist*, vol. 13, no. 2, pp. 4–7, 2008.

[4] K. K. Roggin and M. C. Posner, "Modern treatment of gastric gastrointestinal stromal tumors," *World Journal of Gastroenterology*, vol. 18, no. 46, pp. 6720–6728, 2012.

[5] G. Gatta, J. M. van der Zwan, P. G. Casali et al., "Rare cancers are not so rare: the rare cancer burden in Europe," *European Journal of Cancer*, vol. 47, no. 17, pp. 2493–2511, 2011.

[6] N. Abbassi-Ghadi, K. Bartlam, S. Rasheed, and T. Holme, "A case of obscure gastrointestinal bleeding in a teenager," *Annals of the Royal College of Surgeons of England*, vol. 91, no. 5, pp. 1–3, 2009.

[7] D. A. Sass, K. B. Chopra, S. D. Finkelstein, and P. R. Schauer, "Jejunal gastrointestinal stromal tumor: a cause of obscure gastrointestinal bleeding," *Archives of Pathology and Laboratory Medicine*, vol. 128, no. 2, pp. 214–217, 2004.

[8] S. Daldoul, A. Moussi, W. Triki, R. B. Baraket, and A. Zaouche, "Jejunal GIST causing acute massive gastrointestinal bleeding: role of multidetector row helical CT in the preoperative diagnosis and management," *Arab Journal of Gastroenterology*, vol. 13, no. 3, pp. 153–157, 2012.

[9] M. Bianchi, B. De Pascalis, and M. Koch, "Jejunal GIST: an unusual cause of gastrointestinal bleeding," *Digestive and Liver Disease*, vol. 42, no. 10, p. 744, 2010.

[10] K. Majdoub Hassani, F. Zahid, A. Ousadden, K. Mazaz, and K. Taleb, "Gastrointestinal stromal tumors and shock," *Journal of Emergencies, Trauma, and Shock*, vol. 2, no. 3, pp. 199–202, 2009.

[11] C. D. M. Fletcher, J. J. Berman, C. Corless et al., "Diagnosis of gastrointestinal stromal tumors: a consensus approach," *Human Pathology*, vol. 33, no. 5, pp. 459–465, 2002.

[12] G. D. Demetri, M. von Mehren, C. R. Antonescu et al., "NCCN task force report: update on the management of patients with gastrointestinal stromal tumors," *Journal of the National Comprehensive Cancer Network*, vol. 8, supplement 2, pp. S1–S41, 2010.

[13] B. Nilsson, K. Sjölund, L.-G. Kindblom et al., "Adjuvant imatinib treatment improves recurrence-free survival in patients with high-risk Gastrointestinal Stromal Tumours (GIST)," *British Journal of Cancer*, vol. 96, no. 11, pp. 1656–1658, 2007.

[14] W. C. Teoh, S. Y. Teo, and C. L. Ong, "Gastrointestinal stromal tumors presenting as gynecological masses: usefulness of multidetector computed tomography," *Ultrasound in Obstetrics and Gynecology*, vol. 37, no. 1, pp. 107–109, 2011.

[15] S. Hirasaki, K. Fujita, M. Matsubara et al., "A ruptured large extraluminal ileal gastrointestinal stromal tumor causing hemoperitoneum," *World Journal of Gastroenterology*, vol. 14, no. 18, pp. 2928–2931, 2008.

[16] K. Sandrasegaran, A. Rajesh, J. Rydberg, D. A. Rushing, F. M. Akisik, and J. D. Henley, "Gastrointestinal stromal tumors: clinical, radiologic, and pathologic features," *American Journal of Roentgenology*, vol. 184, no. 3, pp. 803–811, 2005.

[17] J. Y. Blay, S. Bonvalot, P. Casali et al., "Consensus meeting for the management of gastrointestinal stromal tumors. Report of the GIST Consensus Conference of 20-21 March 2004, under the auspices of ESMO," *Annals of Oncology*, vol. 16, no. 4, pp. 566–578, 2005.

[18] J. Paral, I. Slaninka, H. Kalabova, and D. Hadzi-Nikolov, "Gastrointestinal stromal tumors: review on morphology, molecular pathology, diagnostics, prognosis and treatment options," *Acta Gastro-Enterologica Belgica*, vol. 73, no. 3, pp. 349–359, 2010.

[19] S. Zheng, L.-R. Chen, H.-J. Wang, and S.-Z. Chen, "Analysis of mutation and expression of c-kit and PDGFR-α gene in gastrointestinal stromal tumor," *Hepato-Gastroenterology*, vol. 54, no. 80, pp. 2285–2290, 2007.

[20] C. Mucciarini, G. Rossi, F. Bertolini et al., "Incidence and clinicopathologic features of gastrointestinal stromal tumors. A population-based study," *BMC Cancer*, vol. 7, article 230, 2007.

[21] H. J. Yang, T. H. Kim, M. K. Park et al., "A case of primary extragastrointestinal stromal tumor presenting as peritoneal dissemination," *Korean Journal of Gastroenterology*, vol. 56, no. 5, pp. 319–323, 2010.

24

Colopancreatic Fistula: An Uncommon Complication of Recurrent Acute Pancreatitis

Mouhanna Abu Ghanimeh,[1] Omar Abughanimeh,[2] Khalil Abuamr,[3] Osama Yousef,[3] and Esmat Sadeddin[3]

[1]*Henry Ford Health System, 2799 W Grand Blvd, Gastroenterology K-7 Room E-744, Detroit, MI 48202, USA*
[2]*Internal Medicine, Graduate Medical Education, School of Medicine, University of Missouri-Kansas City, 2411 Holmes Street, M2-302, Kansas City, MO 64108, USA*
[3]*Gastroenterology, School of Medicine, University of Missouri-Kansas City, 2411 Holmes Street, Kansas City, MO 64108, USA*

Correspondence should be addressed to Mouhanna Abu Ghanimeh; mouhannaka87@yahoo.com

Academic Editor: Hideto Kawaratani

Colonic complications, including colopancreatic fistulas (CPFs), are uncommon after acute and chronic pancreatitis. However, they have been reported and are serious. CPFs are less likely to close spontaneously and are associated with a higher risk of complications. Therefore, more definitive treatment is required that includes surgical and endoscopic options. We present a case of a 62-year-old male patient with a history of heavy alcohol intake and recurrent acute pancreatitis who presented with a 6-month history of watery diarrhea and abdominal pain. His abdominal imaging showed a possible connection between the colon and the pancreas. A further multidisciplinary workup by the gastroenterology and surgery teams, including endoscopic ultrasound, endoscopic retrograde cholangiopancreatography, and colonoscopy, resulted in a diagnosis of CPF. A distal pancreatectomy and left hemicolectomy were performed, and the diagnosis of CPF was confirmed intraoperatively. The patient showed improvement afterward.

1. Introduction

Acute and chronic pancreatitis are not uncommon [1–3]. Both conditions can be associated with a variety of systemic as well as local complications [3–7]. Colonic complications are uncommon with acute and chronic pancreatitis. However, when they occur, they are usually serious and require further intervention [5–7]. These complications range from a localized ileus to severe colonic ischemia and necrosis with resulting perforation, hemorrhage, or fistula formation [5–9]. Colopancreatic fistulas (CPFs) occur in 3%–10% of patients with severe acute pancreatitis and can occur with chronic pancreatitis as well [5, 8–10]. When CPFs are suspected, computed tomography (CT) scan of the abdomen with or without contrast is a useful initial diagnostic tool [11]. Colonoscopy might also detect many cases [9]. As CPFs are less likely to close spontaneously and are usually associated with a complicated course, a more definitive intervention is typically warranted [5, 8]. Treatment modalities include surgical as well as endoscopic options [12–15].

2. Case Report

A 62-year-old male patient with a history of heavy alcohol intake and recurrent episodes of acute pancreatitis presented with a 6-month history of watery diarrhea, abdominal pain, weight loss and severe electrolyte abnormalities.

The patient had had an extensive workup in the last 3 months prior to presentation. His tissue transglutaminase IgA was 1 unit/ml (normal: < 4 units/ml), stool studies showed normal split fat and were negative for *Clostridium difficile,* ova, and parasites, esophagogastroduodenoscopy (EGD) showed mild gastritis with negative biopsies for *Helicobacter pylori,* and colonoscopy showed uncomplicated internal hemorrhoids. At that time, these tests did not reveal a significant pathology to explain his symptoms.

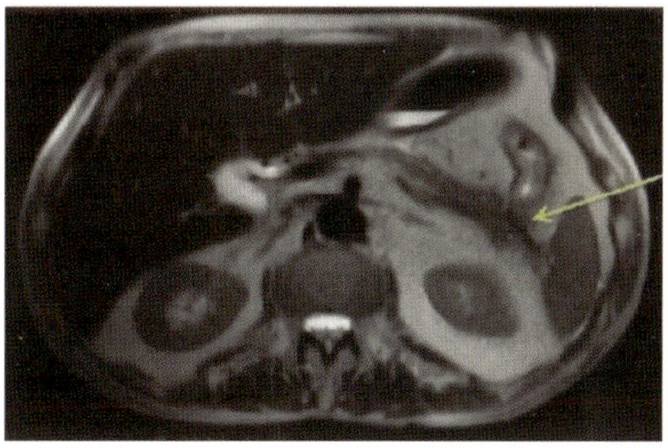

FIGURE 1: MRCP showing cystic foci in the pancreatic tail and colonic wall thickening. No strictures were noted. Green arrow denotes possible connection between the colon and pancreas.

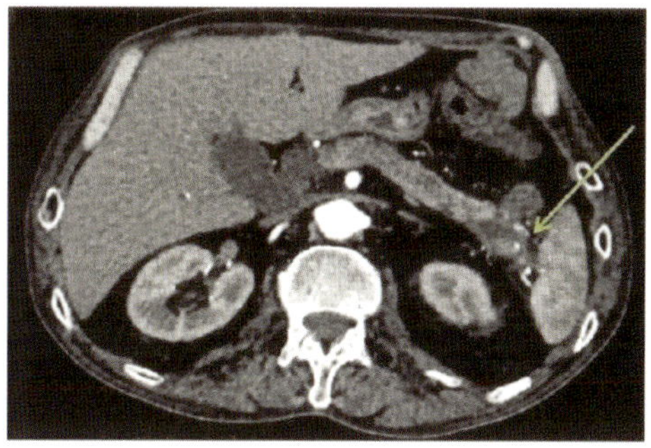

FIGURE 2: CTA showing a pancreatic tail lesion, with a focus of fluid and interval diffuse progression of colonic wall thickening. The pancreatic tail was inseparable from the colon, with a possible connection between the colon and the pancreas. Green arrow denotes possible connection between the colon and pancreas.

Upon evaluation, he appeared to be dehydrated and distressed. An abdominal examination showed mild tenderness to palpation with no rebound tenderness, guarding, or rigidity.

The initial laboratory workup showed the following levels: Na 131 mmol/L (normal: 136–144 mmol/L), Cl 94 mmol/L (normal: 95–105 mmol/L), K 3.0 mmol/L (normal: 3.6–5.1 mmol/L), creatinine 1.5 mg/dl (normal: 0.9–1.2 mg/dl), lipase 81 units/L (normal: 13–60 units/L), hemoglobin 10.9 g/dl (normal: 12–16 g/dl), and WBC 9,600/cmm (normal: 4,000-11,000/cmm). The patient was admitted for fluid and electrolyte replacement, symptomatic control, and additional evaluation of his underlying symptoms.

The CT scan of the abdomen without contrast showed a prominent common bile duct (CBD), dilated gallbladder (GB), and colonic wall thickening that was not thought to be significant initially. Magnetic resonance cholangiopancreatography (MRCP) was performed later (given the abnormalities in GB and CBD) and excluded strictures in the CBD. However, it did show cystic foci in the pancreatic tail and persistent colonic wall thickening [Figure 1]. This finding permitted greater discussion regarding endoscopic ultrasound (EUS) and possible endoscopic retrograde cholangiopancreatography (ERCP).

Prior to the EUS and ERCP, a CT scan angiography of the abdomen (CTA) was performed to rule out mesenteric ischemia. The pancreatic tail lesion was remarkable, with an internal focus of fluid and interval diffuse progression of circumferential colonic wall thickening. The pancreatic tail was inseparable from the colon, with a possible connection between the colon and the pancreas [Figure 2]. The tumor marker CA 19-9 was 36.6 units/ml (normal: <37 units/ml).

An EUS showed an anechoic lesion that was 10 × 11 mm, a possible cystic structure in the pancreatic tail with mild hypoechogenicity in the surrounding parenchyma. Fine-needle aspiration (FNA) was done and revealed ductal and inflammatory cells with Gram-negative rods. This finding increased the suspicion of a colonic connection. A repeated colonoscopy [Figure 3] was significant for a localized edematous area with bluish discoloration 45 cm from the anus that correlated with the area revealed in the CT scan. The surgery team was consulted, and an ERCP was scheduled to define the anatomy of the area, especially preoperatively.

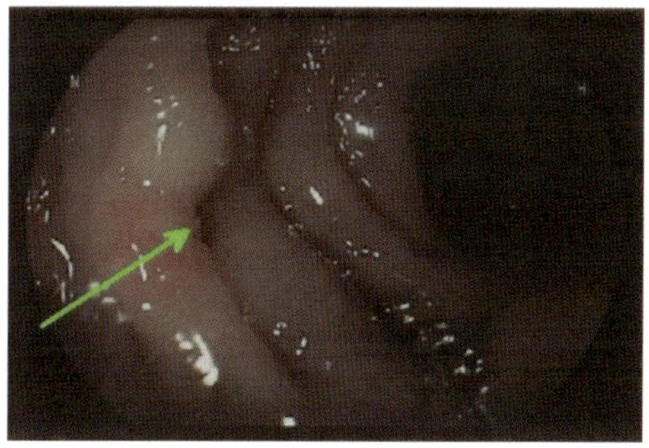

FIGURE 3: Colonoscopy showing the localized edematous area with bluish discoloration 45 cm from the anus that correlated with the area revealed in the CT scan. Green arrow denotes the edematous area on colonoscopy about 45 cm from anus which likely represents fistula's opening.

The ERCP did not show an extravasation of contrast. The surgery team decided to proceed with surgery, as the patient continued to have symptoms. A pancreatectomy, splenectomy, and partial left colectomy were performed. It was possible to visualize the posterior colonic surface near the splenic flexure intraoperatively, which showed a connection between the colon and the pancreas. The patient showed improvement postoperatively, with complete resolution of his symptoms. He continued to attend surgery and gastroenterology clinics.

3. Discussion

Acute pancreatitis is an acute inflammatory condition of the pancreas. It is characterized by abdominal pain and elevated serum levels of pancreatic enzymes, primarily amylase and lipase [1]. Chronic pancreatitis is an enduring and progressive fibroinflammatory process that eventually leads to permanent pancreatic structural damage, resulting in exocrine and endocrine dysfunction [2].

Acute pancreatitis is not uncommon, with a reported annual incidence ranging from 4.9 to 35 per 100,000 individuals [3]. The overall mortality rate of acute pancreatitis is approximately 5%. Acute necrotizing pancreatitis usually is associated with a worse prognosis than acute interstitial pancreatitis. The mortality rate is 17% versus 3%, respectively [4].

Colonic complications are uncommon with acute and chronic pancreatitis [5–7]. However, they have been reported and are potentially serious. Different studies have shown an incidence of 3.3%–6.1% of acute pancreatitis [5, 8]. The incidence increased to 15% among patients with acute severe pancreatitis [5]. These complications are of variable severity. They include but are not limited to a localized ileus, obstruction due to severe edema or inflammation, colonic ischemia with or without necrosis, hemorrhage, and fistula formation [5, 7].

CPFs occur in 3%–10% of patients with severe acute pancreatitis [5, 8–10]. They can occur with chronic pancreatitis as well [8]. The time course between acute pancreatitis and CPF formation is variable, ranging from 10 to 180 days, according to different studies [5, 16]. Due to the anatomical proximity, the left side of the colon is more commonly involved in CPFs [17].

The clinical presentation of CPFs is either colonic symptoms such as bleeding or diarrhea or common symptoms of acute pancreatitis such as pain, nausea, and vomiting [5, 9]. Gastrointestinal bleeding is one of the most common presentations of CPFs, with 60% of patients presenting with it [18].

CT scan of the abdomen with or without contrast is useful in the diagnosis of CPFs and all pancreatic-enteric fistulas in general [11]. Additionally, colonoscopy usually detects many cases, including the patient in this report. However, the patient could have numerous fistulas at the time of surgery [9].

In contrast to upper pancreatic-enteric fistulas, which may close spontaneously, CPFs generally are less likely to close spontaneously [5, 8]. They are associated with a higher risk of complications, including spontaneous or persistent infection, severe hemorrhage, perforation, or overwhelming infections [5, 8]. Therefore, more definitive treatment is recommended, typically with surgery [5, 6, 8, 10].

Surgery usually involves resection of the involved part of the colon with or without a distal pancreatectomy. A diverting ileostomy, to preserve the colon, was reported in less severe cases [5, 6, 10]. Drainage of any abscess in the peripancreatic area or around the fistula is also necessary [10, 16].

Less invasive interventions such as endoscopic treatment have been described in some cases [12–15, 19–23]. However, there are no clear guidelines for the use of these techniques as standard treatment until now [13]. Fibrin glue alone can be used, especially in small fistulas [24]. The use of hemoclips, either via the conventional hemoclips or via an over-the-scope clip system, were described in many case reports with favorable outcomes [13, 19, 20]. Over the scope clip system is a technique that involves mechanical compression of the gastrointestinal tissue which facilitates tissue entrapment [21]. It was introduced by Kirschniak et al. [22] and has been used in management of gastrointestinal bleeding, compression of large vessels, and closure of defects along the gastrointestinal tract [21]. In general, these endoscopic techniques are more suitable to close small defects <10 mm in diameter [19]. Will et al. [23] described a unique endoscopic technique to close the colonic end of the fistula with ligation bands, endoloops, fibrin glue, and hemoclips. This technique involves an endoscopic rendezvous that approached both ends of the fistula simultaneously.

In our case, the radiological evidence of colonic wall thickening and the proximity between the pancreases and the colon raised the suspicion of CPFs. This was supported by the growth of enteric Gram-negative rods in the FNA and the colonoscopic findings. The challenging point in the diagnosis was the failure of the ERCP to show the extravasation of the contrast. Nevertheless, we think that this can be explained by the complexity in the anatomy of the fistula that prevented the contrast from passing. In this case, the multidisciplinary decision was made to proceed with surgery, given the clinical symptoms and all the evidence described above. The direct visualization of the communication between the pancreas and the colon intraoperatively added additional evidence of the presence of CPF. The standard surgical intervention was performed based on the availability of resources and expertise. Hopefully, clear guidelines can be developed so that patients do not have to undergo these invasive procedures.

4. Conclusion

Colonic complications, including CPFs, are uncommon with acute and chronic pancreatitis. However, they are reported and potentially serious. A definitive treatment, typically with surgery, is usually recommended. Less invasive interventions such as endoscopic treatment have been described as well.

Consent

The patient has provided permission to publish these features of his case, and the identity of the patient has been protected.

Disclosure

The case abstract was accepted for poster presentation in the American College of Gastroenterology (ACG) 2015 Annual Scientific Meeting. The abstract was published in a special supplement of the American Journal of Gastroenterology (AJG).

Authors' Contributions

All authors contributed to the manuscript. Mouhanna Abu Ghanimeh and Omar Abughanimeh wrote the manuscript. Khalil Abuamr edited the initial manuscript draft and provided endoscopy images. Osama Yousef and Esmat Sadeddin reviewed, edited, and approved the final manuscript.

References

[1] H. Sarles, *Pancreatitis symposium*, S. K. Basel, Ed., Marseille, France, 1963.

[2] M. L. Steer, I. Waxman, and S. Freedman, "Chronic pancreatitis," *The New England Journal of Medicine*, vol. 332, no. 22, pp. 1482–1490, 1995.

[3] N. J. Talley, G. R. Locke, and Y. A. Saito, "Pancreatitis," in *GI Epidemiology*, N. Talley, S. Locke, and W. Saito, Eds., Blackwell Publishing, Malden, MA, USA, 2007.

[4] P. A. Banks and M. L. Freeman, "Practice guidelines in acute pancreatitis," *American Journal of Gastroenterology*, vol. 101, no. 10, pp. 2379–2400, 2006.

[5] S. R. Mohamed and A. K. Siriwardena, "Understanding the colonic complications of pancreatitis," *Pancreatology*, vol. 8, no. 2, pp. 153–158, 2008.

[6] H. S. Ho, "Gastrointestinal and Pancreatic Complications Associated With Severe Pancreatitis," *JAMA Surgery*, vol. 130, no. 8, p. 817, 1995.

[7] M. C. Aldridge, N. D. Francis, and H. A. F. Dudley, "Colonic complications of severe acute pancreatitis," *British Journal of Surgery*, vol. 76, no. 4, pp. 362–367, 1989.

[8] D. B. Adams, B. R. Davis, and M. C. Anderson, "Colonic complications of pancreatitis," *The American Surgeon*, vol. 60, no. 1, pp. 44–49, 1994.

[9] R. Kochhar, K. Jain, V. Gupta et al., "Fistulization in the GI tract in acute pancreatitis," *Gastrointestinal Endoscopy*, vol. 75, no. 2, pp. 436–440, 2012.

[10] A. Suzuki, S. Suzuki, T. Sakaguchi et al., "Colonic fistula associated with severe acute pancreatitis: Report of two cases," *Surgery Today*, vol. 38, no. 2, pp. 178–183, 2008.

[11] Y. K. Tsou, Y. Y. Chu, and C. H. Lin, "Education and imaging. Gastrointestinal: Spontaneous pancreaticoduodenal fistula associated with acute necrotizing pancreatitis," *Journal of Gastroenterology and Hepatology*, vol. 25, no. 1, p. 217, 2010.

[12] Z. R. Heeter, E. Hauptmann, R. Crane et al., "Pancreaticocolonic fistulas secondary to severe acute pancreatitis treated by percutaneous drainage: successful nonsurgical outcomes in a single-center case series," *Journal of Vascular and Interventional Radiology*, vol. 24, no. 1, pp. 122–129, 2013.

[13] D. M. Gray and D. K. Mullady, "Attempted Endoscopic Closure of a Pancreaticocolonic Fistula with an Over-The-Scope Clip," *JOP*, vol. 13, pp. 712–714, 2012.

[14] S. O. Hwang, T. H. Lee, J. W. Park, S. Park, and S. Kim, "Endoscopic management of multiple colonic fistulae secondary to acute pancreatitis (with video)," *Gastrointestinal Endoscopy*, vol. 71, no. 2, pp. 395–397, 2010.

[15] J. Halttunen, L. Weckman, E. Kemppainen, and M. L. Kylänpää, "The endoscopic management of pancreatic fistulas," *Surgical Endoscopy*, vol. 19, no. 4, pp. 559–562, 2005.

[16] P. Negro, L. DAmore, G. Flati et al., "Colonic involvement in pancreatitis. Six cases more," *International Surgery*, vol. 76, no. 2, p. 122, 1991.

[17] H. Abcarian, M. Eftaiha, A. R. Kraft, and L. M. Nyhus, "Colonic Complications of Acute Pancreatitis," *JAMA Surgery*, vol. 114, no. 9, pp. 995–1001, 1979.

[18] T. V. Berne and H. A. Edmondson, "Colonic fistulization due to pancreatitis," *The American Journal of Surgery*, vol. 111, no. 3, pp. 359–363, 1966.

[19] Y. Igarashi, T. Mimura, Y. Kishimoto et al., "Severe acute pancreatitis with complicating colonic fistula successfully closed using the over-the-scope clip system," *Case Reports in Gastroenterology*, vol. 7, no. 2, pp. 314–321, 2013.

[20] D. Von Renteln, A. Schmidt, M. C. Vassiliou, H.-U. Rudolph, M. Gieselmann, and K. Caca, "Endoscopic closure of large colonic perforations using an over-the-scope clip: A randomized controlled porcine study," *Endoscopy*, vol. 41, no. 6, pp. 481–486, 2009.

[21] T. H. Kothari, G. Haber, N. Sonpal, and N. Karanth, "The over-the-scope clip system—a novel technique for gastrocutaneous fistula closure: the first North American experience," *Canadian Journal of Gastroenterology & Hepatology*, vol. 26, no. 4, pp. 193–195, 2012.

[22] A. Kirschniak, T. Kratt, D. Stüker, A. Braun, M.-O. Schurr, and A. Königsrainer, "A new endoscopic over-the-scope clip system for treatment of lesions and bleeding in the GI tract: first clinical experiences," *Gastrointestinal Endoscopy*, vol. 66, no. 1, pp. 162–167, 2007.

[23] U. Will, F. Meyer, S. Hartmeier, H. Schramm, and H. Bosseckert, "Endoscopic treatment of a pseudocystocolonic fistula by band ligation and endoloop application: Case report," *Gastrointestinal Endoscopy*, vol. 59, no. 4, pp. 581–583, 2004.

[24] J. Karvonen, R. Gullichsen, P. Salminen, and J. M. Grnroos, "Endoscopic treatment of pseudocystocolonic fistula with fibrin glue," *Gastrointestinal Endoscopy*, vol. 72, no. 3, pp. 664-665, 2010.

Acute Clinical Manifestation of Mesenteric Heterotopic Pancreatitis: A Pre- and Postoperative Confirmed Case

Bente M. de Kok,[1] Fleur I. de Korte,[1] Lars E. Perk,[2] Valeska Terpstra,[3] J. Sven D. Mieog,[4] and Frank M. Zijta[1]

[1]*Department of Radiology, Haaglanden Medical Centre, Lijnbaan 32, 2512 VA The Hague, Netherlands*
[2]*Department of Gastroenterology, Haaglanden Medical Centre, Lijnbaan 32, 2512 VA The Hague, Netherlands*
[3]*Department of Pathology, Haaglanden Medical Centre, Lijnbaan 32, 2512 VA The Hague, Netherlands*
[4]*Department of Surgery, Leiden University Medical Centre, Albinusdreef 2, 2333 ZA, Leiden, Netherlands*

Correspondence should be addressed to Bente M. de Kok; bentedekok@hotmail.com

Academic Editor: Shiro Kikuchi

Heterotopic pancreas is a relatively uncommon congenital anomaly, defined as pancreatic tissue in ectopic sites without an anatomic and vascular continuity with the main body of the pancreas. We report the case of a 58-year-old woman who was admitted to the hospital with the clinical suspicion of a mild, acute pancreatitis. Computed tomography, magnetic resonance imaging, transabdominal ultrasound, and endoscopic ultrasound revealed a normal orthotopic pancreas and the suspicion of a large heterotopic pancreas in the small bowel mesentery with signs of acute inflammation. The diagnosis of mesenteric heterotopic pancreatitis was preoperatively confirmed by endoscopic ultrasound-guided fine-needle aspiration and consequently histologically established after surgical resection.

1. Introduction

Heterotopic pancreas, also referred to as ectopic pancreas, aberrant pancreas, or choristoma, is defined as the presence of pancreatic tissue in ectopic sites which lacks an anatomic and vascular continuity with the main body of the orthotopic pancreas. Although it is the most common heterotopia within the gastrointestinal system, it still concerns a relatively uncommon entity with prevalence at autopsy studies ranging from 0.6 to 13.7% [1]. Most prevalent anatomic sites include the stomach, duodenum, and jejunum, whereas a manifestation in the small bowel mesentery is fairly rare. Though the majority of patients are asymptomatic, with lesions being incidentally detected at unrelated surgery or autopsy, patients with heterotopic pancreas may present with clinically significant pathology, identical to the normal pancreas.

2. Case Report

A 58-year-old woman presented to the Emergency Room with an acute, 4-hour history of increasing continuous abdominal pain. The pain was severe and associated with nausea and vomiting. She reported not having a medical history, no history of a similar episode of abdominal pain, no alcohol consumption, and no smoking. Physical examination revealed generalized abdominal pain. The vital signs were stable. Early laboratory values included a normal white blood cell count ($8.8 * 10^9$/L) and a normal C-reactive protein (CRP) level (3 mg/L, reference range 0–8 mg/L). Serum amylase was increased (417 U/L; reference value < 107 U/L). Liver function tests results were within normal ranges. Besides a significantly increased urine amylase (2286 U/L, reference range 0–460 U/L), urinalysis was normal. Additionally, abdominal ultrasound was performed but the diagnostic value was limited because of body habitus. The ultrasound examination revealed a small amount of fluid around the liver. There was no evidence of cholelithiasis. The pancreas was not conclusively visualized. With the suspicion of a mild, acute pancreatitis, based on both clinical and laboratory findings, the patient was admitted to the hospital for conservative treatment and both biochemical and radiologic follow-up.

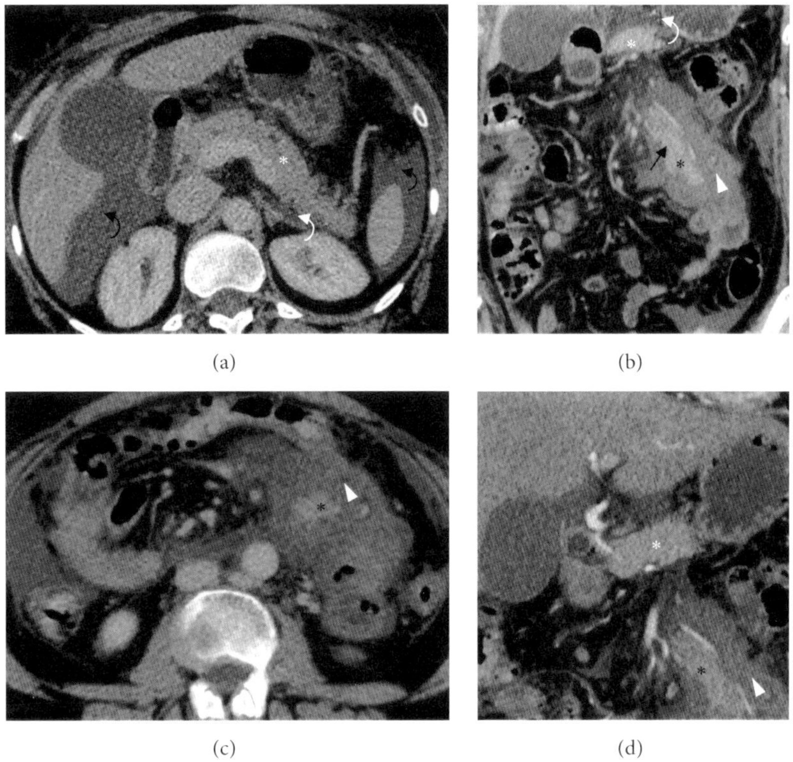

FIGURE 1: CT scan performed at the third day of admission. (a) Axial CT image in the portal venous phase. Normal appearance of the orthotopic pancreas *(white asterisks)*. A nonsignificant small amount of retroperitoneal fluid on the level of the pancreas tail *(white curved arrows)*. Presence of a large amount of free intraperitoneal fluid *(black curved arrows)*. (b-c) Coronal and axial CT image in the portal venous phase. Enhancing soft tissue mass *(black asterisk)* with surrounding mesenteric edema *(white arrowhead)*. Suggestion of a central ductal structure *(black arrow)*. (d) Coronal CT image in the early arterial phase shows a comparable enhancement of the orthotopic and heterotopic pancreas *(resp., white and black asterisks)*.

During admission, the abdominal pain persisted despite pain medication and the level of CRP increased, reaching its maximum of 580 mg/L on day 3. According to the hospital protocol, an abdominal computed tomography (CT) was performed on the third day after onset.

CT revealed a normal morphology and homogenous enhancement of the pancreas, with only a small amount of fluid located around the tail of the gland (Figure 1(a)). The presence of free intraperitoneal fluid was observed in the posterior right subhepatic space, left subphrenic space, paracolic spaces, and pelvis. An enhancing soft tissue mass in the centre of the jejunal mesentery was observed with adjacent increased attenuation of the mesenteric fat and enlarged surrounding lymph nodes. The mass measured up to 8 centimeters in long axis and demonstrated a lobulated morphology. Enhancement characteristics were comparable with normal pancreas enhancement. Also, the presence of a central ductal, tubular structure was suggested (Figures 1(b)–1(d)). Based on both imaging findings and laboratory results, the suspicion of a heterotopic pancreatitis was proposed.

To confirm the hypothesis of heterotopic pancreatitis, an additional targeted ultrasound and magnetic resonance imaging (MRI) of the abdomen were performed. Ultrasound depicted a nonspecific hypoechoic region in the mesentery with a central, lobulated, unsharp delineated, more hyperechoic soft tissue mass (Figure 2(a)). MRI with limited series was performed, including a fat-saturated gradient echo sequence TRUFI (true fast imaging with steady-state free precession) in the coronal plane, an ultrafast gradient echo (VIBE) in the axial plane, and an in-phase and out-of-phase gradient echo sequence in the axial plane. Quality of both axial sequences was limited due to motion-related artefacts in the ill, painful patient. No chemical shift artefacts supporting the heterotopic pancreas-hypothesis were apparent. The coronal TRUFI revealed a mesenteric soft tissue mass with signal characteristics resembling the orthotopic pancreas, surrounding inflammatory changes, and a possible duct (Figure 2(b)); however, these findings were noncontributory for the diagnosis. Additional laboratory findings included a normal carcinoembryonic antigen (CEA) and Cancer Antigen 19.9 level. The Cancer Antigen 125 (CA-125) level was 208 (normal range 0–35 kU/l). Yet both pancreatic cancer and pancreatitis can cause a high level of CA-125; therefore, this was regarded as an unspecific, nondifferentiating finding.

In order to rule out a malignancy and to confirm the diagnosis of heterotopic pancreatic tissue, the gastroenterologist performed an endoscopic ultrasound (EUS) with additional fine-needle aspiration (FNA). EUS performed from

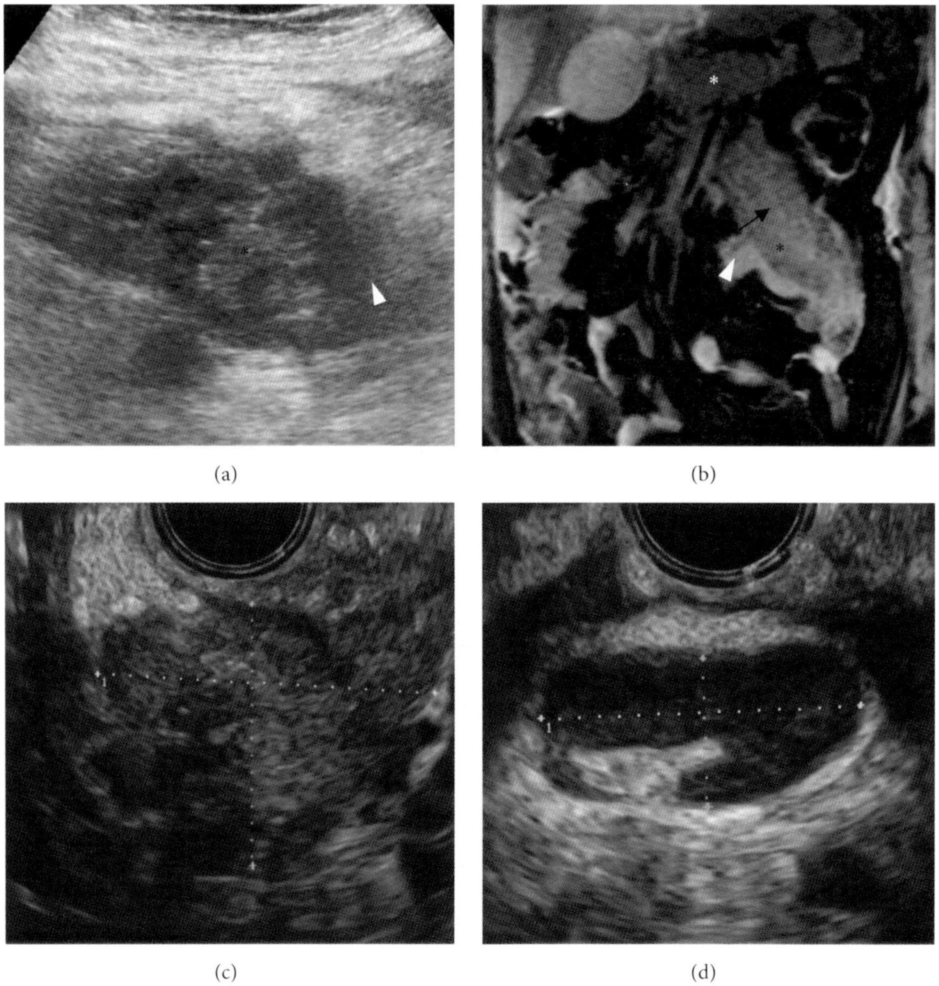

FIGURE 2: (a) Ultrasound image of the mesenteric soft tissue mass *(black asterisks)* with surrounding inflammatory changes *(white arrowhead)*. (b) Coronal TRUFI image depicting the soft tissue mass with signal characteristics according to the orthotopic pancreas *(white asterisk)*. Surrounding, edematous inflammatory changes *(white arrowhead)* and a possible central duct *(black arrow)*. (c) EUS image of the hypoechoic mesenteric soft tissue mass, in the transversal plane measuring approximately 3 × 4 cm. (d). EUS image of an enlarged mesenteric lymph node, with a short axis of 9 mm, demonstrating no suspicious morphological features.

the horizontal part of duodenum showed a hypoechogenic mass of 3 × 4 cm with indistinct delineation and poor vascularisation with adjacent enlarged lymph nodes and inflammatory changes (Figures 2(c) and 2(d)). Endoscopic ultrasound-guided FNA of the soft tissue mass and the largest surrounding lymph node was performed. Cytopathologic examination revealed benign cells; the soft tissue mass was classified as pancreatitis not otherwise specified (NOS). There were no preexisting pancreatic cells distinguishable due to the inflammation; the lymph node was classified as lymphadenitis accordingly.

After one week of conservative treatment, acute clinical findings resolved and laboratory results improved, consequently the patient was discharged from the hospital. A follow-up CT scan of the abdomen, six weeks after admission, revealed the soft tissue mass with substantial regression of inflammatory changes. There were no complications such as cyst formation or necrosis. The orthotopic pancreas was unremarkable (Figure 3).

To conclusively validate the earlier clinical hypothesis and to further analyze the lymph nodes that had increased in size, an additional EUS was executed. EUS performed from the horizontal part of the duodenum depicted the pancreas-like mass with apparent ductal structures (Figure 4). The mass is evidently more hyperechoic than during the episode of inflammation (Figure 2(c)). No definite dominant duct was recognized, and there were no suspicious lymph nodes. Furthermore, FNA of the pancreas-like tissue was repeated. Cytopathologic examination confirmed the hypothesis of heterotopic pancreas showing pancreatic epithelium with both acini and ducts (Figure 5).

The diagnostic findings and the possibility of a resection were discussed with the patient. Given the risk of recurrent episodes of pancreatitis and consequently more challenging surgery and possible malignant degeneration [1–4], the multidisciplinary team advised on a resection of the heterotopic pancreas. The patient followed this advice and underwent surgery. Through a midline incision the

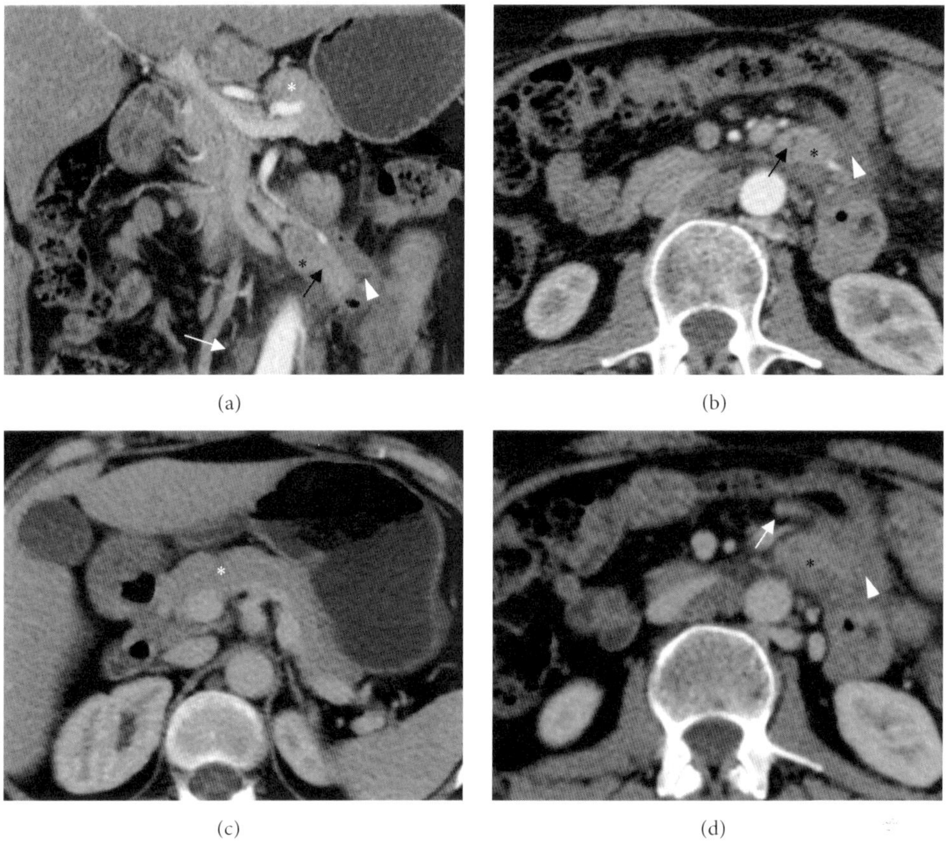

Figure 3: CT scan performed six weeks after admission. (a-b) Coronal and axial image in the arterial phase. (c-d) Axial images in the portal venous phase. Intra-abdominal free fluid is completely resolved. Heterotopic pancreas *(black asterisks)* in the mesentery with attenuation characteristics after intravenous contrast comparable to the orthotopic pancreas *(white asterisks)*. Moreover, presence of a central duct is suggested *(black arrow)*. There is an apparent decrease in inflammatory changes *(white arrowheads)* surrounding the heterotopic pancreas, though several adjacent mesenteric lymph nodes have increased in size *(white arrows)*.

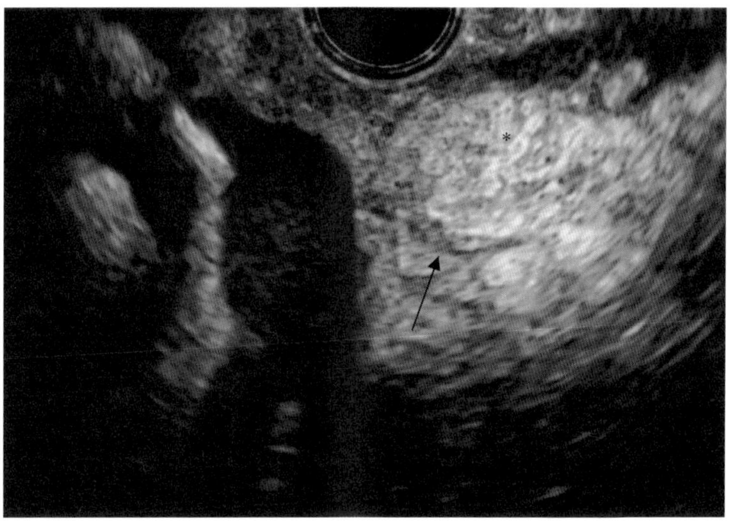

Figure 4: EUS image of the hyperechoic mesenteric soft tissue mass *(black asterisk)* with a hypoechoic, ductal structure *(black arrow)*.

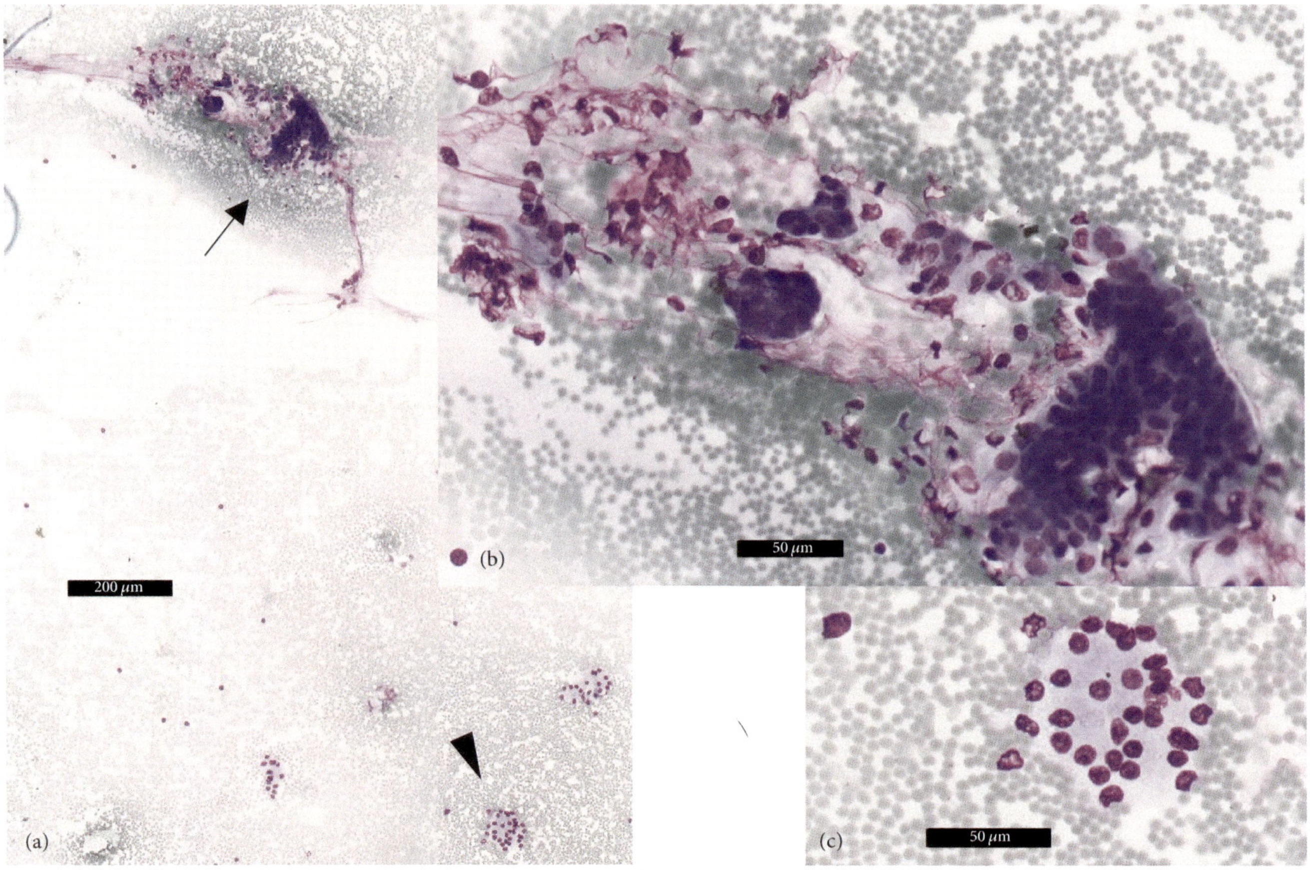

FIGURE 5: Fine-needle aspirate of the mesenteric soft tissue mass, MGG staining. (a) Overview, magnification 50x. Both groups of ductal cells *(black arrow)* and acinar cells *(black arrowhead)* are depicted in this image. (b) Magnification 200x, details of the cylindrical ductal cells. (c) Magnification 200x, details of the acinar pancreatic cells.

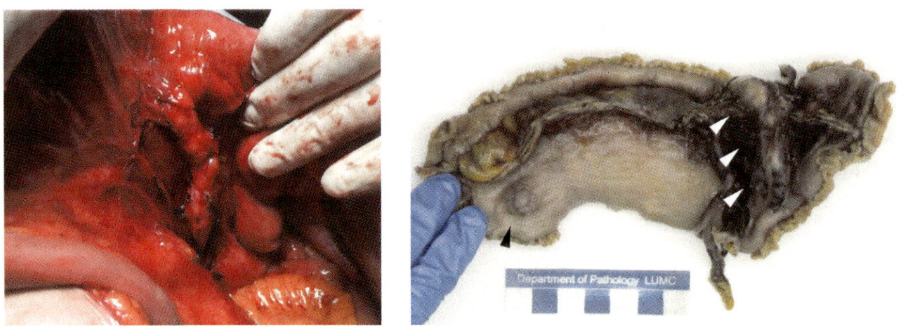

FIGURE 6: (a) Intraoperative view on the proximal jejunum and its mesentery showing the heterotopic pancreas extending centrally. (b) Gross specimen of the segment resection after the jejunum is opened, demonstrating the heterotopic pancreas *(white arrowheads)* connected to the jejunum and the second manifestation of heterotopic pancreas in the serosa of the jejunum *(black arrowhead)*.

heterotopic pancreas was identified in the mesentery of the proximal jejunum approximately 5 cm distally of the ligament of Treitz (Figure 6(a)). The ligament was ligated, and the distal duodenum and proximal jejunum were mobilised. The heterotopic pancreas extended to the central mesenteric root, of which it could be dissected without compromising the mesenteric vascular supply. From a few centimeters of the jejunum, the mesenteric vessels were ligated, and a segment resection of the proximal jejunum was performed. The resection included a second spot of presumed heterotopic pancreas at the antimesenteric side of the jejunum, several centimeters distally of the primary heterotopic pancreas (Figure 6(b)). An enlarged mesenteric lymph node was sent for intraoperative frozen section analysis and was reported as benign. A primary end-to-end anastomosis was constructed. The postoperative course was uneventful. Pathological analysis revealed two locations of heterotopic pancreas of 6.5 cm and 1.5 cm with minimal signs of pancreatitis. The heterotopic pancreas contained acini, ducts, and islet cells.

3. Discussion

Generally considered a developmental anomaly, heterotopic pancreas is defined as anatomically separated pancreatic tissue from the main gland, without vascular or ductal continuity. Most cases of heterotopic pancreas are found in the upper gastrointestinal tract with 70–87% of cases affecting the stomach, duodenum, and jejunum in mostly submucosal localization [1, 5]. Less common sites of origin include Meckel diverticulum, ileum, gallbladder, bile ducts, Fallopian tubes, mediastinum, oesophagus, spleen, omentum, and mesentery [2, 5, 6]. Zhang et al. [7] and Henry et al. [6] report the mesenteric manifestation in, respectively, 3.8% and 5.9% of the heterotopic pancreas.

The exact embryologic basis of heterotopic pancreas is unknown, but there are three apprehended theories. The most widely held theory is the misplacement theory, which states that deposits of pancreatic tissue are "dropped" into the developing gastrointestinal system [2, 8, 9]. This would explain why the majority of cases of heterotopic pancreas are found in other derivatives of the primitive foregut. The two other theories include the metaplasia and the totipotent cell theory, which state the migration with transformation and, respectively, differentiation of endodermal cells into pancreatic tissue [2, 5, 9]. Histologically the heterotopic pancreas mimics the orthotopic pancreas. Gross specimens demonstrate a firm mass with a lobular shape and a well-defined interface with surrounding tissues. Microscopically, the heterotopic mesenteric pancreas infiltrates the bowel wall and extends into the submucosal layer. Four types of heterotopic pancreas are described in the histologic classification system by Fuentes (1973). The first and most common type of heterotopic pancreatic tissue is composed of all the elements of normal pancreas, including acini, ducts, and islet cells. The second, third, and fourth are dominated by, respectively, acini, ducts, and islet cells [2]. Based on histopathologic findings, our patient was classified as a type 1 heterotopic pancreas, containing acini, ducts, and islet cells.

It has been reported that the enhancement pattern of heterotopic pancreas varies depending on the microscopic composition and therefore can differ from the main pancreas. This can cause an unreliable differentiation from other homogenous enhancing tumours, such as gastrointestinal stromal tumour (GIST), carcinoid, lymphoma, or metastasis [10, 11]. Nevertheless, several characteristic CT features of heterotopic mesenteric pancreas resemble the orthotopic pancreas; these include a homogenous, well-enhancing lobulated mass with an elongated appearance. Most mesenteric manifestations have a close relation to the jejunum. The presence of a duct allows differentiation of manifest heterotopic pancreas from other masses [11]. The ductal system communicates with the bowel lumen, which might be difficult to visualize at various imaging modalities. MR cholangiopancreatography (MRCP) is the imaging method of choice to depict an ectopic duct, pathognomonic of ectopic pancreas [5, 12]. Unfortunately, in our patient no MRCP was performed. Possibly partly because of that, the MRI was not fully conclusive. Other contributing factors for the interpretability might have been motion artefacts and the performance in the acute phase, edema impeding identification of an apparent ductal morphology.

Most heterotopic pancreatic lesions exist solitary, in contrast with both the jejunal and mesenteric manifestation in our case, and measure smaller than 3.0 cm. A heterotopic mesenteric manifestation has a mean long axis diameter of 4.4 cm. It typically presents as an elongated lobulated lesion (long- to short-diameter ratio of 3.0) showing a broad base on the jejunal mesenteric side, tapering as it extends centrally into the mesentery [2, 11]. To our knowledge, the heterotopic pancreas in our case is with a long axis diameter of 8 cm on CT, the longest mesenteric pancreas described. In the acute phase, the heterotopic pancreas was swollen due to edema, and the gross specimen measured 6.5 cm. Shin et al. [8] described a patient with a 20 cm diameter heterotopic mass in the jejunal mesentery with a conglomerate of adjacent loops of jejunum, presenting with gastrointestinal bleeding. The article did not appoint the true size of the mass at histologic examination.

Characteristically, the majority of patients are asymptomatic, with lesions being incidentally detected at surgery, endoscopy, or autopsy. Complications of heterotopic pancreas may or may not be related to pathologic conditions of the pancreas itself. Those related might present with inflammation, (pseudo)cyst formation, endocrine (dys)function, or malignant degeneration [3, 4, 7, 9, 10, 13–17]. The pathologically unrelated cases might present with mechanical obstruction, intussusception, or bleeding [2, 8, 13].

Heterotopic pancreatitis is a recognized complication that is usually only detected at microscopy and is rarely diagnosed clinically or radiologically, especially in cases of submucosal manifestations. Usually, the elevation of serum amylase and lipase is modest due to the small volume of pancreatic tissue in the heterotopic tissue [5]. In our case, a relatively large heterotopic volume with clinically significant elevated serum amylase and C-reactive protein levels facilitated a preoperative clinical diagnosis. It must be noted though that the second serosal localization, which was depicted intraoperatively, was not depicted on preoperative imaging.

In case of an asymptomatic patient and histopathologically confirmed diagnosis, a conservative management might be applicable. However, in case of a symptomatic patient or if accurate differentiation from other benign or malignant aetiologies cannot be accurately made, curative resection of the heterotopic pancreas is usually considered [5]. The patient in this case was obviously symptomatic and had been admitted to the hospital for one week. In view of a potential recurrent pancreatitis and the low but not excluded risk of a malignant degeneration, both the patient and the multidisciplinary team decided on surgical resection [3, 4, 9].

4. Conclusion

Heterotopic pancreas is a relatively uncommon congenital anomaly. Most cases concerning solitary lesions were found in the upper gastrointestinal tract in submucosal localization. Though the majority of patients are asymptomatic, patients may present with clinically significant pathology such as inflammation or malignant degeneration, identical to the normal, orthotopic pancreas. We report a case of symptomatic, heterotopic pancreatitis in a patient with heterotopic pancreas tissue in the jejunal serosa and the jejunal mesentery. The clinical diagnosis was made using imaging modalities and cytopathological analysis, that is, ultrasound, CT, MRI, and EUS combined with FNA. Cytopathological examination preoperatively confirmed the diagnosis which is only limitedly reported in current literature. Subsequently it was histopathologically confirmed after complete resection.

Authors' Contributions

Each author had a substantial contribution and met the requirements for authorship. The manuscript has been read and approved by all the authors.

References

[1] E. C. S. Lai and R. K. Tompkins, "Heterotopic pancreas. Review of a 26 year experience," *The American Journal of Surgery*, vol. 151, no. 6, pp. 697–700, 1986.

[2] M. Rezvani, C. Menias, K. Sandrasegaran, J. D. Olpin, K. M. Elsayes, and A. M. Shaaban, "Heterotopic pancreas: Histopathologic features, imaging findings, and complications," *RadioGraphics*, vol. 37, no. 2, pp. 484–499, 2017.

[3] J. C. T. Wong, C. Robinson, E. C. Jones et al., "Recurrent ectopic pancreatitis of the jejunum and mesentery over a 30-year period," *Hepatobiliary & Pancreatic Diseases International*, vol. 10, no. 2, pp. 218–220, 2011.

[4] M. Osanai, N. Miyokawa, T. Tamaki, M. Yonekawa, A. Kawamura, and N. Sawada, "Adenocarcinoma arising in gastric heterotopic pancreas: Clinicopathological and immunohistochemical study with genetic analysis of a case," *Pathology International*, vol. 51, no. 7, pp. 549–554, 2001.

[5] A. K. P. Shanbhogue, N. Fasih, V. R. Surabhi, G. P. Doherty, D. K. P. Shanbhogue, and S. K. Sethi, "A clinical and radiologic review of uncommon types and causes of pancreatitis," *RadioGraphics*, vol. 29, no. 4, pp. 1003–1026, 2009.

[6] C. Henry, T. Prot, S. Maitre, J. Nicolet, E. Bonte, and C. Smadja, "A rare cause of acute abdominal pain: mesenteric heterotopic pancreas complicated by acute pancreatitis," *Gastroenterologie Clinique Et Biologique*, vol. 24, no. 3, pp. 370-371, 2000.

[7] Y. Zhang, X. Sun, J. S. Gold et al., "Heterotopic pancreas: A clinicopathological study of 184 cases from a single high-volume medical center in China," *Human Pathology*, vol. 55, pp. 135–142, 2016.

[8] S. S. Shin, Y. Y. Jeong, and H. K. Kang, "Giant heterotopic pancreas in the jejunal mesentery.," *AJR. American journal of roentgenology*, vol. 189, no. 5, pp. W262–263, 2007.

[9] T. Koshinaga, I. Okabe, and Y. Kurosu, "Unique presentation of heterotopic pancreatic tissue arising from small-bowel mesentery," *Pediatric Surgery International*, vol. 11, no. 2-3, pp. 182–184, 1996.

[10] C.-K. Wang, Y.-T. Kuo, K.-W. Yeung, C.-J. Wu, and G.-C. Liu, "CT appearance of ectopic pancreas: A case report," *Abdominal Imaging*, vol. 23, no. 3, pp. 332-333, 1998.

[11] N. Seo and J. H. Kim, "Characteristic CT features of heterotopic pancreas of the mesentery: 'another pancreas' in the mesentery," *Clinical Imaging*, vol. 38, no. 1, pp. 27–30, 2014.

[12] A. C. Silva, J. C. Charles, B. D. Kimery, J. P. Wood, and P. T. Liu, "MR Cholangiopancreatography in the detection of symptomatic ectopic pancreatitis in the small-bowel mesentery," *AJR. American journal of roentgenology*, vol. 187, no. 2, pp. W195–197, 2006.

[13] H. Canbaz, T. Çolak, D. Düşmez Apa, O. Sezgin, and S. Aydin, "An unusual cause of acute abdomen: Mesenteric heterotopic pancreatitis causing confusion in clinical diagnosis," *The Turkish Journal of Gastroenterology*, vol. 20, no. 2, pp. 142–145, 2009.

[14] J. C. Lee, K. P. Wong, S. S. Lo, C. S. Cheng, and K. Y. Lau, "Acute ectopic pancreatitis," *Hong Kong Medical Journal*, vol. 14, no. 6, pp. 501-502, 2008.

[15] F. C. Deprez, C. Pauls, and B. Coulier, "Heterotopic pancreas revealed by post-traumatic pancreatitis," *Journal Belge de Radiologie*, vol. 95, no. 2, pp. 83–86, 2012.

[16] M. Ginsburg, O. Ahmed, K. A. Rana, R. Boumendjel, A. H. Dachman, and M. Zaritzky, "Ectopic pancreas presenting with pancreatitis and a mesenteric mass," *Journal of Pediatric Surgery*, vol. 48, no. 1, pp. E29–E32, 2013.

[17] S. Fam, D. S. O'Briain, and J. A. Borger, "Ectopic pancreas with acute inflammation," *Journal of Pediatric Surgery*, vol. 17, no. 1, pp. 86-87, 1982.

A Case of Advanced Descending Colon Cancer in an Adult Patient with Intestinal Malrotation

Yoshifumi Nakayama,[1,2] Masaki Akiyama,[1,2] Yusuke Sawatsubashi,[1,2] Noritaka Minagawa,[1] Takayuki Torigoe,[1] and Keiji Hirata[1]

[1] *Department of Surgery 1, School of Medicine, University of Occupational and Environmental Health, 1-1 Iseigaoka, Yahata-nishi-ku, Kitakyushu 807-8555, Japan*
[2] *Department of Gastroenterological and General Surgery, Wakamatsu Hospital of University of Occupational and Environmental Health, 1-17-1 Hamamachi, Wakamatsu-ku, Kitakyushu 808-0024, Japan*

Correspondence should be addressed to Yoshifumi Nakayama; nakayama@med.uoeh-u.ac.jp

Academic Editor: Daniel C. Damin

This report presents an operative case of advanced descending colon cancer in an adult patient with intestinal malrotation. A 63-year-old Japanese male was suffering from left side abdominal pain, abdominal distension, and constipation. An endoscopic examination revealed an advanced tumor in the descending colon. Computed tomography (CT) of the abdomen revealed the thickening of the descending colon wall and superior mesenteric vein rotation. An opaque enema detected severe stenosis of the descending colon. An abdominal X-ray examination revealed the dilation of the colon and small intestine with niveau. At the insertion of an ileus tube, the C-loop of the duodenum was observed to be absent and the small intestine was located on the right side of the abdomen. After the decompression of the bowel contents, laparotomy was performed. Descending colon cancer was observed to have directly invaded the left side of the transverse colon. Left hemicolectomy, lymph node dissection, and appendectomy were performed. The patient had an uneventful recovery and was discharged from the hospital on the 16th day after surgery. This report presents a rare operative case of descending colon cancer in an adult patient with intestinal malrotation.

1. Introduction

Intestinal malrotation can be defined as any deviation from the normal 270-degree rotation of the midgut in a counterclockwise direction during embryonic development [1]. Malrotation or nonrotation of the midgut occurs in approximately 1 in 500 live births [1]. Intestinal malrotation is diagnosed during the first month of life in 85–90% of all cases [2]. Intestinal malrotation is rarely present in adulthood. A barium enema study of 2000 adults demonstrated that the prevalence of malrotation was 0.2% [3]. Synchronous colon cancer in adult patients with intestinal malrotation is extremely rare [4].

This report presents a rare case of descending colon cancer in an adult patient with intestinal malrotation.

2. Case Report

A 63-year-old Japanese male presented with the chief complaints of left side abdominal pain, abdominal distension, and constipation. As the patient's symptoms worsened, he underwent an endoscopic examination, which revealed the presence of an ulcerated tumor of the descending colon. He was referred to the surgical outpatient clinic of our hospital with advanced descending colon cancer.

The laboratory data showed the patient had a white blood cell count of 6,200/mm^3, a hemoglobin level of 8.7 g/dL, a hematocrit level of 25.3%, and a platelet count of 401,000/mm^3. The patient's electrolyte and blood urea nitrogen levels were normal, as was his liver function. His CEA and CA19-9 levels were 1.7 ng/mL and CA19-9 was 21.3 U/mL,

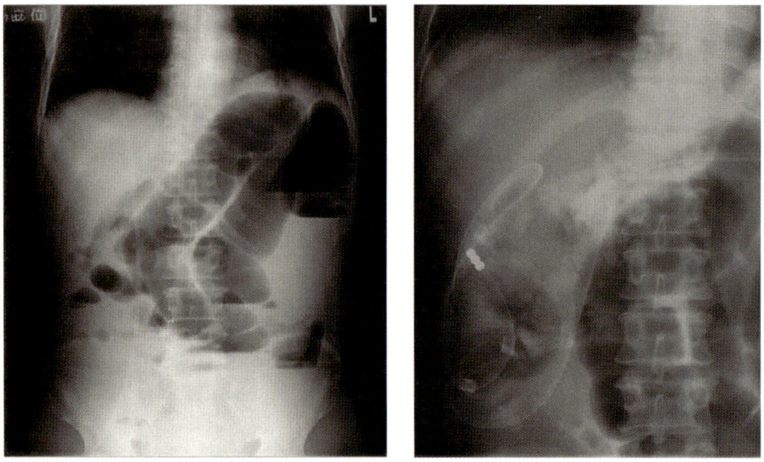

(a) (b)

Figure 1: An abdominal X-ray examination revealed the dilation of the colon and niveau (a). At the insertion of an ileus tube, the C-loop of the duodenum was observed to be absent and the small intestine was located on the right side of the abdomen (b).

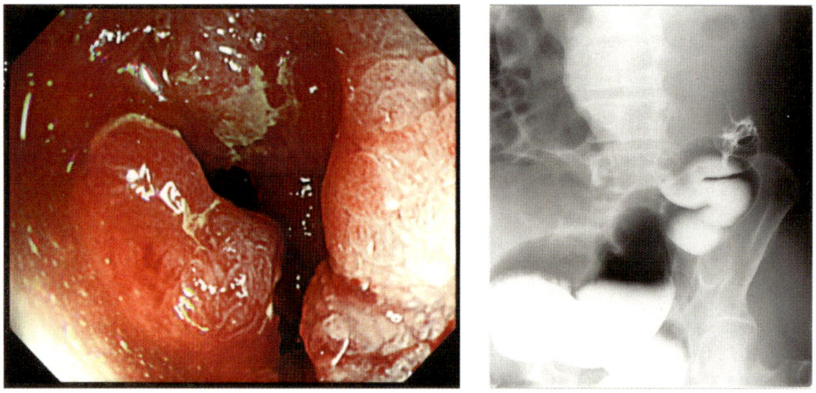

(a) (b)

Figure 2: Colonoscopy revealed an advanced tumor in the descending colon (a). An opaque enema using contrast fluid revealed severe stenosis of the descending colon. The contrast fluid could not pass the stenotic part of the descending colon (b).

respectively. An abdominal X-ray examination revealed a dilated colon and niveau (Figure 1(a)). These findings were consistent with bowel obstruction. Computed tomography (CT) of the abdomen revealed the thickening of the descending colon wall, which was indicative of advanced descending colon cancer (Figure 3(a)); superior mesenteric vein rotation was also observed (Figure 3(b)). Colonoscopy revealed an advanced tumor in the descending colon (Figure 2(a)). The biopsy specimen was found to be moderately differentiated tubular adenocarcinoma. An opaque enema, using contrast fluid, revealed severe stenosis of the descending colon. The contrast fluid could not pass the stenosis (Figure 2(b)). At the insertion of an ileus tube, the C-loop of the duodenum was observed to be absent and the small intestine was located on the right side of the abdomen (Figure 1(b)). After the decompression of the bowel contents, laparotomy was performed. The small intestine was located on the right side of the abdomen. The appendix, cecum, and ascending colon were located in the middle abdomen. Descending colon cancer was observed to have directly invaded the left side of the transverse colon (Figure 4(a)). Left hemicolectomy, lymph node dissection, and appendectomy were performed. A histopathological examination with hematoxylin and eosin staining of the resected lesion revealed moderately differentiated adenocarcinoma (Figure 4(b)). No metastatic regional lymph nodes were identified. However, some lymphatic and venous invasion of the carcinoma cells was observed.

The patient had an uneventful recovery and was discharged from the hospital on the 16th day after surgery. He has been followed up in the outpatient clinic without recurrence for approximately 9 years.

3. Discussion

Given that intestinal malrotation in adults is not common and is usually asymptomatic [3], the clinical importance of intestinal malrotation in adults is less well documented than in children. Most of the clinical symptoms of this disorder are

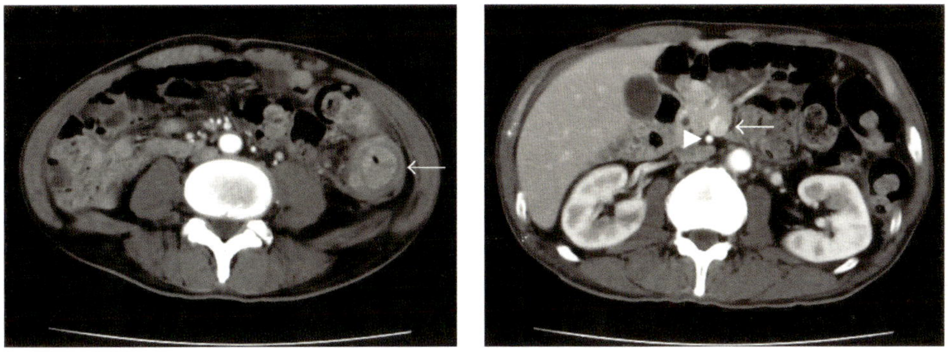

(a) (b)

Figure 3: Computed tomography (CT) of the abdomen revealed thickening of the descending colon wall, which was indicative of advanced descending colon cancer (arrow) (a); superior mesenteric vein rotation was also observed (arrow) (b).

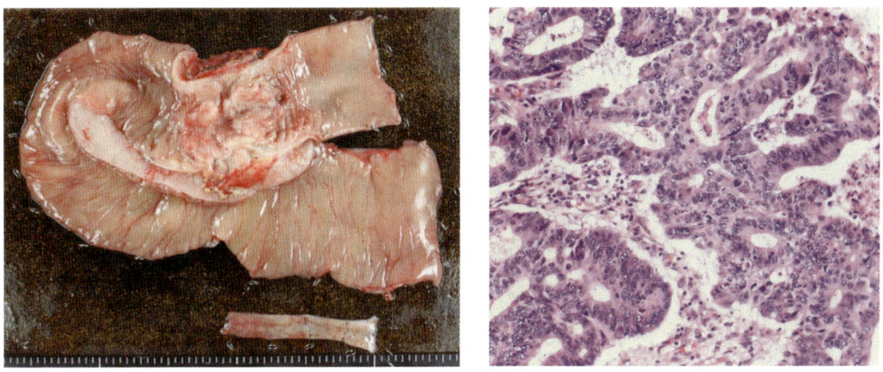

(a) (b)

Figure 4: An operative specimen revealed advanced descending colon cancer with direct invasion of the transverse colon (a). A histopathological examination with hematoxylin and eosin staining confirmed that the lesion was moderately differentiated tubular adenocarcinoma (b).

due to the presence of coincidental intestinal disease. Many cases of adult intestinal malrotation are only discovered coincidentally at surgery for other diseases. In the present case, clinical symptoms of the patient, which included abdominal pain, abdominal distension, and constipation, occurred due to descending colon cancer with bowel obstruction, which was coincidental with the intestinal malrotation.

Intestinal malrotation has been divided into four types: nonrotation type, malrotation type, reversed rotation type, and paraduodenal hernia type, according to the arrest point of development (during embryonic development) anywhere along the rotation of the midgut in a counterclockwise direction [17]. Kato et al. summarized the Japanese literature and reported the frequency of each of the types of adult intestinal malrotation (nonrotation type (53.3%), malrotation type (31.1%), reversed rotation type (6.7%), and paraduodenal hernia type (8.9%)) [18]. The present case seemed to correspond to the nonrotation type, which is the most frequent one. Moreover, in 82.8% of the colorectal cancer patients with intestinal malrotation, the malrotation was classified as nonrotation type [19]. Table 1 shows that nonrotation type malrotation occurred most frequently (75.0%) in colorectal cancer patients with intestinal malrotation.

Table 1 summarized the cases of colon cancer in adult patients with intestinal malrotation that are reported in the English literature, excepting the coexistent cases with situs inversus totalis [4–16]. Most of the patients had right-sided colon cancer (Table 1). Left-sided colon cancer is rare in adult patients with intestinal malrotation. The rate of left-sided colon cancer was 14.3% (Table 1). Anatomical disorders of the placement in this type of intestinal malrotation may be associated with carcinogenesis in the colon. Ren and Lu suggested that malrotation of the gut which may cause chronic bowel obstruction may lead to inflammation and carcinogenesis [8].

There are some problems at the operation in the cases of synchronous colon cancer in adult patients with intestinal malrotation. One of these problems is arterial and venous variations. Before the operation, confirm the presence of arterial and venous variations via enhanced CT. In the case of our patient, superior mesenteric vein rotation (Figure 3(b)) and anomalies were identified. It is important to understand vessel anomalies on CT angiography or enhanced CT scan before surgery [19]. Based on the imaging information, the regional lymph node dissection could be performed along with the arteries.

Table 1: Case reports of colon cancer in adult patient with intestinal malrotation in English literature, which except the coexistent cases with situs inversus totalis.

Number	Citation including year	Age	Sex	Location	Histologic type	Type of IM
1	Gilbert et al., 1990 [5]	55	M	Splenic flexure	Adenoca.	Nonrotation
2	Torreggiani et al., 2001 [6]	86	F	Cecum	Carcinoma	Nonrotation
3	Uchida et al., 2004 [7]	57	M	Transverse colon		Nonrotation
4	Ren and Lu, 2009 [8]	45	M	Ascending colon	Well to mod. diff.	Nonrotation
5	Brillantino et al., 2009 [9]	34	M	Cecum	Well diff.	Nonrotation
6	Michalopoulos et al., 2010 [10]	76	M	Ascending colon	Neoplasm	Reversed rotation
7	Morimoto et al., 2012 [11]	57	M	Cecum	Cancer	Reversed rotation
8	Donaire et al., 2013 [12]	52	M	Right colon	Adenoca.	Nonrotation
9	Hirano et al., 2013 [13]	68	F	Ascending colon	Well diff.	Nonrotation
10	Hirano et al., 2013 [14]	82	F	Transverse colon	Well diff.	Reversed rotation
11	Enomoto et al., 2014 [15]	48	M	Transverse colon	Well to mod. diff.	Nonrotation
12	Lu, 2014 [4]	43	F	Cecum	Adenosquamous ca.	NA
13	Ray et al., 2014 [16]	60	F	Ascending colon	Mod. diff.	NA
14	Our case, 2015	63	M	Descending colon	Mod. diff.	Nonrotation

IM: intestinal malrotation. NA: no assessment.

We herein presented a rare operative case of descending colon cancer in a patient with intestinal malrotation.

Consent

Written informed consent was obtained from the patient for publication of this case report.

Authors' Contribution

Yoshifumi Nakayama contributed to the drafting and the editing of the paper. Masaki Akiyama and Yusuke Sawatsubashi contributed to obtaining the clinical details. Noritaka Minagawa contributed to literature search. Takayuki Torigoe helped in drafting the paper. Keiji Hirata helped in editing of the paper.

References

[1] A. M. Torres and M. M. Ziegler, "Malrotation of the intestine," *World Journal of Surgery*, vol. 17, no. 3, pp. 326–331, 1993.

[2] R. McIntosh and E. J. Donovan, "Disturbances of rotation of the intestinal tract: clinical picture based on observations in twenty cases," *The American Journal of Disease of Children*, vol. 57, no. 1, pp. 116–166, 1939.

[3] JL. Kantor, "Anomalies of the colon," *Radiology*, vol. 23, no. 6, pp. 651–662, 1934.

[4] I. L. Lu, "Adenosquamous carcinoma of the cecum with malrotation and intussusceptions," *Journal of Cancer Research and Practice*, vol. 30, no. 1, pp. 70–74, 2014.

[5] H. W. Gilbert, M. H. Thompson, and C. P. Armstrong, "The presentation of malrotation of the intestine in adults," *Annals of the Royal College of Surgeons of England*, vol. 72, no. 4, pp. 239–242, 1990.

[6] W. C. Torreggiani, F. Thornton, L. Lyburn, C. Brenner, and M. J. Lee, "Malrotation of the bowel resulting in a left-sided caecal carcinoma presenting as a palpable intrahernial mass," *Australasian Radiology*, vol. 45, no. 3, pp. 362–364, 2001.

[7] H. Uchida, Y. J. Kawamura, K. Takegami et al., "Colon cancer complicated by vascular and intestinal anomaly," *Hepato-Gastroenterology*, vol. 51, no. 55, pp. 156–158, 2004.

[8] P.-T. Ren and B.-C. Lu, "Intestinal malrotation associated with colon cancer in an adult: report of a case," *Surgery Today*, vol. 39, no. 7, pp. 624–627, 2009.

[9] A. Brillantino, L. Marano, M. Schettino et al., "Report of a rare case of colon cancer complicated by anomalies of intestinal rotation and fixation: a case report," *Cases Journal*, vol. 2, no. 9, article 6555, 2009.

[10] A. Michalopoulos, V. Papadopoulos, D. Paramythiotis et al., "Colonic cancer in a patient with intestinal malrotation: a case report," *Techniques in Coloproctology*, vol. 14, supplement 1, pp. S65–S66, 2010.

[11] M. Morimoto, H. Horie, H. Kumano, A. Lefor, K. Utano, and Y. Yasuda, "Reversed intestinal malrotation with concurrent cecal carcinoma," *Asian Journal of Endoscopic Surgery*, vol. 5, no. 3, pp. 149–151, 2012.

[12] M. Donaire, J. Mariadason, D. Stephens, S. Pillarisetty, and M. K. Wallack, "Carcinoma of the colon in an adult with intestinal malrotation," *Case Reports in Surgery*, vol. 2013, Article ID 525081, 4 pages, 2013.

[13] Y. Hirano, M. Hattori, D. Yagi, K. Maeda, K. Douden, and Y. Hashizume, "Laparoscopic surgery for the ascending colon cancer associated with malrotation of the midgut," *Indian Journal of Surgery*, vol. 75, no. 1, supplement, pp. 71–73, 2013.

[14] Y. Hirano, M. Hattori, M. Fujita, Y. Nishida, K. Douden, and Y. Hashizume, "The transverse colon cancer with the reversed rotation of the midgut treated with single incision laparoscopic colectomy," *Indian Journal of Surgery*, vol. 75, supplement 1, pp. S195–S198, 2013.

[15] H. Enomoto, H. Kawahara, M. Tomoda, K. Watanabe, T. Akiba, and K. Yanaga, "Laparoscopic surgery for the transverse colon carcinoma associated with non-rotarion type intestinal

malrotation," *Jikeikai Medical Journal*, vol. 61, no. 4, pp. 87–92, 2014.

[16] D. Ray, C. Chattopadhyay, and S. Das, "Malrotation of intestine with carcinoma colon in adult," *Journal of Nepal Medical Association*, vol. 52, no. 8, pp. 727–729, 2014.

[17] C. A. Wang and C. E. Welch, "Anomalies of intestinal rotation in adolescents and adult," *Surgery*, vol. 54, pp. 839–855, 1963.

[18] K. Kato, H. Sakurai, S. Matsuda, and H. Suzuki, "A case of acute appendicitis presenting with left lower abdominal pain associated with malrotation of the intestine," *The Journal of the Japanese Practical Surgeon Society*, vol. 57, no. 10, pp. 2494–2498, 1996 (Japanese).

[19] C. Maeda, E. Hidaka, T. Uchida, T. Omoto, F. Ishida, and S. Kudo, "A case of transverse colon cancer with adult intestinal malrotation," *Journal of Japan Surgical Association*, vol. 74, no. 11, pp. 3103–3107, 2013 (Japanese).

27

Post-ERCP Emphysematous Cholecystitis in a Young Woman: A Rare and Potentially Fatal Complication

Roisin Stack,[1] Joseph McLoughlin,[1] Amy Gillis,[2] and Barbara M. Ryan[1]

[1] *Department of Gastroenterology, Tallaght Hospital and Trinity College, Dublin, Ireland*
[2] *Department of Surgery, Tallaght Hospital and Trinity College, Dublin, Ireland*

Correspondence should be addressed to Roisin Stack; stack.roisin@gmail.com

Academic Editor: Hirotada Akiho

A 45-year-old woman with suspected Functional Biliary Sphincter Disorder (FBSD) developed *Clostridium perfringens* related emphysematous cholecystitis after ERCP. A low index of suspicion for emphysematous cholecystitis in this young, otherwise healthy woman led to a significant delay in making the correct diagnosis, and air in the gallbladder was wrongly attributed to a possible gallbladder perforation. ERCP is associated with significant risks, particularly in patients with FBSD, where diagnostic uncertainty renders the balance of risk versus benefit even more critical. Post-ERCP emphysematous cholecystitis secondary to *Clostridium perfringens* is a rare but potentially fatal complication.

1. Introduction

It is well established that endoscopic retrograde cholangiopancreatography (ERCP) is associated with significant risks. However emphysematous cholecystitis secondary to *Clostridium perfringens* infection is exceedingly rare after ERCP and there are only four such reports in the literature. Emphysematous cholecystitis is generally thought to be an infection of older patients with significant comorbidities and not of young, otherwise healthy individuals.

2. Case Report

A 45-year-old, woman, with a three-year history of severe, intermittent upper abdominal pain, underwent an ERCP and sphincterotomy for suspected Functional Biliary Sphincter Disorder (FBSD) or what would previously have been classified as Sphincter of Oddi Dysfunction (SOD) type II. She was otherwise well with no significant comorbidities. She had previously been extensively investigated: ultrasound, cross sectional abdominal imaging, upper GI endoscopy, endoscopic ultrasound, HIDA scan, and extensive bloods all were normal, apart from intermittent, mildly elevated LFTs. Biliary manometry was not performed. A clinical diagnosis of suspected FBSD was made on the basis of the biliary character of the pain and mildly raised LFTs on a number of occasions. The patient had failed to respond to trials of a number of medications for almost two years. Following extensive discussion and consideration, a decision was made to proceed to elective ERCP.

The patient was given prophylactic 3rd generation cephalosporin preprocedure in line with current guidelines. The ERCP was an uneventful procedure and there was no instrumentation to the pancreatic duct. The CBD was of normal diameter and a sphincterotomy was performed. 100 mg of diclofenac was given PR immediately after procedure. The patient developed upper abdominal pain several hours after procedure and on examination she was mildly tender in the right upper quadrant and epigastrium. She was admitted overnight for observation, was given IV fluids, and was kept fasting. Bloods the following morning were normal apart from a mildly raised CRP of 12 mg/L. The pain had eased and the patient, who was keen to go home, was discharged.

She represented to the emergency department 48 hours after ERCP with severe right upper quadrant pain that radiated to the back. She was pyrexial and her white cell count was 20×10^9/L and CRP was 83 mg/L. Liver function tests and urea and electrolytes were normal. A CT of the abdomen and

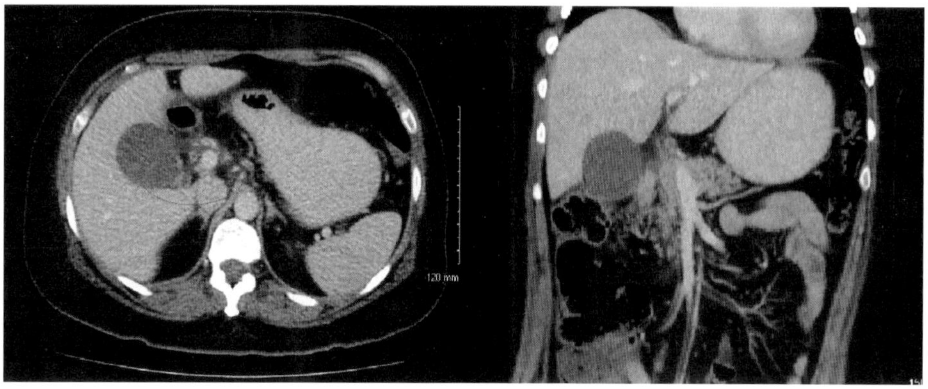

FIGURE 1: CT abdomen pelvis day 2: periportal and pericholecystic fat stranding with hyperaemia of the extrahepatic bile duct and adjacent stranding. Findings are suspicious for an ascending cholangitis and cholecystitis.

pelvis showed periportal and pericholecystic fat stranding with hyperaemia of the extrahepatic bile duct with adjacent stranding (Figure 1). The findings were felt to be consistent with cholecystitis and ascending cholangitis and the patient was commenced on broad-spectrum antibiotics. She failed to settle with antibiotic therapy and the CRP rose to 330 mg/L and the white cell remained elevated at 19×10^9/L. On day 6, a repeat CT abdomen demonstrated air within a distended gall bladder, with persistent pericholecystic fat stranding, extending to involve the hepatic flexure and a peripherally enhancing fluid collection in the right paracolic gutter (Figure 2). The findings were interpreted as complicated cholecystitis with a gallbladder perforation, possibly secondary to ERCP instrumentation. Emphysematous cholecystitis was not considered in the differential diagnosis at this point. An urgent surgical referral was sought and a radiological cholecystostomy tube was inserted at this point rather than emergent surgery. The biliary fluid was sent for culture and sensitivity. On day 7, the patient became increasingly short of breath and a chest X-ray showed a large right-sided pleural effusion and a smaller left-sided effusion. A pleural drain was inserted into the right side.

By day 10, there was limited clinical improvement and the patient was spiking intermittent temperatures. Repeat CT showed an interval reduction in the degree of pericholecystic fat stranding but persistent gallbladder distension and right paracolic collection. In addition, while there was an interval resolution of right pleural effusion, there was also a new interval development of right lower and middle lobe pneumonia. Bacterial culture and sensitivity results from the cholecystostomy biliary fluid were then returned urgently: this showed *Escherichia coli* and *Clostridium perfringens* bacteria, raising concern for a gangrenous gallbladder and emphysematous cholecystitis. Review of the CT scan from day 6 was made at this point and the findings were felt to be more consistent with emphysematous cholecystitis, rather than a gallbladder perforation as had been originally suggested. An emergent open cholecystectomy was performed and this confirmed the presence of a necrotic gallbladder with gas gangrene. The patient remained intermittently febrile for one week but this eventually settled with prolonged IV antibiotics. A repeat CT scan at day 10 after cholecystectomy showed almost complete interval resolution of the right paracolic gutter collection and the patient was discharged home on oral antibiotics on day 11 post-op. At 4 months after cholecystectomy the patient was doing well. Repeat CT of the abdomen and thorax showed resolution of the collections, a clear gallbladder bed, and some residual right basal atelectasis. Eight months after procedures, the abdominal pain has resolved.

3. Discussion

We present a case of acute emphysematous cholecystitis secondary to *Clostridium perfringens* infection following an ERCP in a young healthy woman. Acute emphysematous cholecystitis has been reported in association with a number of pathogens, including *Clostridium perfringens, E. coli,* and *B. fragilis.* Morbidity and mortality rates as high as 50% and 25%, respectively, have been described [1]. *Clostridium perfringens* emphysematous cholecystitis is strongly associated with the presence of diabetes mellitus and older age and is more common in men [1–3].

Clostridial species constitute between 16 and 40% of total gut microbiota and are thought to play an important role in immune regulation within the gut [4]. *Clostridium perfringens* is one of these commensals, although sepsis is rare in clinical practice. A relatively old study found *Clostridium perfringens* colonisation of the gallbladder in up to 19% of surgically removed gallbladders [5]. Whether this is reflective of rates of carriage in the normal population or whether *Clostridium perfringens* colonisation contributes to the development of gallbladder pathology necessitating surgery is not known.

Reports of *Clostridium perfringens* related emphysematous cholecystitis after ERCP are exceedingly rare, and to our knowledge there have only been 4 previously reported cases [6]. One of those four cases had similar features to the current case: a young female with no significant comorbidities who underwent an ERCP for treatment of possible Sphincter of Oddi Dysfunction which was complicated by *Clostridium perfringens* emphysematous cholecystitis requiring a cholecystectomy two days after ERCP [6]. The patient

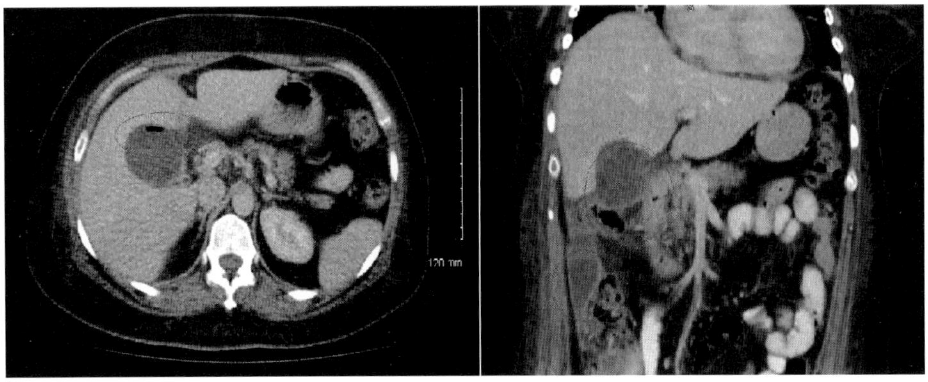

Figure 2: CT abdomen pelvis day 6: air within a distended gall bladder with persistent pericholecystic fat stranding, more marked than on prior imaging and extending to involve the hepatic flexure. New, peripherally enhancing fluid collection extending the inferior tip of the liver along the right paracolic gutter; appearances are suggestive of complicated cholecystitis with a gallbladder perforation.

ultimately required a liver transplantation for secondary biliary cirrhosis. Given the rapid development of post-ERCP *Clostridium perfringens*-related emphysematous cholecystitis in these two patients with suspected FBSD, it is tempting to postulate that both were carriers of *Clostridium perfringens* within their gallbladders prior to the ERCP. Recently one case of post-ERCP gallbladder perforation was described. At the time of surgery several days later a gangrenous gallbladder was described but there was no information regarding the bacterial pathogens [7].

Clostridium perfringens-related emphysematous cholecystitis most commonly presents spontaneously as an acute cholecystitis type picture in elderly, acutely unwell patients, with RUQ pain, raised LFTs, and inflammatory markers [2, 8, 9]. Emphysematous cholecystitis is uncommon and can be difficult to distinguish clinically from typical acute cholecystitis, particularly early in the clinical course. Early CT imaging of the biliary tree is vital for early detection and diagnosis. Ultrasound is not a reliable modality to exclude emphysematous cholecystitis as evidenced by a report of *Clostridium perfringens* related emphysematous cholecystitis: ultrasound imaging of the gallbladder showed gallbladder wall thickening consistent with acute cholecystitis but CT imaging 2 hours later confirmed an emphysematous cholecystitis with perforation and pneumoperitoneum [2]. Plain X-ray imaging has detected radiological signs of EC [10, 11], but the sensitivity is very low.

Sepsis from *Clostridium perfringens* has been associated with other interventions of the biliary tree. One case report describes fulminant sepsis and death at 24 hours after liver biopsy secondary to *Clostridium perfringens* [12]. That patient was under investigation for recurrent cholangitis following previous cholecystectomy and had also undergone an ERCP prior to the liver biopsy. *Clostridium perfringens* sepsis was diagnosed post-mortem.

A high index of suspicion for *Clostridium perfringens* infection is required to ensure early detection and treatment of this potentially fatal infection. In this current case, there was a significant delay in the diagnosis of *Clostridium perfringens*-related emphysematous cholecystitis, which fortunately appears to have had no lasting sequelae for the patient. Air in the gallbladder was erroneously attributed to possible gallbladder perforation per-ERCP. The diagnosis of *Clostridium perfringens*-related cholecystitis was made 10 days after ERCP, whereas the imaging 6 days after the ERCP showed air in the gallbladder. Had there been a higher index of suspicion for emphysematous cholecystitis, despite the fact that the patient did not fit the "typical" demographic for *Clostridium perfringens*-related emphysematous cholecystitis (i.e., being older, being diabetic, and other comorbidities), the diagnosis could have been made earlier.

The diagnosis of FBSD can be difficult. The Rome IV consensus has recently reclassified the previous diagnoses of SOD types I, II, and III [13]. What was previously classified as SOD type I is now thought to represent papillary stenosis, a structural abnormality, and these patients should undergo biliary sphincterotomy. The EPISOD trial showed that patients with so-called Type III SOD do not respond to biliary sphincterotomy and ERCP should be avoided in these patients [14]. Those with previously designated SOD type II are now designated "suspected FBSD" and may benefit from biliary sphincterotomy. The diagnosis of FBSD is based on the presence of biliary type pain and either transient rises in liver enzymes or a dilated bile duct, but not both. ERCP is an invasive procedure and is associated with significant morbidity and mortality. The decision to proceed to ERCP in patients with suspected FBSD should not be taken lightly and the patient should have time to consider the possible complications [13]. The risks of ERCP must always be carefully weighed against potential benefits and noninvasive/medical treatments should be given an adequate trial before deciding to proceed to ERCP. In this case, the patient has been on a number of medications for over a year, without any benefit. A meta-analysis of post-ERCP complications showed a complication rate of 6.85% (95% CI 6.46–7.24%) with rates of 3.5%, 1.5%, 0.60%, and 0.33% respectively, for pancreatitis, infection, perforation, and death [15]. These rates of complication are even higher in the SOD subpopulation [13].

We herein describe the development of a serious, life-threatening *Clostridium perfringens*-related emphysematous, gangrenous cholecystitis in a previously healthy young woman, with suspected FBSD, who underwent a seemingly uneventful ERCP. This is the fifth such case to be described in the literature. One previously reported case also involved a young woman with possible SOD. It is interesting to postulate that functional biliary disorders such as FBSD and functional gallbladder disorder might be related to dysbiosis of the gallbladder/biliary tree.

Consent

The patient has given her written consent for her data to be submitted.

Authors' Contributions

Roisin Stack and Joseph McLoughlin were involved in compilation of the data and drafting of the article. Amy Gillis was involved in management of the case, performed the surgery, and was involved in drafting of the article. Barbara M. Ryan was the senior author and was involved in management of the case and in overseeing the drafting of the article. All authors read and approved the final manuscript.

References

[1] L. G.-S. Tellez, J. A. Rodriguez-Montes, S. F. De Lis, and L. G.-S. Martin, "Acute emphysematous cholecystitis. Report of twenty cases," *Hepato-Gastroenterology*, vol. 46, no. 28, pp. 2144–2148, 1999.

[2] A. E. Mirrakhimov, G. Chandra, P. Voore et al., "Clostridium perfringens bacteremia in an 85-year-old diabetic man," *Case Reports in Gastroenterology*, vol. 8, no. 3, pp. 404–407, 2014.

[3] L. M. Knab, A.-M. Boller, and D. M. Mahvi, "Cholecystitis," *Surgical Clinics of North America*, vol. 94, no. 2, pp. 455–470, 2014.

[4] L. R. Lopetuso, F. Scaldaferri, V. Petito, and A. Gasbarrini, "Commensal Clostridia: leading players in the maintenance of gut homeostasis," *Gut Pathogens*, vol. 5, no. 1, article 23, 2013.

[5] H. R. Magee, "Clostridium perfringens infection of the biliary tract," *Australian and New Zealand Journal of Surgery*, vol. 37, no. 2, pp. 177–183, 1967.

[6] K. Bari, H. R. Aslanian, and J. Pollak, "Emphysematous cholecystitis resulting in secondary biliary cirrhosis: a rare complication of endoscopic retrograde cholangiopancreatography," *ACG Case Reports Journal*, vol. 1, no. 1, pp. 51–54, 2013.

[7] A. H. Mohammad Alizadeh and K. Donboli, "Cholecystectomy for gallbladder perforation after ERCP," *JSM General Surgery: Cases and Images*, vol. 1, no. 2, article 1010, 2016.

[8] H. Miyahara, D. Shida, H. Matsunaga, Y. Takahama, and S. Miyamoto, "Emphysematous cholecystitis with massive gas in the abdominal cavity," *World Journal of Gastroenterology*, vol. 19, no. 4, pp. 604–606, 2013.

[9] P. Kirchhoff, V. Müller, H. Petrowsky, and P.-A. Clavien, "Fatal emphysematous cholecystitis caused by clostridium perfringens," *Surgery*, vol. 141, no. 3, pp. 411–412, 2007.

[10] H. Qandeel, H. Abudeeb, A. Hammad, C. Ray, M. Sajid, and S. Mahmud, "Clostridium perfringens sepsis and liver abscess following laparoscopic cholecystectomy," *Journal of Surgical Case Reports*, vol. 2012, no. 1, p. 5, 2012.

[11] C.-Y. Liao, C.-C. Tsai, W.-H. Kuo et al., "Emphysematous cholecystitis presenting as gas-forming liver abscess and pneumoperitoneum in a dialysis patient: a case report and review of the literature," *BMC Nephrology*, vol. 17, no. 1, article 237, 2016.

[12] C. Claudi, M. Henschel, J. Vogel, M. Schepke, and E. Biecker, "Fulminant sepsis after liver biopsy: a long forgotten complication," *World Journal of Clinical Cases*, vol. 1, no. 1, pp. 41–43, 2013.

[13] P. B. Cotton, G. H. Elta, C. R. Carter, P. J. Pasricha, and E. S. Corazziari, "Gallbladder and sphincter of Oddi disorders," *Gastroenterology*, vol. 150, no. 6, pp. 1420.e2–1429.e2, 2016.

[14] P. B. Cotton, V. Durkalski, J. Romagnuolo et al., "Effect of endoscopic sphincterotomy for suspected sphincter of Oddi dysfunction on pain-related disability following cholecystectomy: the EPISOD randomized clinical trial," *JAMA*, vol. 311, no. 20, pp. 2101–2109, 2014.

[15] A. Andriulli, S. Loperfido, G. Napolitano et al., "Incidence rates of post-ERCP complications: a systematic survey of prospective studies," *American Journal of Gastroenterology*, vol. 102, no. 8, pp. 1781–1788, 2007.

28

Barrett's Oesophagus in an Achalasia Patient: Immunological Analysis and Comparison with a Group of Achalasia Patients

Samuel Torres-Landa,[1] Janette Furuzawa-Carballeda,[2] Enrique Coss-Adame,[3] Miguel A. Valdovinos,[3] Edgar Alejandro-Medrano,[1] Bárbara Ramos-Ávalos,[1] Braulio Martínez-Benítez,[4] and Gonzalo Torres-Villalobos[1]

[1] *Department of Experimental Surgery, Instituto Nacional de Ciencias Médicas y Nutrición Salvador Zubirán, Vasco de Quiroga No. 15, Colonia Belisario Domínguez Sección XVI, 14080 Mexico City, Mexico*

[2] *Department of Immunology and Rheumatology, Instituto Nacional de Ciencias Médicas y Nutrición Salvador Zubirán, Vasco de Quiroga No. 15, Colonia Belisario Domínguez Sección XVI, 14080 Mexico City, Mexico*

[3] *Department of Gastroenterology, Instituto Nacional de Ciencias Médicas y Nutrición Salvador Zubirán, Vasco de Quiroga No. 15, Colonia Belisario Domínguez Sección XVI, 14080 Mexico City, Mexico*

[4] *Department of Pathology, Instituto Nacional de Ciencias Médicas y Nutrición Salvador Zubirán, Vasco de Quiroga No. 15, Colonia Belisario Domínguez Sección XVI, 14080 Mexico City, Mexico*

Correspondence should be addressed to Gonzalo Torres-Villalobos; torresvgm@yahoo.com.mx

Academic Editor: Naohiko Koide

The aim of the study was to characterize the presence of diverse CD4 and CD8 T cell subsets and regulatory cells in peripheral blood and lower oesophageal sphincter (LES) from a young patient with BE/achalasia without treatment versus achalasia group. In order to characterize the circulating cells in this patient, a cytometric analysis was performed. LES tissue was evaluated by double-immunostaining procedure. Five healthy blood donors, 5 type achalasia patients, and 5 oesophagus tissue samples (gastrooesophageal junction) from transplant donors were included as control groups. A conspicuous systemic inflammation was determined in BE/achalasia patient and achalasia versus healthy volunteer group. Nonetheless, a predominance of Th22, Th2, IFN-α-producing T cells, Tregs, Bregs, and pDCregs was observed in BE/achalasia patient versus achalasia group. A low percentage of Th1 subset in BE/achalasia versus achalasia group was determined. A noticeable increase in tissue of Th22, Th17, Th2, Tregs, Bregs, and pDCregs was observed in BE/achalasia versus achalasia group. Th1 subset was lower in the BE/achalasia patient versus achalasia group. This study suggests that inflammation is a possible factor in the pathogenesis of BE/achalasia. Further research needs to be performed to understand the specific cause of the correlation between BE and achalasia.

1. Background

Idiopathic achalasia is a primary oesophageal motor disorder characterized by the loss of oesophageal peristalsis and incomplete relaxation of the lower oesophageal sphincter (LES). The annual incidence and prevalence are 1 case per 100,000 and 10 in every 1,000,000 habitants, respectively [1]. Recent studies have suggested that achalasia has an important local and systemic autoimmune inflammatory response, with a high prevalence of specific autoantibodies against the myenteric plexus, and it has been associated with the presence of Herpes simplex virus type 1 [2]. Clinical manifestations include dysphagia, regurgitation, retrosternal chest pain, weight loss, and heartburn. Diagnosis is established by manometric studies and complementary tests like barium esophagram and esophagogastroduodenoscopy [1].

Barrett's oesophagus (BE) is a disease in which the normal distal squamous epithelial lining is replaced by metaplastic columnar epithelium that can be suspected by endoscopy and confirmed by histopathology [3]. BE/achalasia as cooccurring disease has been reported in up to 14% following treatment of achalasia [4]. However, in untreated patients this cooccurring finding is a rare phenomenon, and to our knowledge there are only 4 studies that have reported this association [5–8].

It is important to mention that the 4 patients previously reported were older (≥40 years), the age being one of the major risk factors for BE due to the long natural history of the disease. In this case report we present the first report of immunological analysis of BE/achalasia in a young patient with no previous surgical or endoscopic treatment, diagnosed with BE.

2. Case Presentation

This case is of a 28-year-old man with a previous history of chronic hypertension, 12 years of tobacco consumption, and 7 years of alcohol consumption every 2 weeks, without any family history of BE. He was referred to our hospital after 1 year of progressive oesophageal dysphagia, associated with regurgitation, retrosternal chest pain, and weight loss of 7 kg. Physical examination was unremarkable, and BMI was 28.37 at the moment of referral (BMI of 30.82 prior to the disease). A barium swallow showed oesophageal dilatation and bird beak sign (Figure 1(a)). A high resolution manometry (HRM) (Figure 1(b)) and panendoscopy were performed. The HRM showed an elevated IRP value of 31.2 mmHg, abnormal relaxation of lower oesophageal sphincter (LES), and aperistalsis with panoesophageal pressurization in >20% of swallows, corresponding with type II achalasia. Hiatal hernia was not reported. Unexpectedly during the endoscopy procedure, irregular Z-line was seen with tong-like protrusions suspicious of BE that was classified as C 0 M1 accordingly with the Prague Classification (Figures 1(c) and 1(d)). Biopsies of suspicious areas were taken and revised by two expert pathologists that reported metaplastic columnar epithelium (Barrett's oesophagus) without dysplasia (Figures 1(e) and 1(f)). The oesophageal 24 h impedance-pH monitoring showed normal acid exposure with 0.2% of pH < 4 and a DeMeester score of 1.1. The patient underwent Heller's myotomy with biopsy of the muscular layer of the oesophagus and Dor fundoplication in November 2015. Transsurgical endoscopy was negative for leakages. Within the first 24 hours the patient developed systemic inflammatory response syndrome. A water-soluble study was performed, which reported a possible leak from the myotomy site. CT scan reported pneumomediastinum without a visible leakage. He underwent a laparoscopic exploration without a visible site of leakage and negative cultures. The patient was treated without any other intervention, only with fasting, and was discharged without any further complications.

2.1. Ethical Considerations. The study was approved by the ethical medical committee in our institution (reference number 1522) and it was according to the principles expressed in the Declaration of Helsinki, 1989. Only patients who gave a written informed consent were recruited for this study. Each participant gave a written consent to publish their individual data.

3. Discussion

3.1. Barrett's Oesophagus and Achalasia. Although achalasia has been related to BE after surgical procedure [4], there is no clear explanation of the cause of this finding in a young patient before myotomy. Nonetheless, it is known that BE has been correlated to acid exposure due to gastric oesophageal reflux disease (GERD) [9]. One of the possibilities of this rare finding could be a chronic acid exposure secondary to GERD prior to the developing of achalasia. Another one could be that, in achalasia patients, food retention and its fermentation lower the pH due to lactic acid production, allowing chronic irritation against the oesophageal epithelium [9]. Although these two hypotheses cannot be confirmed, it is a fact that our patient had many of the risk factors (grade of evidence: II and IIa) for BE [3] including sex, heartburn, smoking, alcohol consumption, and BMI > 30.

3.2. Immunophenotyping of Circulating Regulatory Cell and CD4 Effector T Cell Subpopulations by Flow Cytometry. In a recent publication, our group [2] determined the peripheral blood immunophenotypes of different subtypes of achalasia. In order to characterize the peripheral blood compartment in this patient, we proceeded to follow the same methodology [2]. A group of 5 healthy blood donors and 5 type II achalasia patients, specifically sampled for this study, were included as control groups. A sample of venous blood (10 mL) was obtained from each subject. Peripheral blood mononuclear cells (PBMCs) were isolated by gradient centrifugation on Lymphoprep (Axis-Shield PoC AS, Oslo, Norway). Th22 ($CD3^+/CD4^+/CD161^-/IL\text{-}22^+$), Th17 ($CD3^+/CD4^+/CD161^+/IL\text{-}17A^+$), Th2 ($CD3^+/CD4^+/CD25^+/IL\text{-}4^+$), Th1 ($CD3^+/CD4^+/CD25^+/IFN\text{-}\gamma^+$), IFN-$\alpha$-producing T cells ($CD3^+/CD4^+/CD25^+/IFN\text{-}\alpha^+$ and $CD3^+/CD8^+/CD28^+/IFN\text{-}\alpha^+$), regulatory T cells ($CD3^+/CD4^+/CD25^{hi}/Foxp3^+$, $CD3^+/CD4^+/CD25^{hi}/IL\text{-}35^+$, $CD3^+/CD8^+/CD28^-/Foxp3^+$, and $CD3^+/CD8^+/CD28^-/IL\text{-}35^+$), regulatory B cells ($CD3^+/CD19^+/CD38^{hi}/IL\text{-}10^+$ and $CD3^+/CD19^+/CD38^{hi}/IL\text{-}35^+$), and regulatory plasmacytoid dendritic cells (pDCs; $CD123^{hi}/CD196^+/IDO^+$) were determined. In the cytometric analysis, a conspicuous systemic inflammation was determined in BE/achalasia patient and achalasia group compared with healthy volunteer group (Table 1). Nonetheless, a predominance of Th22, Th2, IFN-α-producing T cells, Tregs, Bregs, and pDCregs was observed in BE/achalasia patient compared with achalasia group. In contrast a low percentage of Th1 subset in BE/achalasia versus achalasia patient group was determined (Table 1). Th17 profile was similar in our BE/achalasia patient compared with achalasia group (Table 1).

3.3. Characterization of Tissue Regulatory Cell and CD4 Effector Cell Subsets by Immunohistochemistry. In order to determine the characteristics of the cellular infiltrate,

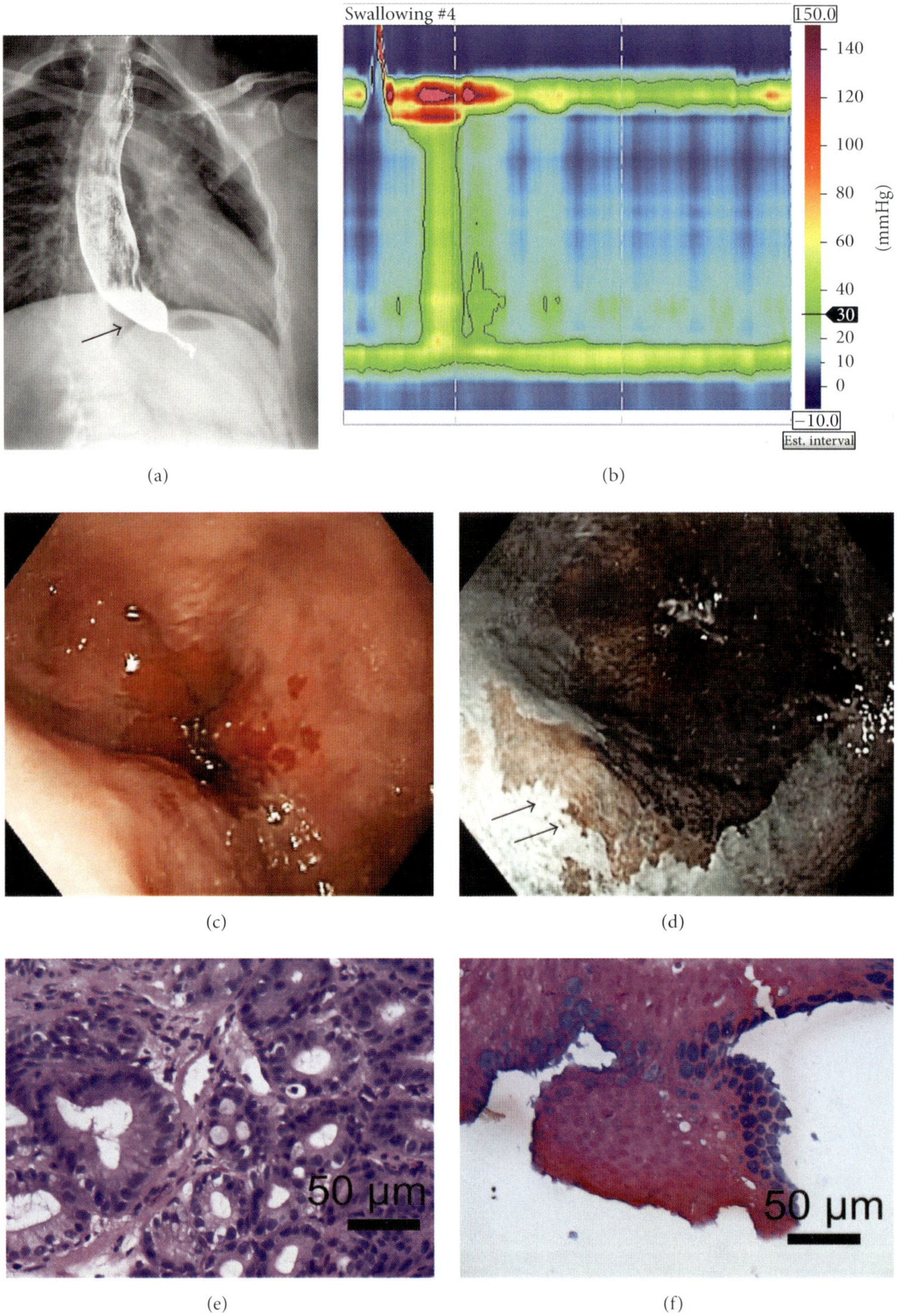

Figure 1: (a) Barium oesophagram that shows dilatation and bird beak sign (arrow). (b) High resolution manometry that shows abnormal relaxation of lower oesophageal sphincter and aperistalsis with panesophageal pressurization in 40% of swallows, corresponding with type II achalasia. (c) Upper endoscopy shows dilated esophagus with mucosal changes consistent with C0 M1 Barrett's oesophagus. (d) Arrows indicate margins of "tongues" of Barrett's metaplasia. (e) Metaplastic columnar epithelium. (f) Photomicrograph that highlights the metaplasia. Original magnification in high field power (100x).

Table 1: Analysis of peripheral blood and tissue immunophenotypes in the present case compared to 5 achalasia patients and 5 control subjects.

	Healthy donors ($n = 5$)	Type II achalasia ($n = 5$)	Patient
		Blood	
Peripheral blood immunophenotypes			
$CD3^+/CD4^+/CD161^-/IL\text{-}22^+$ (%)			
Mean ± SD	1.95 ± 0.53	6.58 ± 2.56	
Median	1.79	4.90	**7.72**
Range	1.39–2.55	2.79–16.70	
$CD3^+/CD4^+/CD161^+/IL\text{-}17A^+$ (%)			
Mean ± SD	1.96 ± 0.80	5.62 ± 1.73	
Median	1.64	4.95	5.42
Range	1.40–3.35	2.72–12.30	
$CD3^+/CD4^+/CD25^+/IL\text{-}4^+$ (%)			
Mean ± SD	1.44 ± 0.65	3.23 ± 0.70	
Median	1.36	3.76	**4.19**
Range	0.52–2.09	1.55–4.99	
$CD3^+/CD4^+/CD25^+/IFN\text{-}\gamma^+$ (%)			
Mean ± SD	1.76 ± 0.97	4.18 ± 1.31	
Median	1.91	3.43	3.6
Range	0.29–2.87	2.15–9.30	
$CD3^+/CD4^+/CD25^+/IFN\text{-}\alpha^+$ (%)			
Mean ± SD	2.26 ± 1.2	4.47 ± 0.85	
Median	1.81	3.73	**5.08**
Range	1.31–4.35	2.11–6.80	
$CD3^+/CD8^+/CD28^+/IFN\text{-}\alpha^+$ (%)			
Mean ± SD	3.05 ± 1.97	3.99 ± 0.47	
Median	2.82	4.28	**5.87**
Range	1.48–6.39	2.54–5.27	
$CD3^+/CD4^+/CD25^{hi}/Foxp3^+$ (%)			
Mean ± SD	5.16 ± 0.78	7.21 ± 0.45	
Median	5.05	7.32	**10.1**
Range	4.00–6.03	5.64–8.35	
$CD3^+/CD4^+/CD25^{hi}/IL\text{-}35^+$ (%)			
Mean ± SD	3.60 ± 0.98	4.08 ± 0.44	
Median	3.64	4.28	9.96
Range	2.50–5.11	2.39–4.88	
$CD3^+/CD8^+/CD28^-/Foxp3^+$ (%)			
Mean ± SD	3.82 ± 0.71	5.39 ± 0.28	
Median	3.95	5.46	**6.72**
Range	3.01–4.77	4.42–6.06	
$CD3^+/CD8^+/CD28^-/IL\text{-}35^+$ (%)			
Mean ± SD	3.37 ± 0.77	4.53 ± 1.28	
Median	3.69	3.02	**12.4**
Range	2.19–4.01	2.12–9.09	
$CD3^+/CD19^+/CD38^+/IL\text{-}10^+$ (%)			
Mean ± SD	6.27 ± 1.07	6.99 ± 0.58	
Median	6.08	6.50	**14.1**
Range	5.07–7.81	4.88–8.09	
$CD3^+/CD19^+/CD38^+/IL\text{-}35^+$ (%)			
Mean ± SD	5.95 ± 0.45	4.31 ± 0.89	
Median	5.88	3.90	**19.2**
Range	5.58–6.70	2.20–7.60	
$CD123^+/CD196^+/IDO^+$ (%)			
Mean ± SD	11.84 ± 1.36	16.82 ± 1.66	
Median	11.50	18.70	**21.2**
Range	10.30–14.00	10.80–19.47	

Table 1: Continued.

	Healthy donors ($n = 5$)	Type II achalasia ($n = 5$)	Patient
		Tissue	
Tissue immunophenotypes			
IL-22-expressing cells (%)			
Mean ± SD	3.83 ± 1.83	17.83 ± 1.47	
Median	4.00	17.50	**23.5**
Range	2.00–7.00	16.00–20.00	
IL-17A-expressing CD4 T cells (%)			
Mean ± SD	1.00 ± 0.68	8.33 ± 1.75	
Median	0.00	7.50	**17.00**
Range	0.00–4.00	7.00–11.00	
IL-4-expressing CD4 T cells (%)			
Mean ± SD	1.33 ± 0.33	6.33 ± 0.75	
Median	1.50	7.00	**14.00**
Range	0.00–2.00	4.00–9.00	
IFN-γ-expressing CD4 T cells (%)			
Mean ± SD	1.50 ± 0.67	15.0 ± 1.27	
Median	1.00	14.5	10.00
Range	0.00–4.00	14.00–17.00	
Foxp3-expressing CD25 T cells (%)			
Mean ± SD	4.33 ± 0.33	7.83 ± 0.48	
Median	4.50	8.00	**11.50**
Range	3.00–5.00	6.00–9.00	
IL-10-expressing CD20 B cells (%)			
Mean ± SD	1.83 ± 1.31	5.33 ± 0.49	
Median	2.00	5.50	**7.5**
Range	1.00–3.00	4.00–7.00	
IDO-expressing CD123 cells (%)			
Mean ± SD	3.67 ± 0.82	6.67 ± 0.33	
Median	3.50	6.50	**8.5**
Range	3.00–5.00	6.00–8.00	

regulatory cells, and interleukin expression present at the lower oesophageal muscle, tissue was stained with specific monoclonal antibodies. Five type II achalasia patients and 5 oesophagus tissue samples (gastrooesophageal junction) from transplant donors were included as a control tissue (Figure 2). Thus, the subpopulation of IL-22-producing cells, $CD4^+/IL\text{-}17A^+$-, $CD4^+/IL\text{-}4^+$-, $CD4^+/IFN\text{-}\gamma^+$-expressing T cells, $CD25^+/Foxp3^+$ regulatory T cells, $CD123^+/IDO^+$ pDCs, and $CD20^+/IL\text{-}10^+$-producing B cells was determined with a simultaneous detection using a Multiview (mouse-HRP/rabbit-AP) immunohistochemistry kit (Enzo Life Sciences, Inc., Farmingdale, NY, USA) [2]. Immunohistochemistry findings showed greater amounts of inflammatory and regulatory cells in BE/achalasia patient and achalasia group compared with control group (Table 1). On the other hand, a noticeable increase in Th22, Th17, Th2, Tregs, Bregs, and pDCregs was observed in BE/achalasia compared to achalasia patient group (Table 1, Figure 2). Th1 subset was lower in the BE/achalasia patient compared with the achalasia group (Table 1, Figure 2).

3.4. Appropriate Treatment and Surveillance. One of the main concerns regarding this patient condition is the posterior risk of developing dysplasia. It has been reported that, due to the high acid exposure presented after Heller's myotomy, a partial fundoplication is now recommended to reduce gastrooesophageal reflux [10]. Although Dor/Toupet fundoplication is more commonly performed on these patients, a significant difference between both partial fundoplications acting as acid barrier has not been reported [11]. The patient underwent an appropriate treatment for his condition although a close surveillance with symptoms, acid exposure, and upper endoscopy could be needed.

Our data suggest that patients with BE/achalasia could have higher inflammation and a higher risk of oesophageal perforation compared with achalasia patients. Moreover, inflammation is considered as the connection of Barrett's carcinogenesis. Key mediators of inflammation in BE have been previously described and include proinflammatory cytokines, chemokines, reactive oxygen species, prostaglandins, and microRNAs [12]. Moons et al. have also demonstrated an increase of Th2 effector cells in BE tissue [13]. Moreover, in serum from BE patients a strong positive association with high level of IL-12p70, IL-8, and leptin and a negative association with IL-10 and IL-1β have been determined. Meanwhile there were no differences between

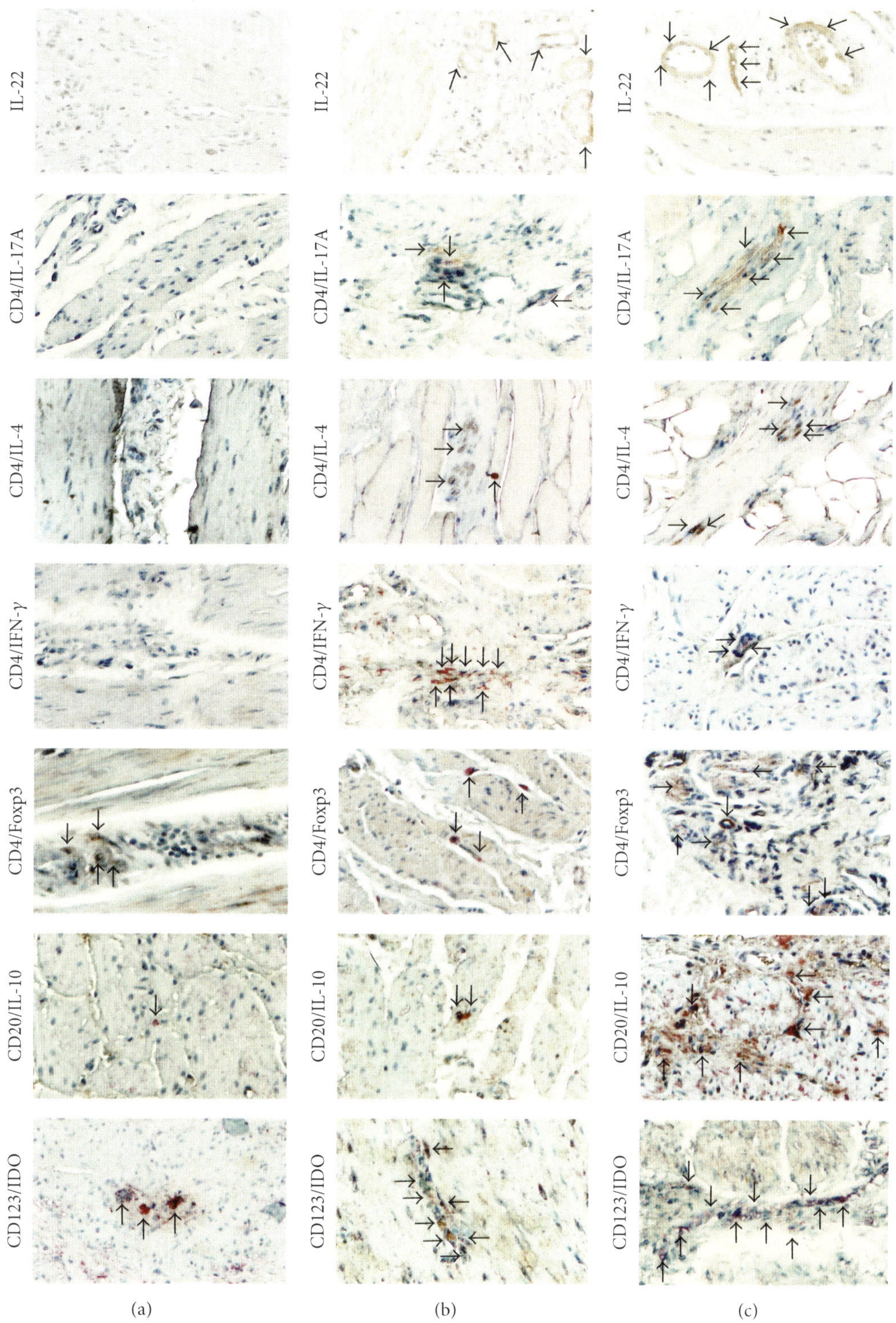

FIGURE 2: CD4 effector T cells and regulatory cells in lower oesophageal sphincter. Representative photomicrograph from control (healthy donor, (a)), type II achalasia (b), and Barrett's oesophagus/type II achalasia patient (c). Arrows depict immunoreactive cells. Original magnification was ×320.

serum controls and BE patients in levels of IFN-γ, TNF-α, adiponectin, or insulin [14]. In the BE/achalasia patient we have shown that Th22, Th17, and Th2 but not Th1 profile interplay at tissue and peripheral cells in BE/achalasia patient. In addition to the presence of proinflammatory cells there is an increase of Treg, IL-10-producing B cell, and pDCreg cell percentage suggesting that proinflammatory and regulatory balance favours the former with the failure of the latter in maintaining homeostasis and conducting more vigorous tissue damage. However this study suggests that inflammation is a possible factor in the pathogenesis of BE/achalasia with the concomitant use of immunosuppressive drugs as probable future treatment for this pathology. It is relevant to highlight the need for a close follow-up to prevent further complications.

4. Conclusion

In conclusion, our preliminary results deserve to be studied in depth to appraise the clinical relevance of these findings. It is also necessary to clarify whether the association of BE and achalasia is an epiphenomenon or might share common pathophysiological pathways.

Abbreviations

AP:	Alkaline phosphatase
BE:	Barrett's oesophagus
BMI:	Body Mass Index
GERD:	Gastric oesophageal reflux disease
HRM:	High resolution manometry
HRP:	Horseradish peroxidase
IFN:	Interferon
IL:	Interleukin
LES:	Lower oesophageal sphincter
PBMCs:	Peripheral blood mononuclear cells
pDCreg:	Regulatory plasmacytoid dendritic cell
Th:	T helper cell
TNF:	Tumour necrosis factor
Treg:	Regulatory T cell.

Consent

Each participant gave a written consent to publish their individual data (only patients who gave a written informed consent were recruited for this study).

Authors' Contributions

Samuel Torres-Landa and Janette Furuzawa-Carballeda are responsible for study concept and design, acquisition of data, analysis and interpretation of data, drafting of the paper, critical revision of the paper for important intellectual content, technical support, and obtained funding. Enrique Coss-Adame, Miguel A. Valdovinos, and Bárbara Ramos-Ávalos performed acquisition of data, analysis and interpretation of data, and critical revision of the paper for important intellectual content. Edgar Alejandro-Medrano and Braulio Martínez-Benítez contributed to acquisition of data, analysis, interpretation of data, and technical and material support. Gonzalo Torres-Villalobos is responsible for study concept and design, acquisition of data, analysis and interpretation of data, drafting of the paper, critical revision of the paper for important intellectual content, statistical analysis, technical support, and study supervision and obtained funding. Samuel Torres-Landa and Janette Furuzawa-Carballeda contributed equally to this work.

Acknowledgments

This work was supported by grant from CONACyT (SALUD-2014-1-233760).

References

[1] M. F. Vaezi, J. E. Pandolfino, and M. F. Vela, "ACG clinical guideline: diagnosis and management of achalasia," *American Journal of Gastroenterology*, vol. 108, no. 8, pp. 1238–1249, 2013.

[2] J. Furuzawa-Carballeda, D. Aguilar-León, A. Gamboa-Domínguez et al., "Achalasia—an autoimmune inflammatory disease: a cross-sectional study," *Journal of Immunology Research*, vol. 2015, Article ID 729217, 18 pages, 2015.

[3] R. C. Fitzgerald, M. di Pietro, K. Ragunath et al., "British Society of Gastroenterology guidelines on the diagnosis and management of Barrett's oesophagus," *Gut*, vol. 63, no. 1, pp. 7–42, 2014.

[4] K. Ravi, D. M. Geno, and D. A. Katzka, "Esophageal cancer screening in achalasia: is there a consensus?" *Diseases of the Esophagus*, vol. 28, no. 3, pp. 299–304, 2016.

[5] D. J. Sprung and S. P. Gibb, "Barrett's esophagus in a patient with achalasia," *American Journal of Gastroenterology*, vol. 80, no. 5, pp. 330–333, 1985.

[6] M. Halland and J. A. Alexander, "A case of esophageal 'double jeopardy'," *Gastroenterology*, vol. 148, pp. 711–712, 2015.

[7] J.-P. Guo, P. B. Gilman, R. M. Thomas, R. S. Fisher, and H. P. Parkman, "Barrett's esophagus and achalasia," *Journal of Clinical Gastroenterology*, vol. 34, no. 4, pp. 439–443, 2002.

[8] P. Cantù, D. Savojardo, D. Baldoli, L. Bonavina, and R. Penagini, "Barrett's esophagus in untreated achalasia: 'Guess who's coming to dinner'first," *Diseases of the Esophagus*, vol. 21, no. 5, p. 473, 2008.

[9] H. L. Smart, P. N. Foster, and D. F. Evans, "Twenty four hour oesophaeal acidity in achalasia before and after pneumatic dilatation," *Gut*, vol. 28, no. 7, pp. 883–887, 1987.

[10] W. O. Richards, A. Torquati, M. D. Holzman et al., "Heller myotomy versus heller myotomy with dor fundoplication for achalasia: a prospective randomized double-blind clinical trial," *Annals of Surgery*, vol. 240, no. 3, pp. 405–415, 2004.

[11] A. Rawlings, N. J. Soper, B. Oelschlager et al., "Laparoscopic Dor versus Toupet fundoplication following Heller myotomy for achalasia: results of a multicenter, prospective, randomized-controlled trial," *Surgical Endoscopy*, vol. 26, no. 1, pp. 18–26, 2012.

[12] A. Poehlmann, D. Kuester, P. Malfertheiner, T. Guenther, and A. Roessner, "Inflammation and Barrett's carcinogenesis," *Pathology Research and Practice*, vol. 208, no. 5, pp. 269–280, 2012.

[13] L. M. G. Moons, J. G. Kusters, E. Bultman et al., "Barrett's oesophagus is characterized by a predominantly humoral inflammatory response," *The Journal of Pathology*, vol. 207, no. 3, pp. 269–276, 2005.

[14] J. M. Garcia, A. E. Splenser, J. Kramer et al., "Circulating inflammatory cytokines and adipokines are associated with increased risk of Barrett's esophagus: a case-control study," *Clinical Gastroenterology and Hepatology*, vol. 12, no. 2, pp. 229.e3–238.e3, 2014.

Acute Gastrointestinal Bleeding in Olmesartan-Associated Collagenous Gastroduodenitis: A Potential Endoscopic Complication

Rachel Hudacko [1] and Lance Siegel [2]

[1] *Orange Pathology Associates, PC, Department of Pathology, Orange Regional Medical Center, 707 East Main St., Middletown, NY 10940, USA*
[2] *Horizon Family Medical Group, Department of Gastroenterology, Orange Regional Medical Center, 707 East Main St., Middletown, NY 10940, USA*

Correspondence should be addressed to Rachel Hudacko; rhudacko@gmail.com

Academic Editor: Chia-Tung Shun

Collagenous gastroenteritis is a rare disease that is known to be associated with the drug olmesartan, an angiotensin II receptor antagonist used to treat hypertension. It is characterized histologically by increased subepithelial collagen deposition with associated inflammation and epithelial injury. Endoscopically, the mucosa appears inflamed and friable and may be nodular or atrophic. We report a case of acute gastric bleeding on direct mucosal contact during endoscopy in a patient with olmesartan-associated collagenous gastroduodenitis to raise awareness of this potential endoscopic complication.

1. Introduction

Collagenous gastroenteritis is a pattern of injury that is characterized histologically by subepithelial collagen deposition >10 μm in thickness with associated mucosal inflammation and epithelial injury [1]. The collagen bands are usually irregular, often entrap small capillaries, and can be highlighted with a trichrome stain. It is a rare disorder that may involve the stomach (collagenous gastritis) and/or small bowel (collagenous enteritis/sprue) and may occasionally coexist with the more common entity, collagenous colitis. The etiology of collagenous gastroenteritis is unknown but is suspected to be immune-mediated and may be associated with certain medications including the antihypertensive drug olmesartan, an angiotensin II receptor antagonist [2]. Several reports in the literature describe cases of olmesartan-associated collagenous duodenitis/sprue [3–5] with fewer reports of olmesartan-associated collagenous gastritis [3, 6] and only rare reports involving both the stomach and small bowel [3]. We herein report a case of olmesartan-associated collagenous gastroduodenitis that was complicated by acute gastrointestinal bleeding during endoscopy.

2. Case Presentation

A 64-year-old woman presented to the gastroenterologist with abdominal pain, unintentional 10 pound weight loss over 3 months, and reflux symptoms. Pertinent medical history included hypertension treated with olmesartan 20 mg once a day for the past 7 years, hyperlipidemia treated with simvastatin, gastroesophageal reflux disease treated with pantoprazole 20 mg twice a day, and osteoporosis treated with denosumab injections every 6 months. Esophagogastroduodenoscopy (EGD) performed in the office showed granular mucosa in the proximal duodenum and nodular mucosa in the stomach with numerous linear ulcers. On withdrawal of the scope from the duodenum, a large amount of fresh blood was noted in the stomach with clotted blood near the cardia. The bleeding was believed to be due to either the underlying gastric ulcers or a Mallory Weiss tear. The patient

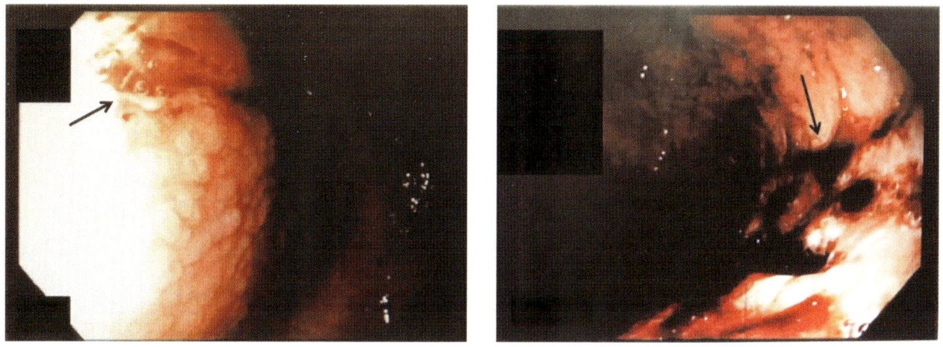

(a) (b)

FIGURE 1: Endoscopic photos of the body of the stomach show diffusely nodular mucosa (a) with deep linear ulcers (arrows) and severe inflammation and hemorrhage (b).

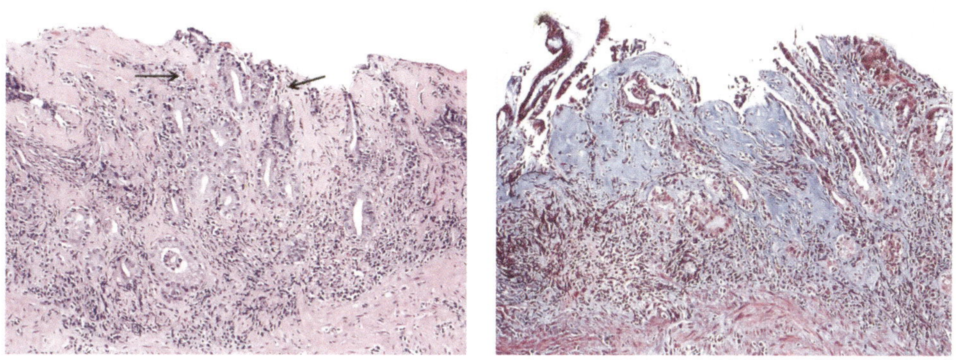

(a) (b)

FIGURE 2: 20x magnification: (a) hematoxylin and eosin-stained section of the gastric body shows a thick, markedly irregular pink band of subepithelial collagen deposition with complete surface erosion. The mucosa is inflamed and atrophic with loss of parietal cells. Arrows indicate entrapped capillaries. (b) Trichrome stain highlights the collagen blue.

was transferred to the emergency department for further evaluation.

On admission, the hemoglobin and hematocrit were normal, and an emergent EGD was performed. The gastric fundus and body appeared atrophic with friable and severely inflamed mucosa and multiple linear ulcers without active bleeding (Figure 1). The antral mucosa appeared erythematous. Biopsies of the stomach and duodenum were performed. The biopsies of the antrum and body showed increased subepithelial collagen deposition confirmed on a trichrome stain, chronic inflammation in the lamina propria, surface epithelial regenerative changes, and erosions, consistent with collagenous gastritis (Figure 2). The gastric body mucosa was atrophic with near-total loss of parietal cells. Immunostain for *H. pylori* organisms was negative, and a Congo red stain for amyloid was negative. The biopsies of the duodenum showed partial villous atrophy and increased subepithelial collagen deposition confirmed on a trichrome stain, consistent with collagenous duodenitis/sprue (Figure 3). The patient was started on high dose acid suppression with pantoprazole 40 mg twice a day, and the olmesartan was discontinued.

Follow-up EGD 7 weeks later showed somewhat atrophic gastric mucosa with few residual linear areas of erythema and complete resolution of the ulcers, inflammation, and mucosal friability (Figure 4). The duodenal mucosa appeared normal. Colonoscopy was unremarkable. Repeat biopsies showed marked improvement of the collagenous gastritis with resolution of the epithelial injury and only rare residual foci of subepithelial collagen. A mild nonspecific chronic inactive gastritis remained present. The biopsies from the duodenum and left colon showed normal mucosa without evidence of collagenous duodenitis or collagenous colitis.

3. Brief Discussion

Olmesartan-associated collagenous gastroenteritis is a rare entity that may be immune-mediated in nature. The length of time of olmesartan use before onset of symptoms varies from less than 1 month to 11 years [7]. When the stomach is solely involved, symptoms include dyspepsia, anemia due to bleeding, weight loss, and diarrhea. When the small intestine is involved, the most common symptoms are watery diarrhea and weight loss due to malabsorption [2]. The

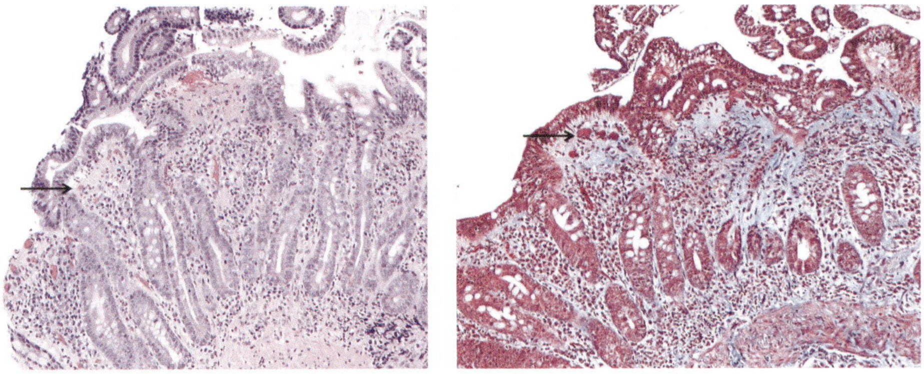

(a) (b)

Figure 3: 20x magnification: (a) hematoxylin and eosin-stained section of the duodenum shows villous shortening/partial atrophy with increased subepithelial collagen deposition (pink). (b) Trichrome stain highlights the collagen blue. Arrows indicate entrapped capillaries.

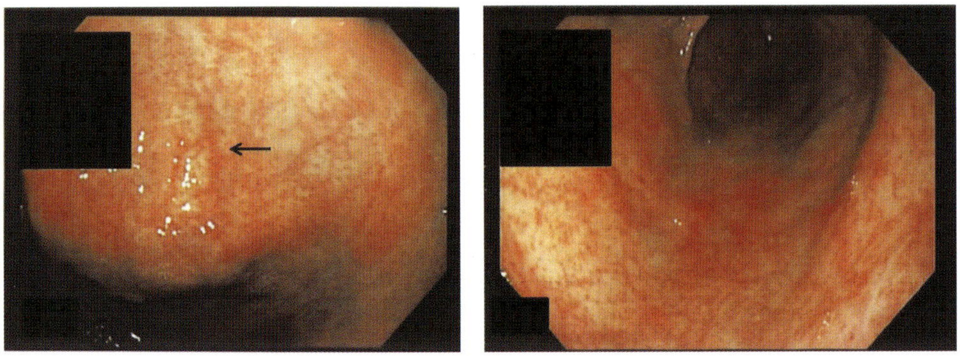

Figure 4: Endoscopic photos of the body of the stomach 7 weeks after cessation of olmesartan show atrophic mucosa with few residual areas of erythema (arrow) and complete resolution of the ulcers.

characteristic endoscopic finding of collagenous gastritis is nodular mucosa. Other findings include erythema, mucosal friability, erosions, ulcers, and atrophy [2, 6]. The endoscopic findings in the small bowel are nonspecific and include pale mucosa, mucosal thickening, and scalloping [2, 4].

The diagnostic histologic feature of collagenous gastroenteritis is band-like layer of subepithelial collagen deposition that is at least 10 μm in thickness and is associated with a chronic inflammatory infiltrate and surface epithelial injury [1]. The deposits can be patchy and irregular and often entrap superficial dilated capillaries [2]. Bleeding results from surface epithelial injury and sloughing which exposes these capillaries.

The majority of cases of olmesartan-associated collagenous gastroenteritis reported in the literature resolved after cessation of the drug [7]. One study reported complete clinical and pathologic resolution of collagenous duodenitis after treatment with the immunosuppressive drugs FK-506 and rapamycin [8]. Our patient had a complete clinical response and near-complete pathologic response at 7-week follow-up after discontinuation of olmesartan.

In summary, we report a case of acute gastric bleeding during endoscopy due to olmesartan-associated collagenous gastroduodenitis. The mechanism of bleeding in this disease is the presence of abnormal subepithelial collagen causing mucosal fragility. Bleeding may be spontaneous and chronic with associated anemia or may be acute and caused by direct contact with instruments during endoscopy, as was believed to be the reason for the acute bleed in this case. Although rare, it is important for endoscopists to be aware of this potential endoscopic complication in patients taking olmesartan.

References

[1] R. B. Colletti and T. D. Trainer, "Collagenous gastritis," *Gastroenterology*, vol. 97, no. 6, pp. 1552–1555, 1989.

[2] O. H. Nielsen, L. B. Riis, S. Danese, R. D. Bojesen, and C. Soendergaard, "Proximal collagenous gastroenteritides: clinical management: a systematic review," *Annals of Medicine*, vol. 46, no. 5, pp. 311–317, 2014.

[3] A. Rubio-Tapia, M. L. Herman, J. F. Ludvigsson et al., "Severe spruelike enteropathy associated with olmesartan," *Mayo Clinic Proceedings*, vol. 87, no. 8, pp. 732–738, 2012.

[4] J. A. Nielsen, A. Steephen, and M. Lewin, "Angiotensin-II inhibitor (olmesartan)-induced collagenous sprue with resolution following discontinuation of drug," *World Journal of Gastroenterology*, vol. 19, no. 40, pp. 6928–6930, 2013.

[5] C. Desruisseaux, M. Bensoussan, E. Désilets et al., "Adding water to the mill: olmesartan-induced collagenous sprue—a case report and brief literature review," *Canadian Journal of Gastroenterology and Hepatology*, vol. 2016, Article ID 4837270, 2 pages, 2016.

[6] C. Ma, J. Y. Park, E. A. Montgomery et al., "A comparative clinicopathologic study of collagenous gastritis in children and adults: The same disorder with associated immune-mediated diseases," *The American Journal of Surgical Pathology*, vol. 39, no. 6, pp. 802–812, 2015.

[7] N. Burbure, B. Lebwohl, C. Arguelles-Grande, P. H. R. Green, G. Bhagat, and S. Lagana, "Olmesartan-associated sprue-like enteropathy: A systematic review with emphasis on histopathology," *Human Pathology*, vol. 50, pp. 127–134, 2016.

[8] S. Scialom, G. Malamut, B. Meresse et al., "Gastrointestinal disorder associated with olmesartan mimics autoimmune enteropathy," *PLoS ONE*, vol. 10, no. 6, article e0125024, 2015.

30

Pneumatosis Cystoides Intestinalis in Patients with Systemic Sclerosis: A Case Report and Review of 39 Japanese Cases

Manabu Kaneko,[1] Shin Sasaki,[1] Shuzo Teruya,[2] Kosuke Ozaki,[1] Kazuhiro Ishimaru,[1] Emi Terai,[1] Hiroshi Nakayama,[1] and Toshiyuki Watanabe[1]

[1] *Department of Surgery, Omori Red Cross Hospital, 4-30-1 Chuo, Ota-ku, Tokyo 143-8527, Japan*
[2] *Department of Internal Medicine, Division of Rheumatology, Omori Red Cross Hospital, 4-30-1 Chuo, Ota-ku, Tokyo 143-8527, Japan*

Correspondence should be addressed to Manabu Kaneko; m.kaneko@fancy.ocn.ne.jp

Academic Editor: Tetsuo Hirata

Pneumatosis cystoides intestinalis (PCI) is a rare gastrointestinal complication of systemic sclerosis (SSc) characterized by intramural accumulation of gas within thin-walled cysts. We report the case of an 82-year-old female patient with pneumoperitoneum due to PCI associated with SSc and review the features of the 39 Japanese cases. The median patient age was 57 years (range 24–83 years) and the male/female ratio was 1 : 12. In the recent decade, 14 out of 15 cases (93.3%) evaluated with CT scans were diagnosed with PCI. The results suggest that CT scan may be a useful diagnostic tool for detecting PCI. PCI in patients with SSc is usually benign and requires only conservative therapy. However, two patients (5.1%) with signs of peritoneal irritation required surgery. When peritoneal irritation secondary to additional pathology is observed, surgical treatment may be warranted; a precise diagnosis for this condition is therefore essential.

1. Introduction

Pneumatosis cystoides intestinalis (PCI) is a rare gastrointestinal complication of systemic sclerosis (SSc). It is characterized by submucosal and/or subserosal collections of free gas, forming cystic lesions within the gastrointestinal tract and neighboring tissues [1, 2]. This complication is usually asymptomatic and detected incidentally through widespread use of computed tomography (CT) in recent years; however, it can be accompanied by abdominal pain and pneumoperitoneum. Clinical presentations and imaging characteristics in this condition may simulate true gastrointestinal perforation. A precise diagnosis is therefore essential, since PCI is generally treated conservatively. An extensive search on PubMed and the Japanese Medical Abstracts Society found 38 Japanese patients diagnosed with PCI accompanied by SSc over a span of 38 years (from 1978 to 2015). We hereby describe a case of SSc complicated by PCI and review the demographic, clinical, diagnostic, and therapeutic features of the 39 Japanese cases.

2. Case Report

An 82-year-old woman was referred to our department for incidental finding of pneumoperitoneum on a chest radiograph during a medical checkup at another hospital. Initial history taking revealed a prior surgical history of only a laparotomy secondary to acute appendicitis approximately 60 years before. During physical examination, the patient was afebrile with a pulse rate of 82 beats per minute and blood pressure of 136/86 mmHg. Abdominal examination revealed a slightly distended but soft, tympanic, and nontender abdomen, without signs of peritoneal irritation. There were no palpable masses. Urgent laboratory investigations showed a slightly low hemoglobin level with normal white blood cell count and C-reactive protein level (Table 1). A plain abdominal radiograph showed free air under the diaphragm bilaterally and small bowel dilatation (Figure 1). Abdominal CT scan revealed massive free air and dilated small intestine with gas inside the bowel wall; however, there was no radiological evidence of a localized point of

Table 1: Laboratory data on admission.

Complete blood count		Blood chemistry		Autoantibody (normal value)	
WBC	4800/μL	TP	7.4 g/dL	Antinuclear (speckled)	1:40 (<×40)
RBC	$332 \times 10^4/\mu$L	Alb	3.9 g/dL	Anti-Scl-70	8.9 (<10)
Hemoglobin	10.3 g/dL	BUN	20.8 mg/dL	Anticentromere	<5.0 (<10)
Hematocrit	32.1%	Cre	1.0 mg/dL		
Platelet	$12.9 \times 10^4/\mu$L	Na	143 mEq/L		
		K	4.4 mEq/L		
		Cl	111 mEq/L		
		T-Bil	0.4 mg/dL		
		AST	20 IU/L		
		ALT	12 IU/L		
		LDH	166 IU/L		
		γ-GTP	9 IU/L		
		CRP	0.00 mg/dL		
		HbA1c	5.4%		

WBC: white blood cell; RBC: red blood cell; TP: total protein; Alb: albumin; BUN: blood urea nitrogen; Cre: creatinine; T-Bil: total bilirubin; AST: aspartate aminotransferase; ALT: alanine aminotransferase; LDH: lactate dehydrogenase; γ-GTP: γ-glutamyl transferase; CRP: C-reactive protein; Na: sodium; K: potassium; Cl: chloride; HbA1c: glycated hemoglobin.

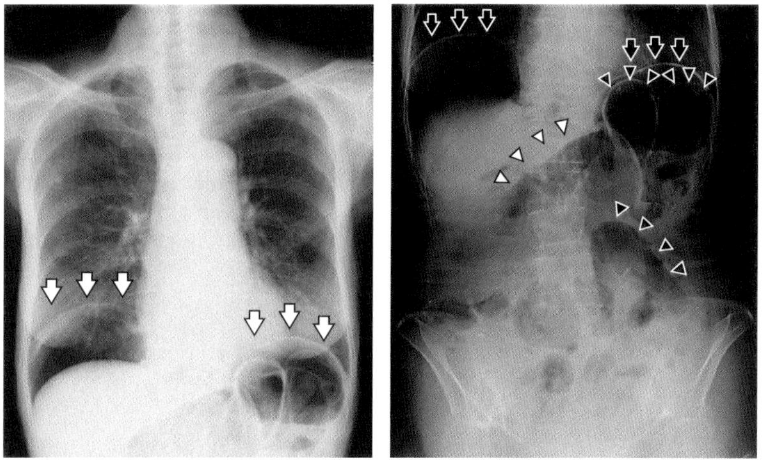

Figure 1: A chest radiograph demonstrating pneumoperitoneum in the subdiaphragmatic regions bilaterally (arrows). A plain abdominal radiograph showing several dilated loops of small intestine (arrowheads).

bowel obstruction and no apparent life-threatening acute causes of PCI (Figure 2). Although autoimmune serological testing showed negative results for antinuclear, anti-Scl-70, and anticentromere antibodies, further detailed history taking revealed that the patient had suffered from Raynaud's phenomenon and was previously diagnosed with SSc approximately 30 years before. She recalled that she was treated and followed up for several years, albeit without detailed information regarding her treatment. A rheumatologist later confirmed that she indeed had limited cutaneous SSc, in view of the presence of sclerodactyly of the fingers, telangiectasia on her face, chest, and hands, and Raynaud's phenomenon, all of which met the criteria for SSc [3]. Her pneumoperitoneum was considered to be due to PCI. As the patient was stable with no life-threatening signs and symptoms, she was treated conservatively with bowel rest and maintenance of fluid levels and subsequently discharged home without surgical intervention. The patient remained well eighteen months after discharge, without any abdominal symptoms.

3. Discussion

PCI is a rare gastrointestinal complication of SSc characterized by intramural accumulation of gas within thin-walled cysts. Air-filled bubble-like lesions are located in the submucosa or the subserosa of the alimentary tract. Although PCI is most commonly seen in the small intestine, it can also be detected in the large intestine or the stomach [2]. When these air-filled cysts rupture, they cause a pneumoperitoneum, which is generally benign in nature.

We searched on PubMed and the Japanese Medical Abstracts Society for case reports, excluding brief reports on clinical images, containing the key words "pneumatosis cystoides intestinalis" and "systemic sclerosis or scleroderma".

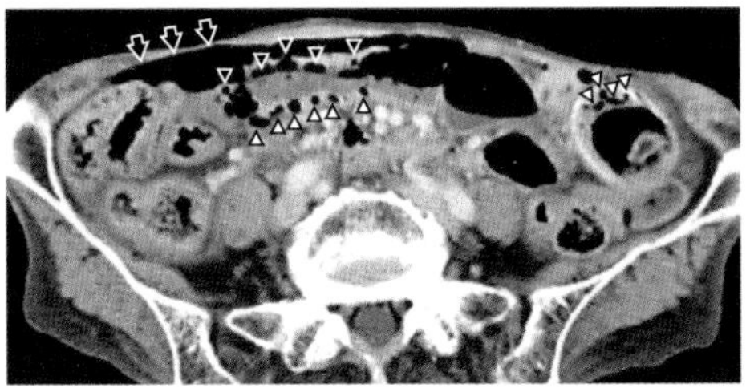

Figure 2: An abdominal computed tomography image demonstrating a large quantity of free air in the abdominal cavity (arrows). Multiple small cysts are seen within the wall of the small bowel (arrowheads), consistent with pneumatosis cystoides intestinalis in this patient with systemic sclerosis.

Of note, 39 cases from Japan (including our case) have been reported in the literature. Of these, 35 cases were reported in Japanese, while the others were in English [4–6] (Table 2). Any symptom that was not described was presumed to be absent. Likewise, any test that was not mentioned was presumed to have not been done. The median patient age was 57 years (range 24–83 years) and the male/female ratio was 1 : 12. Of these, 11 patients (28.2%) had SSc of the diffuse type while 23 (59.0%) had the limited type. The remaining 5 patients (12.8%) had types that could not be assessed. The mean disease duration from onset of SSc symptoms to diagnosis of PCI was 6 years (range 0–30 years). Antinuclear, anticentromere, and anti-Scl-70 antibodies were positive in 33, 7, and 3 patients (84.6%, 18.0%, and 7.7%), respectively. Overlap syndrome was seen in 8 patients with polymyositis (20.5%) and 1 patient with Sjogren's syndrome (2.6%). Small intestinal PCI was detected in 29 patients (74.3%) and large intestinal PCI in 4 patients (10.2%). The symptoms observed, in decreasing order, were abdominal distention ($n = 32$, 82.1%), abdominal pain ($n = 13$, 33.3%), abdominal tenderness ($n = 11$, 28.2%), and nausea or vomiting ($n = 9$, 23.1%), among others. Peritoneal irritation was seen in two patients (5.1%), both of whom required surgery. Pneumoperitoneum was involved in 34 patients (87.2%).

Gastrointestinal manifestation in SSc is characterized by atrophy of the muscularis propria and its replacement by collagen tissue, resulting in disturbances of digestive peristalsis and leading to gastroparesis, bacterial overgrowth of the small intestine, or constipation [7]. The etiology of PCI in patients with SSc is not fully understood. However, there are several possible mechanisms of how gas cysts were produced in the bowel wall. The mechanical theory suggests that increased luminal pressure caused by intestinal obstruction allows gas to penetrate into the submucosal space through a mucosal breakdown [8]. The bacterial theory suggests that gas cysts result from either excess hydrogen gas produced by intraluminal bacterial fermentation or altered partial pressure of nitrogen within the intestinal wall [9]. Finally, it has been advocated that long term use of corticosteroids could possibly induce atrophy of the intestinal mucosa, sometimes resulting in a mucosal break and the subsequent translocation of gas into the submucosal layer [10, 11]. In this review, 24 patients (61.5%) were reported to have received corticosteroid therapy.

Table 2: Demographic data for 39 Japanese cases of SSc with PCI.

Characteristics	Number of patients
Age (years), median (range)	57 (24–83)
Sex	
Female	36 (92.3%)
Male	3 (7.7%)
Types of scleroderma	
Diffuse	11 (28.2%)
Limited	23 (59.0%)
NA	5 (12.8%)
Duration from onset of SSc to onset of PCI (years), median (range)	6 (0–30)
Past corticosteroid therapy	
Present	24 (61.5%)
Autoantibody positivity	
Antinuclear antibody	33 (84.6%)
Anticentromere antibody	7 (18.0%)
Anti-Scl-70 antibody	3 (7.7%)
Negative	6 (15.4%)
Overlap syndrome	
Polymyositis/scleroderma	8 (20.5%)
Sjogren's syndrome/scleroderma	1 (2.6%)
Site of PCI	
Small intestine	27 (69.2%)
Small and large intestine	2 (5.1%)
Large intestine	2 (5.1%)
NA	8 (20.5%)
Symptoms and signs	
Abdominal distention	32 (82.1%)
Abdominal pain	13 (33.3%)
Abdominal tenderness	11 (28.2%)
Nausea/vomiting	9 (23.1%)
Weight loss	8 (20.5%)
Anorexia	8 (20.5%)
Constipation	5 (12.8%)
Fatigue	5 (12.8%)
Diarrhea	5 (12.8%)
Peritoneal irritation sign	2 (5.1%)
Diagnostic modalities	
Upper gastrointestinal series	2 (5.1%)
Plain X-ray film	10 (25.6%)
CT	11 (28.2%)
Plain X-ray film and CT	11 (28.2%)
Exploratory laparotomy	5 (12.8%)
Pneumoperitoneum	
Present	34 (87.2%)
Absent	5 (12.8%)
Treatment	
Antibiotics	13 (33.3%)
Oxygen therapy	9 (23.1%)
Octreotide	2 (5.1%)
Surgery	2 (5.1%)
Treatments other than the above-mentioned ones (symptomatic therapy combined with fluid therapy or elemental diet, etc.)	15 (38.5%)

SSc: systemic sclerosis; PCI: pneumatosis cystoides intestinalis; NA: not available; CT: computed tomography.

PCI may be detected through a variety of different radiographic imaging modalities, such as plain radiographs, contrast studies, CT scan, ultrasound, and magnetic resonance imaging. Among these, CT scan is the best diagnostic modality, with better sensitivity than plain radiographs or ultrasound [12]. In actual clinical settings, CT scan should follow a plain radiograph film with suggestive findings such as radiolucent linear or circular air bubbles in the bowel wall with/without subdiaphragmatic free air. In addition, a CT scan can provide additional information that may suggest the existence of other causes of PCI, such as intestinal volvulus, necrosis, or perforation [7]. In this review, CT scan was reported to be useful for detection of PCI in 22 (56.4%) cases. In the recent decade, particularly, 14 out of 15 cases (93.3%) evaluated with CT scans were diagnosed with PCI.

Treatment of PCI should be based on symptoms; in other words, patients with asymptomatic PCI need no treatment. If there are symptoms, excluding peritoneal irritation, conservative treatment, including one or more of the following, may be initiated: fluid and electrolyte supplementation, total parenteral nutrition, bowel rest, bowel tract decompression, elemental diet, antibiotics (tetracycline, metronidazole, or ampicillin), high concentration or hyperbaric oxygen inhalation therapy, and octreotide infusion [13–16]. Antibiotics are used for small intestinal bacterial overgrowth [17]. The bacterial theory is supported by the observation that benign PCI often responds to dietary changes, antibiotic therapy, and oxygen, which is believed to attenuate the gaseous cysts by decreasing the partial pressure of the nitrogenous gases and by being toxic to the anaerobic gut bacteria [9, 18–21]. In this review, the number of patients who received antibiotics, high concentration oxygen therapy, and hyperbaric oxygen therapy was 13 (33.3%), 7 (17.9%), and 2 (5.1%), respectively. Fifteen patients (38.5%) received other treatments such as fluid therapy, bowel tract decompression, or elemental diet. In our case, the patient did not exhibit any signs of peritonitis or bowel ischemia; therefore, conservative management was selected. Surgical treatment is generally not preferred because the disease is almost always generalized, and operative manipulation of a scleroderma bowel tends to result in prolonged ileus [13]. However, emergency surgical exploration must be taken into consideration when the clinical presentation, laboratory results, or imaging tests indicate peritoneal irritation [22]. In this review, two patients (5.1%) with signs of peritoneal irritation required surgery: one for small bowel volvulus and the other for recurrent peritonitis due to inflammation of the dilated jejunal loops resulting from distal jejunal stricture.

In conclusion, PCI among SSc patients is a rare complication, and its pathology is still not fully understood. In most cases, conservative management is preferable to surgical intervention. However, when peritoneal irritation is observed, surgical treatment may be warranted; a precise diagnosis is therefore essential in deciding whether a patient should be subjected to extensive surgery or treated conservatively. CT scan is a useful diagnostic tool for detecting not only PCI, but also additional pathology.

Consent

Written informed consent was obtained from the patient for publication.

Authors' Contributions

All authors contributed equally to this paper.

References

[1] V. Suarez, I. M. Chesner, A. B. Price, and J. Newman, "Pneumatosis cystoides intestinalis. Histological mucosal changes mimicking inflammatory bowel diseae," *Archives of Pathology and Laboratory Medicine*, vol. 113, no. 8, pp. 898–901, 1989.

[2] W. Sequeira, "Pneumatosis cystoides intestinalis in systemic sclerosis and other diseases," *Seminars in Arthritis and Rheumatism*, vol. 19, no. 5, pp. 269–277, 1990.

[3] F. Van Den Hoogen, D. Khanna, J. Fransen et al., "2013 classification criteria for systemic sclerosis: an american college of rheumatology/European league against rheumatism collaborative initiative," *Arthritis and Rheumatism*, vol. 65, no. 11, pp. 2737–2747, 2013.

[4] T. Kobayashi, M. Kobayashi, M. Naka, K. Nakajima, A. Momose, and M. Toi, "Response to octreotide of intestinal pseudoobstruction and pneumatosis cystoides intestinalis associated with progressive systemic sclerosis," *Internal Medicine*, vol. 32, no. 7, pp. 607–609, 1993.

[5] M. Hamada, M. Kayashima, Y. Morai, T. C. Masuda, K. Urabe, and M. Furue, "Pneumatosis cystoides intestinalis with systemic sclerosis, limited type resulting in a poor prognosis," *American Journal of the Medical Sciences*, vol. 332, no. 2, pp. 100–102, 2006.

[6] A. Sagara, K. Kitagawa, K. Furuichi et al., "Three cases of pneumatosis intestinalis presenting in autoimmune diseases," *Modern Rheumatology*, vol. 22, no. 4, pp. 610–615, 2012.

[7] L. M. Ho, E. K. Paulson, and W. M. Thompson, "Pneumatosis intestinal is in the adult: benign to life-threatening causes," *American Journal of Roentgenology*, vol. 188, no. 6, pp. 1604–1613, 2007.

[8] A. S. Pieterse, A. S.-Y. Leong, and R. Rowland, "The mucosal changes and pathogenesis of pneumatosis cystoides intestinalis," *Human Pathology*, vol. 16, no. 7, pp. 683–688, 1985.

[9] M. D. Levitt and S. Olsson, "Pneumatosis cystoides intestinalis and high breath H_2 excretion: insights into the role of H_2 in this condition," *Gastroenterology*, vol. 108, no. 5, pp. 1560–1565, 1995.

[10] B. H. Smith and L. H. Welter, "Pneumatosis intestinalis," *American Journal of Clinical Pathology*, vol. 48, no. 5, pp. 455–465, 1967.

[11] R. R. Hall, A. Anagnostou, M. Kanojia, and A. Zander, "Pneumatosis intestinalis associated with graft-versus-host disease of the intestinal tract," *Transplantation Proceedings*, vol. 16, no. 6, pp. 1666–1668, 1984.

[12] S. D. St Peter, M. A. Abbas, and K. A. Kelly, "The spectrum of pneumatosis intestinalis," *Archives of Surgery*, vol. 138, no. 1, pp. 68–75, 2003.

[13] G. Lock, A. Holstege, B. Lang, and J. Schölmerich, "Gastrointestinal manifestations of progressive systemic sclerosis," *The American Journal of Gastroenterology*, vol. 92, no. 5, pp. 763–771, 1997.

[14] E. C. Ebert, "Gastric and enteric involvement in progressive systemic sclerosis," *Journal of Clinical Gastroenterology*, vol. 42, no. 1, pp. 5–12, 2008.

[15] J. Vischio, Z. Matlyuk-Urman, and S. Lakshminarayanan, "Benign spontaneous pneumoperitoneum in systemic sclerosis," *Journal of Clinical Rheumatology*, vol. 16, no. 8, pp. 379–381, 2010.

[16] A. Balbir-Gurman, O. R. Brook, I. Chermesh, and Y. Braun-Moscovici, "Pneumatosis cystoides intestinalis in scleroderma-related conditions," *Internal Medicine Journal*, vol. 42, no. 3, pp. 323–329, 2012.

[17] G. Gyger and M. Baron, "Systemic sclerosis: gastrointestinal disease and its management," *Rheumatic Disease Clinics of North America*, vol. 41, no. 3, pp. 459–473, 2015.

[18] C. E. Yale, E. Balish, and J. P. Wu, "The bacterial etiology of pneumatosis cystoides intestinalis," *Archives of Surgery*, vol. 109, no. 1, pp. 89–94, 1974.

[19] R. Reyna, R. T. Soper, and R. E. Condon, "Pneumatosis intestinalis. Report of twelve cases," *The American Journal of Surgery*, vol. 125, no. 6, pp. 667–671, 1973.

[20] N. W. Read, M. N. Al-Janabi, and P. A. Cann, "Is raised breath hydrogen related to the pathogenesis of pneumatosis coli?" *Gut*, vol. 25, no. 8, pp. 839–845, 1984.

[21] T. Florin and B. Hills, "Does counterperfusion supersaturation cause gas cysts in pneumatosis cystoides coli, and can breathing heliox reduce them?" *The Lancet*, vol. 345, no. 8959, pp. 1220–1222, 1995.

[22] P. N. Khalil, S. Huber-Wagner, R. Ladurner et al., "Natural history, clinical pattern, and surgical considerations of pneumatosis intestinalis," *European Journal of Medical Research*, vol. 14, no. 6, pp. 231–239, 2009.

Periampullary Variceal Bleeding: An Atypical Complication of Portal Hypertension

Zahava C. Farkas,[1] Priyanka Chugh,[2] Shalom Frager,[2] Khwaja F. Haq,[1] Muhammad Ali Khan,[3] Shantanu Solanki,[4] Edward Esses,[5] Gregory Veillette,[6] and Roxana Bodin[2]

[1] *Department of Medicine, New York Medical College at Westchester Medical Center, Valhalla, NY, USA*
[2] *Division of Gastroenterology and Hepatobiliary Disease, New York Medical College at Westchester Medical Center, Valhalla, NY, USA*
[3] *Division of Gastroenterology and Hepatobiliary Disease, University of Tennessee Health Science Center, Memphis, TN, USA*
[4] *Internal Medicine, New York Medical College at Westchester Medical Center, Valhalla, NY, USA*
[5] *Department of Radiology, New York Medical College at Westchester Medical Center, Valhalla, NY, USA*
[6] *Department of Hepatobiliary Surgery, New York Medical College at Westchester Medical Center, Valhalla, NY, USA*

Correspondence should be addressed to Zahava C. Farkas; zahava88@gmail.com

Academic Editor: Engin Altintas

Variceal bleeding remains a fatal complication of portal hypertension. Periampullary varices are rare and, due to their location, are difficult to diagnose and treat. Similar to esophagogastric varices, they are the result of high portosystemic pressures secondary to intrahepatic causes such as cirrhosis and extrahepatic causes such as portal or splenic vein thrombosis. We report a case of a periampullary varix resulting in hemobilia during endoscopic retrograde cholangiopancreatography (ERCP).

1. Introduction

A periampullary varix, or dilated venous collateral surrounding the ampulla of vater, is a rare complication of portal hypertension. In our review of the available literature, only 1–3% of variceal bleeding in cirrhotic patients is attributed to duodenal varices with the most common sites being the duodenal bulb followed by the second part of the duodenum [1]. Although the vast majority of gastrointestinal (GI) bleeding occurs from ruptured esophagogastric varices, the portal enteropathy known to occur with portal hypertension makes the small bowel, including the region of the duodenal papilla, a potential source of bleeding.

This rare form of ectopic varix should be considered in patients with portal hypertension who are undergoing an ERCP and in those with upper GI bleeding without obvious stigmata of portal hypertension and a normal upper GI endoscopy. In some patients this may be the first manifestation of underlying portal hypertension, and therefore, maintaining a high clinical suspicion may reduce mortality rates and improve patient outcomes. The following case is presented to emphasize the clinical challenges of a periampullary varix resulting in GI bleeding during an ERCP.

2. Case Report

A 37-year-old woman with chronic portal vein thrombosis and cavernous transformation presented due to a recurrent episode of hematemesis. She had previously undergone multiple esophageal band ligations for esophageal varices seen on esophagogastroduodenoscopy (EGD). Ultrasonography showed elevated portal pressures and magnetic resonance cholangiopancreatography (MRCP) showed portal vein thrombosis. In addition, there were dilated periportal varices (cavernous transformation) exerting mass effect on the extrahepatic common bile duct and severe intrahepatic biliary ductal dilation involving all hepatic segments. Liver enzymes were persistently elevated in a cholestatic pattern: aspartate aminotransferase (AST) 64 U/L, alanine aminotransferase (ALT) 48 U/L, alkaline phosphatase (ALK) 303 U/L, total bilirubin (Tbili) 8.4 mg/dl, albumin 3.8 g/dl, and prothrombin time 11.9 seconds.

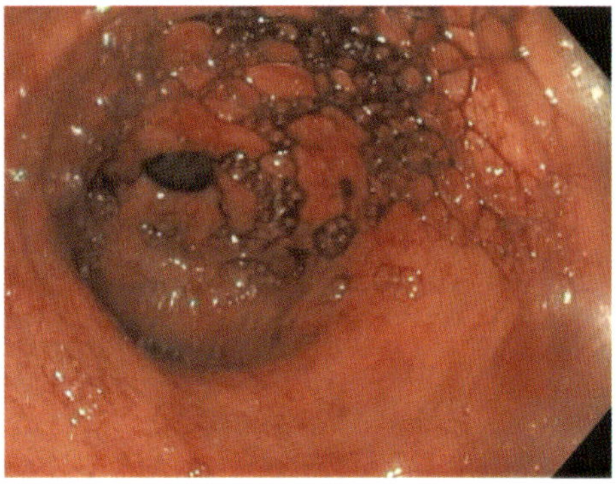

Figure 1: Hemobilia from a ruptured periampullary varix seen during an endoscopic retrograde cholangiopancreatography (ERCP).

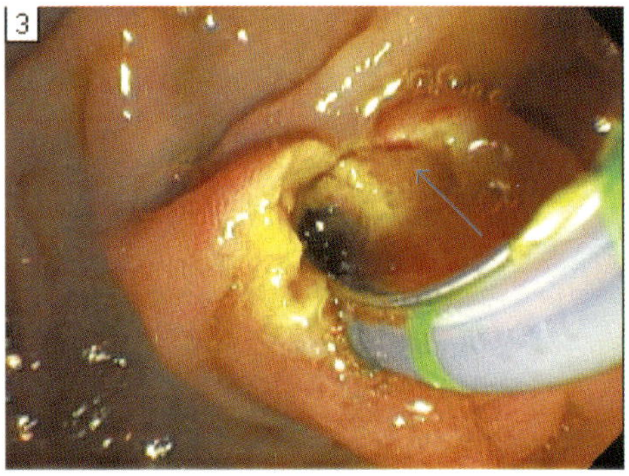

Figure 2: A duodenal varix (blue arrow) seen in the periampullary region on retroflexion during endoscopic retrograde cholangiopancreatography (ERCP).

The liver was noncirrhotic on biopsy. Computed tomography (CT) of the abdomen showed large varices in the porta hepatis and portal vein thrombosis that appeared chronic in nature with cavernous transformation. Operative management with a mesocaval shunt was planned with the hopes of reducing portal pressure and preventing recurrent GI bleeding, portal biliopathy, and secondary cirrhosis. A selective shunt, such as a splenorenal shunt, selects nonintestinal flow to be shunted to the systemic venous drainage and has the advantage of reducing the incidence of encephalopathy. This type of shunt, however, would not have adequately reduced variceal pressures and therefore the decision was made to proceed with a mesocaval shunt.

The patient underwent an ERCP to better assess the biliary anatomy, as part of the preoperative evaluation for a shunt. During the procedure, she developed active hemobilia (Figure 1) from a newly discovered periampullary varix (Figure 2). A biliary covered metal stent was immediately placed, but without hemostasis. Due to ongoing bleeding that required activation of a massive transfusion protocol, an exploratory laparotomy was performed with emergent mesocaval shunt placement (Figures 3 and 4). An 8 mm ringed polytetrafluoroethylene (PTFE) graft was used to create a mesocaval shunt between the proximal superior mesenteric vein (SMV) and the infrarenal inferior vena cava (IVC).

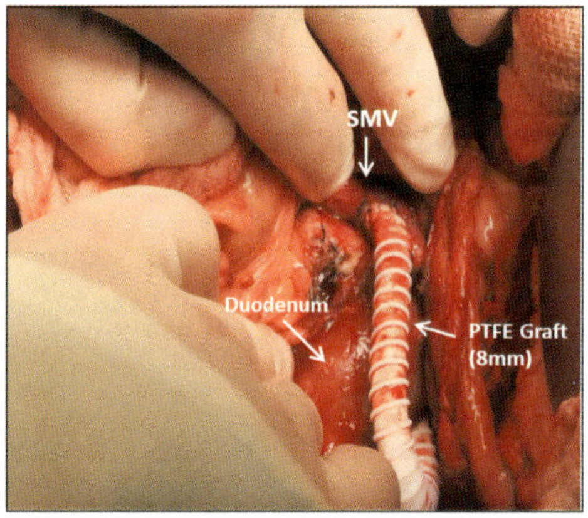

Figure 3: Intraoperative photo demonstrating the mesocaval bypass. An 8 mm ringed polytetrafluoroethylene (PTFE) graft was used to shunt blood flow from the proximal superior mesenteric vein (SMV) to the infrarenal IVC.

Portal pressures decreased by 8 mmHg after shunting and the bleeding stopped. She remained hemodynamically stable and was discharged ten days postoperatively. Follow-up mesocaval shuntogram showed a patent shunt with an outflow pressure of 13 mm Hg at the IVC and a portosystemic pressure gradient of 12 mm Hg. Two months postoperatively, she had an AST of 56 U/L, ALT 51 U/L, ALK 416 U/L, and Tbili 0.9 mg/dl. To date, she has had no episodes of hepatic encephalopathy.

3. Discussion

The second portion of the duodenum contains the major duodenal papilla and receives drainage from the pancreatic and common bile ducts through the ampulla of vater. Venous blood return from this area is through the pancreaticoduodenal vein to the gastroduodenal vein and ultimately into portal circulation through the splenic or superior mesenteric vein [2]. Elevated portal pressures can result in dilated tortuous vessels surrounding the ampulla, known as a periampullary varix. Similar to esophagogastric varices, they are the result of high portosystemic pressures secondary to intrahepatic causes such as cirrhosis and extrahepatic causes such as portal or splenic vein thrombosis.

The above reported case is an example of portal hypertensive biliopathy, defined as changes in the biliary tract in patients with portal hypertension due to extrahepatic portal vein obstruction [3]. Esophagogastric varices are the most common complication of portal hypertension; however, portosystemic venous collaterals can occur anywhere in the GI tract and are known as ectopic varices. These varices are less common and account for between 1% and 5% of all variceal bleeding. Although bleeding from ectopic varices is rare, it is generally massive and life-threatening [4].

Duodenal varices, such as the periampullary varix seen in this case, are most commonly found in the duodenal bulb and second portion of the duodenum. They are especially clinically relevant in patients known to have elevated portal

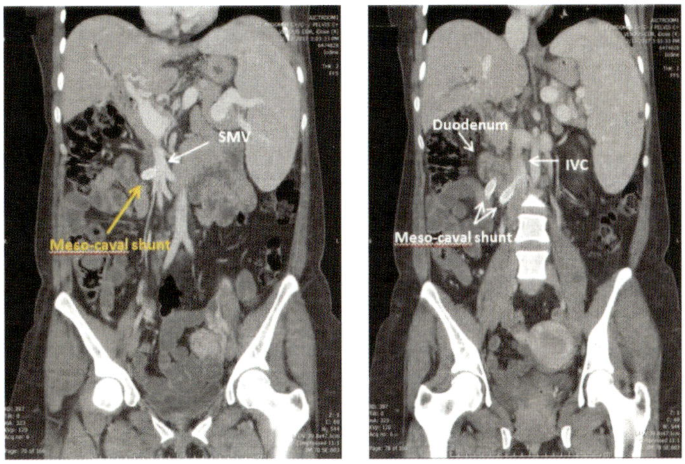

(a) (b)

Figure 4: Coronal view on computed tomography showing the mesocaval shunt (yellow arrow) originating from the SMV and inserting into the infrarenal IVC.

pressures who are undergoing endoscopic intervention such as an ERCP. Appropriate preprocedure planning, using a multidisciplinary team approach, is important as mortality rates from bleeding duodenal varices are reportedly as high as 40% [5, 6].

Endoscopic variceal ligation (EVL) and endoscopic injection sclerotherapy (EIS) are the mainstay of treatment for bleeding esophageal varices; however, there are no widely accepted guidelines for treatment of a duodenal varix [6]. Isolated case reports describe treatment of bleeding duodenal varices using band ligation, injection sclerotherapy, decompressive procedures such as a mesocaval shunt, and surgical procedures like oversewing the varices [7, 8]. Interventional radiology treatment options for duodenal varices include transjugular intrahepatic portosystemic shunt (TIPS), balloon-occluded retrograde transvenous obliteration (BRTO), and percutaneous transhepatic obliteration (PTO). In the above reported case, a mesocaval shunt was performed to decrease pressures and control the bleeding. A mesocaval shunt reduces portal pressures by forming an anastomosis between the superior mesenteric vein and the inferior vena cava, thereby diverting flow away from the portal system.

In conclusion, this case highlights the importance of recognizing more rare complications of portal hypertension such as a periampullary varix. Appropriate foresight into such complications is necessary as bleeding from ectopic varices is often massive and achieving hemostasis is difficult. A multidisciplinary team including a skilled endoscopists, a hepatobiliary surgeon, and an interventional radiologist should be involved early on, in anticipation of these potential complications.

Consent

Informed patient consent was obtained for publication of the case details. Documentation is available upon request.

Disclosure

This manuscript was presented as a poster presentation at the World Congress of Gastroenterology at ACG 2017. This study was carried out at the Department of Medicine and Division of Gastroenterology, New York Medical College at Westchester Medical Center, Valhalla, NY 10595, USA. This article's guarantor is Roxana Bodin, MD.

References

[1] N. H. Zubaidah, J. H. Asraf, L. Lee, and T. Gee, "Idiopathic duodenal varix presenting as a massive upper gastrointestinal bleeding: a case report," *Medical Journal of Malaysia*, vol. 71, no. 5, pp. 294-295, 2016.

[2] M. Hashizume, K. Tanoue, M. Ohta et al., "Vascular anatomy of duodenal varices: angiographic and histopathological assessments," *The American Journal of Gastroenterology*, vol. 88, no. 11, pp. 1942–1945, 1993.

[3] V. Suárez, A. Puerta, L. F. Santos, J. M. Pérez, A. Varón, and R. C. Botero, "Portal hypertensive biliopathy: a single center experience and literature review," *World Journal of Hepatology*, vol. 5, no. 3, pp. 137–144, 2013.

[4] T. Sato, J. Akaike, J. Toyota, Y. Karino, and T. Ohmura, "Clinicopathological features and treatment of ectopic varices with portal hypertension," *International Journal of Hepatology*, vol. 2011, Article ID 960720, 9 pages, 2011.

[5] S. Bhagani, C. Winters, and S. Moreea, "Duodenal variceal bleed: An unusual cause of upper gastrointestinal bleed and a difficult diagnosis to make," *BMJ Case Reports*, vol. 2017, 2017.

[6] A. Helmy, K. A. Kahtani, and M. Al Fadda, "Updates in the pathogenesis, diagnosis and management of ectopic varices," *Hepatology International*, vol. 2, no. 3, pp. 322–334, 2008.

[7] C.-S. Wang, L.-B. B. Jeng, and M.-F. Chen, "Duodenal variceal bleeding—successfully treated by mesocaval shunt after failure of sclerotherapy," *Hepato-Gastroenterology*, vol. 42, no. 1, pp. 59–61, 1995.

[8] J. Kee Ho, N. Mahmoudi, J. Al-Ali, E. Yoshida, and M. Byrne, "Duodenal varices: a rare manifestation of portal hypertension," *The Internet Journal of Gastroenterology*, vol. 5, no. 1, 2006.

32

Isolated Polycystic Liver Disease: An Unusual Cause of Recurrent Variceal Bleed

Mohammad Saud Khan,[1] **Zubair Khan**,[1] **Toseef Javaid**,[1] **Jamal Akhtar**,[2] **Abdelmoniem Moustafa**,[1] **Amos Lal**,[2] **Abhinav Tiwari**,[1] **and Mohammad Taleb**[3]

[1]*Department of Internal Medicine, University of Toledo Medical Center, Toledo, OH, USA*
[2]*Department of Internal Medicine, Saint Vincent Hospital, Worcester, MA, USA*
[3]*Division of Pulmonary, Critical Care and Sleep Medicine, University of Toledo Medical Center, Toledo, OH, USA*

Correspondence should be addressed to Mohammad Saud Khan; mohammad.khan2@utoledo.edu

Academic Editor: Chia-Tung Shun

Isolated polycystic liver disease is a rare disorder. Majority of the patients with isolated polycystic liver disease are asymptomatic with incidental detection of liver cysts on imaging studies done for other purposes. Minority of patients develop symptoms which are mostly secondary to enlarging cysts size and hepatomegaly. Rarely, these patients develop portal hypertension and can present with its clinical manifestations and consequences in the form acute variceal bleeding or recurrent ascites. We present a rare case of 67-year-old female patient with significant history of polycystic liver disease who presented to the hospital with recurrent hematemesis and melena. She underwent esophagogastroduodenoscopy which showed multiple large esophageal varices requiring banding.

1. Introduction

Acute variceal bleeding is most commonly caused by portal hypertension secondary to liver cirrhosis. Polycystic liver disease is a rare etiology for portal hypertension and bleeding varices [1]. Portal hypertension is usually seen in advanced stages of polycystic liver disease. It can result from mechanical pressure of enlarging cysts on vascular structures such as hepatic veins, inferior vena cava, and portal vein or can be caused by secondary fibrosis in the setting of polycystic liver disease [1, 2]. We present a case of a 67 year old female patient with significant history of polycystic liver disease and had recurrent episodes of variceal bleeding requiring multiple banding.

2. Case Report

A 67-year-old Caucasian female patient presented to the hospital with one day history of hematemesis and melena. She had two episodes of bright red emesis and four episodes of dark colored stools the day she presented, followed by a brief syncopal episode lasting for 10-15 seconds. She also complained of epigastric pain. She was diagnosed with polycystic liver disease and portal hypertension one year ago when she presented similarly with hematemesis and melena. At that time, she had an esophagogastroduodenoscopy (EGD) which showed esophageal varices and underwent banding. She denied any history of alcohol use, NSAID ingestion, or peptic ulcer disease. She was gravida 3, para 3, and had tubal ligation following her last pregnancy. She denied use of oral contraceptive pills or hormonal replacement therapy in the past. Her family history was significant for cystic liver disease and chronic liver failure in mother and maternal aunt.

At the time of presentation, she was afebrile (temperature of 98.7°F), tachycardic (heart rate of 110 beats/min), tachypneic (respiratory rate of 18/min), and hypotensive (blood pressure of 97/60 mmHg). Cardiopulmonary examination was normal. Abdominal examination showed mildly distended abdomen with epigastric and right upper quadrant tenderness, and bowel sounds were normal. Extremities showed bilateral 1+ pitting edema. Initial laboratory work showed hemoglobin of 7.7 g/dl, hematocrit of 24%, white blood count of 10.8 cells/mm^3, and platelet count of 162 cells/mm^3. Metabolic panel showed nonanion gap metabolic acidosis with serum bicarbonate of 17 mEq/L, normal serum

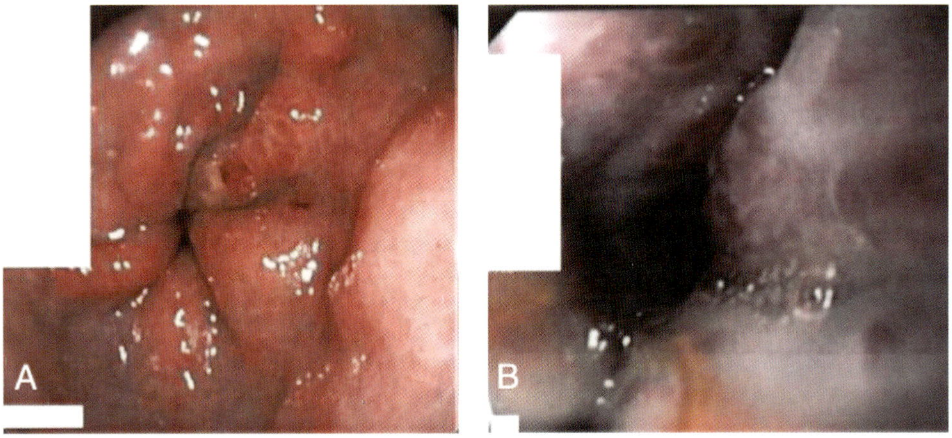

(a) (b)

Figure 1: Endoscopy images showing large esophageal varices.

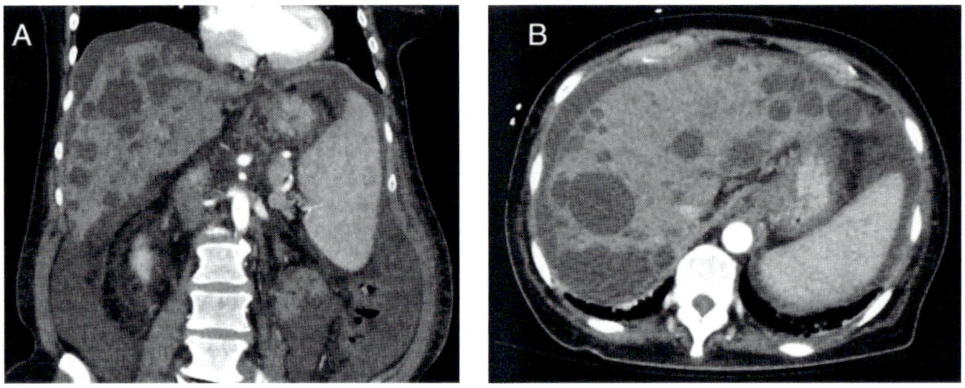

(a) (b)

Figure 2: Computed tomography of abdomen and pelvis (coronal and axial scans) showing polycystic liver disease along with evidence of portal hypertension in form of splenomegaly and ascites.

BUN, and creatinine of 23 mg/dl and 0.57 mg/dl, respectively. Liver panel showed total bilirubin of 2.2 mg/dl, direct bilirubin of 0.4 mg/dl, albumin of 2.5 g/dl, alkaline phosphatase of 51U/L, AST of 22 U/L, and ALT of 16 U/L. Gamma-glutamyltransferase was measured to be 27 U/L and prothrombin time (INR) was measured to be 1.46.

She was aggressively resuscitated with fluids, pressors, and packed red blood cell (PRBC) transfusion. Octreotide and proton pump inhibitor infusions were started. Patient was electively intubated for hemodynamic instability and altered mental status. An EGD was done which showed four columns of large esophageal varices with red wale sign showing stigmata of high risk for bleeding and type 1 gastroesophageal varices (Figure 1). Four bands were successfully applied starting from cardia up to midesophagus. A computed tomography (CT) of abdomen showed multiple cysts in the liver with evidence of portal hypertension in form of splenomegaly, ascites, and esophageal varices (Figure 2). Liver surface was smooth and no thrombus was identified in hepatic veins and inferior vena cava. Bilateral kidneys were normal with no evidence of renal cysts (Figure 3(a)). Vital signs and hemoglobin were monitored closely. Patient was successfully extubated next day and pressors were weaned off. Patient did not have any further episode of hematemesis but continued to have melena. She slowly dropped her hemoglobin requiring transfusions with PRBC. An EGD was repeated which reveled 3 more columns of esophageal varices with intact bands from previous EGD. Four more bands were placed on remaining varices. Following repeat EGD patient's hemoglobin remained stable for rest of her hospital stay. During her hospital stay, she also underwent therapeutic paracentesis with removal of 330 ml of peritoneal fluid for worsening ascites (Figure 3(b)). Peritoneal fluid analysis showed serum ascites albumin gradient (SAAG) of more than 1.1 g/dl, normal white cell count, negative gram stain, and cultures. She was started on propranolol, furosemide, and spironolactone. She was discharged home with recommendations to follow up in outpatient clinic with a plan of repeat EGD in 3-4 weeks.

3. Discussion

Polycystic liver disease (PLD) is an inherited disorder characterized by development of multiple cysts in the liver. It can

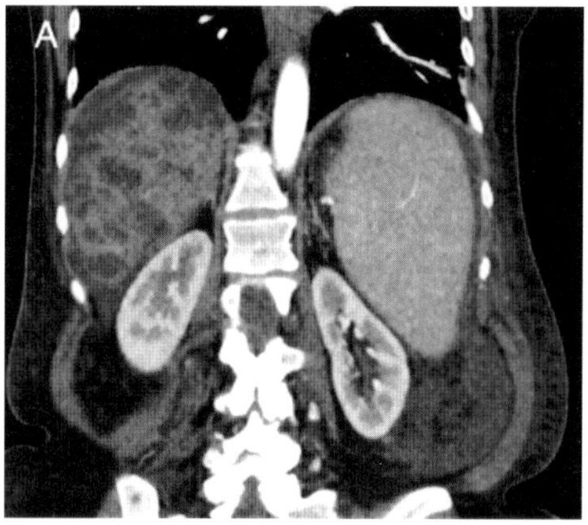

(a)

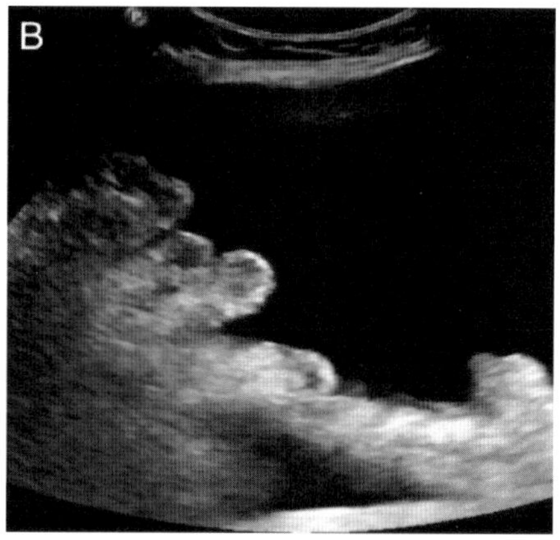

(b)

FIGURE 3: (a) Computed tomography of abdomen and pelvis (coronal view) showing normal architecture and enhancement of bilateral kidneys with no evidence of renal cysts. (b) Abdominal ultrasonographic image showed gross ascites.

occur as an isolated disease or in combination with polycystic kidney disease. Most of the cases of isolated polycystic liver disease are inherited in autosomal dominant pattern and hence it is also referred to as autosomal dominant polycystic liver disease (ADPLD). Isolated PLD is a genetically heterogeneous disorder and in majority of cases (approximately 70-80%) no mutation is identified [2, 3]. In rest minority of the cases (approximately 20-30%) a mutation in either PRKCSH or SEC63 gene is identified [4, 5]. PRKCSH gene is located on short arm of chromosome 19 (19p13.2-13.1) and encodes for a protein called hepatocystin [4]. SEC63 gene located on long arm of chromosome 6 (6q21-q23) [5]. Both these genes encode for proteins which are located within endoplasmic reticulum and play important role in synthesis of glycoproteins. Isolated PLD is a rare with an estimated prevalence of 1/100000 to 1/1000000 [1]. However, this might be underestimation of the true prevalence, as most of the patients have asymptomatic disease and never get diagnosed. More commonly PLD occurs in combination with polycystic kidney disease which is inherited either as autosomal dominant (ADPKD) or as autosomal recessive (ARPKD). Both of them can have liver involvement in the form of formation of multiple cysts in liver.

Liver cysts arise due to malformation of the ductal plate during embryonic development of biliary tract in liver [3]. There is proliferation of biliary ductules which leads to formation of biliary microhamartomas, also called von Meyenburg complexes. These biliary microhamartomas can be subject to progressive dilatation, leading to formation of liver cysts. The extent of liver involvement in PLD varies from few cysts confined to one or more segments to massive cystic enlargement of liver diffusely involving all segments. The severity of disease is seen to be more in females especially with history of multiple pregnancies or prolonged exposure to exogenous estrogen. Females tend to present at early age, have more widespread disease, and are more likely to progress to liver failure [2].

Majority of patients with isolated PLD (more than 80%) are asymptomatic with detection of liver cysts an incidental finding [3]. Minority of the patients develop symptoms which are typically secondary to enlarging size and mass effect of liver cysts. These include abdominal fullness, abdominal discomfort, back pain, anorexia, early satiety, malnutrition, gastroesophageal reflux, and dyspnea. Sometimes, it may present with acute abdominal pain which is secondary to cyst rupture, hemorrhage, or infection. Very rarely, patients of PLD can present with signs and symptoms of portal hypertension as seen in our patient. Portal hypertension is usually seen in advanced stages of PLD and can be caused by a number of processes in polycystic liver disease [1]. Firstly, portal hypertension can result from mechanical pressure from enlarging cysts on hepatic veins or inferior vena cava leading to obstruction in hepatic vein outflow. In some cases of polycystic liver disease, hepatic vein outflow obstruction may occur secondary to hepatic vein thrombosis (Budd-Chiari syndrome) [1, 6]. Secondly, enlarging hepatic cysts can compress on portal vein inflow leading to portal hypertension. Lastly, in advanced stages of disease there may be development of liver fibrosis which might lead to portal hypertension [1]. Portal hypertension leads to development of esophageal varices, splenomegaly, and ascites. Jaundice is an uncommon finding in polycystic liver disease and seen only in advanced stages. Liver functions are usually preserved in majority of patients of PLD and progression to end stage liver disease is rare. The most common laboratory abnormality seen in polycystic liver disease is mild elevation of gamma-glutamyltransferase and alkaline phosphatase [2].

Diagnosis of PLD is established radiologically by imaging studies including ultrasonography, CT, and magnetic resonance imaging. Treatment strategies for PLD include conservative management, invasive approach, and medical therapy [7]. Long-term outcome in majority of patients of PLD is good with normal quality of life. These patients if asymptomatic will require no treatment. In those who are symptomatic or have advance disease, various invasive procedures can be used for management of PLD and include aspiration sclerotherapy, laparoscopic fenestration, surgical deroofing, and segmental hepatic resection [7]. Liver transplantation is considered in patients who suffer tremendous morbidity and medical complications from severe PLD and are unsuitable for segmental hepatic resection or surgical interventions. Although no medical therapy is presently approved for treatment of PLD, recent studies with somatostatin analogues and mTOR inhibitors have been encouraging. When compared to placebo both octreotide and lanreotide (somatostatin analogues) have shown significant reduction in total liver volume in patients with PLD [8, 9]. Similarly, use of sirolimus and everolimus (mTOR inhibitors) has shown significant reduction in polycystic liver volumes suggesting a potential role in the treatment of PLD [10]. However further studies are needed to determine their long-term efficacy and tolerability in PLD. As discussed earlier, development of portal hypertension in PLD may be multifactorial and can be of significant concern in advanced disease. Portal hypertension and its complications such as acute variceal bleeding and recurrent ascites can be difficult to treat in patients of PLD. Somatostatin analogues can potentially serve as useful medical treatment in this regard due to their dual effect on decreasing the portal venous pressure and arresting the variceal bleeding as well reducing the cyst size and total liver volume. Currently, patients of PLD with recurrent complications of portal hypertension are treated with surgical portosystemic shunt creation and/or liver transplantation.

Polycystic liver disease has been considered a contraindication for transjugular intrahepatic portosystemic shunt (TIPPS) creation. Although, the rationale behind this is poorly documented, it is believed that presence of multiple cysts in liver leads to hepatic architectural distortion causing technical difficulties in creation of TIPPS. However, the absolute contraindication of TIPPS in polycystic liver disease has been challenged recently in a number of case reports [11–14]. These case reports have documented successful creation of TIPPS in polycystic liver disease patients warranting reconsideration of this contraindication.

4. Conclusion

Isolated polycystic liver disease is a rare disease and portal hypertension presenting as acute variceal bleeding is an uncommon manifestation of it.

References

[1] W. R. Cnossen and J. P. H. Drenth, "Polycystic liver disease: An overview of pathogenesis, clinical manifestations and management," *Orphanet Journal of Rare Diseases*, vol. 9, no. 1, article no. 69, 2014.

[2] N. Chandok, "Polycystic liver disease: a clinical review," *Annals of Hepatology*, vol. 11, no. 6, pp. 819–826, 2012.

[3] Q. Qian, "Isolated polycystic liver disease," *Advances in Chronic Kidney Disease*, vol. 17, no. 2, pp. 181–189, 2010.

[4] A. Li, S. Davila, L. Furu et al., "Mutations in PRKCSH cause isolated autosomal dominant polycystic liver disease," *American Journal of Human Genetics*, vol. 72, no. 3, pp. 691–703, 2003.

[5] S. Davila et al., "Mutations in SEC63 cause autosomal dominant polycystic liver disease," *Nature Genetics*, vol. 36, no. 6, pp. 575–577, 2004.

[6] W. Uddin, J. K. Ramage, B. Portmann et al., "Hepatic venous outflow obstruction in patients with polycystic liver disease: pathogenesis and treatment," *Gut*, vol. 36, no. 1, pp. 142–145, 1995.

[7] J. P. Drenth et al., "Medical and surgical treatment options for polycystic liver disease," *Hepatology*, vol. 52, no. 6, pp. 2223–2230, 2010.

[8] T. J. Gevers and J. P. Drenth, "Somatostatin analogues for treatment of polycystic liver disease," *Current Opinion in Gastroenterology*, vol. 27, no. 3, pp. 294–300, 2011.

[9] M. C. Hogan, T. V. Masyuk, L. Page et al., "Somatostatin analog therapy for severe polycystic liver disease: Results after 2 years," *Nephrology Dialysis Transplantation* , vol. 27, no. 9, pp. 3532–3539, 2012.

[10] Q. Qian, H. Du, B. F. King et al., "Sirolimus reduces polycystic liver volume in ADPKD patients," *Journal of the American Society of Nephrology*, vol. 19, no. 3, pp. 631–638, 2008.

[11] R. M. Spillane, J. A. Kaufman, J. Powelson, S. C. Geller, and A. C. Waltman, "Successful Transjugular Intrahepatic Portosystemic Shunt Creation in a Patient with Polycystic Liver Disease," *American Journal of Roentgenology*, vol. 169, no. 6, pp. 1542–1544, 1997.

[12] P. F. Bahramipour, S. Festa, R. Biswal, and R. H. Wachsberg, "Transjugular intrahepatic portosystemic shunt for the treatment of intractable ascites in a patient with polycystic liver disease," *CardioVascular and Interventional Radiology*, vol. 23, no. 3, pp. 232–234, 2000.

[13] E. S. Shin and M. D. Darcy, "Transjugular intrahepatic portosystemic shunt placement in the setting of polycystic liver disease: Questioning the contraindication," *Journal of Vascular and Interventional Radiology*, vol. 12, no. 9, pp. 1099–1102, 2001.

[14] D. Y. Sze, N. Strobel, R. Fahrig, T. Moore, S. Busque, and J. K. Frisoli, "Transjugular intrahepatic portosystemic shunt creation in a polycystic liver facilitated by hybrid cross-sectional/angiographic imaging," *Journal of Vascular and Interventional Radiology*, vol. 17, no. 4, pp. 711–715, 2006.

33

Non-*Helicobacter pylori* Gastric Intestinal Metaplasia in Children: A Series of Cases and Review of the Literature

Sandra Mabel Camacho-Gomez,[1] Anas Bernieh,[2] Ali G. Saad,[2] and Neelesh Ajit Tipnis[1]

[1]*Department of Pediatrics, University of Mississippi Medical Center, 2500 North State Street, Jackson, MS 39216, USA*
[2]*Department of Pathology, University of Mississippi Medical Center, 2500 North State Street, Jackson, MS 39216, USA*

Correspondence should be addressed to Neelesh Ajit Tipnis; neeleshtipnis@gmail.com

Academic Editor: I. Michael Leitman

In the pediatric population, Gastric Intestinal Metaplasia (GIM) is a finding with unknown frequency and, more importantly, unknown clinical implications. The relationship between *Helicobacter pylori* (HP) infection and GIM is well documented, as well as an association between duodenogastric reflux and GIM. We present two cases of pediatric patients with GIM along with a review of the literature. The diagnosis of GIM may have adverse clinical implications and should be made with caution in a child. The association of GIM and adenoma/dysplasia and carcinoma is rarely seen in children, primarily because the time required for these to develop takes the individual into adulthood. Treatment, long-term consequences, and surveillance protocols are not well established in the pediatric population. Studies to evaluate the long-term natural history, treatment, and surveillance protocols in children with GIM are needed.

1. Introduction

Gastric Intestinal Metaplasia (GIM) is a finding with unknown frequency and, more importantly, unknown clinical implications in children. We present two cases of pediatric patients with GIM and a review of the literature. We discuss the epidemiology of GIM in patients with *Helicobacter pylori* (HP) gastritis and the potential role of HP gastritis and bile acid reflux in the development of GIM. We discuss histologic risk factors for the progression of GIM to gastric cancer. We also discuss the potential need for the long-term surveillance and natural history studies of GIM in children.

2. Case Report

2.1. Case 1. A 16-year-old female presented to the clinic complaining of progressive worsening of dysphagia to solid foods with sensation of fullness in the chest and sour taste in the mouth but denies heartburn or chest pain. She did not have any weight loss. Her symptoms were unresponsive to PPI therapy started by her primary care physician. There was no family history of gastric cancer. The physical exam was unremarkable and the blood work was normal (including celiac panel, comprehensive metabolic panel, and HP IgG). An esophagram was normal. She underwent esophagogastroduodenoscopy (EGD), which revealed a 4 mm prepyloric nodule (see Figure 1(a)). A rapid urease test for HP was negative. Hematoxylin and eosin-stained sections on the prepyloric nodule biopsy showed antral-type gastric mucosa (see Figures 1(b) and 1(c)). The lamina propria was distended by a chronic inflammatory cell infiltrate consisting of lymphocytes and plasma cells. Numerous mucin producing cells, characteristic of intestinal epithelium, were identified. The features were those of chronic gastritis with intestinal metaplasia of the complete type. No dysplasia was present. No HP organisms were identified on light microscopy and by immunostain. Patient reports improvement in her symptoms after completing a course of double dose PPI therapy. Repeated EGD 1 year after showed resolution of the gastric erosion and persistence of the prepyloric nodule on EGD. Complete type intestinal metaplasia persisted on histologic evaluation.

2.2. Case 2. An 8-year-old female with generalized but not radiated abdominal pain, described as cramping and

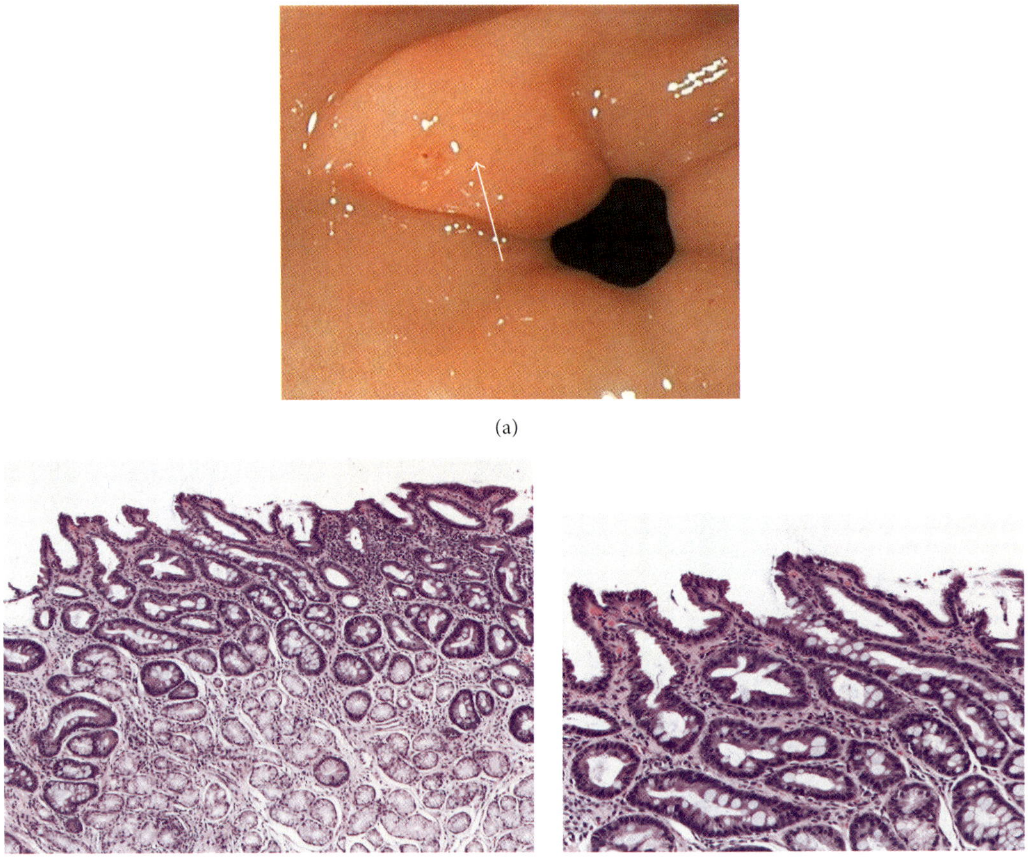

(a)

(b)

(c)

Figure 1: Endoscopic and histologic appearance of gastrointestinal metaplasia in case 1. (a) shows the appearance of a prepyloric nodule with an erosion located on the lesser curvature of the antrum. A cold forceps biopsy was taken from a region adjacent to the erosion (arrow). (b) shows a low power and (c) a high power histopathology image of the prepyloric nodule. The lamina propria is distended by a chronic inflammatory cell infiltrate consisting of lymphocytes and plasma cells. Numerous mucin producing cells, characteristic of intestinal epithelium, are identified. The features are those of chronic gastritis with intestinal metaplasia of the complete type.

sharp for the last one year, presented to our clinic. She reported intermittent nausea associated with nonbloody and nonbilious vomiting. Vomiting was more frequent at night. There was no family history of gastric cancer. The patient had an unremarkable blood work (including complete blood count, chemistry panel, antibodies to HP, and celiac panel). Computed tomography of the abdomen was significant for mesenteric adenopathy. The EGD showed a prepyloric nodule (Figure 2(a)) and bile-lake. Histological examination showed incomplete intestinal gastric metaplasia with irregular mucin droplets and an absent brush border (see Figures 2(b) and 2(c)). Rapid urease testing for HP, as well as immunostains, was negative. She was treated with double dose PPI therapy. Vomiting improved with cyproheptadine. Repeat EGD 6 months later showed resolution of the prepyloric erosion and continued presence of the prepyloric nodule. Histologic examination showed persistence of incomplete gastric intestinal metaplasia without progression to dysplasia.

3. Discussion

GIM is defined as the replacement of gastric columnar cells by cells of intestinal morphology characterized by the presence of mucin-containing goblet, Paneth, and absorptive cells [1]. The intestinal cells are easily distinguished in the gastric mucosa, because they are not present in healthy gastric mucosa [2]. The histopathologic diagnosis of GIM has been found to have high interobserver agreement [3, 4]. No consensus is available about the optimal number or location of biopsies needed in children [5]. In adults, biopsy mapping of the stomach requires at least 5 biopsy specimens: 2 from the antrum within 2 to 3 cm from the pylorus (1 each from the lesser and greater curvatures); 2 from the corpus approximately 8 cm from the cardia (1 each from the lesser and greater curvatures); and 1 from the incisura angularis [6].

The prevalence of GIM in children is largely unknown [7]. Furthermore, endoscopic features of GIM in pediatric patient are poorly defined. A white opaque substance visualized by

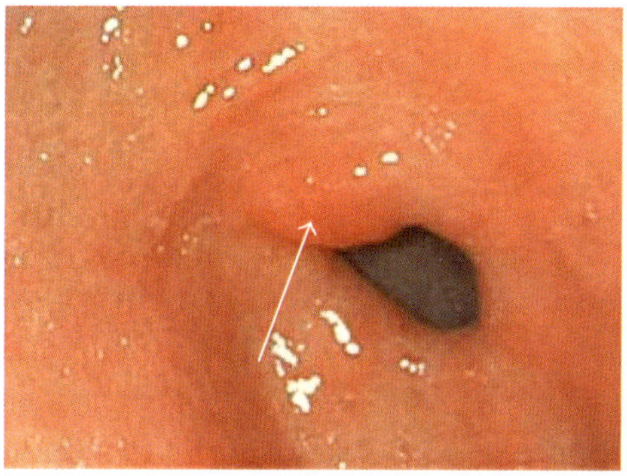

(a)

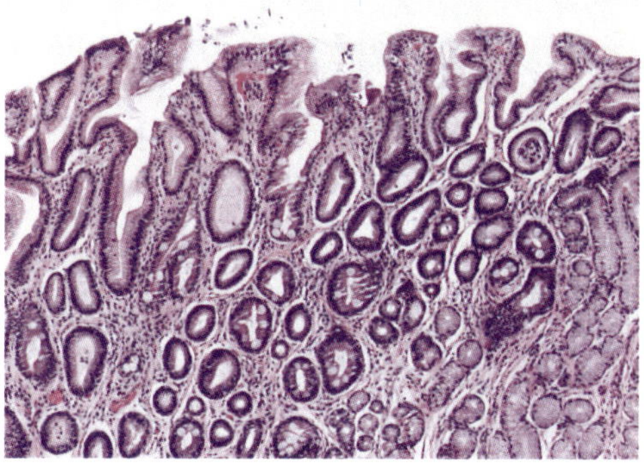

(b)

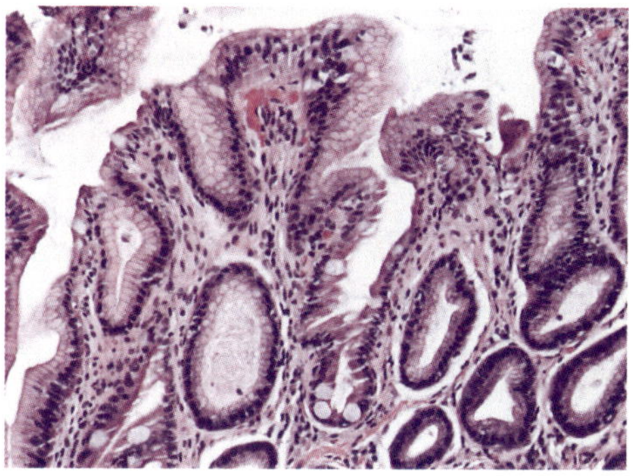

(c)

FIGURE 2: Endoscopic and histologic appearance of gastrointestinal metaplasia in case 2. (a) shows the appearance of a prepyloric nodule with an erosion located on the lesser curvature of the antrum. A cold forceps biopsy was taken from a region adjacent to the erosion (arrow). (b) shows a low power image and (c) shows a high power histopathology image of the prepyloric nodule in case 2. The lamina propria is distended by a chronic inflammatory cell infiltrate, irregular columnar cells filled with mucin, and an absence of brush border is noted, signifying an incomplete type.

magnifying endoscopy with narrow-band imaging (M-NBI) appears to be a useful indicator of the histological diagnosis of GIM [8]. GIM is a common finding on routine endoscopy in adults [9] and is more frequently associated with HP than in children [10]. The frequency of GIM in children related to HP-positive gastritis versus HP-negative gastritis is variable. Shabib et al. [11] reported a frequency of 42% in children with HP-positive gastritis versus 6% in children with HP-negative gastritis. However, Kato et al. [12] documented no difference in the presence of intestinal metaplasia between the study groups of children with and without HP infection. However, no children in a Brazilian cohort of 96 children with HP gastritis were found to have GIM [13].

HP infection causes inflammatory cell infiltration in the gastric mucosa, resulting in atrophy of the foveolar epithelium and long-term mucosal changes such as intestinal metaplasia, which are precursors of gastric cancer [13–15]. HP organisms seem to be the most important member of the gastric microbiota with the highest relative abundance when present, but when it is absent, the stomach has a diverse microbiota [16]. Proteobacteria, Firmicutes, Actinobacteria, Bacteroidetes, and Fusobacteria are the most abundant phyla in both HP-positive and HP-negative patients [16].

Reactive gastropathy represents the second most common cause for the occurrence of age-dependent mucosal alterations [17]. Primary duodenogastric reflux (DGER) could cause gastric mucosal lesions manifested as intestinal metaplasia histologically in children. DGER is probably an independent etiological factor and might play a synergistic role in the pathogenesis of gastric mucosal lesions along with gastric acid and HP infection [18]. Other causes that are associated with GIM in adults include high gastric pH, increased bile acid exposure, smoking [19], and gastric denervation after surgery for benign disease [20].

The diagnosis of intestinal metaplasia can have adverse clinical implications and should be made with caution in a child [21]. The association of GIM with adenoma/dysplasia/carcinoma progression is commonly encountered in adults but is rarely seen in children. Only 10% of gastric cancer cases are found in patients younger than 40 years of age [22]. It is very likely that time plays an important factor the progression of GIM to adenoma. The progression from intestinal metaplasia to gastric adenocarcinoma takes an average of about 7 years in adult studies [23]. Thus, by the time GIM undergoes neoplastic transformation, the patient would become an adult and, therefore, managed in the adult service [5, 10]. The malignant potential of GIM has been shown to vary based on histologic subtype, location, and extent of mucosal involvement [24, 25]. Adults with incomplete GIM subtype versus complete GIM subtype, diffuse involvement of the antrum and gastric body versus antrum alone, and greater than 20% extension of mucosal involvement between endoscopic sampling had a greater risk of gastric cancer [25, 26]. Family history of gastric cancer on initial evaluation was associated with increased risk of subsequent gastric cancer in adult patients [9, 23, 24].

Treatment, long-term consequences, and surveillance protocols of GIM are not well established in the pediatric population. Contrary to our first case presented, a case report of a 15-year-old with GIM located inside the cryptic antral epithelium showed complete resolution following 3 months of PPI treatment [27]. In adults, as a pragmatic behavior, yearly endoscopic evaluation would appear justified in all GIM patients with at least one of these conditions: (1) IM extension > 20% mucosal involvement between endoscopies; (2) the presence of incomplete type IM; (3) first-degree relative of gastric cancer patients; and (4) smokers [24]. Controversy exists regarding whether routine surveillance should be performed in individuals with GIM in low HP prevalence regions such as the United States [28]. In patients with few risk factors, surveillance every 2-3 years could be proposed [24].

We believe it is important to report pediatric patients with GIM and, more importantly, ensure a long-term follow-up into adulthood in order to better understand the natural history of this disease and early detection of dysplasia, should it occur. We presented herein an overview of the current knowledge on the detection and surveillance of patients with GIM. However, the treatment, long-term consequences, and surveillance protocols are not well stablished in pediatric patients likely due to the limited literature available and the need for consensus on the follow-up of this histopathological finding. At present, GIM is frequently disregarded in clinical practice or results in widely varying follow-up frequency or treatment. These uncertainties require further research in the pediatric population.

Disclosure

An earlier version of this work was presented as a poster at Clinical Vignette Abstracts NASPGHAN 2017.

References

[1] A. C. de Vries, J. Haringsma, and E. J. Kuipers, "The detection, surveillance and treatment of premalignant gastric lesions related to *Helicobacter pylori*infection," *Helicobacter*, vol. 12, no. 1, pp. 1–15, 2007.

[2] B. C. Morson, "Intestinal metaplasia of the gastric mucosa," *British Journal of Cancer*, vol. 9, no. 3, pp. 365–376, 1955.

[3] L. G. Capelle, A. C. de Vries, J. Haringsma et al., "The staging of gastritis with the OLGA system by using intestinal metaplasia as an accurate alternative for atrophic gastritis," *Gastrointestinal Endoscopy*, vol. 71, no. 7, pp. 1150–1158, 2010.

[4] M. F. Dixon, R. M. Genta, J. H. Yardley et al., "Classification and grading of gastritis: the updated Sydney system," *The American Journal of Surgical Pathology*, vol. 20, no. 10, pp. 1161–1181, 1996.

[5] G. Dimitrov and F. Gottrand, "Does gastric atrophy exist in children?" *World Journal of Gastroenterology*, vol. 12, no. 39, pp. 6274–6279, 2006.

[6] M. Dinis-Ribeiro, M. Areia, A. C. De Vries et al., "Management of precancerous conditions and lesions in the stomach (MAPS): guideline from the European Society of Gastrointestinal Endoscopy (ESGE), European Helicobacter Study Group (EHSG), European Society of Pathology (ESP), and the Sociedade Portuguesa de Endoscopia Digestiva (SPED)," *Endoscopy*, vol. 44, no. 1, pp. 74–94, 2012.

[7] Y. Elitsur and W. E. Triest, "Is duodenal gastric metaplasia a consequence of Helicobacter pylori infection in children?" *American Journal of Gastroenterology*, vol. 92, no. 12, pp. 2216–2219, 1997.

[8] T. Kanemitsu, K. Yao, T. Nagahama et al., "Extending magnifying NBI diagnosis of intestinal metaplasia in the stomach: the white opaque substance marker," *Endoscopy*, vol. 49, no. 6, pp. 529–535, 2017.

[9] K. M. Reddy, J. I. Chang, J. M. Shi, and B. U. Wu, "Risk of gastric cancer among patients with intestinal metaplasia of the stomach in a us integrated health care system," *Clinical Gastroenterology and Hepatology*, vol. 14, no. 10, pp. 1420–1425, 2016.

[10] R. H. Riddell, "Pathobiology of Helicobacter pylori infection in children," *Canadian Journal of Gastroenterology & Hepatology*, vol. 13, no. 7, pp. 599–603, 1999.

[11] S. M. Shabib, E. Cutz, B. Drumm, and P. M. Sherman, "Association of gastric metaplasia and duodenitis with Helicobacter pylori infection in children," *American Journal of Clinical Pathology*, vol. 102, no. 2, pp. 188–191, 1994.

[12] S. Kato, S. Nakajima, Y. Nishino et al., "Association between gastric atrophy and Helicobacter pylori infection in Japanese children: a retrospective multicenter study," *Digestive Diseases and Sciences*, vol. 51, no. 1, pp. 99–104, 2006.

[13] M. A. Carvalho, N. C. Machado, E. V. P. Ortolan, and M. A. M. Rodrigues, "Upper gastrointestinal histopathological findings in children and adolescents with nonulcer dyspepsia with helicobacter pylori infection," *Journal of Pediatric Gastroenterology and Nutrition*, vol. 55, no. 5, pp. 523–529, 2012.

[14] N. Uemura, S. Okamoto, S. Yamamoto et al., "Helicobacter pylori infection and the development of gastric cancer," *The New England Journal of Medicine*, vol. 345, no. 11, pp. 784–789, 2001.

[15] M. I. Filipe, F. Potet, W. V. Bogomoletz et al., "Incomplete sulphomucin-secreting intestinal metaplasia for gastric cancer. Preliminary data from a prospective study from three centres," *Gut*, vol. 26, no. 12, pp. 1319–1326, 1985.

[16] T. Alarcón, L. Llorca, and G. Perez-Perez, "Impact of the microbiota and gastric disease development by Helicobacter pylori," *Current Topics in Microbiology and Immunology*, vol. 400, pp. 253–275, 2017.

[17] A. Sonnenberg and R. M. Genta, "Changes in the gastric mucosa with aging," *Clinical Gastroenterology and Hepatology*, vol. 13, no. 13, pp. 2276–2281, 2015.

[18] M. Ma, J. Chen, Y.-Y. Zhang, Z.-Y. Li, M.-Z. Jiang, and J.-D. Yu, "Pathogenic effects of primary duodenogastric reflux on gastric mucosa of children," *Chinese Journal of Pediatrics*, vol. 46, no. 4, pp. 257–262, 2008.

[19] M. Nakamura, K. Haruma, T. Kamada et al., "Duodenogastric reflux is associated with antral metaplastic gastritis," *Gastrointestinal Endoscopy*, vol. 53, no. 1, pp. 53–59, 2001.

[20] M. Ohira, T. Toyokawa, K. Sakurai et al., "Current status in remnant gastric cancer after distal gastrectomy," *World Journal of Gastroenterology*, vol. 22, no. 8, pp. 2424–2433, 2016.

[21] A. G. Weinberg, "The significance of small intestinal epithelium in gastric antral biopsies in children," *Pediatric and Developmental Pathology*, vol. 15, no. 2, pp. 101–106, 2012.

[22] A. Kokkola and P. Sipponen, "Gastric carcinoma in young adults," *Hepato-Gastroenterology*, vol. 48, no. 42, pp. 1552–1555, 2001.

[23] O. O. Olaofe, D. Sabageh, and A. O. Komolafe, "A review of the clinicopathologic characteristics of intestinal metaplasia in gastric mucosal biopsies," *Pan African Medical Journal*, vol. 23, article 77, 2016.

[24] A. Zullo, C. Hassan, A. Romiti et al., "Follow-up of intestinal metaplasia in the stomach: when, how and why," *World Journal of Gastrointestinal Oncology*, vol. 4, no. 3, pp. 30–36, 2012.

[25] M. Rugge, A. Meggio, G. Pennelli et al., "Gastritis staging in clinical practice: the OLGA staging system," *Gut*, vol. 56, no. 5, pp. 631–636, 2007.

[26] S. Silva and M. I. Filipe, "Intestinal metaplasia and its variants in the gastric mucosa of portuguese subjects: a comparative analysis of biopsy and gastrectomy material," *Human Pathology*, vol. 17, no. 10, pp. 988–995, 1986.

[27] N. Kalach, S. Papadopoulos, E. Asmar et al., "In french children, primary gastritis is more frequent than helicobacter pylori gastritis," *Digestive Diseases and Sciences*, vol. 54, no. 9, pp. 1958–1965, 2009.

[28] P. Correa, M. B. Piazuelo, and K. T. Wilson, "Pathology of gastric intestinal metaplasia: clinical implications," *American Journal of Gastroenterology*, vol. 105, no. 3, pp. 493–498, 2010.

34

Isolated Pancreatic Tuberculosis Mimicking Pancreatic Cancer: A Diagnostic Challenge

Abhishek Bhurwal,[1] Muhammad Masoodul Haq,[1] Sunil Sapru,[1] Matthew Tortora,[2] and Dhanasekaran Ramasamy[3]

[1]*Department of Internal Medicine, Saint Barnabas Medical Center, RWJBarnabas Health, West Orange, NJ, USA*
[2]*Department of Pathology, Saint Barnabas Medical Center, RWJBarnabas Health, West Orange, NJ, USA*
[3]*Department of Internal Medicine, Division of Gastroenterology, Saint Barnabas Medical Center, RWJBarnabas Health, West Orange, NJ, USA*

Correspondence should be addressed to Abhishek Bhurwal; abhishek.bhurwal@gmail.com

Academic Editor: Gregory Kouraklis

Isolated pancreatic tuberculosis is an exceedingly rare condition, even in areas of the world where the disease is highly prevalent. Abdominal tuberculosis is a common form of extrapulmonary tuberculosis but involvement of the pancreas is very rare. We report a case of isolated pancreatic tuberculosis presenting as a pancreatic mass in a patient with persistent abdominal pain and jaundice. Clinically and radiologically, the mass mimicked a malignant pancreatic tumor with a vastly different prognostic implication and therapeutic approach. Endoscopic ultrasound with fine-needle aspiration (EUS-FNA) can provide valuable diagnostic information in this scenario. After the tissue showed evidence of acid-fast bacilli and the cultures showed growth of *Mycobacterium tuberculosis*, antituberculosis therapy was initiated. Conservative management is usually successful in alleviating symptoms and leading to a cure. The excellent response to ATT makes it imperative that these patients are diagnosed early and managed appropriately to avoid unnecessary surgery and associated morbidity.

1. Background

Isolated pancreatic tuberculosis is an exceedingly rare condition, even in areas of the world where the disease is highly prevalent [1]. The diagnosis is often a challenge as the symptoms and radiological appearance often mimic pancreatic cancer. Endoscopic ultrasound with fine-needle aspiration (EUS-FNA) can provide valuable diagnostic information [2]. The excellent response to antitubercular therapy makes it imperative to diagnose pancreatic tuberculosis early and avoid unnecessary interventions. We report one such case of isolated pancreatic tuberculosis presenting as a pancreatic mass where cytological diagnosis prevented untoward surgical resection.

2. Case Report

A previously healthy 38-year-old gentleman began to experience episodes of intermittent abdominal pain five days prior to presentation. The abdominal pain was predominantly in the epigastrium, nonradiating, and occasionally associated with nausea. He did not have any episodes of vomiting or diarrhea. Over the course of next five days, he noticed yellowing of his eyes and urine which prompted him to visit the emergency room. Patient denied any history of fever, night sweats, weight loss, or decreased appetite. Family history was unremarkable. He migrated to the United States at the age of 33 from the Philippines. He had received BCG vaccination during childhood but had no previous history of treatment for tuberculosis. He denied any sick contacts or travel within the last few years. He worked as a pharmacist. He denied smoking and alcohol or intravenous drug use.

The patient appeared well nourished with icteric sclera. Physical examination revealed a temperature of 38°C, blood pressure 110/55 mmHg, heart rate 85 beats per minute, respiratory rate 18 breaths per minute, and oxygen saturation 95% on room air. Cardiopulmonary examination was normal.

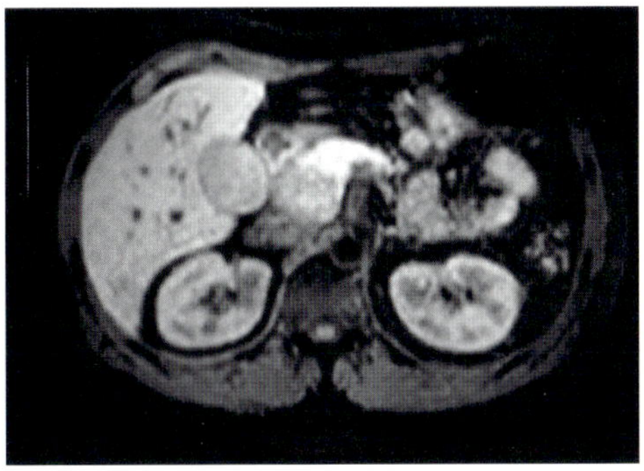

FIGURE 1: Initial MRCP showing pancreatic head mass with nonenhancing areas in the center.

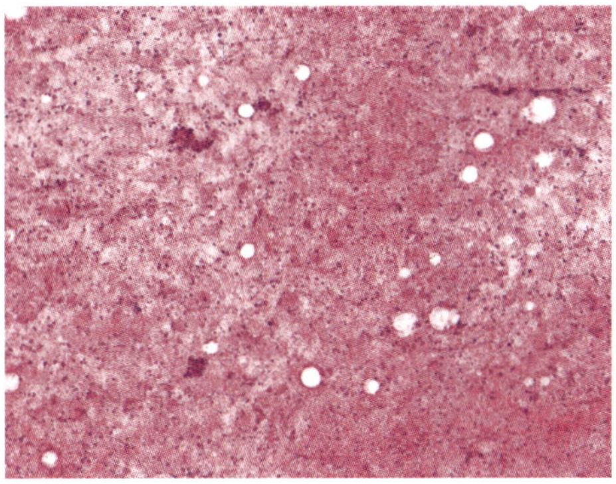

FIGURE 2: Necrotic material on the needle aspiration smear (H&E stain).

FIGURE 3: Scattered acid-fast bacilli on the cell block preparation (acid-fast stain).

Abdominal examination revealed tenderness in the epigastric region with no guarding or rigidity. However, no palpable mass could be appreciated.

Routine laboratory investigations showed normochromic normocytic anemia with Hb 12.3 gm/dl. Total bilirubin was 2.9 mg/dl while aspartate aminotransferase 167 U/L, alanine aminotransferase 443 U/L, and alkaline phosphatase were 424 U/L, respectively. Serum lipase and amylase were not elevated.

The chest radiograph at the time of admission was normal. Subsequently, he underwent an abdominal computed tomography (CT) scan which revealed a 3.8 × 2.7 cm solid mass posterolateral to the pancreatic head, suggestive of peripancreatic lymphadenopathy. Magnetic resonance imaging (MRCP) showed a 4.1 × 2.6 cm mass in the pancreatic head encasing the portal vein with multiple central areas of nonenhancement (Figure 1). There was a 1.5 cm segment of narrowing in the mid common bile duct with mild dilation of the intrahepatic ducts. The pancreatic duct was not dilated.

The differential diagnosis included malignant pancreatic tumor, autoimmune pancreatitis, neuroendocrine tumor, and gastrointestinal stromal tumor. Endoscopic ultrasound (EUS) with fine-needle aspiration (FNA) was performed which showed a heterogeneous hyperechoic pancreatic lesion which on histopathology revealed areas of coagulation necrosis, lymphocytes, and epithelioid histiocytes suggestive of granulomatous inflammation (Figure 2).

3. Discussion

Granulomatous inflammation in the pancreas is an unusual occurrence and has rarely been described in the literature [6]. It can be seen in mycobacterial infections, fungal infections, sarcoidosis, inflammatory bowel disorder, Wegner's disease, malignancy, and foreign body retention after procedures [6]. In our patient, fungal infection was unlikely with negative HIV and no immunosuppression, along with no evidence of systemic involvement. He did not have any prior ERCP or other procedures to suspect foreign body retention in the pancreas. Absence of sinus disease, bland urinalysis, and no kidney involvement ruled out Wegner's disease. Crohn's disease was unlikely due to absence of bowel involvement. Our patient did not have any febrile episodes, night sweats, weight loss, or exposure to sick contacts and there was no pulmonary involvement to suggest mycobacterial infection. His only risk factor was that he was born in Philippines.

Even though our initial suspicion was low, the tissue showed evidence of acid-fast bacilli and the cultures showed growth of *Mycobacterium tuberculosis* (Figure 3). After the diagnosis of tuberculosis was confirmed by AFB stain and cultures, he was started on antitubercular therapy. He was treated with isoniazid, rifampin, pyrazinamide, and ethambutol for 4 months followed by isoniazid and rifampin for 10 months. He tolerated the regimen well. Repeat laboratory investigations such as total bilirubin level and liver chemistries (AST, ALT, and ALP) were also normal. Repeat MRI performed at 5 months of treatment did not reveal any discrete pancreatic lesion (Figure 4).

Tuberculosis is a common occurrence in certain endemic zones of Asia and Africa [7]. Even though, tuberculosis primarily affects the lungs, isolated abdominal tuberculosis is not rare with incidence ranging from 0.59% to 12% [1, 8]. Pancreatic tuberculosis was first described by Auerbach in 1944 [9]. Since then, most of the medical literature on this rare disease is limited to case reports or small case series.

The possible mechanisms of isolated pancreatic tuberculosis are as follows [10]:

(i) Hematogenous dissemination to the pancreas from an occult lesion in the lungs or abdomen

Table 1: It is showing cases of isolated pancreatic tuberculosis in the Western World along with the case characteristics and management strategies and outcomes over the last 5 years.

Study, year	Patient characteristics	Therapy and outcomes
Patel et al., 2013 [3]	(i) 41-year-old female (ii) CT, 5.1 cm × 2.8 cm multiloculated solid lesion in the head of the pancreas (iii) EUS, 4.3 cm × 2.5 cm hypoechoic, homogenous mass lesion with a cystic component within the pancreatic head	RIPE for 2 months and then IR for 7 months
Salahuddin and Saif, 2014 [4]	(i) 59-year-old male (ii) MRCP, dilated common bile duct, dilated pancreatic duct, and enlarged lymph nodes in the porta hepatis, peripancreatic and perigastric regions (iii) EUS, ahypoechoic mass measuring 3 by 4 cm was seen in the pancreatic head	Antitubercular therapy (RIPE) for 18 months
Waintraub et al., 2016 [5]	(i) 31-year-old male (ii) MRI, periportal lymphadenopathy indenting pancreatic head and uncinate process and compressing CBD (iii) EUS, irregular, hypoechoic mass with poorly defined borders in the pancreatic head. Anechoic lesion in the pancreatic tail, suggestive of a cyst or pseudocyst.	Antitubercular therapy

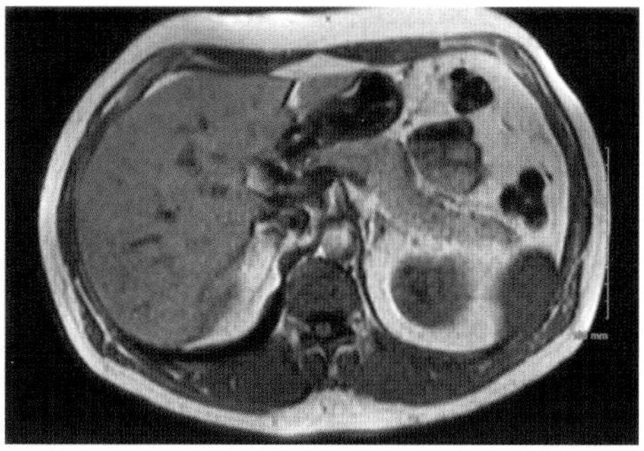

Figure 4: Follow-up imaging at 5 months showing resolution with no discrete pancreatic head mass.

(ii) Direct spread from contiguous lymph nodes

(iii) Reactivation of a dormant bacilli in an old tubercular lesion in an immunosuppressive state.

Pancreatic tuberculosis most commonly presents with nonspecific symptoms such as abdominal pain, jaundice, vomiting, anorexia, or weight loss. It usually involves the head and uncinate process of the pancreas. Most of the cases have been described in young people, especially females, often with a past history of TB or coming from endemic zone of active tuberculosis [11]. Table 1 shows recently published case reports of isolated pancreatic tuberculosis in the United States. Our case is only the fourth case of isolated pancreatic tuberculosis in the Western hemisphere over the last 5 years [3–5].

The diagnosis of pancreatic tuberculosis is a challenge because of the rarity of the disease and nonspecific signs and symptoms of the disease. Ultrasound and CECT are often used for initial evaluation. Focal hypoechoic lesions or cystic lesions are usually seen on ultrasonography [12]. CT may reveal hypodense lesions mostly in the head of the pancreas [13]. There might be diffuse enlargement of the pancreas or presence of enlarged peripancreatic lymph nodes [13]. There are no specific features on imaging and even the evidence of vascular invasion does not differentiate malignancy from pancreatic tuberculosis [10].

The suspicion of malignancy leads to an unwarranted resection as many cases are diagnosed after surgical resection [14]. Therefore, high index of suspicion is warranted to diagnose the condition early to prevent unnecessary surgical intervention and associated morbidity. EUS-FNA, CT/US guided biopsy or surgical biopsy provides valuable histopathological diagnosis [2]. The presence of caseating granulomatous inflammation and acid-fast bacilli is suggestive of tuberculosis. Cultures for mycobacteria take up to 6 weeks to grow and are used to confirm the diagnosis. Once the diagnosis is confirmed, medical management (antitubercular therapy (ATT)) is the mainstay of the therapy. ATT consists of multidrug chemotherapy and is usually recommended for 6 to 12 months [15]. The disease responds well to the treatment.

In summary, isolated pancreatic tuberculosis is an uncommon presentation of tuberculosis. The clinical presentation and the radiological finding of a pancreatic mass may be suggestive of a malignant pancreatic tumor with a vastly different prognostic implication and therapeutic approach. The diagnosis of isolated pancreatic TB requires a high index of suspicion. It should be considered in patients presenting with pancreatic mass especially in immunocompromised patients. EUS-FNA is an excellent investigation to detect pancreatic tuberculosis promptly and prevents unnecessary surgical procedures. Patients respond well to conservative management and antitubercular therapy.

References

[1] C. S. Pramesh, A. A. Heroor, S. G. Gupta et al., "Pancreatic tuberculosis: An elusive diagnosis," *HPB*, vol. 5, no. 1, pp. 43–45, 2003.

[2] A. A. Riaz, A. Singh, P. Robshaw, and A. M. Isla, "Tuberculosis of the pancreas diagnosed with needle aspiration," *Infectious Diseases*, vol. 34, no. 4, pp. 303-304, 2002.

[3] D. Patel, D. Loren, T. Kowalski, and A. A. Siddiqui, "Pancreatic tuberculosis mimicking malignancy diagnosed with endoscopic ultrasound-guided fine needle aspiration," *Endoscopic Ultrasound*, vol. 2, no. 1, pp. 38–40, 2013.

[4] A. Salahuddin and M. W. Saif, "Pancreatic tuberculosis or autoimmune pancreatitis," *Case Reports in Medicine*, vol. 2014, Article ID 410142, 5 pages, 2014.

[5] D. J. Waintraub, L. S. D'Souza, E. Madrigal, M. Harshan, and G. I. Ascunce, "A Rare Case of Isolated Pancreatic Tuberculosis," *ACG Case Reports Journal*, vol. 3, no. 4, article e91, 2016.

[6] J. Stürmer and V. Becker, "Granulomatous pancreatitis - granulomas in chronic pancreatitis," *Virchows Archiv A Pathological Anatomy and Histopathology*, vol. 410, no. 4, pp. 327–338, 1987.

[7] K. Floyd and A. Pantoja, "Financial resources required for tuberculosis control to achieve global targets set for 2015," *Bulletin of the World Health Organization*, vol. 86, no. 7, pp. 568–576, 2008.

[8] Y. Rong, W. Lou, and D. Jin, "Pancreatic tuberculosis with splenic tuberculosis mimicking advanced pancreatic cancer with splenic metastasizes: a case report," *Cases Journal*, vol. 1, no. 1, p. 84, 2008.

[9] O. Auerbach, "Acute Generalized Miliary Tuberculosis," *American Journal of Pathology*, vol. 20, no. 1, pp. 121–136, 1944.

[10] Q. Liu, Z. He, and P. Bie, "Solitary pancreatic tuberculous abscess mimicking prancreatic cystadenocarcinoma: A case report," *BMC Gastroenterology*, vol. 3, article no. 1, 2003.

[11] F. Xia, T.-P. Poon, S.-G. Wang, P. Bie, X.-Q. Huang, and J.-H. Dong, "Tuberculosis of pancreas and peripancreatic lymph nodes in immunocompetent patients: experience from China," *World Journal of Gastroenterology*, vol. 9, no. 6, pp. 1361–1364, 2003.

[12] D. L. Morris, L. S. Wilkinson, and N. A. Mokhtar, "Case report: Emphysematous tuberculous pancreatitis diagnosis by ultrasound and computed tomography," *Clinical Radiology*, vol. 48, no. 4, pp. 286-287, 1993.

[13] F. Pombo, M. J. Díaz Candamio, E. Rodriguez, and S. Pombo, "Pancreatic tuberculosis: CT findings," *Abdominal Imaging*, vol. 23, no. 4, pp. 394–397, 1998.

[14] S. S. Saluja, S. Ray, S. Pal et al., "Hepatobiliary and pancreatic tuberculosis: a two decade experience," *BMC Surgery*, vol. 7, article 10, 2007.

[15] P. Chaudhary, U. Bhadana, and M. P. Arora, "Pancreatic Tuberculosis," *Indian Journal of Surgery*, vol. 77, no. 6, pp. 517–524, 2015.

35

A Case of Unresolved and Worsening Retroperitoneal Abscess

Raghav Bansal,[1] Mohamed Barakat,[2] Soohwan Chun,[1] Sonam Rosberger,[3] Joel Baum,[1] and Melik Tiba[1]

[1]*Division of Gastroenterology and Hepatology, Icahn School of Medicine at Mount Sinai, Elmhurst Hospital Center, Elmhurst, NY, USA*
[2]*Department of Internal Medicine, Icahn School of Medicine at Mount Sinai, Queens Hospital Center, Jamaica, NY, USA*
[3]*Department of Radiology, Icahn School of Medicine at Mount Sinai, Elmhurst Hospital Center, Elmhurst, NY, USA*

Correspondence should be addressed to Mohamed Barakat; mo_barakat@hotmail.com

Academic Editor: Olga I. Giouleme

Retroperitoneal abscess is a rare condition which is difficult to diagnose and treat because of its insidious onset. Herein, we present a case of retroperitoneal abscess secondary to a perforation that occurred during an ERCP. A 54-year-old female patient was admitted to an outside hospital with gallstone pancreatitis and underwent ERCP with sphincterotomy followed by laparoscopic cholecystectomy. An abdominal CT scan was performed at the outside hospital 10 days later for worsening abdominal pain which showed multiple loculated pockets in the right upper and lower quadrant. Her condition improved after IV antibiotics and percutaneous drainage. Her symptoms recurred a month later and she presented to our hospital. Repeat abdominal CT scan at our hospital revealed recurrence of her abscesses. Multiple drains were placed and the abscess cavity was washed out without much improvement. EGD revealed a small mucosal defect in the distal portion of the duodenal bulb which was closed successfully using an over-the-scope clip. Repeat CT scan after 8 weeks from the endoscopic closure showed near complete resolution of the abscess. ERCP-associated perforation is a rare complication and can be challenging to diagnose and treat; prompt recognition is mandatory for favorable prognosis. Our patient was managed successfully via nonsurgical approach.

1. Introduction

Retroperitoneal abscess is a rare condition which is difficult to diagnose and treat because of its insidious onset and nonspecific clinical manifestations. Retroperitoneal abscess may result from a variety of causes, such as pyelonephritis, pancreatitis, retroperitoneal appendicitis, diverticulitis, peptic ulcer disease, perforated cancer, inflammatory bowel disease, spinal infection, trauma, and postinstrumentation. Herein, we report a unique case of retroperitoneal abscess in a 54-year-old female and its management.

2. Case Report

A 54-year-old female patient was admitted to an outside hospital with gallstone pancreatitis and underwent endoscopic retrograde cholangiopancreatography (ERCP) with sphincterotomy followed by laparoscopic cholecystectomy. A hepatobiliary scan (HIDA) was performed on postoperative day 5 for worsening abdominal pain and failed to reveal any evidence of bile leak or obstruction. Abdominal computed tomography (CT) scan with i.v. contrast revealed normally enhancing pancreas along with multiple loculated pockets in the right upper and lower quadrant. The patient was started on i.v. antibiotics and a total of 800 ml of fluid was aspirated via percutaneous drainage. The patient's condition eventually improved and she was discharged home with a Jackson Pratt (JP) catheter in place. Her symptoms recurred after 1 month and she presented to our hospital.

The initial computed tomography (CT) abdomen at our hospital revealed a loculated air and fluid filled, rim enhancing collection in the right retroperitoneum extending to the pelvis measuring approximately $20.8 \times 6.7 \times 5.3$ cm with a JP drain (Figure 1). Another loculated 2.5×1.9 cm collection was seen in the region of the gallbladder fossa and right extraperitoneal perivesical component measuring

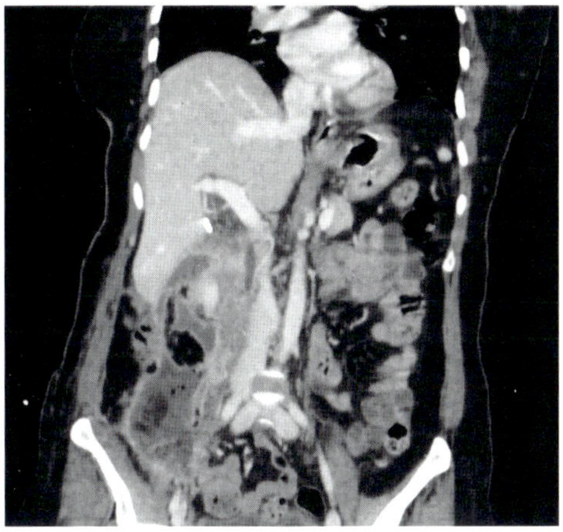

Figure 1: Coronal abdominal CT scan image showing retroperitoneal abscess.

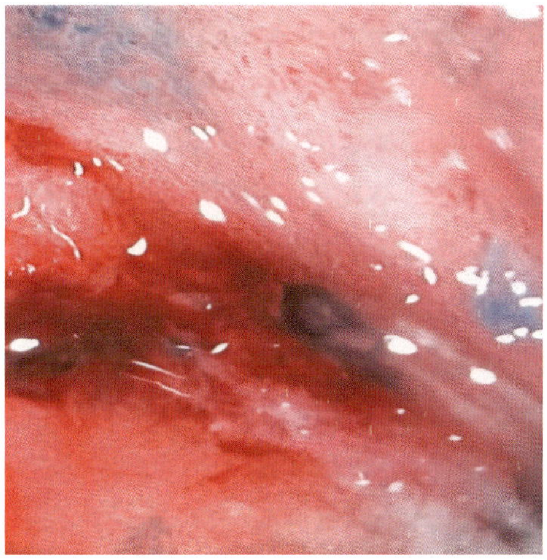

Figure 2: Fistulous opening in the duodenum.

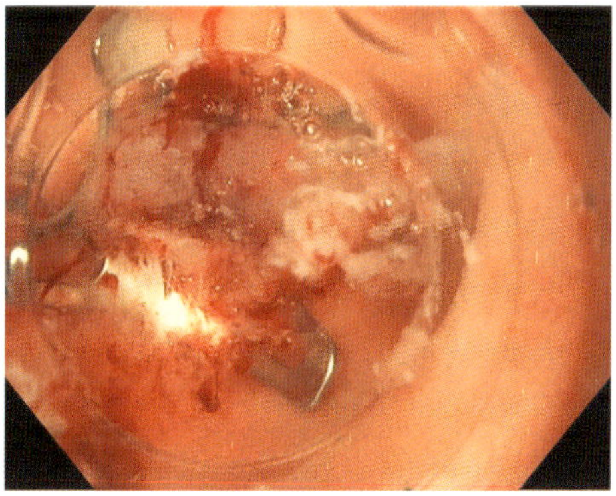

Figure 3: Endoscopic closure of luminal perforation of the duodenum with OVESCO over-the-scope clip.

8.0 × 2.4 cm. The drain was suspected to be clogged and was subsequently replaced with a new JP catheter. The pancreas appeared normal on imaging.

Culture from the abscess grew multiple bacteria: *Haemophilus parainfluenzae*, *Streptococcus anginosus*, *Pseudomonas aeruginosa*, and *Eikenella corrodens*. The presence of multiple gut-derived bacteria was concerning for possible gastrointestinal tract injury during either ERCP or laparoscopic cholecystectomy. There was no obvious evidence of extraluminal air or oral contrast extravasation on imaging. Given patient's overall stable condition, the abscess was managed conservatively with broad spectrum intravenous antibiotics (piperacillin and tazobactam) and percutaneous drainage.

At 2 weeks, repeat CT scan of the abdomen and pelvis showed no significant change in size of the abscess with persistence of multiple loculations. The patient subsequently underwent surgical drainage and wash-out. However, another repeat CT scan of the abdomen and pelvis two weeks later showed recurrence of the retroperitoneal abscess. Amylase and lipase levels were tested in the fluid drained from the abscess and were found to be elevated to 1335 units/L and 1655 units/L, respectively. Both magnetic resonance cholangiopancreatography (MRCP) and HIDA scan did not show any evidence of biliopancreatic ductal disruption and was confirmed with a normal cholangiogram during repeat ERCP. At this point, a nonhealing gastrointestinal tract perforation was strongly suspected. Finally, an upper endoscopy was performed after 12 weeks of initial admission revealed a small mucosal defect in medio-posterior wall of distal portion of the duodenal bulb that was draining pus intermittently, suspicious for the site of perforation (Figure 2). Methylene blue was injected through one of the JP catheters and was noted to be intravasating into the lumen via the defect, confirming communication with the retroperitoneal abscess. An OVESCO over-the-scope clip (12/6T) was used to close the defect and a second injection of methylene blue via the catheter did not show further luminal drainage (Figure 3).

The patient's condition improved gradually with significant reduction in size of the abscess at 6 weeks from the clip placement. Repeat CT scan after 8 weeks from the endoscopic closure showed near complete resolution of the abscess (Figure 4).

3. Discussion

ERCP-associated perforation is a rare complication that occurs in less than 1% of cases [1]. It is associated with significant morbidity and mortality; prompt recognition is central to the management as earlier intervention is associated with improved survival [2]. Our case reflects significantly delayed recognition of a probable post-ERCP perforation and highlights the importance of having high index of suspicion despite negative radiographic studies.

ERCP-associated perforation has been traditionally classified into four types according to Stapfer classification, based on its location and mechanism of injury [3, 4]. Type 1 refers to the perforation occurring in lateral (more often) or medial wall of duodenum caused by the side-viewing duodenoscope. Type 2 perforation occurs in periampullary region, most frequently due to sphincterotomy or precut papillotomy.

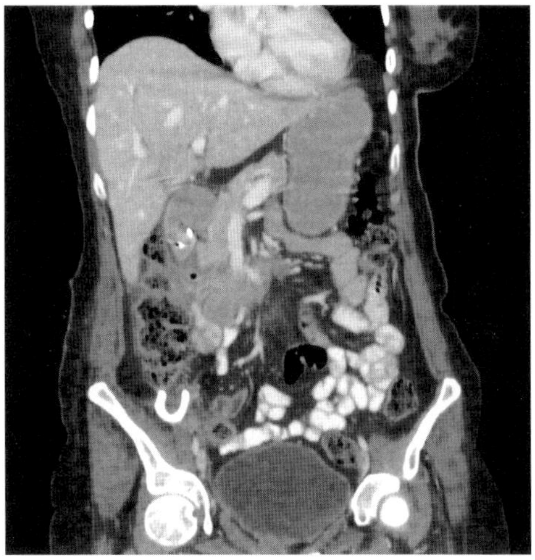

Figure 4: Coronal abdominal CT scan images after the closure of the fistula.

Type 3 refers to disruption of the biliary or pancreatic duct due to instrumentation such as with a guidewire or during stone extractions. Type 4 is a retroperitoneal microperforation, occurring in the setting of excessive insufflation while manipulating the sphincter.

Emergent surgical intervention is required for patients who have signs of peritonitis and intraperitoneal air, suggestive of an intraperitoneal perforation. Patients with retroperitoneal perforation will lack peritoneal signs, present less acutely, and may allow medical management as an initial approach. Perforations associated with retroperitoneal collections generally carry a worse prognosis [4, 5]. Type 1 perforations often tends to result in a large defect with intraperitoneal leakage and has been traditionally managed surgically [6]. Type 2 perforations are the most common, small, and retroperitoneal and can be initially managed medically with intravenous antibiotics and nasogastric tube decompression with or without percutaneous drainage [6, 7]. Type 3 perforations are often recognized during the procedure via fluoroscopy and managed with the placement of biliary or pancreatic plastic stents. Type 4 perforations are often asymptomatic, found incidentally, and typically do not require invasive intervention.

Various treatment algorithms have been suggested based on the type of perforation. Kumbhari et al. [7] proposed surgery as the best initial approach for Type 1 perforation, whereas for Type 2 lesion, surgical intervention was suggested only for refractory patients after a trial of maximal medical therapy. Endoscopic repair has been reported successful and can be attempted in stable patients with both Type 1 and Type 2 perforation. Endoscopic clip placement may suffice for a small Type 1 lesion; larger lesions have been successfully closed with adjunctive use of an endoloop, fibrin glue, and over-the-scope stitch system and more recently with use of an over-the-scope clip [2, 7–11]. Endoscopic band ligation has also been used successfully for closure and may be useful for a defect in a difficult location, given the ease of its application [8].

For Type 2 perforation, biliary plastic stent placement has been performed for biliary diversion and was suggested for a large defect at index endoscopy [12]. More recently, fully covered self-expanding metal stent has been used successfully at both index and repeat (within a few days) endoscopy [13, 14]. Larger final diameter and greater opposing force may confer improved seal at the perforation site. Repeat endoscopy for removal of the stent was successful without increased risk of stent migration in most cases, when performed within 1 month. [14]. Though the scope clips have been used for Type 2 perforation, their application can be challenging using side-viewing endoscope [15]. OTSC similarly may not be ideal for its application, given the acute angulation and potential risk of ampullary orifice closure [15]. Types 3 and 4 lesions were recommended to be managed nonsurgically, in agreement with other previous authors.

Multidetector computed tomography (MDCT) scan is considered highly sensitive in detecting gastrointestinal perforation, whether intraperitoneal or extraperitoneal [16, 17]. Extraluminal air is the most common and consistent finding of gastrointestinal perforation; MDCT is able to detect tiny bubbles of air that plain film may fail to show in as high as 50% of the cases. Focal bowel wall defect with an abrupt adjacent wall thickening and surrounding stranding may be seen. Direct visualization of oral contrast extravasation is an infrequent finding. Based on the focus of abnormality and distribution of the extraluminal air, MDCT can often localize the site of retroperitoneal perforation. For example, right para-renal collection of retroperitoneal air indicates perforation in duodenum or ascending colon, whereas left para-renal collection indicates defect in descending or sigmoid colon: bilateral distribution can be seen in rectal perforation. Our patient had right-sided para-renal distribution of the retroperitoneal abscess but had no evidence of extraluminal air or focal bowel wall abnormalities on imaging, thus making the diagnosis challenging.

Our patient had perforation in distal portion of the duodenal bulb, far from the native ampulla: thus, a Type 1 perforation. The diagnosis was delayed in our case due to lack of typical findings of perforation on the CT scans and contained nature of the perforation.

Elevated pleural amylase level is frequently used to guide the diagnosis in the case of esophageal perforation [18]; however, the relationship between elevated retroperitoneal amylase and/or lipase level and duodenal perforation is unclear. Croce et al. [19] in a case series reported an increase in amylase concentration in bile in a patient with a duodenal perforation resulting from cholecystectomy. Significantly elevated levels of amylase and lipase in our patient likely reflected leakage of the enzymes from the duodenal lumen into the retroperitoneal space via the area of perforation similar to the previously reported case. It is important to exclude other etiologies that can give rise to elevated amylase and lipase in the retroperitoneal collection, such as pancreatic duct disruption or fluid collection in patients with severe pancreatitis. Some bacteria and fungi produce amylase and/or lipase and can cause elevation of the enzymes in an infected collection making it less specific, in the setting of an abscess.

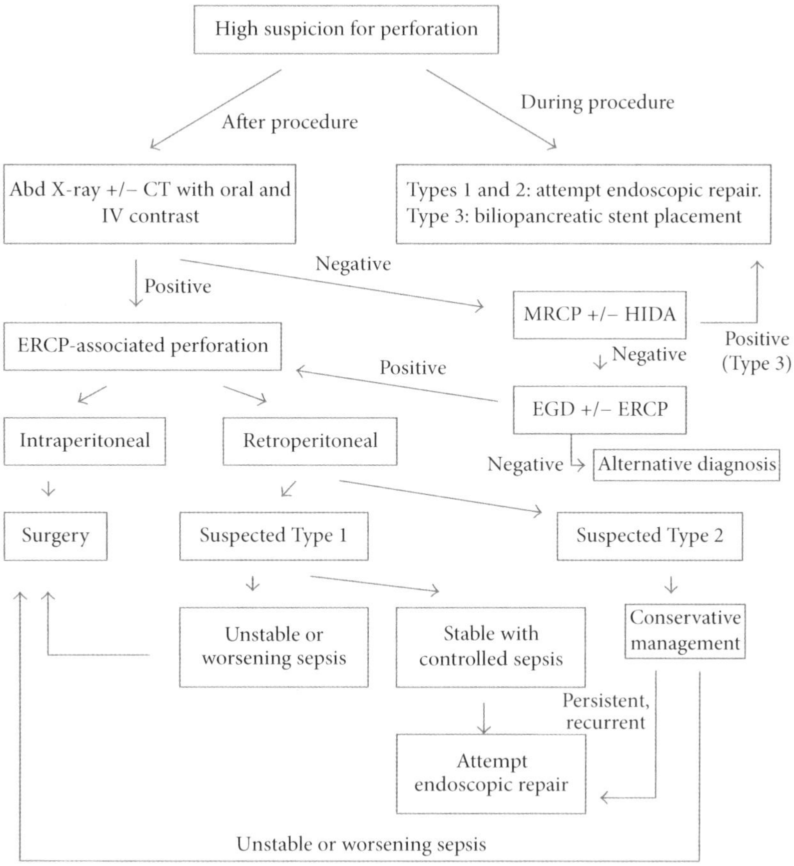

FIGURE 5: The proposed treatment algorithm for ERCP-associated perforation.

It is unknown whether degree of the enzyme elevation is relevant in differentiating the underlying etiologies.

Many of the ERCP-associated perforations are found during the index procedure. The vast majority of the initially unrecognized perforations are further diagnosed via imaging studies. Delayed diagnosis is rare but may occur in patients with small and contained retroperitoneal perforation. Endoscopy is not only seldom required but also is not a routinely recommended diagnostic tool for perforation, given concern for worsening of clinical condition and delay in definitive management. Upon upper endoscopy, an obvious luminal defect may be found; however, small defects may also be unnoticed and thus require a careful examination.

Endoscopic repair with fibrin glue, clips, and over-the-scope clip or stitch with or without biliopancreatic stents has been described for both Type 1 and Type 2 perforations [8–11]. In majority of the cases, the repair was performed during the same index procedure. Jin et al. suggested endoscopic repair to be considered if the diagnosis was made within 6 hours [2]. Artifon et al. showed in their randomized control trial of 23 patients that endoscopic repair within 12 hours was able to close the defect as safely and effectively as a surgical approach [20]. The study did not characterize the perforations based on Stapfer classification; however, it was mentioned that approximately 40% were intraperitoneal. Majority of defects were less than 10 mm; however, up to 9% were larger than 20 mm. Despite the literature, some endoscopists might not feel comfortable pursuing an endoscopic repair for ERCP-associated perforations.

High index of suspicion is required for a prompt diagnosis of ERCP-associated perforations. We propose an algorithm for the work-up and management of ERCP-associated perforations (Figure 5). Overall clinical stability and unremarkable work-up influenced our decision to perform diagnostic and therapeutic endoscopy. Endoscopic repair should be considered even if the diagnosis is significantly delayed—in our case, 10 weeks from the index ERCP.

Disclosure

This case was presented at the World Congress of Gastroenterology at ACG 2017 Meeting poster session in Orlando, Florida.

References

[1] A. Andriulli, S. Loperfido, G. Napolitano et al., "Incidence rates of post-ERCP complications: a systematic survey of prospective

studies," *American Journal of Gastroenterology*, vol. 102, no. 8, pp. 1781–1788, 2007.

[2] Y. J. Jin, S. Jeong, J. H. Kim et al., *Clinical Course and Proposed Treatment Strategy for ERCP-Related Duodenal Perforation: a Multicenter Analysis Endoscopy*, vol. 45, 2013.

[3] T. J. Howard, T. Tzujen, G. A. Lehman et al., "Classification and management of perforations complicating endoscopic sphincterotomy," *Surgery*, vol. 126, no. 4, pp. 658–663, 1999.

[4] M. Stapfer, R. R. Selby, S. C. Stain et al., "Management of duodenal perforation after endoscopic retrograde cholangiopancreatography and sphincterotomy," *Annals of Surgery*, vol. 232, no. 2, pp. 191–198, 2000.

[5] M. G. Sarr, E. K. Fishman, F. D. Milligan, S. S. Siegelman, and J. L. Cameron, "Pancreatitis or duodenal perforation after peri-Vaterian therapeutic endoscopic procedures: Diagnosis, differentiation, and management," *Surgery*, vol. 100, no. 3, pp. 461–466, 1986.

[6] R. Cirocchi, M. D. Kelly, E. A. Griffiths et al., "A systematic review of the management and outcome of ERCP related duodenal perforations using a standardized classification system," *The Surgeon*, 2017.

[7] V. Kumbhari, A. Sinha, A. Reddy et al., "Algorithm for the management of ERCP-related perforations," *Gastrointestinal Endoscopy*, vol. 83, no. 5, pp. 934–943, 2016.

[8] S. M. Park, "Recent advanced endoscopic management of endoscopic retrograde cholangiopancreatography related duodenal perforations," *Clinical Endoscopy*, vol. 49, no. 4, pp. 376–382, 2016.

[9] T. H. Baron, C. J. Gostout, and L. Herman, "Hemoclip repair of a sphincterotomy-induced duodenal perforation," *Gastrointestinal Endoscopy*, vol. 52, no. 4, pp. 566–568, 2000.

[10] M. Mutignani, F. Iacopini, S. Dokas et al., "Successful endoscopic closure of a lateral duodenal perforation at ERCP with fibrin glue," *Gastrointestinal Endoscopy*, vol. 63, no. 4, pp. 725–727, 2006.

[11] G. S. Raju and L. Gajula, "Endoclips for GI endoscopy," *Gastrointestinal Endoscopy*, vol. 59, no. 2, pp. 267–279, 2004.

[12] G. A. Paspatis, J.-M. Dumonceau, M. Barthet et al., "Diagnosis and management of iatrogenic endoscopic perforations: European Society of Gastrointestinal Endoscopy (ESGE) position statement," *Endoscopy*, vol. 46, no. 8, pp. 693–711, 2014.

[13] W. Y. Park, K. Bum Cho, E. Soo Kim, and K. Sik Park, "A case of ampullary perforation treated with a temporally covered metal stent," *Clinical Endoscopy*, vol. 45, no. 2, pp. 177–180, 2012.

[14] J. Canena, M. Liberato, D. Horta, C. Romão, and A. Coutinho, "Short-term stenting using fully covered self-expandable metal stents for treatment of refractory biliary leaks, postsphincterotomy bleeding, and perforations," *Surgical Endoscopy*, vol. 27, no. 1, pp. 313–324, 2013.

[15] B. Odemis, E. Oztas, U. B. Kuzu et al., "Can a fully covered self-expandable metallic stent be used temporarily for the management of duodenal retroperitoneal perforation during ERCP as a part of conservative therapy?" *Surgical Laparoscopy Endoscopy & Percutaneous Techniques*, vol. 26, no. 1, pp. e9–e17, 2016.

[16] A. Furukawa, M. Sakoda, M. Yamasaki et al., "Gastrointestinal tract perforation: CT diagnosis of presence, site, and cause," *Abdominal Imaging*, vol. 30, no. 5, pp. 524–534, 2005.

[17] H. K. Sung, S. S. Sang, Y. J. Yong, H. H. Suk, W. K. Jin, and K. K. Heoung, "Gastrointestinal tract perforation: MDCT findings according to the perforation sites," *Korean Journal of Radiology*, vol. 10, no. 1, pp. 63–70, 2009.

[18] R. W. Light, "Exudative pleural effusions secondary to gastrointestinal diseases," *Clinics in Chest Medicine*, vol. 6, no. 1, pp. 103-11, 1985.

[19] E. Croce, M. Golia, R. Russo, M. Azzola, S. Olmi, and G. De Murtas, "Duodenal perforations after laparoscopic cholecystectomy," *Surgical Endoscopy*, vol. 13, no. 5, pp. 523–525, 1999.

[20] E. L. A. Artifon, M. K. Minata, M. A. B. Cunha et al., "Surgical or endoscopic management for post-ERCP large transmural duodenal perforations: a randomized prospective trial," *Revista de gastroenterologia del Peru : organo oficial de la Sociedad de Gastroenterologia del Peru*, vol. 35, no. 4, pp. 313–317, 2015.

36

Isolated Retropancreatic Tuberculous Lymphadenitis Mimicking Carcinoma: A Diagnostic Challenge

H. Kuriry,[1] R. Alenezi,[2] A. Alghamdi,[3] and A. M. Swied[1]

[1] *Gastroenterology Division, Department of Medicine 1443, King Abdulaziz Medical City, P.O. Box 22490, Riyadh 11426, Saudi Arabia*
[2] *Department of Medicine 1443, King Abdulaziz Medical City, P.O. Box 22490, Riyadh 11426, Saudi Arabia*
[3] *Gastroenterology Division, Department of Medicine, King Fahad Medical City, P.O. Box 59046, Riyadh 11525, Saudi Arabia*

Correspondence should be addressed to H. Kuriry; h.kuriry@live.com

Academic Editor: Gregory Kouraklis

Tuberculosis as a cause of obstructive jaundice is a rare entity with only a few cases reported in the literature. Patients with this condition usually present with a protracted illness, jaundice, and weight loss, which may be confused with malignancies. We are reporting unusual case of isolated enlarged tuberculous lymph node compressing the common bile duct in the retropancreatic region and causing obstructive jaundice in an immunocompetent patient which to the best of our knowledge is the first case of isolated retropancreatic tuberculous lymphadenitis in Saudi Arabia.

1. Introduction

The extrapulmonary tuberculosis (EPTB) represents around 10–25% of all TB cases and this proportion varies between countries. EPTB as cause of obstructive jaundice is a rare entity with only a few cases reported in the literature. Patients with this condition usually present with a protracted illness, jaundice, and weight loss, which may be confused with malignancies.

2. Case Report

Our patient is 20-year-old male who is healthy before complaining of a gradual onset right upper quadrant abdominal pain for one month. It was associated with nausea, vomiting, and decreased appetite, yellowish discoloration of the sclera, itching, pale stool, and dark urine. There was no fever, weight loss, or change in bowel habits. There was no history of gallstones or similar previous episodes. He gave a history of contact with a pulmonary TB patient (his aunt) 4 years ago without precaution. His past medical and surgical histories were unremarkable. There was no family history of liver, pancreatic disease, or malignancies. He denied any history of smoking, alcohol consumption, drug abuse, or high-risk sexual exposure.

The patient initially was investigated in another hospital, where he was labeled as a case of a peripancreatic mass with common bile duct compression, and endoscopic retrograde cholangiopancreatography (ERCP) with sphincterotomy and insertion of a plastic biliary stent were done three weeks before seeking our opinion.

In our hospital, he was well, alert, and oriented, not jaundiced; his body mass index was 29.7. Abdominal examination showed soft abdomen and no palpable lymph node or masses. Chest examination was unremarkable.

His complete blood count was normal. Biochemical investigation revealed raised total bilirubin (20.8 mmol/L) with conjugated hyperbilirubinemia (13.6 mmol/L) and raised hepatic enzymes, including AST (57 IU/L), ALT (131 IU/L), and alkaline phosphatase (103 IU/L). All the viral markers and tumor markers (CA 19.9, AFP, and CEA) were negative. ESR was 28 mm/hr and tuberculosis quantiferon was positive.

Abdomen ultrasound showed hypoechoic peripancreatic soft tissue mass with minimal vascularity measuring 4.8 × 3.2 cm, no pancreatic mass, and common bile duct stent seen likely relieving obstruction caused by the mass; there is no

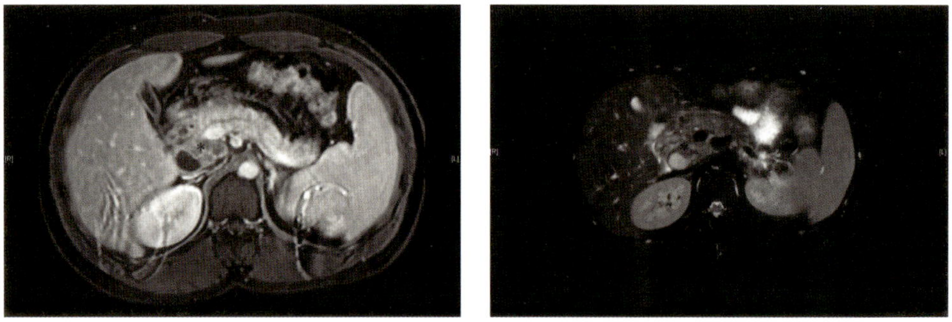

(a) (b)

Figure 1: Axial abdominal MRI. (a) T1 MRI with contrast in arterial phase and (b) T2 MRI. Demonstrating a multiloculated complex cystic mass at the posterior aspect of the pancreatic head with heterogeneous content and enhancing septations (asterisk). It measures 4.7 × 4 cm with mild mass effect on the portal vein and no definite communication with common bile duct or pancreatic duct.

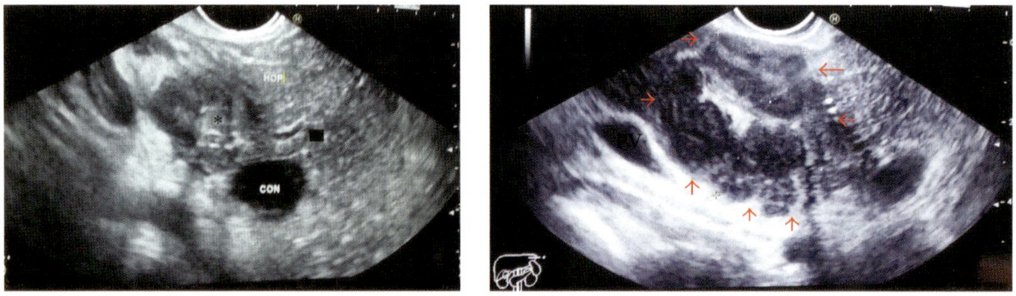

(a) (b)

Figure 2: EUS showed a large hypoechoic mass mixed with hyperechoic spots and septate, measuring 4 × 4.7 cm, sets in the retropancreatic area with no fluid content noted with significant mass effect on the common bile duct. Superior mesenteric artery visualized and portal vain patent.

intrahepatic duct dilatation. Abdomen MRI showed complex cystic mass at the posterior aspect of the pancreatic head with no intra-abdominal lymphadenopathy (Figure 1). Chest X-ray was normal.

The patient subsequently underwent endoscopic ultrasound (EUS) with fine needle aspiration which showed large hypoechoic mass mixed with hyperechoic spots and septations, measuring 4 × 4.7 cm, sets in the retropancreatic area (Figure 2).

Cytopathological examination showed necrotizing granulomatous lymphadenitis. No fungi or acid-fast bacilli on special staining were seen. TB PCR for *M. tuberculosis* complex was positive (Figure 3).

Antituberculous therapy with isoniazid, rifampicin, pyrazinamide, and ethambutol regimen was initiated. In follow-up, he has gained 4 kg of his weight and normalized his liver enzymes after one month of treatment. Patient completed 9 months of anti-TB therapy without complication, stent then was removed, and his bilirubin level stayed within the normal range in subsequent follow-up.

3. Discussion

Tuberculosis (TB) is a major global health problem, causing morbidity and mortality. Worldwide, it is the second leading cause of death from an infectious disease. The extrapulmonary TB represents around 10–25% of all TB cases and this proportion varies between countries [1].

Abdominal tuberculosis is a common extrapulmonary TB site and known to be a diagnostic challenge. It can involve the gastrointestinal tract, peritoneum, lymph nodes, or any intraabdominal organ [1]. The most frequent form of abdominal TB is tuberculous lymphadenopathy, which is related to the disease nature of spreading through lymphatic system [2].

The mesenteric, periportal region and peripancreatic lymph node are commonly involved [2]. TB rarely involves the pancreas [3]. Pancreatic and peripancreatic tuberculosis are difficult to diagnose and often misdiagnosed as pancreatic carcinoma.

The initial symptoms of abdominal TB are variable and depend on the area involved. Commonly patients presented with abdominal pain followed by fever and weight loss. Jaundice was reported in less than thirty percent of the cases [4] and usually it is secondary to involvement of the head of the pancreas, compression of the bile duct by enlarged lymph nodes in the porta hepatis, tubercular stricture of the biliary tree, or a tubercular mass of the retroperitoneum [5].

The definitive diagnosis of abdominal tuberculous lymphadenopathy is based on histopathological and microbiological evidence of tuberculosis. It is usually seen by

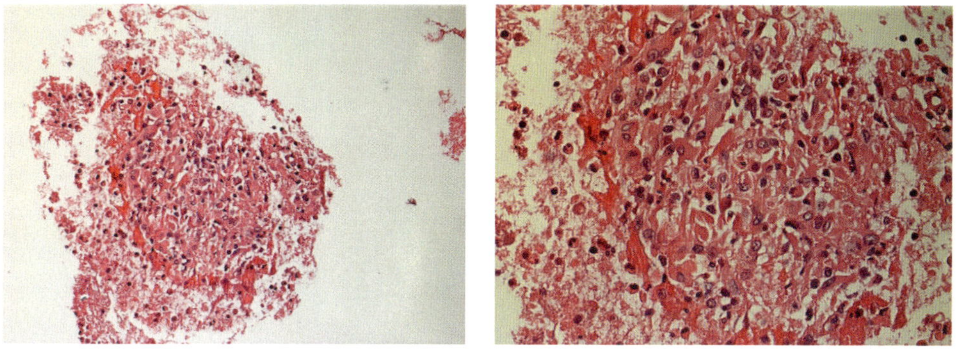

(a) (b)

FIGURE 3: The histological finding of hematoxylin and eosin staining. (a) Low power sections (100x) and (b) high power section (400x) revealed mixed population of lymphoid cells. In addition, there are aggregates of epithelioid cells, forming granulomas; some showed central necrosis occasional multinucleated giant cells are also seen. On immunohistochemistry, the lymphoid cells are a mixture of both B and T lymphocytes forming germinal centers. No Reed-Sternberg cells are seen.

abdominal CT as hypodense mass or masses with peripheral enhancement, with irregular borders and a multilocular appearance [6]. This is highly suggestive of TB but is not pathognomonic feature.

Recently, endoscopic ultrasound (EUS) has emerged as a safe and accurate tool for imaging and sampling of intra-abdominal pathology. It can differentiate pancreatic and peripancreatic masses as well as identifying abdominal lymphadenopathy that may have been missed on cross-sectional imaging. In addition, EUS guided fine needle aspiration and biopsy can also be performed [7].

In our case, EUS has a major role in the diagnosis. It allows us to assess and visualize the mass adequately and distinguish it from the surrounding structures. In addition to that, we are able to obtain a tissue biopsy in the same setting and avoid unnecessarily invasive surgical procedure.

The diagnostic accuracy of EUS-FNA of pancreatic/peripancreatic TB has been determined in several studies. In a series of 21 consecutive patients with pancreatic/peripancreatic TB EUS-FNA showed 13 (61.9%) had granulomatous inflammation on histopathological examination, 66.7% were positive on a TB PCR assay, Ziehl-Neelsen staining was positive in 26.7%, and 37.5% had positive cultures for *Mycobacterium tuberculosis* [8].

The classical cytological patterns of TB lymphadenitis are Langerhans giant cells, caseating necrosis, granulomatous inflammation, and calcification [9].

Multiple studies have shown that the cytological patterns influence the positivity of AFB stain. In a series of three hundred and eighteen lymph nodes aspirate of clinically suspected tuberculous patients showed the highest AFB positivity was seen in smears revealing necrosis without epithelioid granulomas (85.5%) while the lowest was seen in smears showing epithelioid granulomas without necrosis (3.2%) [9]. Similar result is shown by Bezabih et al. [10].

Drug treatment is the most important modality and follows standard regimens and principles. Six to nine months of therapy is probably adequate for most sites. Most of the pancreatic and peripancreatic tuberculosis cases respond well to antituberculous treatment [4]. The most common regimen was isoniazid, rifampicin, pyrazinamide, and ethambutol [4].

4. Conclusion

Isolated peripancreatic tuberculous lymphadenitis is extremely rare. It is a diagnostic challenge and for that a high index of suspicion is needed and should be considered in the context of the peripancreatic or pancreas head mass in the endemic area especially in a young adult.

Consent

Informed consent was obtained from the present patient.

References

[1] American Thoracic Society, "Diagnostic standards and classification of tuberculosis in adults and children," *American Journal of Respiratory and Critical Care Medicine*, vol. 161, no. 4, pp. 1376–1395, 2000.

[2] H. M. Peto, R. H. Pratt, T. A. Harrington, P. A. LoBue, and L. R. Armstrong, "Epidemiology of extrapulmonary tuberculosis in the United States, 1993–2006," *Clinical Infectious Diseases*, vol. 49, no. 9, pp. 1350–1357, 2009.

[3] H. Vafa, M. Arvanitakis, C. Matos et al., "Pancreatic tuberculosis diagnosed by EUS: one disease, many faces," *Journal of the Pancreas*, vol. 14, no. 3, pp. 256–260, 2013.

[4] F. Xia, T.-P. Poon, S.-G. Wang, P. Bie, X.-Q. Huang, and J.-H. Dong, "Tuberculosis of pancreas and peripancreatic lymph nodes in immunocompetent patients: experience from China," *World Journal of Gastroenterology*, vol. 9, no. 6, pp. 1361–1364, 2003.

[5] R. Colovic, N. Grubor, R. Jesic et al., "Tuberculous lymphadenitis as a cause of obstructive jaundice: a case report and literature

review," *World Journal of Gastroenterology*, vol. 14, no. 19, pp. 3098–3100, 2008.

[6] T. Sinan, M. Sheikh, S. Ramadan, S. Sahwney, and A. Behbehani, "CT features in abdominal tuberculosis: 20 years experience," *BMC Medical Imaging*, vol. 2, article 3, 2002.

[7] J. D. Boujaoude, K. Honein, C. Yaghi, C. Ghora, G. Abadjian, and R. Sayegh, "Diagnosis by endoscopic ultrasound guided fine needle aspiration of tuberculous lymphadenitis involving the peripancreatic lymph nodes: a case report," *World Journal of Gastroenterology*, vol. 13, no. 3, pp. 474–477, 2007.

[8] T. J. Song, S. S. Lee, D. H. Park et al., "Yield of EUS-guided FNA on the diagnosis of pancreatic/peripancreatic tuberculosis," *Gastrointestinal Endoscopy*, vol. 69, no. 3, pp. 484–491, 2009.

[9] P. Nidhi, T. Sapna, M. Shalini, and G. Kumud, "FNAC in tuberculous lymphadenitis: experience from a tertiary level referral centre," *Indian Journal of Tuberculosis*, vol. 58, no. 3, pp. 102–107, 2011.

[10] M. Bezabih, D. W. Mariam, and S. G. Selassie, "Fine needle aspiration cytology of suspected tuberculous lymphadenitis," *Cytopathology*, vol. 13, no. 5, pp. 284–290, 2002.

37

A Perplexing Case of Abdominal Pain That Led to the Diagnosis of Zollinger-Ellison Syndrome

Adrienne Lenhart,[1] Mona Hassan,[2] Alireza Meighani,[1] Omar Sadiq,[1] and Yousuf Siddiqui[2]

[1]*Department of Internal Medicine, Henry Ford Hospital, Detroit, MI 48202, USA*
[2]*Division of Gastroenterology and Hepatology, Henry Ford Hospital, Detroit, MI 48202, USA*

Correspondence should be addressed to Adrienne Lenhart; alenhar2@hfhs.org

Academic Editor: Naohiko Koide

Zollinger-Ellison syndrome (ZES) is a rare clinical disorder, characterized by hypersecretion of gastric acid and multiple ulcers distal to the duodenal bulb. This occurs via the release of gastrin by neuroendocrine tumors known as gastrinomas. Patients with ZES present with nonspecific GI symptoms, which often leads to a delay in diagnosis. Our patient is a 55-year-old female with chronic abdominal pain, nausea, and diarrhea. She underwent EGD, EUS, MRCP, CT scans, and cholecystectomy, which did not reveal the cause of her symptoms. Repeat EGD showed a cratered ulcer in the second portion of the duodenum, suspicious for ZES. Serum gastrin was initially only moderately elevated while on PPI therapy, but chromogranin A was also elevated. Repeat gastrin level after stopping PPI therapy was 1639 pg/mL. Somatostatin receptor scintigraphy was obtained, which showed two small lesions in the gastrinoma triangle. She subsequently underwent a Whipple pancreaticoduodenectomy and pathology was positive for four microscopic foci of a neuroendocrine tumor. She reported improvement in her symptoms after surgery. This case highlights the need for increased awareness of ZES in patients with unexplained GI complaints and emphasizes the use of multiple modalities in the diagnosis of ZES.

1. Introduction

Zollinger-Ellison syndrome (ZES) is a rare clinical disorder, characterized by hypersecretion of gastric acid into the proximal gastrointestinal (GI) tract. The syndrome results from increased secretion of the hormone gastrin by duodenal or pancreatic neuroendocrine tumors, known as gastrinomas [1–4]. The incidence of ZES is rare, ranging from 0.1 to 3 per million in the population each year [1, 5–7]. Patients with gastrinomas are usually diagnosed between the ages of twenty and fifty years old, but cases have been reported in both younger and elderly patients [8]. Around 80% of gastrinomas are sporadic in nature, while approximately 20–30% have been found in association with multiple endocrine neoplasia, type 1 (MEN-1) [9].

The majority of gastrinomas originate in the duodenum, and only around 25% of gastrinomas arise from within the pancreas [8]. However, pancreatic tumors are typically more aggressive and are more likely to metastasize to the lymph nodes, liver, and/or bone than are duodenal tumors [10, 11]. Around 80% of gastrinomas are detected within the gastrinoma triangle, defined as the interface between the confluence of the cystic duct and common bile duct, the junction of the second and third portions of the duodenum, and the junction of the neck and body of the pancreas [12, 13]. Patients with ZES typically present with nonspecific GI symptoms, such as abdominal pain, nausea, vomiting, and chronic diarrhea [2]. Subsequent endoscopic evaluation usually reveals multiple peptic ulcerations distal to the duodenal bulb.

The diagnosis of ZES requires confirmation of hypergastrinemia, and a serum gastrin level over 1000 pg/mL in the setting of gastric pH <2 is virtually diagnostic [1, 8, 14]. Secretin stimulation testing can also be used to differentiate patients with gastrinomas from other causes of hypergastrinemia, such as atrophic gastritis, renal failure, or vagotomy. Once the diagnosis of a gastrinoma has been established, localization and staging of the tumor are sought through endoscopic ultrasound (EUS), contrast enhanced computed tomography (CT), magnetic resonance imaging (MRI), or somatostatin receptor scintigraphy (SRS). We present a rare case of a gastrinoma that highlights the challenges present in making the diagnosis of ZES and illustrates the importance of increased awareness of this syndrome in patients with chronic GI complaints.

2. Case

The patient is a 55-year-old Caucasian female with a past medical history of type 2 diabetes, depression, gastroesophageal reflux disease (GERD), and chronic pancreatitis. She had been followed up in the Gastroenterology Clinic for several years, secondary to a history of intermittent, epigastric abdominal pain, nausea, nonbloody emesis, and chronic diarrhea. However, despite extensive testing, a clear etiology of her ailments had not been determined. She initially underwent esophagogastroduodenoscopy (EGD) and EUS that were consistent with erythematous gastropathy and duodenopathy, with pancreatic parenchymal and ductal changes suggestive of chronic pancreatitis. However, no pancreatic masses were visualized on EUS. Magnetic resonance cholangiopancreatography (MRCP) was also unremarkable at that time. Gastric biopsies were consistent with chronic gastritis and staining for *H. pylori* was negative.

She was hospitalized several times in the interim period with recurrent abdominal pain, presumed to be secondary to GERD and acute on chronic pancreatitis. HIDA scan was consistent with biliary dyskinesia with an ejection fraction of 8% after infusion of cholecystokinin, and she subsequently underwent laparoscopic cholecystectomy. She was started on pancreatic enzyme supplementation in addition to proton pump inhibitor (PPI) therapy, with initial mild improvement in her symptoms. However, she was again hospitalized several months after her cholecystectomy for similar complaints. She underwent repeat EGD, which showed a nonbleeding, deep ulceration at the gastroesophageal junction (LA Grade D), diffuse erythematous mucosa throughout the entire stomach, and a 2 cm deeply cratered ulcer in the second portion of the duodenum (D2) (Figure 1). Gastric and duodenal biopsies were consistent with severe, active chronic gastritis and duodenitis without evidence of malignancy.

These findings were suspicious for ZES, and appropriate workup was pursued. Serum gastrin level was moderately elevated at 762 pg/mL while on PPI therapy, and chromogranin A was also elevated at 164 ng/mL. Carcinoembryonic antigen (CEA) and carbohydrate antigen 19-9 (CA 19-9) levels were unremarkable. She underwent repeat EUS and CT abdomen/pelvis with contrast, which again did not reveal any pancreatic or duodenal masses. Serum gastrin level was then reevaluated after temporarily discontinuing PPI therapy several months later, and this time it was significantly elevated at 1,639 pg/mL. She subsequently had a SRS scan performed, which revealed two small lesions within the gastrinoma triangle (Figure 2).

She was evaluated by surgical oncology and subsequently underwent a Whipple pancreaticoduodenectomy. Pathology of the pancreas returned positive for four microscopic foci

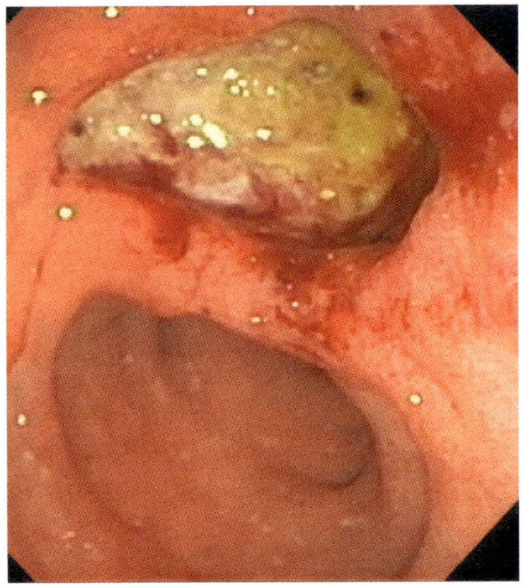

Figure 1: EGD showing 2 cm deeply cratered ulcer in the second portion of the duodenum, suspicious for ZES.

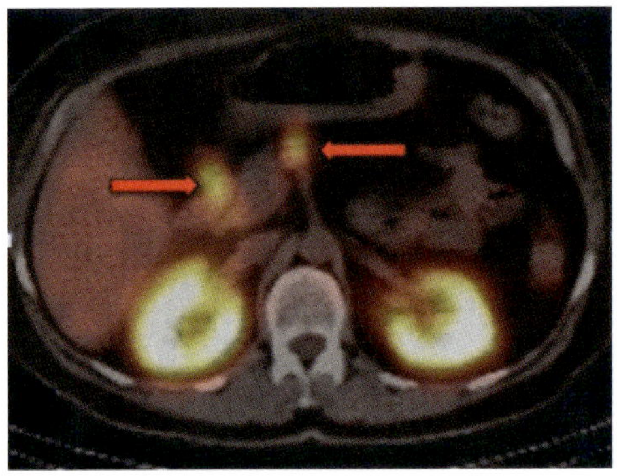

Figure 2: Somatostatin receptor scintigraphy (SRS) showing two small foci of moderately intense abnormal radiotracer uptake within the gastrinoma triangle.

(the largest being 0.1 cm) of a well-differentiated neuroendocrine tumor with metastasis to two peripancreatic lymph nodes (Figure 3). There was also evidence of pancreatic intraepithelial neoplasia, focal chronic pancreatitis, and focal biliary intraepithelial neoplasia. The duodenum and stomach were without significant abnormalities. She is currently maintained on PPI therapy and pancreatic enzyme supplements and has reported improvement in her oral intake and GI symptoms after the surgery.

3. Discussion

ZES is characterized by hypersecretion of gastrin and resultant severe peptic ulcer disease (PUD) [1–4]. The rare nature of ZES can lower clinical suspicion for the disorder and ultimately result in a delay in diagnosis, with studies showing the mean time from symptom onset to diagnosis of around 5.9 years [2]. The most common clinical symptoms of nausea, vomiting, and epigastric pain are nonspecific and may lead physicians to first suspect more common disorders such as

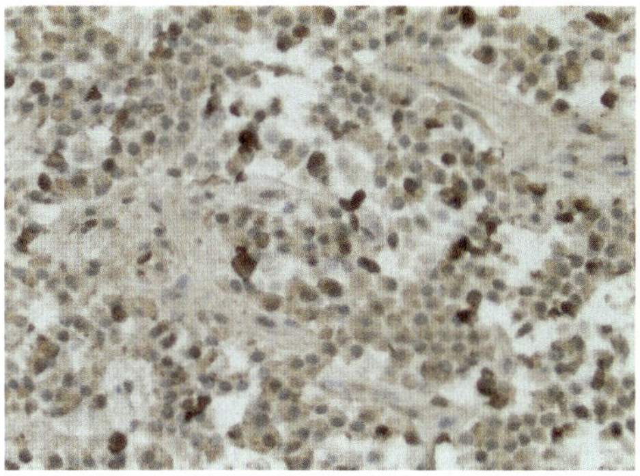

FIGURE 3: Pathology of pancreatic neuroendocrine tumor with positive staining for gastrin.

PUD, GERD, or chronic pancreatitis. However, the symptoms seen in ZES may often be more severe and more refractory to standard medical therapy than are the symptoms seen with PUD caused by nonsteroidal medications or *H. pylori*. This should consequently raise clinicians' suspicion for an alternative diagnosis. In addition, ZES is often characterized by chronic diarrhea (secondary to the high osmotic load of gastric acid as well as malabsorption caused by inactivation of pancreatic enzymes), which would be uncommon with other causes of PUD. These concepts were illustrated in our patient, who was initially diagnosed with GERD and chronic pancreatitis, despite the presence of diarrhea and having recurrent symptoms while on PPI therapy and pancreatic enzyme replacements. If ZES had been entertained earlier in her clinical course, excessive testing may have been avoided, she may have been diagnosed at an earlier stage of disease, and she may have had quicker relief of symptoms.

As previously mentioned, ZES is often suspected when endoscopic evaluation reveals multiple peptic ulcerations or ulcers distal to the first portion of the duodenum in the presence of hypergastrinemia. While gastrin level was elevated in our patient, there were several factors that made the diagnosis of ZES interesting and challenging in this case. For instance, the initial serum gastrin value was less than 1000 pg/mL, which is a nonspecific finding and can be present in other causes of hypergastrinemia other than gastrinomas [8]. In addition, our patient was on PPI therapy at the time of initial testing, which can stimulate a rise in serum gastrin levels secondary to suppression of the normal negative feedback loop to gastrin secretion [15]. It is therefore recommended that patients withhold from PPI therapy for several weeks prior to testing serum gastrin levels [16]. However, despite the only moderately elevated gastrin level while on a PPI, our patient was also noted to have a high serum chromogranin A level, a protein which is elevated in a majority of patients with gastrinomas and often correlates with tumor volume [17]. Chromogranin A levels are not usually elevated in patients with hypergastrinemia secondary to other causes such as chronic atrophic gastritis. Therefore, despite only having a modestly high gastrin level, the elevated chromogranin A level increased clinical suspicion for a gastrinoma in our patient. Serum gastrin was subsequently reevaluated several weeks after discontinuation of her PPI, at which time levels more than doubled.

Once the diagnosis of ZES is established via endoscopy and elevated serum gastrin, imaging should be undertaken to localize the gastrinoma and carry out an evaluation for metastasis. CT and MRI are both highly accurate in detecting lesions greater than 3 cm; however, accuracy decreases for tumors that are smaller than 2 cm in size (studies have reported around 42–56% sensitivity of CT scans and 25–83% sensitivity for MRI) [18, 19]. Gastrinomas express receptors for somatostatin, allowing SRS scans to be utilized for tumor detection with a higher sensitivity than CT/MRI (reported to be around 80–85%) [13, 19]. Recently, EUS has also become an important imaging study and allows for the identification of pancreatic tumors as small as 2–5 mm in diameter, with sensitivity reaching up to 87% [19–21]. Our patient underwent extensive imaging with CT, MRI, and EUS before the tumor was finally identified using SRS. While the reasons why her gastrinoma was not initially detected are not completely known, a large component may be secondary to the very small size of the tumors, as the largest measured only 0.1 cm. This emphasizes that the use of multiple imaging modalities, including SRS, may be imperative in the diagnosis of a gastrinoma.

4. Conclusion

In conclusion, this case provides a unique example of ZES that highlights the importance of increased awareness of this disorder in patients who present with chronic GI symptoms. This case also supports the use of chromogranin A to either increase or decrease clinical suspicion for a gastrinoma when serum gastrin levels are only moderately elevated. In addition, this case emphasizes the use of multiple endoscopic and imaging modalities in the ultimate diagnosis of ZES.

Consent

Informed consent was obtained from the patient described in this case report.

Disclosure

Dr. Adrienne Lenhart (resident) is the primary author of this manuscript. All others are coauthors. Dr. Yousuf Siddiqui is the staff physician in addition to being a coauthor. This case report was presented as a poster presentation at the 2016 Annual American College of Gastroenterology (ACG) meeting in Las Vegas, Nevada.

References

[1] D. C. Metz and R. T. Jensen, "Gastrointestinal neuroendocrine tumors: pancreatic endocrine tumors," *Gastroenterology*, vol. 135, no. 5, pp. 1469–1492, 2008.

[2] P. K. Roy, D. J. Venzon, H. Shojamanesh et al., "Zollinger-Ellison syndrome. Clinical presentation in 261 patients," *Medicine*, vol. 79, no. 6, pp. 379–411, 2000.

[3] R. T. Jensen, B. Niederle, E. Mitry et al., "Gastrinoma (duodenal and pancreatic)," *Neuroendocrinology*, vol. 84, no. 3, pp. 173–182, 2006.

[4] R. M. Zollinger and E. H. Ellison, "Primary peptic ulcerations of the jejunum associated with islet cell tumors of the pancreas," *Annals of Surgery*, vol. 142, no. 4, pp. 709–723, 1955.

[5] B. Eriksson, K. Ouberg, and B. Skogseid, "Neuroendocrine pancreatic tumors clinical findings in a prospective study of 84 patients," *Acta Oncologica*, vol. 28, no. 3, pp. 373–377, 1989.

[6] J. G. Stage and F. Stadil, "The clinical diagnosis of the Zollinger-Ellison syndrome," *Scandinavian Journal of Gastroenterology. Supplement*, vol. 53, pp. 79–91, 1979.

[7] M. H. Kulke, L. B. Anthony, D. L. Bushnell et al., "NANETS treatment guidelines: well-differentiated neuroendocrine tumors of the stomach and pancreas," *Pancreas*, vol. 39, no. 6, pp. 735–752, 2010.

[8] M. J. Berna, K. M. Hoffmann, J. Serrano, F. Gibril, and R. T. Jensen, "Serum gastrin in Zollinger-Ellison syndrome: I. Prospective study of fasting serum gastrin in 309 patients from the national institutes of health and comparison with 2229 cases from the literature," *Medicine*, vol. 85, no. 6, pp. 295–330, 2006.

[9] J. A. Norton, "Neuroendocrine tumors of the pancreas and duodenum," *Current Problems in Surgery*, vol. 31, no. 2, pp. 89–156, 1994.

[10] H. C. Weber, D. J. Venzon, J.-T. Lin et al., "Determinants of metastatic rate and survival in patients with zollinger-ellison syndrome: A Prospective Long-Term Study," *Gastroenterology*, vol. 108, no. 6, pp. 1637–1649, 1995.

[11] F. Yu, D. J. Venzon, J. Serrano et al., "Prospective study of the clinical course, prognostic factors, causes of death, and survival in patients with long-standing Zollinger-Ellison syndrome," *Journal of Clinical Oncology*, vol. 17, no. 2, pp. 615–630, 1999.

[12] B. E. Stabile, D. J. Morrow, and E. Passaro Jr., "The gastrinoma triangle: operative implications," *The American Journal of Surgery*, vol. 147, pp. 25–31, 1984.

[13] E. H. Morrow and J. A. Norton, "Surgical management of Zollinger-Ellison syndrome; state of the art," *Surgical Clinics of North America*, vol. 89, no. 5, pp. 1091–1103, 2009.

[14] F. Gibril and R. T. Jensen, "Zollinger-Ellison syndrome revisited: diagnosis, biologic markers, associated inherited disorders, and acid hypersecretion," *Current Gastroenterology Reports*, vol. 6, no. 6, pp. 454–463, 2004.

[15] G. Cadiot, C. Vissuzaine, D. Pospai, P. Ruszniewski, F. Potet, and M. Mignon, "Influence of long-term treatment with proton pump inhibitors on serum gastrin levels and fundic mucosa. Preliminary results," *Gastroenterologie Clinique et Biologique*, vol. 19, no. 10, pp. 811–817, 1995.

[16] W. S. Dhillo, C. N. Jayasena, C. J. Lewis et al., "Plasma gastrin measurement cannot be used to diagnose a gastrinoma in patients on either proton pump inhibitors or histamine type-2 receptor antagonists," *Annals of Clinical Biochemistry*, vol. 43, no. 2, pp. 153–155, 2006.

[17] F. R. E. Nobels, D. J. Kwekkeboom, W. Coopmans et al., "Chromogranin A as serum marker for neuroendocrine neoplasia: comparison with neuron-specific enolase and the α-subunit of glycoprotein hormones," *Journal of Clinical Endocrinology and Metabolism*, vol. 82, no. 8, pp. 2622–2628, 1997.

[18] I. Epelboym and H. Mazeh, "Zollinger-Ellison syndrome: classical considerations and current controversies," *The Oncologist*, vol. 19, no. 1, pp. 44–50, 2014.

[19] K. J. Klose and J. T. Heverhagen, "Localisation and staging of gastrin producing tumours using cross-sectional imaging modalities," *Wiener Klinische Wochenschrift*, vol. 119, no. 19-20, pp. 588–592, 2007.

[20] M. K. Kim, "Endoscopic ultrasound in gastroenteropancreatic neuroendocrine tumors," *Gut and Liver*, vol. 6, no. 4, pp. 405–410, 2012.

[21] T. Rösch, C. J. Lightdale, J. F. Botet et al., "Localization of pancreatic endocrine tumors by endoscopic ultrasonography," *New England Journal of Medicine*, vol. 326, no. 26, pp. 1721–1726, 1992.

Endoscopic Treatment of Colonic Duplication Cyst: A Case Report and Review of the Literature

Rajat Garg, [1] **Louis D. Saravolatz**, [2] **and Mohammed Barawi**[3]

[1] *Department of Internal Medicine, St. John Hospital and Medical Center, Detroit, MI, USA*
[2] *Department of Medicine, St. John Hospital and Medical Center, Detroit, MI, USA*
[3] *Division of Gastroenterology and Hepatology, St. John Hospital and Medical Center, Detroit, MI, USA*

Correspondence should be addressed to Rajat Garg; drgargrajat@gmail.com

Academic Editor: Engin Altintas

Colonic duplication cysts are a rare congenital abnormality commonly presenting before two years of age. In adults, it has been rarely reported, most often as an incidental finding. We report a case of 42-year-old female complaining of constipation and lower abdominal pain. Patient's CT scan of the abdomen showed a cystic lesion at hepatic flexure and the diagnosis was confirmed endoscopically using endoscopic ultrasound (EUS). The cyst was treated employing hot snare to expose the cyst cavity. On our literature search, there have been no reported cases of colonic duplication cyst treated endoscopically. We here discuss incidence, diagnosis, characteristics, and treatment of duplication cysts with special emphasis on endoscopic therapy.

1. Introduction

Duplication cyst was first described by Fitz in 1884 for the remnant of omphalomesenteric duct [1]. They are rare congenital cysts commonly presenting before two years of age and rarely reported in adults. We report a case of colonic duplication cyst diagnosed endoscopically and treated using endoscopic ultrasound (EUS).

2. Case Report

A 42-year-old female with no past medical history presented with the complaints of constipation and lower abdominal pain for four months. There was no history of anorexia, weight loss, or hematochezia. Examination was negative for any masses or organomegaly. The patient had colonoscopy performed which was negative for any polyps and showed a large submucosal lesion at the hepatic flexure. The lesion showed vascular congestion and was tattooed with India ink. The patient was then referred to an advanced endoscopist for further evaluation. Computed tomography (CT) scan of the abdomen with contrast revealed a 20 mm moderately enhancing cystic lesion at the hepatic flexure (Figure 1).

On repeat colonoscopy, a tattooed subepithelial intraluminal transparent mass lesion was seen at the hepatic flexure (Figure 2). A 12 MHz mini-EUS probe was passed through the biopsy channel of the colonoscope which revealed a 14 mm subepithelial anechoic cystic lesion lined by mucosa consistent with colonic duplication cyst (Figure 3). Hot snare was used to unroof and expose the cyst cavity (Figure 4(a)). Clear fluid was seen gushing from the mass with flattening of the lesion after drainage (Figure 4(b)). The patient had an uneventful recovery and was discharged home with outpatient follow-up. Pathologic evaluation showed normal colonic mucosa without any dysplastic changes (Figure 5).

3. Discussion

Colonic duplication cysts are a rare entity encountered in the pediatric age group and even less common in adults. They are hollow, epithelium lined, cystic, spherical, or tubular structures attached to gastrointestinal tract. Several theories have been postulated regarding their occurrence but no single theory can explain all the duplication cysts [2]. There are four theories to explain the development of duplication cysts: aberrant luminal recanalization theory as suggested by

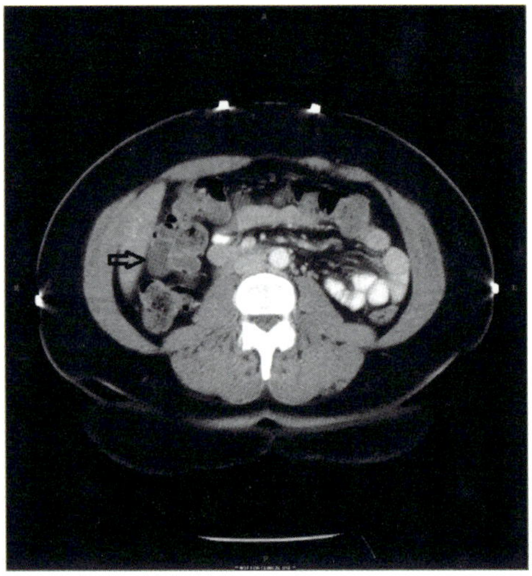

Figure 1: Computed tomographic image showing moderately enhancing cystic lesion at hepatic flexure (arrow).

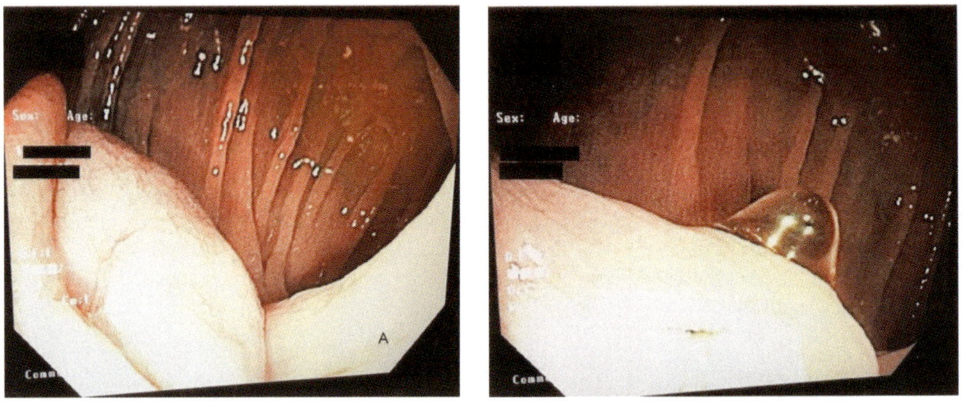

(a) (b)

Figure 2: Intraluminal mass at hepatic flexure (a) and transparent appearance (b).

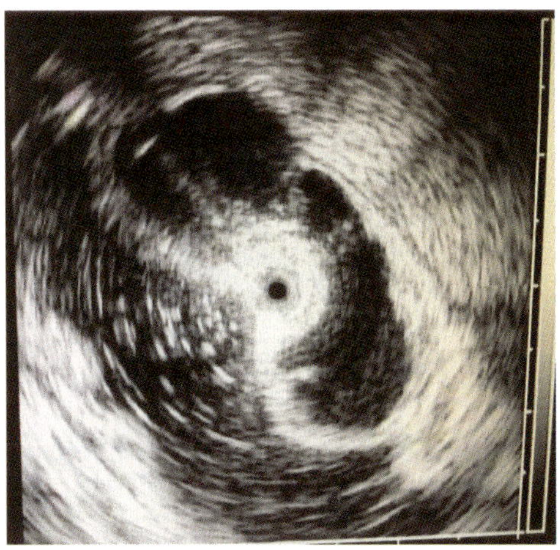

Figure 3: 12 MHz EUS images showing subepithelial anechoic lesion lined by mucosa.

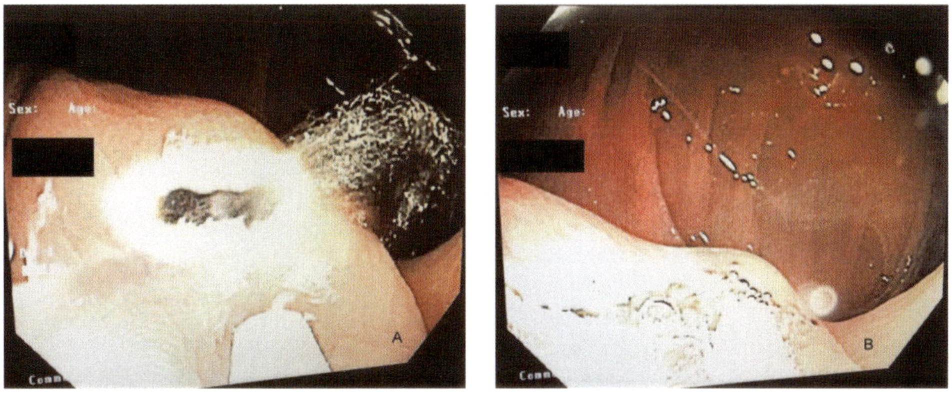

(a) (b)

Figure 4: Fluid drainage after unroofing the cyst cavity (a) and flattening of lesion after drainage (b).

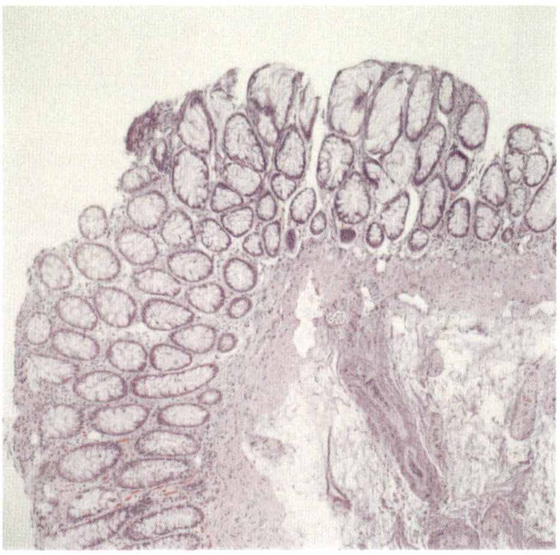

Figure 5: Normal colonic mucosa with thermal cautery artifact.

Bremer, the diverticular theory of Lewis and Thyng, the split notochord theory that explains the formation of neurenteric duplications and associated vertebral anomalies, and the intrauterine vascular accident theory which is also the most accepted one postulating that vascular accidents in utero are responsible for these anomalies. Its actual incidence is unknown due to the rarity of publications of this disease but its estimated incidence is 1 in 4500 [3].

Duplication cysts can occur anywhere from the oral cavity to the rectum. They are named according to the location in the gastrointestinal tract. In the largest case series of 96 pediatric patients, the most common site was ileum (35%) followed by esophagus (21%) and colon (20%) [2]. Another case series that reported only 6.8% of total duplication cyst involves colon [4]. Male sex is more affected than females with a ratio of 1.5 : 1. Caucasians (80%) are more affected than African Americans (20%).

Duplication cysts can be cystic (80%) or tubular (20%) and commonly occur on the mesenteric side of bowel sharing a common blood supply with native bowel. The majority of duplication cysts communicate with bowel with only a few cases reported of noncommunicating duplication cyst [5]. Most adult colonic cysts are asymptomatic and remain undiagnosed over many years; however, the most common presentation is abdominal pain [2, 4, 6, 7]. Cases of duplication cysts causing volvulus, intussusception, rectal bleeding, ischemic bowel, constipation, and obstruction have been described in the literature [8–10]. Due to such variable presentations, diagnosis of duplication is rarely made preoperatively and often made intraoperatively or on pathologic examination.

The wall of duplication cysts is comprised of two layers: the outer muscular layer and the inner mucosal layer. Duplication cysts can also have ectopic tissue of two origins most commonly heterotopic gastric mucosa, which can ulcerate leading to bleeding and less commonly pancreatic tissue [6]. Ectopic gastric tissue has been reported in case series with an incidence of 2–5% [2, 4, 7]. In addition, malignant degeneration has been reported to occur in duplication cysts most commonly in adults. Malignant degeneration has been reported in few case reports and can be anywhere from dysplasia to metastatic adenocarcinoma [11, 12]. Two cases of squamous cell cancer arising from these cysts have been reported in the literature [13]. Despite few reports of malignancy arising from colonic duplication cysts, it still remains extremely rare and only discovered incidentally. In the largest case series of duplication cysts in adults, dysplastic changes were found in 2 of 7 patients: one patient had high-grade dysplasia, and the other patient had low-grade dysplasia [7].

Despite the advancement of imaging modalities, diagnosis of duplication cysts is difficult and often made postoperatively on pathologic examination. Ultrasound (US) and CT scan are commonly used in making a diagnosis of duplication cyst. US may reveal a fluid filled complex cyst with internal echoes. Duplication cysts are characterized by typical inner echogenic mucosa and outer hypoechoic muscular layer. On US, the presence of peristalsis in the cyst is an important feature as it is not seen in any other cystic lesions. Contrast studies will demonstrate a filling defect or communication with the bowel. CT scan may reveal a cystic mass with rarely reported calcified focus [14]. As in our case, colonoscopy with EUS can assist in diagnosing duplication cyst if other studies are normal and the cyst is communicating with the colon. EUS has been reported as safe and accurate for diagnosis of duplication cysts and is commonly employed for diagnosing duodenal and foregut duplication cysts but rarely used for colonic duplication cysts [15]. The typical appearance of duplication cyst on sonographic examination is a "muscular rim sign" manifesting as inner echogenic mucosa and outer hypoechoic muscle layer; however, these changes are sometimes not present due to some degree of involution and degeneration [16]. If a typical inner echogenic mucosal and outer hypoechoic muscle layer can be seen on US, the diagnosis of duplication cyst can be established. In our case, EUS revealed an anechoic lesion lined by mucosa leading to the diagnosis of duplication cyst.

There are no standardized guidelines or consensus for the treatment of duplication cysts. Surgical resection is classically done for the cyst as they are found incidentally or intraoperatively [4, 16]. Duodenal duplication cysts have long been effectively treated endoscopically commonly using needle knife papillotomy with reported good long-term outcomes [17, 18]. Resection of the cyst roof using a snare is sufficient to relieve the symptoms. Due to the concerns of malignancy and incidental diagnosis, en bloc surgical resection is usually recommended for the colonic duplication cyst; however, endoscopic therapy can effectively treat patient's symptoms while avoiding potential extensive surgery and its related complications as surgical resection often involves resection of some part of native bowel due to cyst's intimate attachment with the bowel. One must be cautious in concluding that there is no malignancy with a biopsy of the cystic endothelium alone and further surveillance must be incorporated to determine if malignancy is still present. There are less than twenty cases reported in English language of malignant changes associated with colonic duplication cysts [14]. Moreover, avoiding irritation from cyst secretions theoretically can prevent dysplastic degeneration. Random biopsies should be done to rule out potential premalignant and malignant changes and, if possible, inner layer of the cyst should be biopsied as well. Endoscopic surveillance with random biopsies after 6 and 12 months of treatment as recommended for duodenal duplication cyst should be done to monitor the response to therapy and any premalignant or malignant changes [18].

Our patient had EUS findings consistent with a colonic duplication cyst and the biopsy was negative for any dysplasia; thus effective drainage was established using hot snare resulting in resolution of the patient's symptoms. There is a chance that malignant cells might be missed on biopsy, if they were present in cystic endothelium and the drainage secretion. For the above reason, we reiterated the role of endoscopic surveillance every 6 months for at least one year. There is no data on extended follow-up. If there is any abnormal pathology on regular follow-up in first year, then multidisciplinary and individualized approach should be taken. If the pathology is negative for any malignant/dysplastic changes in first year, there is low likelihood of malignant transformation in the future; however, caution should be exercised in case any gastrointestinal symptoms appear or recur. From our literature search, there has been no reported case of colonic duplication cyst treated endoscopically. EUS guided drainage of colonic duplication cyst is an effective approach for diagnosis and treatment of colonic duplication cysts provided that the lesion can be easily accessed and random biopsies can be done to rule out any premalignant or malignant changes. This case highlights the potential of endoscopic therapy for the diagnosis and management of colonic duplication cysts and may be considered to avoid potentially extensive surgery.

Disclosure

An earlier version of this work was presented as an abstract at World Congress of Gastroenterology at ACG2017 Meeting Abstracts, Orlando, FL, American College of Gastroenterology.

References

[1] R. H. Fitz, "Persistent omphalo-mesenteric remains; their importance in the causation of intestinal duplication, cyst-formation, and obstruction," *The American Journal of the Medical Sciences*, vol. 1, no. 7, pp. 30–57, 1884.

[2] G. W. Holcomb III, A. Gheissari, J. A. O'Neill Jr., N. A. Shorter, and H. C. Bishop, "Surgical management of alimentary tract duplications," *Annals of Surgery*, vol. 209, no. 2, pp. 167–174, 1989.

[3] J. Schalamon, J. Schleef, and M. E. Höllwarth, "Experience with gastro-intestinal duplications in childhood," *Langenbeck's Archives of Surgery*, vol. 385, no. 6, pp. 402–405, 2000.

[4] P. S. Puligandla, L. T. Nguyen, D. St-Vil et al., "Gastrointestinal duplications," *Journal of Pediatric Surgery*, vol. 38, no. 5, pp. 740–744, 2003.

[5] M. Gümüş, M. Kapan, H. Gümüş, A. Önder, and S. Girgin, "Unusual Noncommunicating Isolated Enteric Duplication Cyst in Adults," *Gastroenterology Research and Practice*, vol. 2011, pp. 1–3, 2011.

[6] S. T. Ildstad, D. J. Tollerud, R. G. Weiss, D. P. Ryan, M. A. McGowan, and L. W. Martin, "Duplications of the alimentary tract. Clinical characteristics, preferred treatment, and associated malformations," *Annals of Surgery*, vol. 208, no. 2, pp. 184–189, 1988.

[7] N. Mourra, N. Chafai, B. Bessoud, V. Reveri, A. Werbrouck, and E. Tiret, "Colorectal duplication in adults: Report of seven cases and review of the literature," *Journal of Clinical Pathology*, vol. 63, no. 12, pp. 1080–1083, 2010.

[8] C. Fotiadis, M. Genetzakis, I. Papandreou, E. P. Misiakos, E. Agapitos, and G. C. Zografos, "Colonic duplication in adults: report of two cases presenting with rectal bleeding," *World Journal of Gastroenterology*, vol. 11, no. 32, pp. 5072–5074, 2005.

[9] C. Reiser-Erkan, M. Erkan, E. Ulbrich, J. Nährig, and J. Kleeff, "Cystic colon duplication causing intussusception in a 25-year-old man: Report of a case and review of the literature," *BMC Surgery*, vol. 10, article no. 19, 2010.

[10] C. Fenelon, M. R. Boland, B. Kenny, P. Faul, and S. Tormey, "A colonic duplication cyst causing bowel ischaemia in a 74-year-old lady," *Journal of Surgical Case Reports*, vol. 2016, no. 8, p. rjw147, 2016.

[11] G. Blank, A. Königsrainer, B. Sipos, and R. Ladurner, "Adenocarcinoma arising in a cystic duplication of the small bowel: case report and review of literature," *World Journal of Surgical Oncology*, vol. 10, article 55, 2012.

[12] H. Hsu, M.-K. Gueng, Y.-H. Tseng, C.-C. Wu, P.-H. Liu, and C. C.-C. Chen, "Adenocarcinoma arising from colonic duplication cyst with metastasis to omentum: A case report," *Journal of Clinical Ultrasound*, vol. 39, no. 1, pp. 41–43, 2011.

[13] W. F. Hickey and J. M. Corson, "Squamous cell carcinoma arising in a duplication of the colon: Case report and literature review of squamous cell carcinoma of the colon and of malignancy complicating colonic duplication," *Cancer*, vol. 47, no. 3, pp. 602–609, 1981.

[14] Y. Inoue and H. Nakamura, "Adenocarcinoma arising in colonic duplication cysts with calcification: CT findings of two cases," *Abdominal Imaging*, vol. 23, no. 2, pp. 135–137, 1998.

[15] S. S. Ríos, J. L. Noia, I. A. Nallib et al., "Adult gastric duplication cyst: diagnosis by endoscopic ultrasound-guided fine-needle aspiration (EUS-FNA)," *Revista Española de Enfermedades Digestivas*, vol. 100, no. 9, pp. 586–590, 2008.

[16] R. Liu and D. G. Adler, "Duplication cysts: diagnosis, management, and the role of endoscopic ultrasound," *Endoscopic Ultrasound*, vol. 3, no. 3, pp. 152–160, 2014.

[17] M. Gjeorgjievski, P. Manickam, G. Ghaith, and M. S. Cappell, "Safety and efficacy of endoscopic therapy for nonmalignant duodenal duplication cysts," *Medicine (United States)*, vol. 95, no. 22, Article ID e3799, 2016.

[18] F. Antaki, A. Tringali, P. Deprez et al., "A case series of symptomatic intraluminal duodenal duplication cysts: presentation, endoscopic therapy, and long-term outcome (with video)," *Gastrointestinal Endoscopy*, vol. 67, no. 1, pp. 163–168, 2008.

Adenocarcinoma In Situ Arising from Brunner's Gland Treated by Endoscopic Mucosal Resection

Masaya Iwamuro,[1,2] Sayo Kobayashi,[3] Nobuya Ohara,[4,5] Seiji Kawano,[1] Yoshiro Kawahara,[6] and Hiroyuki Okada[1]

[1] *Department of Gastroenterology and Hepatology, Okayama University Graduate School of Medicine, Dentistry and Pharmaceutical Sciences, Okayama 700-8558, Japan*
[2] *Department of General Medicine, Okayama University Graduate School of Medicine, Dentistry and Pharmaceutical Sciences, Okayama 700-8558, Japan*
[3] *Department of Internal Medicine, Fukuyama City Hospital, Fukuyama 721-8511, Japan*
[4] *Department of Pathology, Okayama University Graduate School of Medicine, Dentistry and Pharmaceutical Sciences, Okayama 700-8558, Japan*
[5] *Department of Pathology, Kagawa Rosai Hospital, Marugame 763-8502, Japan*
[6] *Department of Endoscopy, Okayama University Hospital, Okayama 700-8558, Japan*

Correspondence should be addressed to Masaya Iwamuro; iwamuromasaya@yahoo.co.jp

Academic Editor: Gregory Kouraklis

An 86-year-old Japanese man was presented to our hospital for further investigation of duodenal adenocarcinoma. The tumor was endoscopically resected. Pathological analysis revealed coexistence of gastric foveolar metaplasia and a surrounding hyperplastic Brunner's gland, in addition to an adenocarcinoma component. Immunostaining for MUC5AC and MUC6 confirmed the diagnosis of adenocarcinoma in situ arising from Brunner's gland hyperplasia. This case suggests that although detailed preoperative evaluation is required to determine the depth of tumor invasion, endoscopic resection may be a promising option for the treatment of adenocarcinomas arising from Brunner's gland hyperplasia.

1. Introduction

Brunner's glands exist in the submucosa of the duodenum, typically in the duodenal bulb and the second portion of the duodenum proximal to the sphincter of Oddi. Although the role of Brunner's glands in digestion is controversial, it is hypothesized that a mucus-rich, bicarbonate-containing, alkaline secretion produced by Brunner's glands aids in neutralizing the acidic content of chyme and gastric acid, providing an alkaline milieu to optimize intestinal absorption and lubricate the intestinal walls [1, 2]. Brunner's gland hyperplasia and hamartoma are two representative lesions that are occasionally identified during esophagogastroduodenoscopic examination [1, 3–5]. It has been reported that Brunner's gland hyperplasia and hamartoma account for approximately five per cent of all duodenal masses [2, 6]. Moreover, in rare instances, adenocarcinoma may also arise from Brunner's glands [7–12].

We recently encountered a patient with a sessile polyp in the second portion of the duodenum that was successfully resected by endoscopic mucosal resection and diagnosed as adenocarcinoma in situ arising from the Brunner's gland. In this report, we focus mainly on the pathological characteristics of the adenocarcinoma and review previously reported cases of this disease.

2. Case Report

An 86-year-old Japanese man underwent esophagogastroduodenoscopy for the investigation of anemia. An acute gastric mucosal lesion was identified in the stomach that was

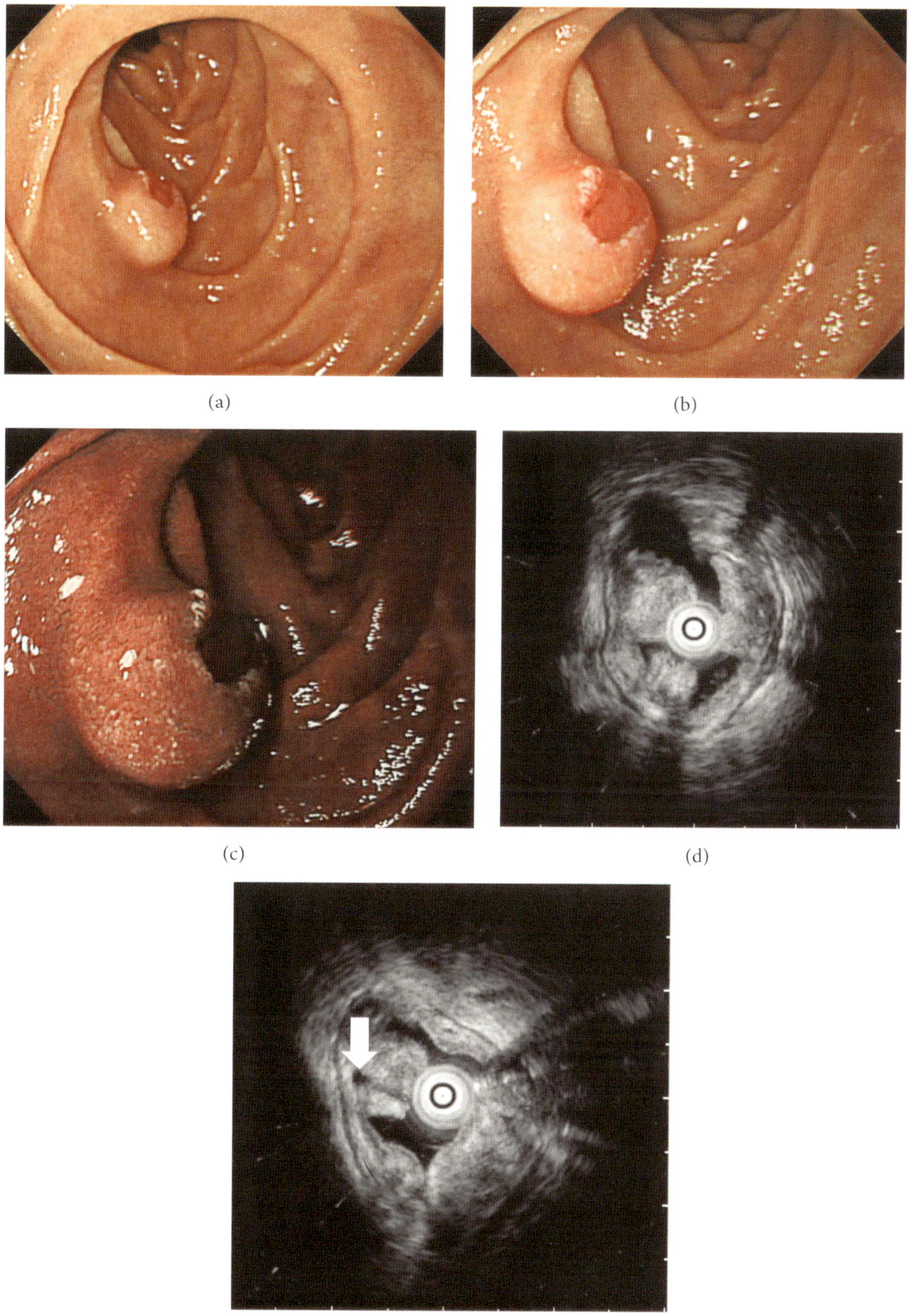

(a) (b) (c) (d) (e)

Figure 1: Endoscopic images. Esophagogastroduodenoscopy shows a solitary submucosal tumor in the duodenal second portion. The top of the tumor is slightly depressed, showing a reddish color on white light imaging (a, b) and a brownish color on narrow band imaging (c). Endoscopic ultrasonography reveals that the hypoechoic mass is mainly confined to the mucosal layer (d). A small cystic area is also seen (white arrow) (e).

thought to be the cause of his anemia. In addition, a solitary submucosal tumor approximately 10 mm in diameter was found in the second portion of the duodenum (Figure 1). The top of the tumor was slightly depressed, showing a reddish color. Histological analysis of the biopsied samples obtained from the reddish part of the tumor revealed adenocarcinoma. The patient was referred to our hospital for further investigation and treatment.

The patient had been consuming medication for atrial fibrillation, diabetes mellitus, and constipation but had

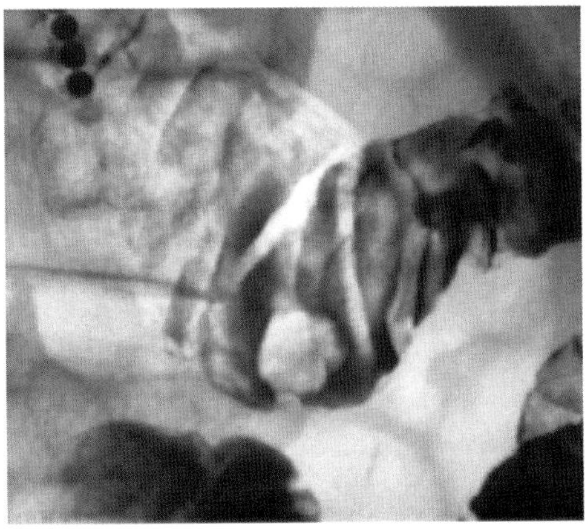

FIGURE 2: Hypotonic duodenography image. A submucosal tumor with bridging folds is seen in the inferior duodenal angle.

no history of gastroduodenal disease. A physical examination revealed conjunctival pallor and arrhythmia, but there were no abnormalities in his abdomen. Laboratory findings revealed decreased levels of red blood cells (4.03 $\times 10^6/mm^3$), hemoglobin (10.6 g/dL), hematocrit (34.2%), serum iron (20 μg/dL), and ferritin (29.6 ng/mL). The levels of carcinoembryonic antigen and carbohydrate antigen 19-9 were within the normal range. The patient tested positive for *Helicobacter pylori* infection.

Hypotonic duodenography showed a submucosal tumor with bridging folds in the inferior duodenal angle (Figure 2). Endoscopic ultrasonography revealed a hypoechoic mass mainly confined to the mucosal layer (Figure 1(d)). A small cystic area was also identified on ultrasonography (Figure 1(e)). Based on the imaging and pathological studies, we diagnosed the duodenal tumor as adenocarcinoma arising from Brunner's glands. Due to the advanced age and multiple underlying disorders, the risks of general anesthesia, artificial ventilation, and radical surgical resection were considered too high. Moreover, endoscopic ultrasonography indicated that the tumor appeared to be resectable using the endoscopic mucosal resection technique. Therefore, we performed endoscopic treatment rather than surgical resection (Figure 3). Hyaluronic acid solution (MucoUp®, Johnson & Johnson K. K., Tokyo, Japan) was injected into the duodenal submucosa using a 23 G injection needle (TOP Co., Tokyo, Japan). Subsequently the tumor was resected with a bipolar snare (Zeon Medical Inc., Tokyo, Japan). The resected area was closed by metallic clips (Olympus Medical Systems Co., Tokyo, Japan). There were no procedure-related adverse events during or after the endoscopic resection.

Pathological analysis of the resected specimen revealed proliferation of Brunner's glands (Figures 4(a) and 4(b)). Gastric foveolar metaplasia was also identified (Figure 4(a), blue square, and Figure 4(c)). Atypical cells with pleomorphic macronuclei containing dense chromatin forming an irregular glandular structure were identified towards the lumen in the superficial layer (Figure 4(a), red square, and Figure 4(d)). Immunohistochemical studies revealed that proliferated Brunner's glands were positive for MUC6 (Figure 5(a), white arrow) and negative for MUC5AC (Figure 5(b), white arrow). In contrast, most of the cells with gastric foveolar differentiation (Figures 5(a) and 5(b), arrowhead) and atypical cells (Figures 5(a) and 5(b), black arrow) were positive for MUC5AC but negative for MUC6. However, both gastric foveolar metaplasia and atypical cells partly showed dual positivity for MUC5AC and MUC6, particularly in the deeper layers (Figures 5(a) and 5(b), arrowhead). Some atypical cells showed relatively higher positivity for Ki-67 staining (Figure 5(c), arrows). Consequently, a diagnosis of adenocarcinoma in situ arising from Brunner's glands was made. Components of the adenocarcinoma, gastric foveolar metaplasia, and Brunner's gland hyperplasia were completely resected by endoscopic mucosal resection.

3. Discussion

Adenocarcinoma arising from Brunner's glands is quite uncommon. The first case was reported in 1894 by Pic [13]. Ohta et al. reviewed 25 previously reported cases and revealed that the mean age was 66.5 years (39 to 85 years) and the male to female ratio was 19 : 6 [14]. Adenocarcinoma arising from Brunner's glands is most frequently found in the second (50.0%) or first (45.8%) portions of the duodenum, followed by the third portion (4.2%). Macroscopically, it has been described as "a pedunculated and lobulated polyp" [11], "a protruding lesion with a surface depression" [9], "an elevated submucosal-tumor-like lesion with a shallow central depression" [9], "a sessile tumor with a slight central depression," and "a fungating ulcerated tumor" [15]. Overall, macroscopic features of adenocarcinoma arising from Brunner's glands vary from submucosal tumor-like lesions with a shallow central depression (52.0%) to polypoid (12.0%), sessile (12.0%), and type 2 tumors (12.0%) [14]. Kamei et al. hypothesized the progression process of this disease as follows [7]: appearance as a submucosal tumor or polypoid form in the early stages with subsequent tumor growth and type 2 tumor formation. Such morphological changes during tumor progression over a 40-month period have been described by Itsuno et al. [15]. The present case showed a submucosal tumor with a shallow central depression, which is the typical morphology of early-stage adenocarcinoma arising from Brunner's glands.

In the present case, pathological analysis of the resected specimen showed three components: Brunner's gland hyperplasia, gastric foveolar metaplasia, and adenocarcinoma in situ. Although the histogenesis of gastric metaplasia in the duodenal mucosa has not been fully revealed, several studies have suggested Brunner's glands as a region where gastric metaplasia may originate [11, 16–18]. During the repair process following duodenal ulceration, gastric foveolar-type cells emerge in the regenerative cell zone in Brunner's glands next to the ulcerated surface [11]. Immunostaining analysis with gastric foveolar-type mucin (MUC5AC) and pyloric/Brunner's gland-type mucin (MUC6) demonstrated that, in the present patient, Brunner's gland hyperplastic region was positive for MUC6 and negative for MUC5AC. Conversely, the cells with gastric foveolar differentiation and adenocarcinoma were positive for MUC5AC. Both gastric foveolar metaplasia and adenocarcinoma were negative for

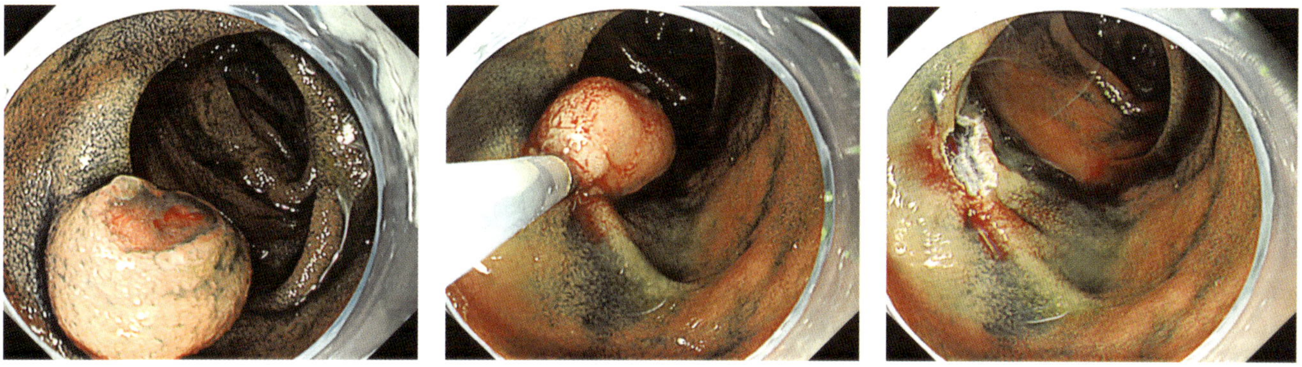

(a) (b) (c)

FIGURE 3: Esophagogastroduodenoscopy images during endoscopic mucosal resection. A duodenal tumor is seen after indigo carmine spraying (a). After injection of hyaluronic acid solution into the duodenal submucosa, the tumor is completely resected with a bipolar snare (b, c).

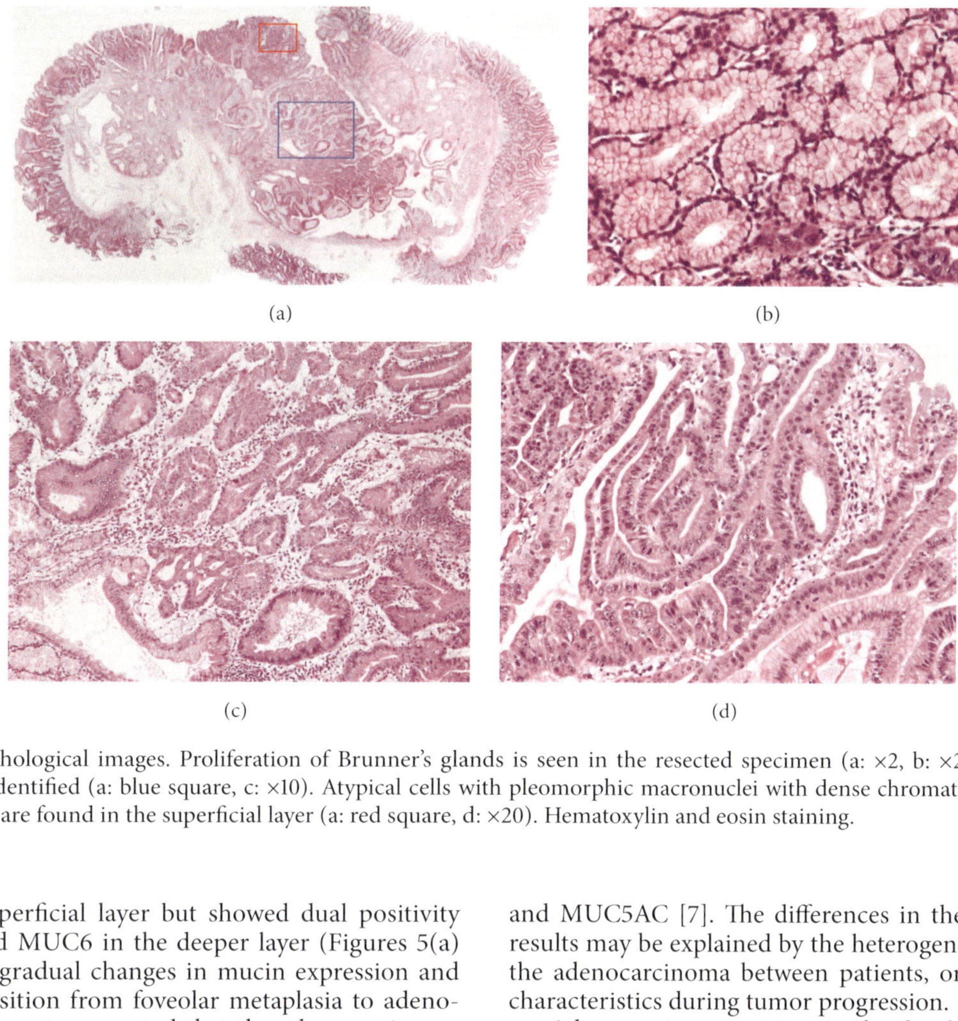

FIGURE 4: Histopathological images. Proliferation of Brunner's glands is seen in the resected specimen (a: ×2, b: ×20). Gastric foveolar metaplasia is also identified (a: blue square, c: ×10). Atypical cells with pleomorphic macronuclei with dense chromatin forming irregular glandular structure are found in the superficial layer (a: red square, d: ×20). Hematoxylin and eosin staining.

MUC6 in the superficial layer but showed dual positivity for MUC5AC and MUC6 in the deeper layer (Figures 5(a) and 5(b)). These gradual changes in mucin expression and the seamless transition from foveolar metaplasia to adenocarcinoma components suggested that the adenocarcinoma emerged via gastric foveolar metaplasia, which originated in Brunner's gland cells. A similar expression pattern of mucin was previously described by Kitagori et al. and Kushima et al. [9, 11]. However, Kamei et al. reported a case of adenocarcinoma arising from Brunner's gland hyperplasia in which the adenocarcinoma component was negative for both MUC6 and MUC5AC [7]. The differences in the immunostaining results may be explained by the heterogeneity of cells within the adenocarcinoma between patients, or alteration of cell characteristics during tumor progression.

Adenocarcinoma arising in the duodenum is most frequently treated by pancreatoduodenectomy (36.0%), partial duodenectomy with gastrectomy (28.0%), or partial duodenectomy (16.0%) [14]. Endoscopic treatments such as endoscopic mucosal resection [12] and endoscopic polypectomy [11] have been reported in 12% of patients. In the present case, the tumor was completely resected in one piece

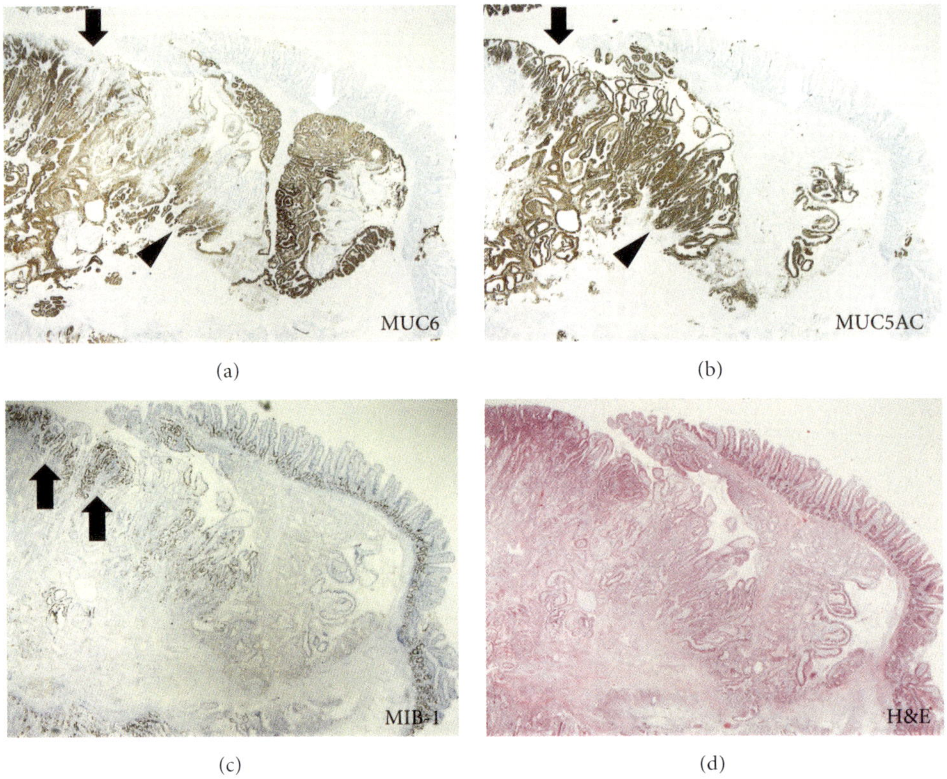

FIGURE 5: Immunohistochemical images. Proliferated Brunner's glands are positive for MUC6 (a, white arrow) and negative for MUC5AC (b, white arrow). In contrast, most of the cells with gastric foveolar differentiation (a, black arrowhead; b, black arrowhead) and atypical cells (a, black arrow; b, black arrow) are positive for MUC5AC but are negative for MUC6. Both gastric foveolar metaplasia and atypical cells partly show dual positivity for MUC5AC and MUC6, particularly in the deeper layer (a, arrowhead; b, arrowhead). Some atypical cells showed relatively higher positivity for Ki-67 staining (c, hematoxylin and eosin staining, arrows).

by endoscopic mucosal resection, similar to that described in previous reports. As shown in the pathological image (Figure 4(a)), the tumor consisted mainly of hyperplastic Brunner's gland cells, rather than gastric foveolar metaplasia or adenocarcinoma components. This structure enabled curative endoscopic resection of the adenocarcinoma.

In conclusion, we treated a patient with adenocarcinoma in situ in the duodenum by endoscopic mucosal resection. Pathological analysis revealed coexistence of gastric foveolar metaplasia and surrounding hyperplastic Brunner's glands, suggesting that the adenocarcinoma arose from Brunner's gland hyperplasia. Although there is no doubt that detailed preoperative evaluation of the depth of tumor invasion is mandatory, endoscopic resection may still be a possible option for the treatment of adenocarcinoma arising from Brunner's gland hyperplasia.

References

[1] T. Nakabori, S. Shinzaki, T. Yamada et al., "Atypical duodenal ulcer and invagination caused by a large pedunculated duodenal Brunner's gland hamartoma," *Gastrointestinal Endoscopy*, vol. 79, no. 4, pp. 679–680, 2014.

[2] N. D. Patel, A. D. Levy, A. K. Mehrotra, and L. H. Sobin, "Brunner's gland hyperplasia and hamartoma: imaging features with clinicopathologic correlation," *American Journal of Roentgenology*, vol. 187, no. 3, pp. 715–722, 2006.

[3] B. Muezzinoglu, H. Ustun, B. Demirhan, and F. Hilmioglu, "Brunner's gland adenoma: case report," *New Zealand Medical Journal*, vol. 108, no. 992, p. 14, 1995.

[4] P. Chattopadhyay, A. K. Kundu, S. Bhattacharyya, and A. Bandyopadhyay, "Diffuse nodular hyperplasia of Brunner's gland presenting as upper gastrointestinal haemorrhage," *Singapore Medical Journal*, vol. 49, no. 1, pp. 81–83, 2008.

[5] M. Iwamuro, T. Tanaka, S. Ando et al., "Endoscopic resection of a pedunculated Brunner's gland hamartoma of the duodenum," *Case Reports in Gastrointestinal Medicine*, vol. 2016, Article ID 6707235, 5 pages, 2016.

[6] T. W. Botsford, P. Crowe, and D. W. Crocker, "Tumors of the small intestine. A review of experience with 115 cases including a report of a rare case of malignant hemangio-endothelioma," *The American Journal of Surgery*, vol. 103, no. 3, pp. 358–365, 1962.

[7] K. Kamei, T. Yasuda, T. Nakai, and Y. Takeyama, "A case of adenocarcinoma of the duodenum arising from brunner's gland," *Case Reports in Gastroenterology*, vol. 7, no. 3, pp. 433–437, 2013.

[8] H. S. Choi, B. Keum, Y.-T. Jeen, and H. J. Chun, "Complete en bloc resection of an adenocarcinoma involving Brunner's gland by using endoscopic submucosal dissection," *Digestive and Liver Disease*, vol. 45, no. 5, p. e7, 2013.

[9] K. Kitagori, S.-I. Miyamoto, and T. Sakurai, "Adenocarcinoma derived from Brunner's gland," *Clinical Gastroenterology and Hepatology*, vol. 8, no. 4, p. A26, 2010.

[10] M. Koizumi, N. Sata, K. Yoshizawa, K. Kurihara, and Y. Yasuda, "Carcinoma arising from Brunner's gland in the duodenum after 17 years of observation—a case report and literature review," *Case Reports in Gastroenterology*, vol. 1, no. 1, pp. 103–109, 2008.

[11] R. Kushima, M. Stolte, K. Dirks et al., "Gastric-type adenocarcinoma of the duodenal second portion histogenetically associated with hyperplasia and gastric-foveolar metaplasia of Brunner's glands," *Virchows Archiv*, vol. 440, no. 6, pp. 655–659, 2002.

[12] K. Akino, Y. Kondo, A. Ueno et al., "Carcinoma of duodenum arising from Brunner's gland," *Journal of Gastroenterology*, vol. 37, no. 4, pp. 293–296, 2002.

[13] A. Pic, "Contribution a l'etude du cancer primitif du duodenum," *Revue de Medicine*, vol. 14, pp. 1081–1101, 1894.

[14] Y. Ohta, K. Saitoh, T. Akai, M. Uesato, T. Ochiai, and H. Matsubara, "Early primary duodenal carcinoma arising from Brunner's glands synchronously occurring with sigmoid colon carcinoma: report of a case," *Surgery Today*, vol. 38, no. 8, pp. 756–760, 2008.

[15] M. Itsuno, K. Makiyama, K. Omagari et al., "Carcinoma of duodenal bulb arising from the Brunner's gland," *Gastroenterologia Japonica*, vol. 28, no. 1, pp. 118–125, 1993.

[16] A. M. Hanby, R. Poulsom, G. Elia, S. Singh, J. M. Longcroft, and N. A. Wright, "The expression of the trefoil peptides pS2 and human spasmolytic polypeptide (hSP) in 'gastric metaplasia' of the proximal duodenum: implications for the nature of 'gastric metaplasia'," *Journal of Pathology*, vol. 169, no. 3, pp. 355–360, 1993.

[17] K. C. Liu and N. A. Wright, "The migration pathway of epithelial cells on human duodenal villi: the origin and fate of 'gastric metaplasia' cells in duodenal mucosa," *Epithelial Cell Biology*, vol. 1, no. 2, pp. 53–58, 1992.

[18] J. H. Kim, J. W. Choi, Y. S. Seo et al., "Inverted cystic tubulovillous adenoma involving Brunner's glands of duodenum," *World Journal of Gastroenterology*, vol. 13, no. 23, pp. 3262–3264, 2007.

A Case of Hepatic Portal Venous Gas: Hypothesis of a Transient Direct Communication between a Penetrating Antral Gastric Ulcer and Mesenteric Varices

Hassan M. Ghoz,[1] Shamlan M. Sheikh,[1] Kanika Khandelwal,[1] Joseph Fiore,[2] Nicholas James,[3] and Joel Weinstock[4]

[1] *Division of Internal Medicine, Steward Carney Hospital, Tufts School of Medicine, Dorchester, MA, USA*
[2] *Division of Gastroenterology and Hepatology, Steward Carney Hospital, Tufts School of Medicine, Dorchester, MA, USA*
[3] *Division of Pulmonology and Critical Care, Steward Carney Hospital, Tufts School of Medicine, Dorchester, MA, USA*
[4] *Division of Gastroenterology and Hepatology, Tufts Medical Center, Tufts School of Medicine, Boston, MA, USA*

Correspondence should be addressed to Hassan M. Ghoz; hassanghoz@gmail.com

Academic Editor: Yoshihiro Moriwaki

Hepatic portal venous gas (HPVG) is a rare radiological sign that usually signifies an acute intra-abdominal process, most commonly bowel ischemia and sepsis. Few reports described an association with underlying gastric pathologies. We report a 60-year-old patient who presented with melena and chills and was discovered to have a gastric ulcer that appeared to have penetrated into a mesenteric varix. This, in turn, likely caused development of HPVG associated with fungemia. Treatment with a proton pump inhibitor and bowel rest was sufficient to resolve symptoms and the HPVG.

1. Background

Hepatic portal venous gas (HPVG) is a radiologic finding that usually denotes serious intra-abdominal pathology [1]. Intestinal ischemia and sepsis account for the majority of cases [2]. However, underlying gastric pathologies such as peptic ulcer disease and acute gastric dilation rarely can cause HPVG [3]. We are reporting a case of HPVG developing in a patient with mesenteric varices and a penetrating antral gastric ulcer. It is hypothesized that the ulcer penetrated a varix allowing introduction of gas into the portal system and fungemia.

2. Case Report

A 60-year-old Vietnamese male presented with malaise, fever, and chills for 2 days. Review of system revealed that he has been having dark loose stools for 2 days. The patient denied any abdominal pain. There was no significant past medical history and the patient was not taking any medications. The patient denied any recent NSAIDs use. He lived independently with his wife, smoked 0.5 pack-years of cigarettes for the past 20 years, and drinks a couple of beers on weekends. There was no history of any recreational drug use. On arrival to the ER, the patient was febrile (102.3 F), hypotensive (79/50 mmHg), and tachycardic (107 beats per minute). On physical exam, the patient appeared pale. All other general, cardiovascular, respiratory, abdominal, neurological, and extremity exams were benign. Stool guaiac was positive. His initial hemoglobin and hematocrit were 11.8 gm/dL and 34%, respectively, and remained stable during this hospitalization. White blood count and platelets levels were within the normal limit. His chemistries were significant for elevated aspartate aminotransferase (AST) of 55 U/L and alkaline phosphatase of 336 U/L. Alanine aminotransferase, lipase, lactic acid, creatinine, and blood urea nitrogen were normal. No recreational drugs were detected on urine toxicology screen. Nasogastric decompression through NG tube yielded 1 L of coffee ground fluid. Blood cultures were drawn. IV fluids and empiric antibiotics (levofloxacin and

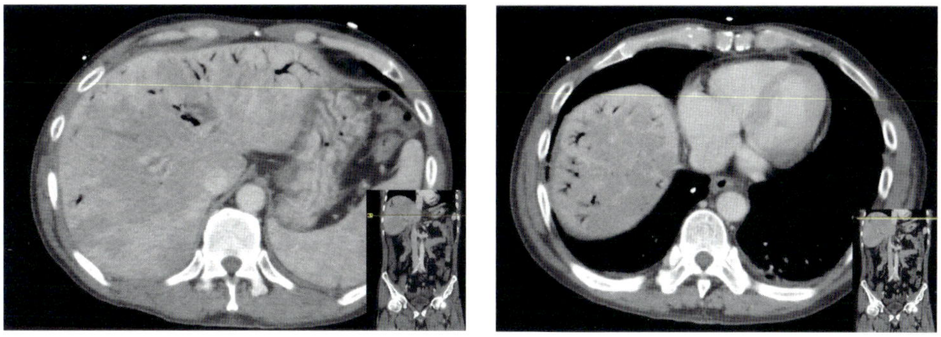

(a) (b)

FIGURE 1: CT scan of the abdomen showing diffuse portal venous gas at different levels of the hepatic parenchyma.

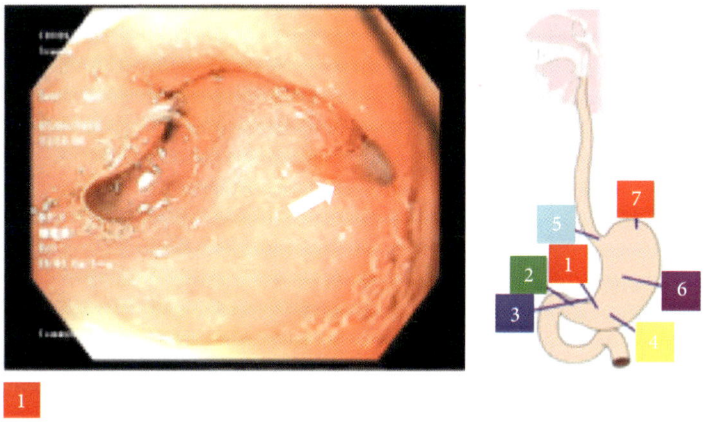

FIGURE 2: Endoscopic image showing the penetrating ulcer in the posterior wall of the gastric antrum.

metronidazole) for possible intra-abdominal source were started as per sepsis protocol. The patient was admitted to the ICU for sepsis and upper GI bleed. He was also started on IV pantoprazole. CT scan of the abdomen/pelvis was done to perform an evaluation for possible intra-abdominal source. It showed extensive portal and mesenteric venous gas (Figures 1(a) and 1(b)). Also, it showed multiple collaterals at porta hepatis (Figure 4). Subsequently, an endoscopy was performed which revealed a normal esophagus and a 7 mm (largest diameter), nonbleeding, penetrating ulcer in the posterior wall of the gastric antrum (Figure 2). There was no evidence of gastric or esophageal varices. The patient was managed for upper gastrointestinal bleeding with intravenous proton pump inhibitor and bowel rest. A repeat CT scan performed 4 days later revealed interval resolution of previously visualized portal venous gas (Figures 3(a) and 3(b)). The patient's blood cultures yielded *Candida albicans* for which he was treated with antifungal therapy. Echocardiogram and eye examination were normal. *Helicobacter pylori* serum IgG antibody came back positive, and the patient was started on amoxicillin and clarithromycin. Other laboratory and serological panels (autoimmune, viral, tumor markers, ceruloplasmin, and iron levels) were within normal limits. Although the gastric ulcer was found to be nonbleeding, in the setting of multiple collaterals seen on CT abdomen, there was a concern of rebleeding. The patient was evaluated for a transjugular intrahepatic portosystemic shunt (TIPS) procedure to decrease the pressure in the portal system and thus decrease the likelihood of rebleeding from the mesenteric varices. His portal vein pressure was found to be only 16 mmHg, which did not indicate the need for a TIPS procedure. However, the pre-TIPS portal venogram showed acute thrombosis of mesenteric varices that were not amendable for intervening with coiling and also showed that the main portal vein was moderately stenotic from prior portal vein thrombosis. Furthermore, multiple small branches of the left and right portal veins were occluded with multiple enlarged collateral vessels. The patient was started on anticoagulation and discharged home 13 days after his admission.

3. Discussion

HPVG is a radiologic sign first described in 1955 by Wolfe and Evens in infants with necrotizing enterocolitis [4]. Since then, HPVG has been described in adults with bowel pathologies that disrupt the intestinal mucosa such as bowel ischemia, inflammatory bowel disease, and diverticulitis [5–7]. A proposed explanation for this association is that damage to the mucosal surface facilitates infiltration of intraluminal

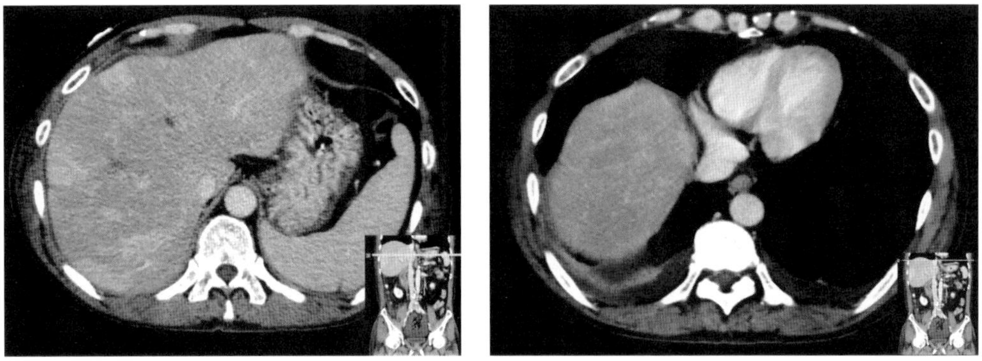

(a) (b)

Figure 3: CT scan of the abdomen showing resolution of the portal venous gas.

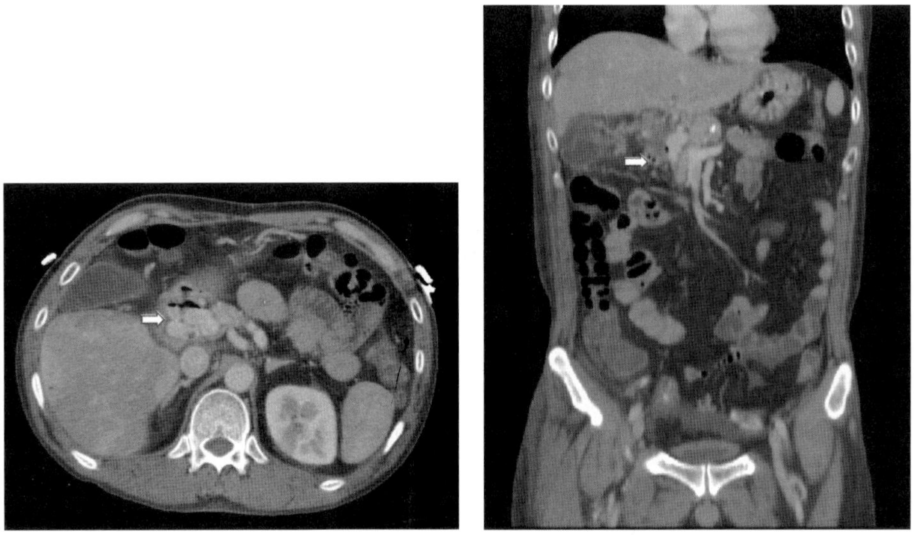

Figure 4: CT scan (coronal and axial views) showing multiple venous collaterals at the porta hepatis.

gas into the portal venous system [2]. In cases with intact mucosa, the presence of a gas forming organism should be suspected. Mechanical distention solely could disrupt the intestinal mucosal barriers offering a possible explanation to the association of bowel obstruction and paralytic ileus with HPVG [8, 9].

HPVG rarely is reported with gastric pathologies like perforated gastric ulcer, acute gastric dilation [3], and gastric cancer [8] and following gastric endoscopy and dilation [10]. There are few reported cases of HPVG developing with peptic ulcer disease [1, 2, 11].

Endoscopic examination of our patient revealed a non-bleeding, penetrating ulcer in the posterior wall of the gastric antrum secondary to *H. pylori* infection. We hypothesize that the penetrating peptic ulcer was the initial pathology and this could have led to a direct communication of the luminal contents with a mesenteric varix. Another possibility could be that venous bowel ischemia signified by the presence of chronic portal vein thrombosis with collaterals could have been present and led to the evolution of the portal venous gas as described by previous few reports [12, 13]. CT scan findings in addition to normal lactic acid levels, lack of significant gastrointestinal symptoms, and relatively benign abdominal examination excluded the more common intestinal pathologies leading to HPVG such as ischemia, diverticulitis, and inflammatory bowel disease.

HPVG is a sign that denotes a life-threatening condition but does not necessarily indicate a need for surgical intervention [11]. Management of HPVG is directed towards the underlying etiology. Resolution of HPVG is a sign of clinical improvement [14, 15]. In our case, the patient was managed with intravenous proton pump inhibitors for the gastric ulcer with complete bowel rest. Antibiotics initially were started for empiric coverage of the presumed intra-abdominal source of infection, which were switched to an antifungal agent once blood cultures grew *Candida albicans*.

We describe another case of HPVG that is associated with peptic ulcer disease in which we hypothesize that the ulcer might have allowed the entrance of luminal gas and fungus into an enlarged mesenteric varix. We also demonstrated the resolution of HPVG following treatment of the gastric ulcer with an intravenous proton pump inhibitor and bowel rest.

Consent

Informed consent was obtained from the patient in agreement with publishing the paper.

References

[1] H. Kinoshita, M. Shinozaki, H. Tanimura et al., "Clinical features and management of hepatic portal venous gas: four case reports and cumulative review of the literature," *Archives of Surgery*, vol. 136, no. 12, pp. 1410–1414, 2001.

[2] P. R. Liebman, M. T. Patten, J. Manny, J. R. Benfield, and H. B. Hechtman, "Hepatic-portal venous gas in adults: etiology, pathophysiology and clinical significance," *Annals of Surgery*, vol. 187, no. 3, pp. 281–287, 1978.

[3] M. M. Sevinc, E. Kinaci, S. Bayrak, A. H. Yardimci, E. Cakar, and H. Bektaş, "Extraordinary cause of acute gastric dilatation and hepatic portal venous gas: chronic use of synthetic cannabinoid," *World Journal of Gastroenterology*, vol. 21, no. 37, pp. 10704–10708, 2015.

[4] J. N. Wolfe and W. A. Evans, "Gas in the portal veins of the liver in infants; a roentgenographic demonstration with postmortem anatomical correlation," *The American Journal of Roentgenology, Radium Therapy, and Nuclear Medicine*, vol. 74, no. 3, pp. 486–488, 1955.

[5] F. A. Birnberg, R. M. Gore, B. Shragg, and A. R. Margulis, "Hepatic portal venous gas: a benign finding in a patient with ulcerative colitis," *Journal of Clinical Gastroenterology*, vol. 5, no. 1, pp. 89–91, 1983.

[6] B. H. Katz and S. S. Schwartz, "Portal venous gas following a barium enema in a patient with Crohn's colitis—a benign finding," *Diseases of the Colon & Rectum*, vol. 29, no. 1, pp. 49–51, 1986.

[7] J. F. Wiot and B. Felson, "Gas in the portal venous system," *The American Journal of Roentgenology, Radium Therapy, and Nuclear Medicine*, vol. 86, pp. 920–929, 1961.

[8] W. Wiesner, K. J. Mortelé, J. N. Glickman, H. Ji, and P. R. Ros, "Portal-venous gas unrelated to mesenteric ischemia," *European Radiology*, vol. 12, no. 6, pp. 1432–1437, 2002.

[9] T. E. Quirke, "Hepatic-portal venous gas associated with ileus," *American Surgeon*, vol. 61, no. 12, pp. 1084–1086, 1995.

[10] K. Seeger and S. R. Achem, "Hepatic portal venous gas: an unusual complication following upper endoscopy and dilation," *ACG Case Reports Journal*, vol. 1, no. 3, pp. 128–130, 2014.

[11] A. L. Nelson, T. M. Millington, D. Sahani et al., "Hepatic portal venous gas: the ABCs of management," *Archives of Surgery*, vol. 144, no. 6, pp. 575–581, 2009.

[12] W. Wiesner, K. J. Mortelé, J. N. Glickman, H. Ji, and P. R. Ros, "Pneumatosis intestinalis and portomesenteric venous gas in intestinal ischemia: correlation of CT findings with severity of ischemia and clinical outcome," *American Journal of Roentgenology*, vol. 177, no. 6, pp. 1319–1323, 2001.

[13] W. Wiesner, B. Khurana, H. Ji, and P. R. Ros, "CT of acute bowel ischemia," *Radiology*, vol. 226, no. 3, pp. 635–650, 2003.

[14] H. Patel, H. Shaaban, N. Shah, and W. Baddoura, "A rare case report of spontaneous resolution of hepatic portal venous gas associated with cocaine-induced intestinal ischemia," *Annals of Medical and Health Sciences Research*, vol. 5, no. 2, pp. 136–138, 2015.

[15] C. G. Lee, H. W. Kang, M. K. Song et al., "A Case of hepatic portal venous gas as a complication of endoscopic balloon dilatation," *Journal of Korean Medical Science*, vol. 26, no. 8, pp. 1108–1110, 2011.

41

Protein Loosing Enteropathy Secondary to Strongyloidiasis: Case Report and Review of the Literature

Weam El Hajj,[1] Gilbert Nakad,[2] and Antoine Abou Rached[1]

[1] *Department of Internal Medicine, Gastroenterology Division, Faculty of Medical Sciences, Lebanese University, Hadath Campus, P.O. Box 3, Hadath, Beirut 2903 1308, Lebanon*

[2] *Department of General Surgery, Faculty of Medical Sciences, Lebanese University, Hadath Campus, P.O. Box 3, Hadath, Beirut 2903 1308, Lebanon*

Correspondence should be addressed to Antoine Abou Rached; abourachedantoine@gmail.com

Academic Editor: Tetsuo Hirata

Strongyloidiasis is a helminthic disease which affects millions around the world resulting in a significant burden in certain high risk groups. It is rarely reported in the Lebanese population probably due to the low index of suspicion in common practice. We are reporting a case of strongyloidiasis that was found in an elderly patient presenting initially with dyspnea followed by skin rash, protein loosing enteropathy, diarrhea, and abdominal pain while on corticosteroid therapy. The diagnosis was suspected based on clinical presentation in addition to peripheral eosinophilia. We will also describe the upper and lower endoscopic aspects of the disease, as well as histologic findings on duodenal and colonic biopsies.

1. Introduction

Intestinal nematode infections are frequently encountered worldwide with a net predominance in the hot and humid tropical and subtropical areas. Strongyloidiasis is among the most important helminthic infections affecting humans and it may manifest clinically as mild or asymptomatic disease persisting for decades, but also it can have life-threatening manifestations. In Lebanon, it is an unusual infection and is not frequently reported in the literature. We are hereby reporting a case of strongyloidiasis in a Lebanese patient presenting in a picture of diarrhea and refractory hypoalbuminemia after two months' history of unexplained dyspnea and skin rash.

2. Case Presentation

This is a case of 77-year-old male patient who presented for lower limbs edema and abdominal pain with diarrhea of 1-month duration.

The patient was an ex-smoker and nonalcoholic. His past surgical history included cholecystectomy and prostatectomy. His medical history was significant for hypertension controlled on Bisoprolol and Irbesartan, dyslipidemia treated with Atorvastatin, and a transient cerebral ischemic attack 5 months prior to presentation for which he was put on aspirin and clopidogrel. At that time, he was incidentally found to have peripheral eosinophilia of 1050 eos/mm^3 (13.7% of total leukocytes) without going into further investigations. As family history, he had a brother diagnosed with Non-Hodgkin Lymphoma who died few months earlier after a prolonged hospitalization for unexplained dyspnea, attributed later on to a *Strongyloides stercoralis* infection detected in his bronchoalveolar lavage only one day before his death.

His history went back to 3 months prior to presentation when he was admitted to another hospital for dyspnea, cough, and high grade fever that started few days after inadvertent inhalation of pesticides while working in his garden. CT chest was done and showed bilateral patchy interstitial infiltrates suspicious of allergic pneumonitis (Figure 1). Bronchoscopy was also done and showed normal bronchial mucosa. Bronchoalveolar lavage (BAL) analysis showed an inflammatory smear and the culture detected few Alcaligenes spp. Blood culture was negative. So patient was considered having pulmonary infection on top of allergic pneumonitis

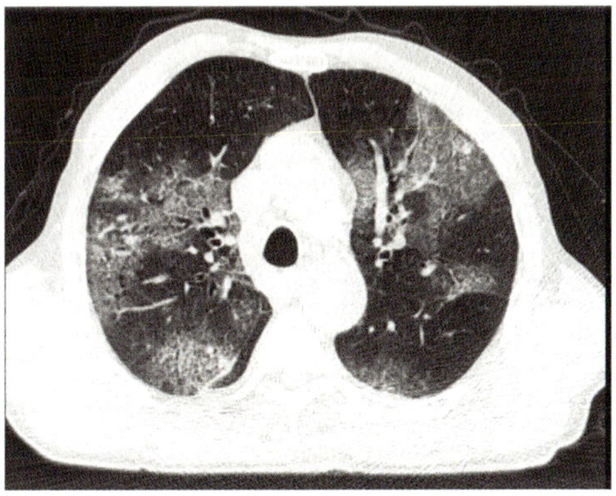

Figure 1: Chest CT scan done during the first admission showing bilateral patchy asymmetric interstitial lung disease suspicious of allergic alveolitis or eosinophilic pneumonitis.

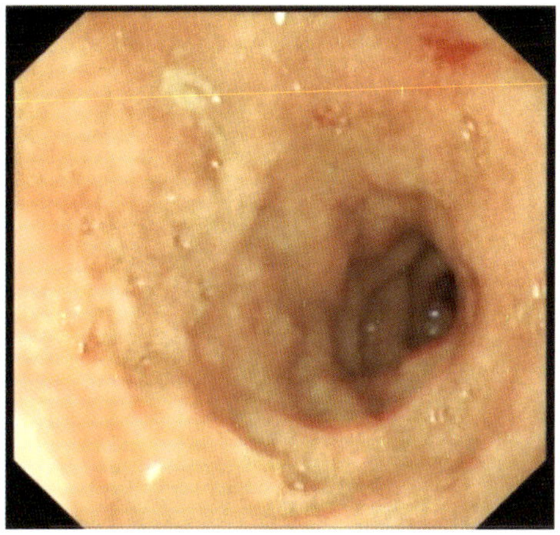

Figure 2: Duodenal bulb showing edematous nodular mucosa with erythematous spot.

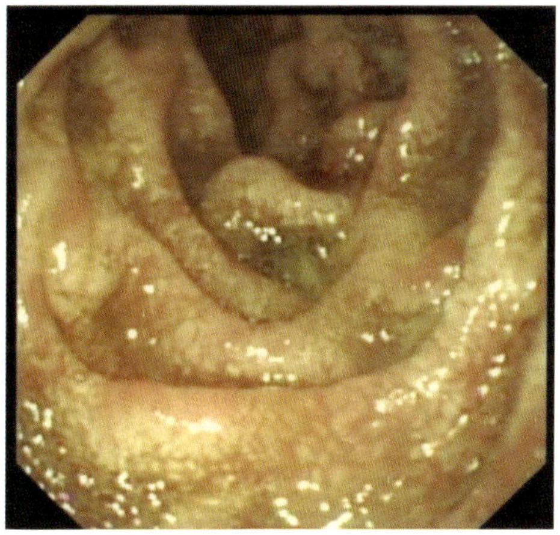

Figure 3: Second duodenum showing edematous mucosa with erosions and white villi.

and was discharged home on levofloxacin and prednisone 1 mg/kg for 1 week to be tapered down over 3 weeks thereafter. Although his dyspnea and chest infiltrates were improving during steroids tapering, our patient developed severe diffuse pruritic skin rash that persisted for about 10 days and he started experiencing a progressively increasing epigastric discomfort associated with diarrhea. In addition, he noted an increasing bilateral lower limbs edema. After stopping steroids, his skin rash disappeared but without improvement of other symptoms.

His diarrhea was watery and nonmucoid accompanied sometimes by fine streaks of blood and having a variable frequency between 1 and 7 episodes per day. It was associated with moderate to severe left lower quadrant abdominal pain not related to food, as well as epigastric pain and many episodes of postprandial vomiting. He also reported a decreased PO intake and a significant weight loss of 12 kg over the last 2 months. His lower limbs edema was progressively increasing, even after stopping steroids. He had no significant dyspnea or cough and no urinary symptoms.

On physical examination, the patient's heart rate was 80 beats per minute, blood pressure was 110/70 mmHg, and temperature was 37°C. He was looking ill without scleral icterus or palpable cervical lymph nodes. His chest auscultation was unremarkable. His abdomen was soft with moderate epigastric and left lower quadrant tenderness and normal bowel sounds. Lower limbs examination showed severe 4+ pitting edema extending from the ankles till the knees. There were no skin rashes and the neurological exam was unremarkable.

Initial tests showed a white blood cell count of 8200 per mm^3 with 14% eosinophils, hemoglobin around 10 g/dL, MCV around 84 fL, creatinine level around 2 mg/dL, and sodium level of 127 meq/L, total serum proteins were 4.5 g/dL with albumin of 1.8 g/dL, liver enzymes were normal, and International Normalized Ratio (INR) was slightly prolonged (1.5). Direct fecal examination was done once and showed no parasites. Stools culture turned out to be negative. Chest X-ray was within normal limits. Twenty-four-hour urine collection revealed only 180 mg of proteins.

In view of his unexplained eosinophilia associated with diarrhea and abdominal pain, together with his history of dyspnea and skin rash that flared up while on steroids and his brother's history of strongyloidiasis, we strongly suspected an underlying strongyloides infection. Thus, we requested strongyloides serology test and upper and lower endoscopies. Upper endoscopy showed severe edematous bulboduodenitis with areas of erosions and whitish villi (Figures 2 and 3) and lower endoscopy showed multiple patchy erythematous lesions separated by areas of normal mucosa that appeared all over the colon, predominantly in the cecum, and in the ileum (Figures 4 and 5). Duodenal biopsy showed severe erosive duodenitis with eosinophilic infiltration and strongyloides larvae (Figures 6(a) and 6(b)). Colonic and ileal biopsies showed severe eosinophilic inflammatory changes without parasitic detection. Serology test showed antistrongyloides antibody titer of 4.5 (normal <1.2). So patient was diagnosed to have strongyloidiasis.

Ivermectin was started at a dose of 200 mcg/kg/day. Patient's diarrhea and abdominal pain disappeared within 3 days. However, patient was still having high eosinophil count

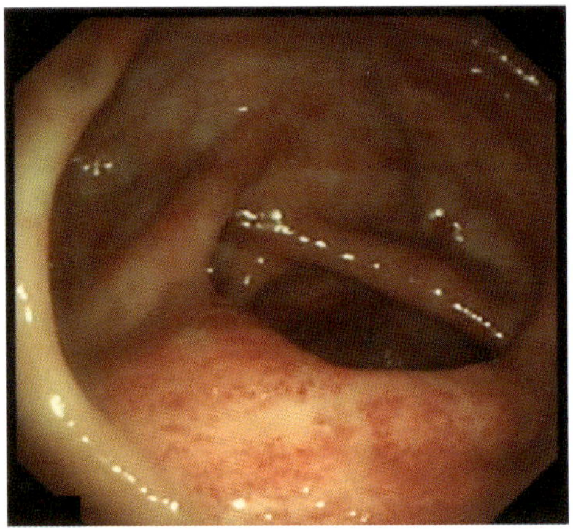

Figure 4: Cecal base showing patchy erythematous and petechial mucosa predominantly over the Ileocecal valve.

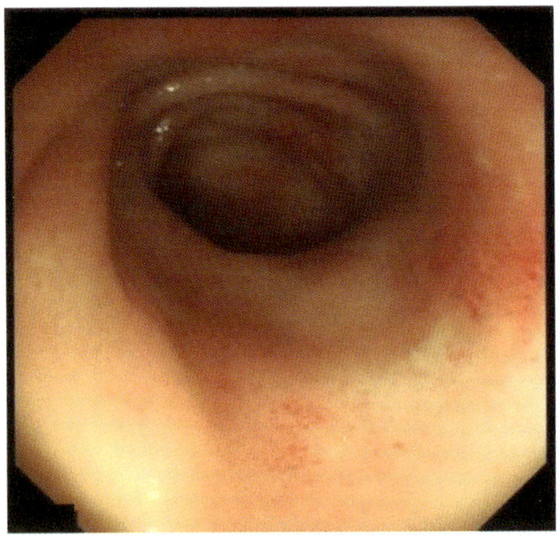

Figure 5: Terminal Ileum showing patchy erythematous lesions.

after 1 week. Since then, we extended Ivermectin course to 2 weeks until disappearance of eosinophilia. Stool test was obtained 2 weeks after initiating treatment and turned out to be negative. Albumin level was progressively increasing to 3.1 g/dL in about 1 month.

3. Discussion

Strongyloidiasis is a helminthic disease caused by *Strongyloides stercoralis* (*S. stercoralis*), a soil transmitted nematode. It affects 30–100 million people globally [1] being hyperendemic (>5%) or endemic (1–5%) in many tropical and subtropical areas including Sub-Saharan Africa, Latin and South America, and South-East Asia and sporadic (<1%) in other temperate areas [2]. In the MENA region, its prevalence varies between countries and it was found to be more frequent in Israel (94%) and Sudan (3.7%) according to community based surveys and in Iraq (24.2%), Kuwait (16.3%), Saudi Arabia (12.5%), and Egypt (11.1%) according to hospital based surveys [3, 4]. In contrast, in Lebanon, *S. stercoralis* is still considered as a rare infection with a reported prevalence of 0.1–0.5% [5, 6] but such values are believed to underestimate the true frequency of the disease due to the low sensitivity of single fecal analysis commonly used in practice as well as the rarity of case reports and studies targeting specifically strongyloidiasis prevalence, in addition to the predominance of subclinical and poorly symptomatic disease manifestations.

S. stercoralis is acquired by contact with contaminated soil, human waste, or sewage. Hence, conditions such as poor hygiene and crowding, as well as some occupations such as farming and coal mining, may increase the risk of infection. Such factors exist in some Lebanese populations, notably in the Northern Province, the hometown of our patient and his brother, where previous studies found a higher rate of parasitosis in general [6].

The filariform larvae, infectious form of the parasite, invade the skin of the affected individuals through which they migrate to the lungs either by hematogeneous or lymphatic spread. Then, they ascend up in the tracheobronchial tree until being swallowed into the GI tract where they mature. The adult female produces eggs that develop into noninfectious rhabditiform larvae. These larvae may mature again into infectious form resulting in a cycle of autoinfection, which enables the parasite to persist for decades after initial infection. However, any state of immunosuppression, most importantly steroid use [7], or other immunosuppressive drugs use, malignancies, AIDS, HTLV-1 infection, advanced age, or malnutrition may increase the parasite burden and accelerate the autoinfectious process inducing a hyperinfection syndrome which might develop into severe disseminated disease thereafter [8]. In our patient, advanced age and prednisone therapy precipitated the infectious flare up.

In acute infection, patients may exhibit a local skin rash followed by dyspnea and cough due to larvae migration into the lungs. During chronic autoinfection, patients may remain asymptomatic or may experience mild waxing and waning gastrointestinal, respiratory, or dermatologic symptoms with peripheral eosinophilia. Hyperinfection syndrome may have a wide range of clinical manifestations that increase in severity in parallel with the parasitic dissemination rate. Gastrointestinal symptoms are common including diarrhea, abdominal pain, and vomiting. Prolonged malabsorption and protein loosing enteropathy may also be present leading to severe hypoalbuminemia and refractory peripheral edema [9]. Pulmonary manifestations may include dyspnea and cough with lung infiltrates mimicking Loeffler Syndrome or even ARDS in severe cases [10, 11]. Skin involvement may present as pruritic rash that has sometimes a pathognomonic migratory serpiginous aspect termed "larva currens." More severe disseminated disease may involve the CNS, the pancreas, the liver, and the heart, and it may be associated with Gram negative septicemia secondary to simultaneous bacterial seeding through the GI tract [8].

Our patient's hyperinfective syndrome was manifested clinically by gastrointestinal involvement including protein loosing enteropathy with diarrhea and abdominal pain in addition to skin involvement. Whether respiratory symptoms were related to strongyloidiasis or to another infection and pesticides inhalation is uncertain, but the improvement of dyspnea and chest infiltrate while on steroids and the absence

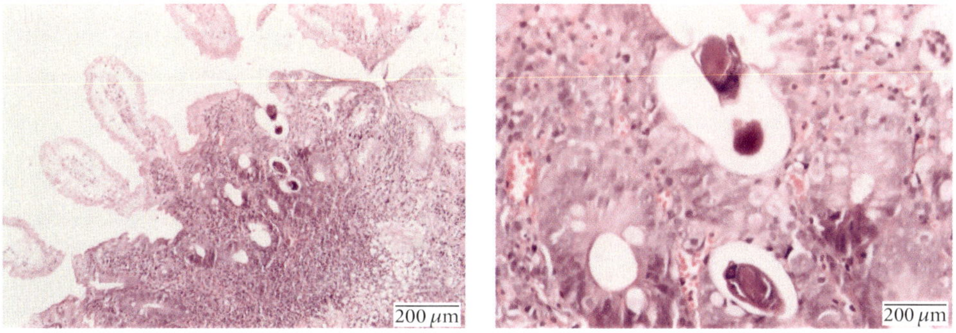

(a) (b)

FIGURE 6: Duodenal biopsy showing preserved villi with dystrophic glands, multiple ulcerations, and eosinophilic infiltration. *Parasitic larvae* are also seen either superficial or encrusted into the mucosa compatible with strongyloidiasis.

of larvae on BAL examination argued against pulmonary strongyloidiasis manifestations.

Peripheral eosinophilia is a strong indicator of the infection in high risk population [12] but it is not sufficiently sensitive to be used as a sole screening test in chronic uncomplicated infection [13] due to its intermittent presence. On the other hand, it might be absent in disseminated disease especially in patients under steroid therapy [14]. Eosinophilia was documented in our patient 5 months before developing the hyperinfection syndrome but it was underappreciated at that time due to the low suspicion index of infection in our population.

Strongyloides larvae are generally passed in stools one month after initial infection. Higher parasitic load is observed during hyperinfection and disseminated disease where larvae detection by stool, sputum, bronchoalveolar lavage, and skin lesions examination is highly sensitive [15]. However, in chronic disease, single direct fecal examination only detects about 30% of infections [16]. Repeated stool test increases such sensitivity that may reach about 100% when 7 samples are used [17]. Other methods such as Formol-Ether Concentration Technique (FECT), the Baermann method, the Harada-Mori filter paper technique, and agar plate culture (APC) were suggested to improve fecal larvae detection rate. Of those, the APC technique is the most suitable having 89% sensitivity [18].

Serologic tests are also useful for strongyloidiasis diagnosis as was shown in our case. Enzyme-Linked Immuno-Sorbent Assay (ELISA) method is highly sensitive for antibody detection [19] but it has a low predictive value in high risk population due to the possible cross reactivity with other helminthes. A newer recombinant antigen based serologic method, the luciferase immunoprecipitation system (LIPS), decreased such confounding factor and improved serologic test reliability [20].

Enterotest or String test is also sensitive for larvae detection but is cumbersome for patients [21]. Molecular testing using PCR for DNA detection on stools samples also appears efficient [22].

Gastrointestinal endoscopy with biopsies may also play a role in the diagnosis. Many endoscopic features were described in the literature including edema and erythematous spots in the duodenum as well as loss of vascular pattern and ulcerations with patchy erythema in the colon but none are pathognomonic for strongyloidiasis [23]. Our reported duodenal endoscopic findings were similar to those reported by Kishimoto et al. study [24] concerning edematous mucosa and notably the white villi which may be a good endoscopic marker for strongyloidiasis in endemic regions. As *S. stercoralis* colonizes the duodenum, duodenal biopsies are the most accurate for larvae detection [23], and this finding was also illustrated in our case where only duodenal specimen showed the strongyloides larvae.

Uncomplicated infection is treated preferably with Ivermectin 200 mcg/kg given for 2 doses (over either 2 consecutive days or 2 weeks apart). Albendazole, Mebendazole, and Thiabendazole are possible alternatives. In hyperinfection syndrome and disseminated disease, same therapeutic modalities and notably Ivermectin can also be used but the appropriate duration of treatment still not well determined. It was suggested to give Ivermectin until getting symptomatic improvement with negative test for larvae for at least 2 weeks (duration of autoinfectious cycle) [25].

Posttreatment eradication should be confirmed to prevent further autoinfectious cycles. Improved eosinophilia, repeated stools examination in 2 weeks, and decreased antibody titer after 6 to 12 months may be useful methods for monitoring in this setting [26, 27].

Prognosis of strongyloidiasis is generally good but mortality rate may be as high as 71% in disseminated disease [14] and it may increase with concomitant bacteremia and severe immunosuppression [28].

4. Conclusion

We presented a case of strongyloidiasis, which is one of the most neglected helminthic infections worldwide and particularly in Lebanon, where we possibly have some underappreciated endemic areas. Index of suspicion should be raised in certain circumstances including peripheral eosinophilia and unexplained intermittent diarrhea or asthma-like symptoms or skin rashes. As it may cause serious burden in certain subgroups, further investigations should focus on implementing appropriate control programs.

Acknowledgment

The authors would like to thank Dr. Saad Khairallah for his cooperation in providing them with the pathology slides photos and their description.

References

[1] A. Olsen, L. van Lieshout, H. Marti et al., "Strongyloidiasis—the most neglected of the neglected tropical diseases?" *Transactions of the Royal Society of Tropical Medicine and Hygiene*, vol. 103, no. 10, pp. 967–972, 2009.

[2] F. M. Paula and J. M. Costa-Cruz, "Epidemiological aspects of strongyloidiasis in Brazil," *Parasitology*, vol. 138, no. 11, pp. 1331–1340, 2011.

[3] M. B. Rokni, W. M. Lotfy, P. J. Hotez, and N. R. de Silva, "Soil-transmitted helminth (STH) infections in the MENA region," in *Neglected Tropical Diseases—Middle East and North Africa*, M. A. McDowell and S. Rafati, Eds., Neglected Tropical Diseases, chapter 1, pp. 1–21, Springer, Vienna, Austria, 2014.

[4] F. Schär, U. Trostdorf, F. Giardina et al., "Strongyloides stercoralis: global distribution and risk factors," *PLoS Neglected Tropical Diseases*, vol. 7, no. 7, Article ID e2288, 2013.

[5] G. F. Araj, U. M. Musharraheh, A. Haydar, A. Ghawi, R. Itani, and R. Saliba, "Trends and prevalence of intestinal parasites at a tertiary care center in Lebanon over a decade," *Journal Medical Libanais*, vol. 59, no. 3, pp. 143–148, 2011.

[6] B. R. Saab, U. Musharrafieh, N. T. Nassar, M. Khogali, and G. F. Araj, "Intestinal parasites among presumably healthy individuals in Lebanon," *Saudi Medical Journal*, vol. 25, no. 1, pp. 34–37, 2004.

[7] N. Suvajdžić, I. Kranjčić-Zec, V. Jovanović, D. Popović, and M. Čolović, "Fatal strongyloidosis following corticosteroid therapy in a patient with chronic idiopathic thrombocytopenia," *Haematologia*, vol. 29, no. 4, pp. 323–326, 1999.

[8] P. B. Keise and T. B. Nutman, "Strongyloides stercoralis in the immunocompromised population," *Clinical Microbiology Reviews*, vol. 17, no. 1, pp. 208–217, 2004.

[9] P. L. Ho, W. K. Luk, A. C. L. Chan, and K. Y. Yuen, "Two cases of fatal strongyloidiasis in Hong Kong," *Pathology*, vol. 29, no. 3, pp. 324–326, 1997.

[10] S. Ahmed, S. Rashid, N. Ammannagari, and W. Cheungpasitporn, "Chasing Eosinophilia in Loeffler's syndrome: a case of strongyloidiasis in upstate New York," *North American Journal of Medical Sciences*, vol. 5, no. 3, article 248, 2013.

[11] A. M. Newberry, D. N. Williams, W. M. Stauffer, D. R. Boulware, B. R. Hendel-Paterson, and P. F. Walker, "Strongyloides hyperinfection presenting as acute respiratory failure and gram-negative sepsis," *Chest*, vol. 128, no. 5, pp. 3681–3684, 2005.

[12] P. Román-Sánchez, A. Pastor-Guzmán, S. Moreno-Guillén, R. Igual-Adell, S. Suñer-Generoso, and C. Tornero-Estébanez, "High prevalence of Strongyloides stercoralis among farm workers on the Mediterranean coast of Spain: analysis of the predictive factors of infection in developed countries," *The American Journal of Tropical Medicine and Hygiene*, vol. 69, no. 3, pp. 336–340, 2003.

[13] S. Sudarshi, R. Stümpfle, M. Armstrong et al., "Clinical presentation and diagnostic sensitivity of laboratory tests for *Strongyloides stercoralis* in travellers compared with immigrants in a non-endemic country," *Tropical Medicine and International Health*, vol. 8, no. 8, pp. 728–732, 2003.

[14] C. S. Lam, M. K. H. Tong, K. M. Chan, and Y. P. Siu, "Disseminated strongyloidiasis: a retrospective study of clinical course and outcome," *European Journal of Clinical Microbiology and Infectious Diseases*, vol. 25, no. 1, pp. 14–18, 2006.

[15] D. Buonfrate, A. Requena-Mendez, A. Angheben et al., "Severe strongyloidiasis: a systematic review of case reports," *BMC Infectious Diseases*, vol. 13, article 78, 2013.

[16] A. A. Siddiqui and S. L. Berk, "Diagnosis of *Strongyloides stercoralis* infection," *Clinical Infectious Diseases*, vol. 33, no. 7, pp. 1040–1047, 2001.

[17] P. B. Nielsen and M. Mojon, "Improved diagnosis of strongyloides stercoralis by seven consecutive stool specimens," *Zentralblatt fur Bakteriologie Mikrobiologie und Hygiene A*, vol. 263, no. 4, pp. 616–618, 1987.

[18] L. C. Polanco, L. A. Gutiérrez, and J. C. Arias, "Diagnosis of strongyloides stercoralis infection: meta-analysis on evaluation of conventional parasitological methods (1980–2013)," *Revista Española de Salud Pública*, vol. 88, no. 5, pp. 581–600, 2014.

[19] S. M. Carroll, K. T. Karthigasu, and D. I. Grove, "Serodiagnosis of human strongyloidiasis by an enzyme-linked immunosorbent assay," *Transactions of the Royal Society of Tropical Medicine and Hygiene*, vol. 75, no. 5, pp. 706–709, 1981.

[20] A. J. Krolewiecki, R. Ramanathan, V. Fink et al., "Improved diagnosis of *Strongyloides stercoralis* using recombinant antigen-based serologies in a community-wide study in northern Argentina," *Clinical and Vaccine Immunology*, vol. 17, no. 10, pp. 1624–1630, 2010.

[21] A. K. J. Goka, D. D. K. Rolston, V. I. Mathan, and M. J. G. Farthing, "Diagnosis of *Strongyloides* and hookworm infections: comparison of faecal and duodenal fluid microscopy," *Transactions of the Royal Society of Tropical Medicine and Hygiene*, vol. 84, no. 6, pp. 829–831, 1990.

[22] H. Moghaddassani, H. Mirhendi, M. Hosseini, M. B. Rokni, G. Mowlavi, and E. Kia, "Molecular diagnosis of strongyloides stercoralis infection by PCR detection of specific DNA in human stool samples," *Iranian Journal of Parasitology*, vol. 6, no. 2, pp. 23–30, 2011.

[23] B. F. Thompson, L. C. Fry, C. D. Wells et al., "The spectrum of GI strongyloidiasis: an endoscopic-pathologic study," *Gastrointestinal Endoscopy*, vol. 59, no. 7, pp. 906–910, 2004.

[24] K. Kishimoto, A. Hokama, T. Hirata et al., "Endoscopic and histopathological study on the duodenum of *Strongyloides stercoralis* hyperinfection," *World Journal of Gastroenterology*, vol. 14, no. 11, pp. 1768–1773, 2008.

[25] R. Mejia and T. B. Nutman, "Screening, prevention, and treatment for hyperinfection syndrome and disseminated infections caused by *Strongyloides stercoralis*," *Current Opinion in Infectious Diseases*, vol. 25, no. 4, pp. 458–463, 2012.

[26] M. R. Loutfy, M. Wilson, J. S. Keystone, and K. C. Kain, "Serology and eosinophil count in the diagnosis and management of strongyloidiasis in a non-endemic area," *American Journal of Tropical Medicine and Hygiene*, vol. 66, no. 6, pp. 749–752, 2002.

[27] M. Montes, C. Sawhney, and N. Barros, "Strongyloides stercoralis: there but not seen," *Current Opinion in Infectious Diseases*, vol. 23, no. 5, pp. 500–504, 2010.

[28] H. Z. El Masry and J. O'Donnell, "Fatal stongyloides hyperinfection in heart transplantation," *Journal of Heart and Lung Transplantation*, vol. 24, no. 11, pp. 1980–1983, 2005.

Primary Pancreatic Burkitt's Lymphoma: A Case Report and Review of the Literature

Venkata Rajesh Konjeti,[1] Gerald M. Hefferman,[2] Sravanthi Paluri,[1] and Prerna Ganjoo[3]

[1] *Virginia Commonwealth University, Richmond, VA, USA*
[2] *Alpert Medical School of Brown University, Providence, RI, USA*
[3] *Nephrology Associates, East Providence, RI, USA*

Correspondence should be addressed to Venkata Rajesh Konjeti; rajesh.konjeti@gmail.com

Academic Editor: Hideto Kawaratani

Primary pancreatic lymphoma (PPL) is of very rare occurrence as an extra nodal site of Non-Hodgkin's lymphoma (NHL). It represents less than 1% of NHL. Out of which Burkitt lymphoma of pancreas is of a rare presentation. It usually occurs in children and presenting in adults is uncommon. The prevalence of pancreatic Burkitt lymphoma is not known as the incidence is significantly low. Clinical features of PPL are predominantly nonspecific and can become difficult with associated inflammation of pancreas. Differentiation of lymphoma to adenocarcinoma is important as chemotherapy is the main stay of treatment in lymphoma. We report a case of 68-year-old female who presented with nonspecific symptoms and was found to have obstructive jaundice secondary to pancreatic head neoplasm which was proved to be pancreatic Burkitt lymphoma which is a rare presentation.

1. Introduction

Non-Hodgkin lymphomas (NHL) are a diverse group of malignancies arising from lymphoid tissue. It is the 8th most common cancer in men and 11th most common cancer in women. It accounts for about 4% of all cancers. The most frequent sites for extra nodal lymphomas, which constitute about 20% to 30% of all lymphomas (peripheral T-cell NHL, 70% to 80%; follicular, 8% to 10%), are the stomach, skin, oral cavity and pharynx, small intestine, and central nervous system (CNS) [1, 2]. Of these primary pancreatic lymphoma is an uncommon extra nodal site of NHL. It accounts for 0.2–2% [3, 4], out of which Burkitt's lymphoma is very rare. There are very few (approximately 20) case reports that are reported in the literature. Most of these are reported in children [5–7]. Identification of Burkitt's lymphoma from others is very crucial as chemotherapy is the mainstay of treatment in pancreatic lymphoma. We report a case of primary pancreatic lymphoma in an adult patient with very low Ca19-9 level.

2. Case Report

Patient is a 68-year-old thin female wit PMH of chronic Hepatitis C (acquired through blood transfusion for postpartum hemorrhage), essential hypertension, hypothyroidism, and diverticulosis presented to PCP with belching and abdominal bloating for 4 weeks. She also reported unintentional weight loss of 5 lbs (97 to 92 lbs) over the last few months. Otherwise, complete ROS were negative. Her physical exam was positive for icterus only. Otherwise, the rest of the exam including abdomen was unremarkable without any palpable organomegaly. She was sent to ER for evaluation of abnormal blood work. After getting admitted to the hospital, her lab work showed CHEM 7: Na 134/K 4.1/creatinine 0.87/glucose 66; ALT 133/AST 207/ALP 203/Alb 3.5/total bilirubin 12.1 (direct bilirubin-8); CBC WBC 11.7/Hb 12.4/platelet 288; CA 19-9 level is 57.

Further workup included the following.

TABLE 1

Antibody	Result
CD10 (M; 56C6; DAKO)	Positive in lesional cells
CD20 (M; L26; Vector)	Positive in lesional cells
CD3 (P; DAKO)	Negative in lesional cells
Bcl-2 (M; 124; DAKO)	Negative in lesional cells
Bcl-6 (M; PG-B6p; DAKO)	Positive in lesional cells
C-myc (RM; Y69; Epitomics)	Focal weak positivity (control is also weak)
Ki- 67 (M; MIB1; DAKO)	>90% positive
TdT (terminal deoxynucleotidyl transferase) (M; SEN28; Vector)	Negative

Abdominal US. There is heterogeneous mass in right lobe of liver with enlarged adjacent pancreatic head containing 2.8 cm hypoechoic mass.

CT Abdomen and Pelvis with Contrast. There is periportal solid 7.5 × 4.9 × 12.7 cm mass which obstructs the central hepatic ducts and encases the main portal vein; it is difficult to separate the lesion from liver and pancreatic parenchyma.

ERCP. This is a limited study as the duct could not be cannulated. A small duodenal mucosal tear was seen and managed with clips.

EGD. There is firm gastric extrinsic compression in stomach body.

Subsequently a 10 Fr transpapillary biliary drain was placed by IR on 5/9→ findings of long smooth stenosis from right and left hepatic ducts to the papilla. Biliary ductal brushings were sent for cytology.

Patient was started on Zosyn and finished 7-day treatment course. Her hospital course was complicated by continued leakage around the drain site and unsuccessful drainage which lead to internalization of biliary stents. During that time biopsy of the pancreatic head was also obtained. CBD brushing cytology showed atypical lymphocytes suspicious for malignant lymphoma. FNA of pancreatic head showed Burkitt's lymphoma. Pancreatic head biopsy resulted in high grade B-cell lymphoma consistent with Burkitt's lymphoma. The histological/immunohistochemical and cytogenetic features of the mass are described as follows.

2.1. Histological Features. The pancreatic head mass needle biopsy morphologically showed sheets of medium-to-large size lymphoid cells with scant-to-moderate amounts of azurophilic cytoplasm, round-to-irregular nuclei with fine basophilic chromatin. Macrophages containing karyorrhectic debris are identified in the background. Immunohistochemically, the lesional cells are positive for CD20, CD10, and bcl-6. A subset shows rare c-myc positivity (control is also weak). They are negative for CD3, TdT, and bcl-2. Ki-67 displays a proliferation index >95%. These morphologic and immunohistochemical features are diagnostic for a high grade B-cell lymphoma and most consistent with Burkitt's lymphoma.

2.2. Immunohistochemistry. See Table 1.

2.3. Cytogenetic Results. (1) FISH showed no fusion of regions MYC and IGH of chromosomes 8 and 14, respectively.

(2) FISH showed no fusion of IGH and BCL2 regions of chromosomes 14 and 18, respectively.

(3) FISH revealed a splitting of the signal for MYC (8q24.1) in 91% of interface cells examined. This is indicative of MYC rearrangement, most likely a translocation.

(4) FISH did not reveal splitting or other rearrangements of 3q27 (BCL6).

Subsequently oncology team was involved and patient had a bone marrow biopsy done which showed B-cell lymphoma. PET scan showed peritoneal carcinomatosis and malignant ascites. Patient was started on chemotherapy regimen consisting of etoposide, prednisone, vincristine (Oncovin), and doxorubicin hydrochloride (hydroxydaunorubicin hydrochloride). After her first dose of chemotherapy she became encephalopathic and MRI of brain at that time showed possible involvement of base of skull and she was started on intrathecal methotrexate. Lumbar puncture was done subsequently and the CSF analysis was negative for infection and malignancy.

She received total of two cycles of chemotherapy and was admitted to hospital with sepsis and bacteremia. She deteriorated very quickly during that hospitalization and family opted for hospice and patient passed away in the hospice.

3. Discussion

The increasing use and sensitivity of cross-sectional imaging in identifying pancreatic lesions has led to a corresponding increase in the detection pancreatic tumors. While pancreatic ducal adenocarcinoma represents the majority of such cases, other, less common pancreatic neoplasms comprise an important fraction of pancreatic cancers. Primary pancreatic lymphoma (PPL) represents a significant class within these less common diagnoses [8]. Patients with either neoplasm may present with similar clinical manifestations; however, as the effective treatments for adenocarcinomas and lymphomas differ greatly, it is critical that an accurate diagnosis be made [9].

PPLs are extremely rare, comprising less than 2% of extra nodal malignant lymphomas and 0.5% of pancreatic tumors [3, 4], although nearly one-third of non-Hodgkin's lymphoma patients will ultimately develop some form of pancreatic involvement [10]. Diffuse large-cell lymphomas comprise the bulk of PPLs [8]. A less common form, Burkitt's lymphoma, is exceptionally rare, with fewer than 20 reported cases worldwide as of 2013 [11].

There are three subtypes of Burkitt's lymphoma: endemic, sporadic, and immunodeficiency- associated. The endemic form, described by Irish surgeon Denis Burkitt, is endemic to Papua New Guiney and Sub-Saharan Africa [12], mainly involves the mandible and maxilla, and is uniformly associated with Epstein-Barr virus (EBV) infection. The sporadic form is rare, with an incidence of 0.2–0.3 per 100,000 people per year globally, accounting for 30% of pediatric lymphomas and less than 1% of adult non-Hodgkin's lymphomas in the United States and Europe. These sporadic- form neoplasms are EBV associated at a rate of only 10–20% [13]. The immunodeficiency-associated variant of the disease, a common neoplasm of HIV infected patients, is generally EBV-negative outside of Africa and strongly associated with EBV within the continent [14].

Histologically, Burkitt's lymphoma presents with monomorphic, medium-sized B-cells with many mitotic figures and basophilic cytoplasm. High rates of apoptosis with benign histiocytic phagocytosis of apoptotic debris may lead to a starry-sky growth pattern [15]. The neoplastic B-cells of Burkitt's lymphoma have several clinically useful distinguishing immunophenotypic features. They are positive for the following: IgM surface immunoglobulin, surface light chains, CD10, CD19, CD20, CD22, CD43, CD79a, HLA-DR, and BCL-6. Additionally, Epstein-Barr virus-associated forms will express the EBV/C3d receptor, CD21. The neoplasms are negative for the following: CD5, CD23, BCL-2, and TdT [13]. Ki-67 expression in these tumors, a proxy measurement for growth fraction [11], approaches 100% [13].

Dysregulation of the MYC gene is a defining molecular marker of Burkitt's lymphoma. This is primarily a consequence of translocations between the MYC gene on chromosome 8 and the IgH gene on chromosome 14 [t(8;14)(q24;q32)], although MYC-κ light chain and MYC-λ light chain translocations [t(2;8)(p12;q24) and t(8;22)(q24;q11), resp.] are also described [13, 16]. Importantly, the absence of a MYC translocation does not rule out a diagnosis of Burkitt's lymphoma; in up to 10% of cases, fluorescence in situ hybridization is negative for these translocations. In these instances, MYC activation may be the result of miRNA deregulation or other causes [17].

Clinical symptoms of PPL are often non-specific [9] and can be made more difficult by inflammation of the pancreas [18]. As a consequence, clinical presentation may be of little help in distinguishing Burkitt's lymphoma from other pancreatic tumors [4, 19]. However, since treatments for pancreatic adenocarcinoma and other lymphomas of the pancreas differ significantly, differentiation of Burkitt's lymphoma from other pancreatic neoplasms is crucial [4, 9, 18]. Diagnosis can typically be made following nonsurgical biopsy of the tumor lesion [4, 11, 20].

Unlike pancreatic adenocarcinoma, which is treated surgically, chemotherapy has been shown to be the most efficacious first-line treatment for PPL [3, 8]. Common chemotherapeutic regimens directed against PPL include CVP (cyclophosphamide, vincristine, and prednisone), MACOP-B (methotrexate, adriamycin, cyclophosphamide, vincristine, prednisone, and bleomycin), and CHOP (cyclophosphamide, doxorubicin, vincristine, and prednisone). The further addition of rituximab, a monoclonal antibody targeting the CD20 B-cell antigen, to the CHOP regimen (R-CHOP) has been shown to enhance complete response rate, event-free survival, and overall survival in patients with diffuse large B-cell lymphoma. The role of radiation therapy in PPL remains poorly defined [3].

Multiple intensive chemotherapeutic approaches have demonstrated excellent efficacy in the treatment of Burkitt's lymphoma more generally; however, due to the relative lack of randomized trials directed towards the treatment of the disease, an optimal initial therapeutic approach has not been clearly defined [13]. This limitation is further compounded in the primary pancreatic form of the disease by its relative rarity. However, present chemotherapeutic approaches, comprising doxorubicin, alkylators, vincristine, and etoposide in combination with directed therapy targeting the prevention and eradication of CNS disease, have shown excellent outcomes. These treatments, described in detail by Jacobson and LaCasce, include CODOX-M/IVAC, the cancer and leukemia group-B regimen, hyperCVAD with and without rituximab, the lymphoma malign B regimen, and DA-REPOCH [13].

To conclude, PPLs are a class of rare cancers affecting the pancreas, of which Burkitt's lymphoma comprises an exceptionally rare subset. However, as efficacious treatments for the disease exist and differ markedly from that of pancreatic adenocarcinoma, it is important that PPLs more generally and Burkitt's lymphoma in particular be included in the differential when evaluating a probable pancreatic neoplasm.

References

[1] I. Joly, A. David, M. J. Payan, J. Sahel, and H. Sarles, "A case of primary Non-Hodgkin lymphoma of the pancreas," *Pancreas*, vol. 7, no. 1, pp. 118–120, 1992.

[2] E. Federico, M. Falconi, G. Zuodar, G. Falconieri, and F. Puglisi, "B-cell lymphoma presenting as acute pancreatitis," *Pancreatology*, vol. 11, no. 6, pp. 553–556, 2011.

[3] M. W. Saif, "Primary pancreatic lymphomas," *Journal of the Pancreas*, vol. 7, no. 3, pp. 262–273, 2006.

[4] W. J. Yoon, Y. B. Yoon, Y. J. Kim, J. K. Ryu, and Y.-T. Kim, "Primary pancreatic lymphoma in Korea-A single center experience," *Journal of Korean Medical Science*, vol. 25, no. 4, pp. 536–540, 2010.

[5] J. Amodio and J. E. Brodsky, "Pediatric burkitt lymphoma presenting as acute pancreatitis: MRI characteristics," *Pediatric Radiology*, vol. 40, no. 5, pp. 770–772, 2010.

[6] F. Glória Silva, M. Paiva, A. Tavares et al., "Paediatric Burkitt lymphoma presenting as acute pancreatitis," *Acta Médica Portuguesa*, vol. 21, no. 5, pp. 515–520, 2008.

[7] I. R. Francis and G. M. Glazer, "Burkitt's lymphoma of the pancreas presenting as acute pancreatitis," *Journal of Computer Assisted Tomography*, vol. 6, no. 2, pp. 395–397, 1982.

[8] M. M. Mortenson, M. H. G. Katz, E. P. Tamm et al., "Current diagnosis and management of unusual pancreatic tumors," *The American Journal of Surgery*, vol. 196, no. 1, pp. 100–113, 2008.

[9] Y. J. Wang, C. M. Jeng, Y. C. Wang, P. P. Chang, and T. H. Wang, "Primary pancreatic Burkitt's lymphoma mimicking carcinoma with obstructive jaundice and very high CA19-9," *European Journal of Gastroenterology & Hepatology*, vol. 18, no. 5, pp. 537–540, 2006.

[10] S. S. Nistala, N. R. Sawalakhe, N. R. Thiruvengadam, and P. M. Rathi, "A rare case of primary pancreatic Burkitt lymphoma in a young Indian male. Case report and review of the literature," *Journal of the Pancreas*, vol. 10, no. 6, pp. 686–689, 2009.

[11] S. Nakaji, N. Hirata, S. Yoshimura et al., "A case of primary pancreatic Burkitt's lymphoma diagnosed by EUS-guided FNA," *Gastrointestinal Endoscopy*, vol. 77, no. 6, pp. 958-959, 2013.

[12] J.-K. Oh and E. Weiderpass, "Infection and cancer: global distribution and burden of diseases," *Annals of Global Health*, vol. 80, no. 5, pp. 384–392, 2014.

[13] C. Jacobson and A. La Casce, "How I treat Burkitt lymphoma in adults," *Blood*, vol. 124, no. 19, pp. 2913–2920, 2014.

[14] C. Bellan, S. Lazzi, G. De Falco, A. Nyongo, A. Giordano, and L. Leoncini, "Burkitt's lymphoma: new insights into molecular pathogenesis," *Journal of Clinical Pathology*, vol. 56, no. 3, pp. 188–192, 2003.

[15] S.-S. Chuang, H. Ye, M.-Q. Du et al., "Histopathology and immunohistochemistry in distinguishing Burkitt lymphoma from diffuse large B-cell lymphoma with very high proliferation index and with or without a starry-sky pattern: a comparative study with EBER and FISH," *American Journal of Clinical Pathology*, vol. 128, no. 4, pp. 558–564, 2007.

[16] L. M. Boxer and C. V. Dang, "Translocations involving c-myc and c-myc function," *Oncogene*, vol. 20, no. 40, pp. 5595–5610, 2001.

[17] M. P. Menon, S. Pittaluga, and E. S. Jaffe, "The histological and biological spectrum of diffuse large B-cell lymphoma in the World Health Organization classification," *Cancer Journal*, vol. 18, no. 5, pp. 411–420, 2012.

[18] F. Carbonetti, E. Iannicelli, M. Federici et al., "Primary pancreatic Burkitt lymphoma presenting as acute pancreatitis," *Journal of Gastrointestinal Cancer*, vol. 45, supplement 1, pp. 265–269, 2014.

[19] M. S. Cappell, F. Yao, K. C. Cho, and C. A. Axiotis, "Lymphoma predominantly involving the pancreas," *Digestive Diseases and Sciences*, vol. 34, no. 6, pp. 942–947, 1989.

[20] B. Kessel, E. Moisseiev, A. Korin et al., "Burkitt's lymphoma: an unusual cause of obstructive jaundice," *Asian Journal of Surgery*, vol. 28, no. 4, pp. 301–304, 2005.

43

Extensive Causative Esophagitis Caused by Thermal Injury: A Case Report and Review of the Literature

Cherng Harng Lim,[1] Hsu-Heng Yen,[1] Wei-Wen Su,[1] Cherng-Jyr Lim,[2] Hao-Chien Tsai,[3] and Shi-Ting Chen[3]

[1] *Division of Gastroenterology and Hepatology, Department of Internal Medicine, Changhua Christian Hospital, Changhua City, Taiwan*
[2] *Department of Emergency Medicine, Cathay General Hospital, Changhua City, Taiwan*
[3] *Nursing Department, Changhua Christian Hospital, Changhua City, Taiwan*

Correspondence should be addressed to Cherng-Jyr Lim; chad_911@hotmail.com

Academic Editor: Yoshihiro Moriwaki

Esophagus thermal injury is a rare case that can be easily overlooked by practitioners. We herein present a case of thermally induced diffuse corrosive esophagitis with complaints of dysphagia and retrosternal chest pain after having steamed pork. A thorough disease course was demonstrated by serials of endoscopy images and video. A comprehensive review of articles and a concise overview of esophageal thermal injury clinical manifestation, disease process, typical endoscopy features, pharmacomanagement option, and outcomes will be conducted in this article.

1. Introduction

Acute esophagus thermal injury (ETI) is considered a reversible esophagus injury as a result of ingestion of hot foods and hot beverage or iatrogenic causes, leading to dysphagia, odynophagia, and retrosternal burning sensation. The endoscopic presentation of ETI varies and can mimic the features of chemical related corrosive injury, infection, and inflammation esophagitis which might need histopathology to be excluded. One of the distinct esophagogastroduodenoscopy (EGD) features is alternating white and reddish mucosa bands along the esophagus, resembling candy-cane appearance [1].

Herein, we report a case of diffuse corrosive esophagitis which was inflicted by steamed pork meat. Medical treatment and a series of images, videos regarding the endoscopic manifestation and healing process, were highlighted in this report. A total of 13 articles published in English literatures from 1982 to 2015 were reviewed for the purpose of analyzing the clinical manifestations, endoscopic features, histology findings, treatment options, and prognosis of ETI.

2. Manuscript

A 50-year-old gentleman presented to emergency department with progressive swallowing difficulty and retrosternal chest pain (pain score: 7/10) for about 20 hours. On arrival, his body temperature was 35.8°C, blood pressure was 155/99 mmHg, and pulse rate was 76 beats/minute. The chest radiography appeared normal and electrocardiogram showed normal sinus rhythm. Laboratory studies were within the reference ranges. There was no relevant medical history reported at that time. Esophagogastroduodenoscopy (EGD) demonstrated a diffuse mucosa erosion almost encircling the whole lumen, along with longitudinal, whitish, exuding, merely detached membranes extending from upper third to lower third of esophagus. Distal part of esophagus showed edematous, corrosive mucosa with spontaneous bleeding, without involving esophagogastric junction and gastric mucosa (Figure 1). Histopathology studies of esophagus biopsy reported ulcer with granulation tissue and inflammatory cell infiltration. There was absence of fungal pseudohyphae and viral inclusion bodies. Meanwhile, he acknowledged that he had swallowed a piece of hot steamed pork

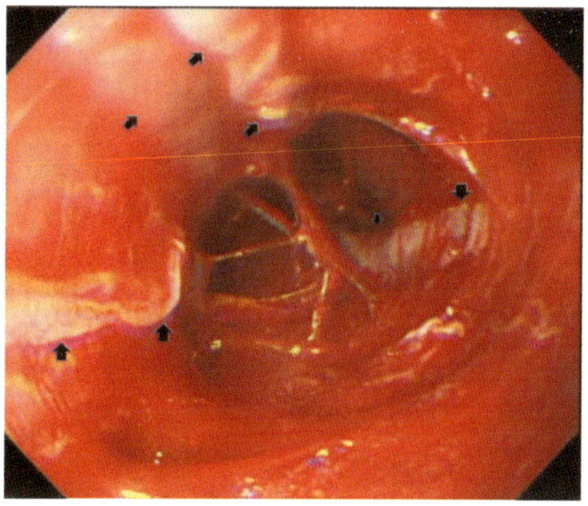

FIGURE 1: Initial endoscopy view (postthermal injury day 1). A diffuse corrosive surface with longitudinal thin, exuding, white merely scaling membranes (arrow), intervening with friable, spontaneous bleeding mucosa.

about 20 hours before. Subsequently, he felt progressive burning and pain sensation over his retrosternal area, particularly swallowing or drinking water. On the next day, his dysphagia symptom worsened making him unable to consume anything, even water. One episode of tarry stool on the day he visited the emergency department was noted. He denied consuming any caustic substances including detergents, pesticide, lye, or other chemical substances. This information was verified by his family members. In light of his medical history, endoscopy finding, and histology features, a diagnosis of corrosive esophagitis inflicted by thermal injury was made. Intravenous proton pump inhibitor (PPI, esomeprazole 80 mg/day) and sucralfate suspension (4 g/day) were prescribed to protect esophagus mucosa and avoid secondary acid reflux injury. During his hospitalization, generalized skin rash was noticed; drug allergy to esomeprazole was suspected; thus esomeprazole was changed to histamine-2 receptor antagonists (H2RA, Famotidine 40 mg/day), along with peripheral parenteral nutrition administration. Follow-up EGD on the 5th day showed alternating irregular white bands with hyperemic mucosa which bled easily on touching throughout the involved esophagus. After a week of treatment, his symptom improved gradually, cool liquid diet was tried initially, and normal diet was resumed on the 10th day of admission. He was discharged on his 11th day of admission and kept on Lansoprazole treatment for 1 month. Subsequent EGD follow-up on 10th and 30th day revealed marked improvement of mucosa. After 5 months of follow-up he was totally free of the aforementioned symptoms without any delayed complication.

3. Discussion

Acute ETI is a rare esophageal disease which can occur after consuming hot liquid and solid substances or iatrogenic insults. The prevalence of ETI has not yet been identified and is not easily reported [2]. It is more common in Eastern population owing to food culture. There was no direct evidence regarding coagulation abnormalities or any underlying diseases correlated with ETI. We conducted a search on PubMed and Medline Database with following terms: "(esophagus) AND (thermal injury OR burn injury OR candy-cane)"; all links and bibliography reference articles were explored and iatrogenic related ETI were excluded; a total of 18 cases were retrieved from 13 published English literatures (Tables 1, 2, and 3).

Based on our reviewed data, acute ETI caused by hot drinks and foods comprised 55% (10/18) and 40% (7/18), respectively. There was only 1 case reported in the literatures inflicted by smoking freebase cocaine. Majority of the patients, up to 72%, presented with odynophagia and/or dysphagia, 39% presented with chest discomfort, and only a small number presented with epigastric pain, dyspnea, hematemesis, melena, and so forth (Table 1). The clinical presentations often depend on the involved area. Six out of 18 of the cases with proximal esophagus involvement had the symptoms of hematemesis, dyspnea, or hoarseness.

Endoscopic features of ETI vary greatly, ranging from mild erythema to blister or ulcerative lesion, as with the affected area. It can be localized, linear, or diffused which can mimic variety of esophageal disorders such as chemically induced corrosive esophagitis, infectious esophagitis, inflammation caused by radiation, and pill esophagitis. However, there is one particular endoscopic characteristic unique to ETI referred to as candy-cane esophagus [1], but this only occurs in 22% of patients. According to our reviewed data, the most common presentation was longitudinal lesion (78%), as a result of thermal tract flow along esophagus, either manifested as pseudomembranous alone (8/14), erythematous (8/14), ulcerative (4/14), or mixed mucosa (7/14) (Table 2). Through our case study, we postulated that the early stages of ETI resemble first- or second-degree (partial-thickness) skin burns, which either appear as hyperemic mucosa or whitish exuding blisters depending on the depth of injury, configured in a longitudinal pattern. Peeling or rupture of blisters may result in a longitudinal mucosa erosion or ulcer. Subsequent edematous change may attribute to temporary intraluminal stenosis. Mucosa regeneration can be observed after blister exfoliation, leaving an erythematous mucosa band. In contrast to previous article [5], our case showed that the whitish exuding blisters, which withstand from previous insult, gradually turned into pseudomembranous lesion (Figure 2). Alternation of the erythematous mucosa band and the pseudomembrane lesions formed the "candy-cane" appearance. As the erythematous mucosa bands heal they will leave scar tracts along the esophagus [7] (Figure 3). This healing process is clearly demonstrated in our case (watch the *video* in Supplementary Material available online at https://doi.org/10.1155/2017/8243567). Moreover, the endoscopic features have direct correlation with the depth and severity of thermal injury which in turn depends on the following factors: material properties (size, temperature, and form), exposure duration, and time to endoscopy. On the other hand, about 33% of the cases had evidence of oral and upper airway involvement in endoscopy, and 2 of the cases were complicated with airway obstruction [8]. Therefore, the oral cavity, laryngopharynx, and vocal cord should be investigated simultaneously during endoscopy. Interestingly,

TABLE 1: Summary of clinical manifestation in ETI published cases.

Number	Age/gender	Material	Clinical manifestation		
			Odynophagia, dysphagia	Chest discomfort	Other
1	22/M	Microwave heated jelly roll	√		
2 [2]	21/F	Microwave heated lasagna	√	√	
3 [1]	66/M	Hot beverages	√	√	
4 [1]	72/F	Hot soups			Melena
5 [3]	20/M	Hot hamburger	√		
6 [4]	55/M	Smoking freebase cocaine			Melena, diaphoresis, hypotension
7 [5]	30/F	Hot tea	√	√	Hematemesis
8 [6]	69/M	Hot tea	√	√	Epigastric discomfort
9 [7]	53/M	Hot prawn	√	√	
10	79/M	Microwaved lasagna	√		Drooling, hoarseness
11	45/F	Hot tea	√		Hematemesis
12	52/M	Stew		√	
13	29/M	Hot water	√		
14	57/F	Hot water			Anemia
15	54/M	Hot tea	√		
16 [8]	28/M	Hot coffee	√		Dyspnea
17 [9]	47/F	Hot dumpling	√	√	
18 [10]	19/M	Hot tea			Hematemesis

M, male; F, female; N/A, not applicable.

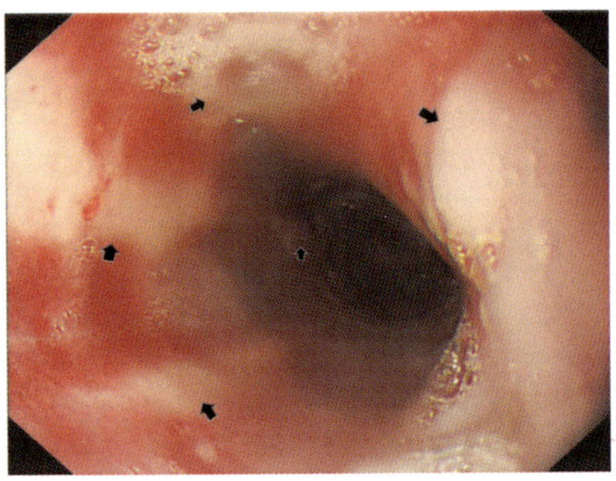

FIGURE 2: Second endoscopy view (postthermal injury day 5). Alternating geographic, longitudinal, geographic, whitish pseudomembranous (arrow) and inflamed, erythematous mucosa.

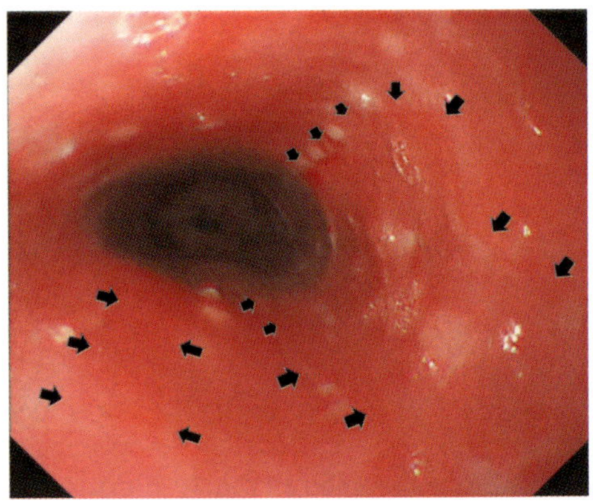

FIGURE 3: Third endoscopy view (postthermal injury day 10). Several healing hyperemic mucosa scar tracts along esophagus (arrow).

none of the cases ever reported gastric mucosa involvement directly to thermal injury. In addition, no perforation or severe blood loss events were mentioned in our collected articles.

Esophagus biopsy is not mandatory in ETI; less than half of the cases underwent biopsy via EGD (Table 2). Moreover, the histopathological findings of ETI in acute stage were unspecific, including necrosis, inflammatory cell infiltration, parakeratosis hyperplasia, and granulation tissue. Thermal involvement beyond submucosa layer was demonstrated in one case with evidence of fibrosis from submucosa to adventitia layer resulting in delayed esophagus stricture [8]. We reasonably infer that depth of thermal insult is one of the major determinants of outcome and manifestation in clinical aspect, yet solely using biopsy via EGD for histopathology evaluation is inadequate owing to its limited specimen size. The main purpose of biopsy in this aspect is to provide useful information contributing to excluding other diseases, particularly those with atypical endoscopy features.

The clinical course of ETI was considered relatively benign and reversible. Most cases were treated successfully with conservative treatment, such as avoiding further thermal insult (17%) and antisecretory treatment, such as PPIs (67%) and H2RAs (11%) or in combination with sucralfate suspension (33%) to prevent further injury from reflux gastric acid. The treatment duration in each case was inconsistent,

TABLE 2: Summary of endoscopy manifestation and treatment in ETI published cases.

Number	Timeline	Image presentation: Esophagus Apparatus/length/circumferences (i) Finding	Image presentation: Other Area/finding	Histology
1	3 days	EGD/28–38 cm from incisors/partial (i) Multiple linear erythematous	N/A	N/A
2 [2]	3 days	Esophagogram/mid to distal/partial (i) Longitudinally linear collection and filling defect	N/A	N/A
3 [1]	1 month	EGD/upper to lower/whole (i) Candy-cane appearance	N/A	necrotic, anucleated, nonviable epithelium
4 [1]	3 weeks	EGD/upper to lower/whole (i) Candy-cane appearance	N/A	Necrotic anucleated nonviable epithelium
5 [3]	12 days	EGD/30 cm from incisor/partial (i) Single longitudinal ulcer	N/A	N/A
6 [4]	2 days	EGD/distal/whole (i) Candy-cane appearance	Heart/Transient cardiac ischemia;	parakeratosis, squamous hyperplasia, inflammatory cell infiltration
7 [5]	7 days	EGD/full length/partial (i) Pseudomembranous mucosa band with hyperemic mucosa	N/A	Ulcer with granulation tissue
8 [6]	1 week 10 days	EGD/full length/whole (i) Diffuse pseudomembranous mucosa and erosion (ii) Linear plaque, lower esophagus small fibrotic changes	Oral cavity/whitish plaque, erosion	
9 [7]	3 days 8 days	EGD/full length/partial (i) Longitudinal ulcer band EGD/full length/partial (i) Pseudomembranous mucosa band		Ulcer with activated endothelial cell
10	1 day	EGD /full length/N/A (i) Erythema and swelling mucosa	Pharyngeal, laryngeal & vocal cord/inflammation	N/A
11	7 days 14 days	EGD/hypopharynx to 25 cm from incisors/partial (i) Pseudomembranous mucosa in geographic shape (ii) Candy-cane appearance	arytenoid folds/edematous mucosa	Ulceration with inflammation, atypia epithelial

Table 2: Continued.

Number	Timeline	Image presentation: Esophagus Apparatus/length/circumferences (i) Finding	Other Area/finding	Histology
12	7 days	EGD/middle to distal esophagus/partial (i) Longitudinal pseudomembrane and erosion	N/A	N/A
13	Same day 7 days	EGD/upper to middle/whole (i) Pseudomembrane and hyperemic mucosa (ii) Whitish fibrosis and edematous hyperemic mucosa	N/A	N/A
14	Few days	EGD/lower esophagus/N/A (i) Friable mucosa, fibrosis, and edema	Oral cavity/pseudomembrane mucosa	N/A
15	1 day	ED/34 cm from incisor/partial (i) Focal ulcer	N/A	necrosis with white cells and cellular debris
16 [8]	N/A 40 days 5 months + 53 days	EGD/N/A/N/A (i) Failed to pass through (ii) Healing of edematous mucosa EGD/19 cm from incisor to distal/whole (i) Circumference stenosis	Laryngopharyngeal/edematous mucosa N/A	Fibrosis over submucosa and muscularis propria and adventitia
17 [9]	1 day	EGD/upper to middle (30 cm from incisor)/partial/ (i) Longitudinal pseudomembrane	Pharynx/pseudomembrane mucosa	N/A
18 [10]	N/A	EGD/N/A/N/A (i) Diffuse ulcerations with candy-cane appearance	N/A	N/A

EGD, esophagogastroduodenoscopy; N/A, not applicable.

Table 3: Summary of treatment and follow-up duration in ETI published cases.

Number	Medication	Time to resolve	Follow-up duration
1	Avoid	Symptom resolves in 2 days	2 days
2 [2]	H2RA (Famotidine) for 1 month	Symptom improves in 1 week	N/A
3 [1]	Avoid	N/A	N/A
4 [1]	Avoid	N/A	N/A
5 [3]	PPI (omeprazole) for 1 month	Clinical improvement in 1 month	2 months
6 [4]	PPI for 1 month	N/A	12 months
7 [5]	PPI (Pantoprazole) for 4 weeks	N/A	2 months
8 [6]	PPI (Pantoprazole)	Symptom improves in 3 days	11 days
9 [7]	PPI (Pantoprazole) for 1 month	Symptom improves in 8 days	2 months
10	Steroid (dexamethasone) + intubation	Clinical improves in 2 days	2 days
11	PPI (Lansoprazole) + sucralfate	N/A	2 weeks
12	H2R A (ranitidine) + sucralfate for 3 weeks	Endoscopic improvement in 3 weeks	3 weeks
13	PPI (Lansoprazole) + sucralfate	Symptom improves in 1 week	1 week
14	PPI (Lansoprazole) + sucralfate	Endoscopic improvement in 1 week	1 week
15	PPI (Lansoprazole) + sucralfate	Endoscopic improvement in 1 week	1 month
16 [8]	PPI + tracheostomy	N/A	10 months
17 [9]	Esophagus reconstruction	N/A	
18 [10]	PPI (Lansoprazole)	Symptom improves in 2 days	2 months
1	PPI (esomeprazole) + sucralfate	Endoscopic improvement in 1 month	1 month

H2RA, histamine-2 receptor antagonist; PPI, proton pump inhibitor; N/A, not applicable.

ranging from 0 to 1 month (Table 3). There is no consensus yet as to the grading of ETI, optimum treatment options, and duration of treatment. Individualized treatments are still favored, based on depth, extending of thermal injury, and organ involvement which contribute to overall outcomes. On the other hand, airway obstruction is one deadly complication as there were two published cases that required intubation and tracheotomy to obtain airway [8]. Therefore airway evaluation and protection should be the first priority before undergoing further endoscopy examination. Steroid had been applied in one of the cases for the purpose of ameliorating trachea edema. In fact, there was no direct evidence supporting their use in thermal injury [11, 12], but exposing the risk of infection and delayed wound healing. Concomitant transient ischemic heart event [4] was reported in ETI induced by smoking freebase cocaine, albeit more likely due to cocaine itself.

The prognosis of ETI is generally favorable and is directly related to the depth and severity of thermal injury. One ETI case developed delayed esophageal stenosis requiring esophagus reconstruction [8]. Whether there is an association between acute ETI and esophageal cancer is not known. Although more studies have pointed out that "long term" consuming high-temperature beverages or food may lead to esophageal cancer as a result of impairing mucosa barrier and chronic inflammation [13], speaking of "long term" is related to amount, duration, and temperature of consumption; thus whether it can apply for those after one episode of acute thermal insult is not well described. None of the published ETI cases have ever reported to have esophageal cancer, yet the average follow-up duration was 2.4 months (range from 2 days to 12 months). Therefore, further investigation regarding the association of carcinogenesis might need substantial studies with long term follow-up to clarify.

In conclusion, ETI can easily be overlooked by practitioners due to its rarity. Often times, patients left out important clues for diagnosis during history taking. By recognizing the distinctive features of endoscopic findings in ETI, treating physician can obtain relevant history and make the correct diagnosis easily. For atypical cases, a prompt investigation of etiology is required; further biopsies might be needed to exclude other possibilities. Meanwhile, airway evaluation should be assessed by endoscopist other than gastrointestinal tract alone. The endoscopic grading system for ETI is yet to be standardized which is relevant to treatment strategies and prognosis.

References

[1] S. K. Dutta, K. Y. Chung, and B. S. Bhagavan, "Thermal injury of the esophagus," *New England Journal of Medicine*, vol. 339, no. 7, pp. 480-481, 1998.

[2] B. R. Javors, D. E. Panzer, and I. S. Goldman, "Acute thermal injury of the esophagus," *Dysphagia*, vol. 11, no. 1, pp. 72–74, 1996.

[3] R. Eliakim, "Thermal injury from a hamburger: a rare cause of odynophagia," *Gastrointestinal Endoscopy*, vol. 50, no. 2, pp. 282-283, 1999.

[4] M. E. Cohen and J. G. Kegel, "Candy cocaine esophagus," *Chest*, vol. 121, no. 5, pp. 1701–1703, 2002.

[5] E. K. Choi, H. L. Gin, H.-Y. Jung et al., "The healing course of thermal esophageal injury: a case report," *Gastrointestinal Endoscopy*, vol. 62, no. 1, pp. 158–160, 2005.

[6] G. Hoon, W. Y. Hyeon, H. J. Sung et al., "Esophageal thermal injury by hot adlay tea," *Korean Journal of Internal Medicine*, vol. 22, no. 1, pp. 59–62, 2007.

[7] W. C. Chung, C. N. Paik, J. H. Jung, J. D. Kim, K.-M. Lee, and J. M. Yang, "Acute thermal injury of the esophagus from solid food: clinical course and endoscopic findings," *Journal of Korean Medical Science*, vol. 25, no. 3, pp. 489–491, 2010.

[8] T. Kitajima, K. Momose, S. Lee et al., "Benign esophageal stricture after thermal injury treated with esophagectomy and ileocolon interposition," *World Journal of Gastroenterology*, vol. 20, pp. 9205–9209, 2014.

[9] C.-H. Wu, M.-J. Bair, I.-T. Lin, Y.-K. Lee, and H.-L. Chen, "Early endoscopic finding of esophageal thermal injury after having spicy hot pot," *Advances in Digestive Medicine*, vol. 2, no. 3, pp. 111–113, 2015.

[10] A. AC and J. Rajma, "Candy cane appearance of the esophagus caused by acute thermal injury," *Clinical Gastroenterology and Hepatology*, vol. 14, no. 10, A19 pages, 2016.

[11] S. I. Cha, C. H. Kim, J. H. Lee et al., "Isolated smoke inhalation injuries: Acute respiratory dysfunction, clinical outcomes, and short-term evolution of pulmonary functions with the effects of steroids," *Burns*, vol. 33, no. 2, pp. 200–208, 2007.

[12] D. N. Herndon, R. E. Barrow, H. A. Linares et al., "Inhalation injury in burned patients: effects and treatment," *Burns*, vol. 14, no. 5, pp. 349–356, 1988.

[13] F. Islami, P. Boffetta, J.-S. Ren, L. Pedoeim, D. Khatib, and F. Kamangar, "High-temperature beverages and foods and esophageal cancer risk—a systematic review," *International Journal of Cancer*, vol. 125, no. 3, pp. 491–524, 2009.

Shigella sonnei Bacteremia Presenting with Profound Hepatic Dysfunction

Oluwaseun Shogbesan,[1] Andrew Rettew,[2] Bilal Shaikh,[3] Abdullateef Abdulkareem,[1] and Anthony Donato[1]

[1]*Department of Internal Medicine, Reading Health System, Spruce Street and 6th Avenue, West Reading, PA 19610, USA*
[2]*Department of Hematology and Oncology, Banner University Medical Center, Tuscon, AZ, USA*
[3]*St Francis Medical Center, Cape Girardeau, MO, USA*

Correspondence should be addressed to Oluwaseun Shogbesan; oluwaseun.shogbesan@readinghealth.org

Academic Editor: Warwick S. Selby

Worldwide, Shigellosis is a significant public health issue, associated with nearly one million deaths annually. About half a million cases of *Shigella* infection are reported annually in the United States. *Shigella* bacteremia is uncommon and generally seen in children and immunocompromised adults. We present a case of a *Shigella sonnei* bacteremia with marked hepatic derangement in a 27-year-old previously healthy homosexual male with history of Roux-en-Y gastric bypass, who presented to the emergency room with a 4-day history of loose watery stool, abdominal cramps, nausea and vomiting, and yellow skin of 2-day duration. He reports similar diarrhea illness in two close contacts in preceding days. On examination, he was fully oriented but dehydrated, icteric, and febrile. Laboratory data revealed WBC of 2200/μL, elevated AST and ALT (201 IU/L, 73 IU/L resp.), normal alkaline phosphatase, elevated total and direct bilirubin of 8.2 mg/dL and 4.4 mg/dL, albumin of 3.2 g/dL, INR of 2.9, prothrombin time of 31.7, and platelet of 96,000/μL. Workup for infectious, autoimmune and medication-induced hepatitis, Wilson's disease, and hemochromatosis was negative. Abdominal ultrasound and computed tomography of the abdomen showed hepatic steatosis and right-sided colitis. Stool and blood cultures were positive for *Shigella sonnei*. He was treated with ciprofloxacin with improvement in liver function. Follow-up blood test 4 months later was within normal limits.

1. Introduction

Worldwide, *Shigella* is a common food-borne bacterial cause of dysentery and rarely causes bacteremia in the immunocompromised host [1, 2]. Infection is more common in developing countries and areas with poor hygiene and contaminated water sources, but sexual transmission has been reported among men who have sex with men (MSM) [1, 3–6]. We report a case of *Shigella* bacteremia in a homosexual male complicated by hepatic dysfunction.

2. Case Report

A 27-year-old African American male with a history of morbid obesity status post-Roux-en-Y gastric bypass 9 years prior presented with painful nonbloody mucoid diarrhea, icterus, and dark urine of four-day duration. He described recent travel with family to a beach resort in the United States during which he noted that two family members had developed a self-limited diarrheal illness. Three days after exposure, he noted abdominal cramps followed by hourly watery yellow stools without blood. He also had intermittent nausea and an episode of bilious vomiting and reports not eating since onset of diarrheal illness. He noticed a 17-pound weight loss over 1 week. He had no fevers, chills, or rash. There was no preceding history of eating uncooked fish or meats and he had no tick exposure. Medication history included Lisinopril and Amlodipine, and he denied any new medications or alcohol use. He admitted to homosexual intercourse.

He was acutely ill-looking with icteric sclera and dry mucus membranes. Vitals signs showed low-grade fever of

100.2°F and pulse rate of 126 beats per minute. Cardiac, lung, and skin examinations were unremarkable. Abdomen was diffusely tender with hyperactive bowel sounds without peritoneal signs.

Laboratory data was remarkable for leukopenia of 2200/μL, hemoglobin of 12.7 g/dL, normal platelet of 158,000/μL, sodium of 128 meq/L and potassium of 3.2 meq/L, acute kidney injury with creatinine of 1.59 mg/dL (baseline of 0.63 mg/dL), BUN of 41 mg/dL, and anion gap of 19. After intravenous hydration, hemoglobin dropped to 10.1 g/dL and platelet to 96,000/μL. Sodium, BUN, and creatinine also improved with rehydration. He was also noted to have elevated transaminases AST 201 IU/L and ALT 73 IU/L, elevated total bilirubin of 8.2 mg/dL, direct bilirubin of 4.4 mg/dL, normal alkaline phosphatase of 66 IU/L, albumin of 3.2 g/dL, normal lipase of 40 U/L, and elevated lactate of 3.5 meq/L. INR was elevated to 1.8; however, he had normal haptoglobin 236 mg/dL (36–195 mg/dL) and LDH 177 IU/L (normal: 94–202 IU/L). Hepatitis panel was negative. Patient also tested negative for HIV, CMV, EBV, and Parvovirus B19 infection. Tylenol level was normal. Urinalysis showed moderate bilirubinuria. Stool study was positive for *Shigella sonnei* but was otherwise negative for bacteria, ova, or parasites. *Rickettsia rickettsii* IgM was positive and he was treated with Doxycycline. Other workup for tick-borne infection including Lyme, *Babesia*, *Ehrlichia*, and *Anaplasma* was negative. Autoimmune workups including ANA, antismooth muscle, liver/kidney microsome, and mitochondrial antibodies were negative. Alpha-1 antitrypsin and ceruloplasmin were also normal.

Abdominal ultrasound showed a diffusely increased heterogeneous liver echogenicity with underlying hepatomegaly consistent with hepatic steatosis. Hepatoportal duplex showed patent portal vein and hepatic artery. Computed tomography of the abdomen and pelvis was significant for hepatic steatosis, hepatomegaly, mild right colitis, and absence of gallstones. Magnetic resonance cholangiopancreatography (MRCP) was unremarkable with normal intra- and extrahepatic biliary tree.

During his hospital course, bilirubin trended up to 9 mg/dL and INR peaked at 2.9. Patient was not encephalopathic. Given impending hepatic failure, recommendation was made to transfer the patient to a transplant center but he declined. He was treated with N-acetylcysteine. Blood culture initially reported as Gram-negative rods presumptively *Escherichia coli (E. coli)* was later confirmed to be *Shigella sonnei*. Urine culture remained negative. He was treated with ciprofloxacin based on sensitivity results with an improvement in diarrhea frequency and downward trend in transaminases. He remained stable and was discharged home on Day 8. He was doing well 4 months later with normal cell counts, normal liver, and kidney function.

3. Discussion

Shigella has a low infectious dose, requiring as low as 10 organisms for infection, and it is easily transmitted from person to person [20]. Outbreaks are common in day care centers, institutions, and urban areas with crowded living conditions [6]. In the United States and other developed countries, transmission is usually fecal-oral from symptomatic patient and fecal contamination of raw vegetable has been identified in outbreaks [3, 6]. Average incubation period is three days and patients typically presents with small volume watery to mucoid diarrhea, abdominal pain, vomiting, fever, and bloody diarrhea.

Shigella sonnei is responsible for three-quarters of all cases in the US, while *Shigella flexneri* is predominant in developing countries [1, 21, 22]. Complications range from rare intestinal complications of toxic megacolon, intestinal obstruction to systemic complications of hypovolemia, seizures, hyponatremia, and leukemoid reaction.

This case is unique for several reasons, first because *Shigella* bacteremia is uncommon in adults and even less common in the absence of underlying immunosuppression [23, 24]. Our patient was not immunocompromised and extensive workup to detect underlying predisposition was negative. Patient did have a history of Roux-en-Y gastric bypass and possibility of underlying nutritional deficiency cannot be conclusively excluded. Morduchowicz et al. reported 27 cases of *Shigella* bacteremia of which 16 had an underlying predisposing condition [12]. Appannanavar et al. also reported a case of bacteremia in a renal transplant patient and two other cases in postrenal transplant are reported in literature [8, 25, 26]. Hawkins et al. presented a total of 9 cases of *Shigella* bacteremia in adults with underlying predisposing comorbidities including the use of immunosuppressant, diabetes mellitus, alcohol liver disease, HIV/AIDS, and malignancy [16]. Similar to our case, Huynh et al. presented an otherwise healthy male without identified comorbidities; he was a MSM [19].

Increasing cases of Shigellosis have been reported among MSM [4, 19]. In a case series of 466 cases of *Shigella* bacteremia, two-thirds of reported cases in adult males were in MSM [19]. Outbreak of *Shigella* among MSM has also been reported in Europe, USA, and Australia [27–31]. There is no increase in incidence of *Shigella* bacteremia among HIV infected individuals, although increased mortality has been noted in HIV-positive patients with *Shigella* bacteremia [1].

Additionally, to our knowledge, this is the first reported case of hepatic manifestation of Shigellosis in an adult. Our patient had coagulopathy with bilirubinemia, elevated transaminases, and thrombocytopenia but was not encephalopathic and thus not by definition in fulminant liver failure. Workup for viral hepatitis, toxin or drug hepatitis, autoimmune hepatitis, Wilson's disease, malignant, or vascular etiology was negative in the setting of *Shigella* bacteremia. His underlying fatty liver disease might have played a role. Despite the absence of encephalopathy, our patient was considered for referral to transplant center given rising bilirubin and INR concerning for impending fulminant hepatic failure. Guided by evidence of increased transplant free survival in hepatic failure, he was treated with N-acetylcysteine when he declined transfer. Of note, liver function improved with treatment of *Shigella* infection. A case of fulminant hepatic failure in a three-and-a-half-year-old boy with *Shigella* bacteremia also made clinical and biochemical improvement with Shigellosis treatment [32].

TABLE 1: Reported cases of adult *Shigella sonnei* bacteremia.

Author	Comorbidity	Outcome
Winter and Harding 1962 [7]	None	Recovery
Netter et al., 1974 [8]	Renal transplant	Recovery
O'Connor and O'Callaghan 1981 [9]	Marrow Aplasia	Death
Roncoroni et al., 1984 [10]	(1) CKD	Recovery
	(2) None	Death
Alkan et al., 1985 [11]	Metastatic adenocarcinoma	Death
Morduchowicz et al., 1987 [12]	(1) None	Recovery
	(2) Diabetes mellitus	Recovery
Dronda et al., 1988 [2]	Diabetes mellitus	Recovery
Christensen et al., 1990 [13]	Congenital antithrombin III deficiency, postsplenectomy	Recovery
Seymour et al., 1994 [14]	(1) AIDS	Death
	(2) Alcoholic liver disease	Recovery
Kenet et al., 1994 [15]	Metastatic breast cancer	Death
Hawkins et al., 2007 [16]	(1) Multiple myeloma	Recovery
	(2) Diabetes mellitus	Recovery
Liu et al., 2009 [17]	Lung cancer	Death
Markham et al., 2012 [18]	AIDS	Recovery
Huynh et al., 2015 [19]	None	Recovery

Our patient tested positive for *Rickettsia rickettsii* IgM and this was considered to be a false positive result in the absence of prominent fever and classical rash which is seen in 90% of cases. Also our patient did not have other common features of Rocky Mountain spotted fever (RMSF) including headaches, myalgia, and arthralgia and no preceding tick exposure. In advance cases of RMSF, elevations in serum aminotransferases and bilirubin and prolongation of prothrombin time are possible; it was however considered an unlikely explanation in our index case. False positive *Rickettsia* IgM is known to occur in presence of other bacteria pathogen due to cross reactivity to similar lipopolysaccharide [33, 34].

Huynh et al. reported a case of *Shigella* bacteremia in 34-year-old MSM in which a positive blood culture was initially reported as *E. coli* [19]. *E. coli* and *Shigella* both Enterobacteriaceae are genomically similar with identical O-antigens and similar virulence determinants [35, 36]. Rapid testing methods such as the natrix-assisted laser desorption ionization-time of flight mass spectrometry (MALDI-TOF MS) used in many diagnostic microbiology laboratories cannot distinguish between both [37, 38]. In patients with discordant *Shigella* stool culture and *E. coli* bacteremia, conventional and serologic testing is required to correctly identify *Shigella* and prevent an unnecessary search for an additional infection source.

We found 18 reported adult cases of *Shigella sonnei* bacteremia in literature. 14 of the 18 patients had an underlying immunocompromising comorbidity including diabetes mellitus, AIDS, malignancy, and postorgan transplantation (Table 1). One of the 4 patients without an identified comorbidity was a MSM similar to our case. All 3 patients with underlying solid organ malignancy died during the course of *Shigella* bacteremia. Over all, there were 6 deaths, 5 of which had significant underlying comorbidities.

Shigellosis is often self-limited and infection tends to clear spontaneously in most individuals. In severe cases with complications, including bacteremia, treatment is indicated. First-line treatment is with fluoroquinolones. However, given increasing antibiotic resistance, particularly strains acquired from Asia and Africa, susceptibility testing is important [3, 39, 40]. Of note, reduced susceptibility and/or resistance to ciprofloxacin has been reported in the United States [21].

Acknowledgments

Valerie Schaeffer helped in retrieving articles.

References

[1] K. H. Keddy, A. Sooka, P. Crowther-Gibson et al., "Systemic shigellosis in South Africa," *Clinical Infectious Diseases*, vol. 54, no. 10, pp. 1448–1454, 2012.

[2] F. Dronda, F. Parras, J. L. Martinez, and F. Baquero, "Shigella sonnei bacteremia in an elderly diabetic patient," *European Journal of Clinical Microbiology & Infectious Diseases*, vol. 7, no. 3, pp. 404–405, 1988.

[3] K. L. Kotloff, J. P. Winickoff, B. Ivanoff et al., "Global burden of Shigella infections: implications for vaccine development and implementation of control strategies," *Bulletin of the World Health Organization*, vol. 77, no. 8, pp. 651–666, 1999.

[4] R. L. Serafino Wani, S. A. Filson, M. A. Chattaway, and G. Godbole, "Invasive shigellosis in MSM," *International Journal of STD and AIDS*, vol. 27, no. 10, pp. 917–919, 2016.

[5] J. Z. Hines, T. Pinsent, K. Rees et al., "Shigellosis outbreak among men who have sex with men and homeless persons — Oregon, 2015-2016," *Morbidity and Mortality Weekly Report*, vol. 65, no. 31, pp. 812–813, 2016.

[6] W. H. Mosley, B. Adams, and E. D. Lyman, "Epidemiologic and sociologic features of a large urban outbreak of Shigellosis," *JAMA*, vol. 182, no. 13, pp. 1307–1311, 1962.

[7] B. V. Winter and H. B. Harding, "Shigella sonnei bacteremia: case report and review of the literature," *JAMA*, vol. 180, no. 11, pp. 927–931, 1962.

[8] E. Neter, C. Merrin, M. J. Surgalla, and Z. Wajsman, "Shigella sonnei bacteremia unusual antibody response from immunosuppressive therapy following renal transplantation," *Urology*, vol. 4, no. 2, pp. 198–200, 1974.

[9] H. J. O'Connor and U. O'Callaghan, "Fatal *Shigella sonnei* septicaemia in an adult complicated by marrow aplasia and intestinal perforation," *Journal of Infection*, vol. 3, no. 3, pp. 277–279, 1981.

[10] A. J. Roncoroni, H. M. Bianchini, N. Frega, and A. Avagnina, "Septicemia caused by Shigella sonnei," *Medicina*, vol. 44, no. 3, pp. 332–333, 1984.

[11] M. Alkan, E. Salzstein, and A. Simu, "Four cases of shigella septicemia in Israel," *European Journal of Clinical Microbiology*, vol. 4, no. 4, pp. 417–418, 1985.

[12] G. Morduchowicz, D. Huminer, Y. Siegman Igra, M. Drucker, C. S. Block, and S. D. Pitlik, "Shigella bacteremia in adults: a report of five cases and review of the literature," *Archives of Internal Medicine*, vol. 147, no. 11, pp. 2034–2037, 1987.

[13] P. Christensen, J. Renneberg, and E. Wallmark, "Shigella sonnei sepsis after splenectomy and portacaval shunt," *European Journal of Clinical Microbiology & Infectious Diseases*, vol. 9, no. 2, pp. 148–149, 1990.

[14] C. Seymour, H. M. Crowe, and M. E. Wilson, "Comparative virulence of blood and stool isolates of Shigella sonnei," *Journal of Clinical Microbiology*, vol. 32, no. 3, pp. 835–838, 1994.

[15] G. Kenet, F. Salomon, Z. Samra, J. Pinkhas, Y. Sidi, and N. Arber, "Fatal Shigella sepsis in a neutropenic patient," *Mount Sinai Journal of Medicine*, vol. 61, no. 4, pp. 367–368, 1994.

[16] C. Hawkins, B. Taiwo, M. Bolon, K. Julka, A. Adewole, and V. Stosor, "Shigella sonnei bacteremia: two adult cases and review of the literature," *Scandinavian Journal of Infectious Diseases*, vol. 39, no. 2, pp. 170–173, 2007.

[17] C.-Y. Liu, Y.-T. Huang, C.-H. Liao, S.-C. Chang, and P.-R. Hsueh, "Rapidly fatal bacteremia caused by *Shigella sonnei* without preceding gastrointestinal symptoms in an adult patient with lung cancer," *Clinical Infectious Diseases*, vol. 48, no. 11, pp. 1635–1636, 2009.

[18] K. B. Markham, C. Backes, and P. Samuels, "Bacteremia and intrauterine infection with Shigella sonnei in a pregnant woman with AIDS," *Archives of Gynecology and Obstetrics*, vol. 286, no. 3, pp. 799–801, 2012.

[19] A. Huynh, C. McGrath, D. Johnson, and L. M. Burrell, "*Shigella sonnei* bacteraemia occurring in a young man with shigellosis," *BMJ Case Reports*, vol. 2015, 2015.

[20] H. L. Dupont, M. M. Levine, R. B. Hornick, and S. B. Formal, "Inoculum size in shigellosis and implications for expected mode of transmission," *Journal of Infectious Diseases*, vol. 159, no. 6, pp. 1126–1128, 1989.

[21] S. Sivapalasingam, J. M. Nelson, K. Joyce, M. Hoekstra, F. J. Angulo, and E. D. Mintz, "High prevalence of antimicrobial resistance among *Shigella* isolates in the United States tested by the national antimicrobial resistance monitoring system from 1999 to 2002," *Antimicrobial Agents and Chemotherapy*, vol. 50, no. 1, pp. 49–54, 2006.

[22] S. Livio, N. A. Strockbine, S. Panchalingam et al., "Shigella isolates from the global enteric multicenter study inform vaccine development," *Clinical Infectious Diseases*, vol. 59, no. 7, pp. 933–941, 2014.

[23] M. J. Struelens, D. Patte, A. Kabir, A. Salam, S. K. Nath, and T. Butler, "Shigella septicemia: prevalence, presentation, risk factors, and outcome," *Journal of Infectious Diseases*, vol. 152, no. 4, pp. 784–790, 1985.

[24] A. J. Trevett, B. O. Ogunbanjo, S. Naraqi, and J. D. Igo, "Shigella bacteraemia in adults," *Postgraduate Medical Journal*, vol. 69, no. 812, pp. 466–468, 1993.

[25] S. B. Appannanavar, K. Goyal, R. Garg, P. Ray, M. Rathi, and N. Taneja, "Shigellemia in a post renal transplant patient: a case report and literature review," *Journal of Infection in Developing Countries*, vol. 8, no. 2, pp. 237–239, 2014.

[26] M. Severn and J. Michael, "Shigella septicaemia following renal transplantation," *Postgraduate Medical Journal*, vol. 56, no. 662, pp. 852–853, 1980.

[27] R. Keay, G. Singh, M. Abdul-Latif, M. Rayment, and M. Nelson, "Shigella flexneri enteritis in risk-taking HIV-infected MSM," *Journal of Infection*, vol. 68, no. 1, pp. 103–104, 2014.

[28] M. L. Borg, A. Modi, A. Tostmann et al., "Ongoing outbreak of Shigella flexneri serotype 3a in men who have sex with men in England and Wales, data from 2009–2011," *Eurosurveillance*, vol. 17, no. 13, 2012.

[29] M. R. Nelson, D. C. Shanson, D. Hawkins, and B. G. Gazzard, "Shigella in HIV infection," *AIDS*, vol. 5, no. 8, pp. 1031–1032, 1991.

[30] U. Marcus, P. Zucs, V. Bremer et al., "Shigellosis—a re-emerging sexually transmitted infection: outbreak in men having sex with men in Berlin," *International Journal of STD and AIDS*, vol. 15, no. 8, pp. 533–537, 2004.

[31] B. O'Sullivan, V. Delpech, G. Pontivivo et al., "Shigellosis linked to sex Venues, Australia," *Emerging Infectious Diseases*, vol. 8, no. 8, pp. 862–864, 2002.

[32] Z. Abidin, N. Iyngkaran, and S. D. Puthucheary, "Fulminant hepatic failure and shigella bacteremia," *Medical Journal of Malaysia*, vol. 38, no. 2, pp. 112–113, 1983.

[33] B. La Scola and D. Raoult, "Laboratory diagnosis of rickettsioses: current approaches to diagnosis of old and new rickettsial diseases," *Journal of Clinical Microbiology*, vol. 35, no. 11, pp. 2715–2727, 1997.

[34] J. H. McQuiston, C. Wiedeman, J. Singleton et al., "Inadequacy of IgM antibody tests for diagnosis of Rocky Mountain spotted fever," *American Journal of Tropical Medicine and Hygiene*, vol. 91, no. 4, pp. 767–770, 2014.

[35] F. Yang, J. Yang, X. Zhang et al., "Genome dynamics and diversity of Shigella species, the etiologic agents of bacillary dysentery," *Nucleic Acids Research*, vol. 33, no. 19, pp. 6445–6458, 2005.

[36] J. R. Johnson, "*Shigella* and *Escherichia coli* at the crossroads: machiavellian masqueraders or taxonomic treachery?" *Journal of Medical Microbiology*, vol. 49, pp. 583–585, 2000.

[37] A. Bizzini, C. Durussel, J. Bille, G. Greub, and G. Prod'hom, "Performance of matrix-assisted laser desorption ionization-time of flight mass spectrometry for identification of bacterial

strains routinely isolated in a clinical microbiology laboratory," *Journal of Clinical Microbiology*, vol. 48, no. 5, pp. 1549–1554, 2010.

[38] S. A. Neville, A. LeCordier, H. Ziochos et al., "Utility of matrix-assisted laser desorption ionization-time of flight mass spectrometry following introduction for routine laboratory bacterial identification," *Journal of Clinical Microbiology*, vol. 49, no. 8, pp. 2980–2984, 2011.

[39] H. Kruse, S. Kariuki, N. Søli, and Ö. Olsvik, "Multiresistant shigella species from african AIDS patients: antibacterial resistance patterns and application of the e-test for determination of minimum inhibitory concentration," *Scandinavian Journal of Infectious Diseases*, vol. 24, no. 6, pp. 733–739, 1992.

[40] S. Ashkenazi, I. Levy, V. Kazaronovski, and Z. Samra, "Growing antimicrobial resistance of Shigella isolates," *Journal of Antimicrobial Chemotherapy*, vol. 51, no. 2, pp. 427–429, 2003.

Delayed Awareness of the History of Barium Examination: Perforated Barium Appendicitis

Susumu Saigusa,[1] Masaki Ohi,[2] Satoshi Oki,[2,3] Takashi Ichikawa,[2,3] Minako Kobayashi,[2] Yasuhiro Inoue,[2] and Chikao Miki[1]

[1] *Department of Surgery, Iga City General Hospital, 831 Shijuku-cho, Iga, Mie 518-0823, Japan*
[2] *Department of Gastrointestinal and Pediatric Surgery, Mie University Hospital, 2-174 Edobashi, Tsu, Mie 514-8507, Japan*
[3] *Department of Surgery, Wakaba Hospital, 28-13 Minami-Chuo, Tsu, Mie 514-0832, Japan*

Correspondence should be addressed to Susumu Saigusa; saigusas@yahoo.co.jp

Academic Editor: Naohiko Koide

A 41-year-old man presented to our hospital with lower abdominal pain and a high-grade fever. Physical examination revealed rebound tenderness and guarding in the lower abdomen. Abdominal X-ray examination showed a radiopaque object in the right lower quadrant of the abdomen. Abdominal computed tomography (CT) demonstrated that the object had a strong artifact with over 10,000 Hounsfield units, as well as ascites around the terminal ileum. We diagnosed acute peritonitis with a suspicion of the perforation due to unknown foreign body and performed an emergency laparotomy. Operative findings showed a contained perforation of a phlegmonous appendicitis, and appendectomy was performed. The resected specimen demonstrated that the appendix contained a fecalith, and histopathological examination showed the crystal structure of barium sulfate in the lumen of the appendix. Unfortunately, we did not obtain the history of screening for gastric cancer using a barium examination one month prior to our appendectomy. Our experience demonstrates the importance of establishing a history of barium examinations of the gastrointestinal tract in a patient with a radiopaque object in the right lower quadrant of the abdomen for early diagnosis of barium appendicitis. Additionally, early diagnosis of barium appendicitis may affect the selection of surgical procedures.

1. Introduction

Barium appendicitis is a rare clinical entity and a known complication of barium examinations [1, 2]. The pathogenesis of barium appendicitis is unclear, however, and several mechanisms have been reported [3]. Radiographic differential diagnoses for a radiopaque object in the right lower quadrant of the abdomen include right ureteral lithiasis, colonic diverticulum with a calcified fecalith, and a foreign body. The shape and radiopaque density of an object on imaging is misleading and may not suggest barium appendicitis [4–6]. Therefore, comprehensive examination including medical history, physical examination, laboratory findings, and radiological imaging is required for the early diagnosis of barium appendicitis. We report a case wherein preoperative diagnosis of barium appendicitis was difficult due to the shape, location, and strength of the artifact of the object on CT.

2. Case Presentation

A 41-year-old man presented to our hospital with lower abdominal pain and a high-grade fever. Physical examination revealed rebound tenderness and guarding in the lower abdomen. Abdominal X-ray examination showed a radiopaque object suggestive of a foreign body in the right lower quadrant of the abdomen (Figure 1(a)). Abdominal contrast-enhanced computed tomography (CT) showed that the object had strong artifact with more than 10,000 Hounsfield units, as well as ascites around a thickened terminal ileum (Figures 1(b) and 1(c)). On laboratory investigation, C reactive protein (CRP) level was elevated at 13.55 mg/dl (normal range < 0.45 mg/dl), and white blood cell count was 9900/μl. We performed an emergency laparotomy given the patient's evidence of peritonitis on physical exam. Operative findings showed a contained perforation of a phlegmonous

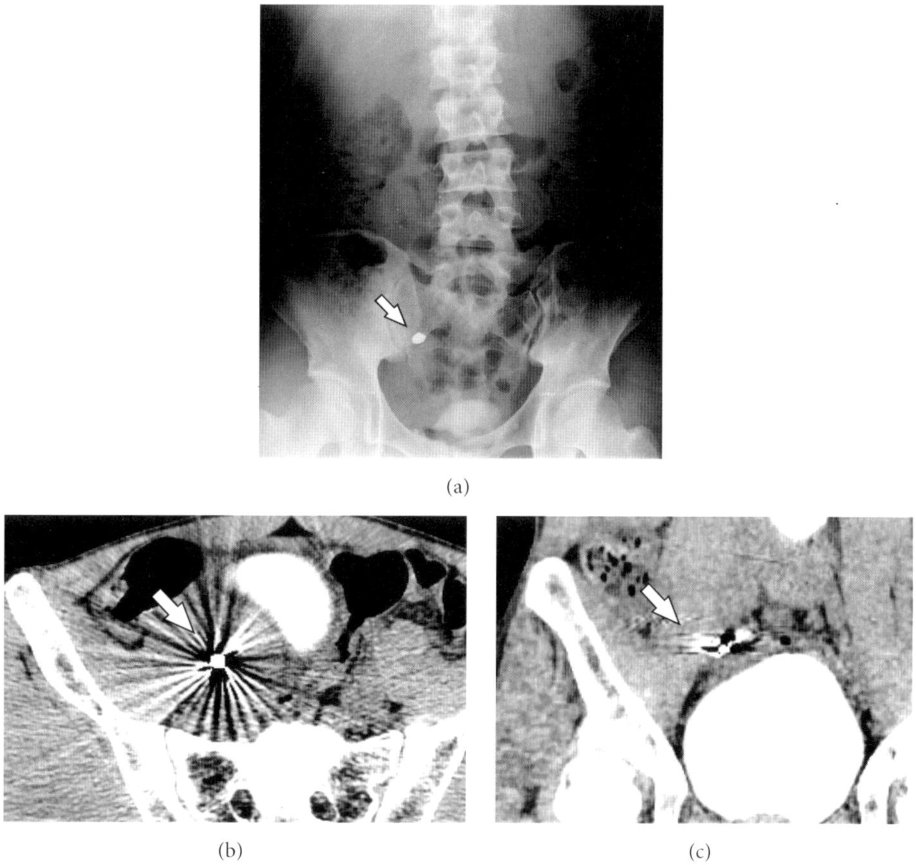

FIGURE 1: Abdominal X-ray examination. Radiopaque object consistent with a metallic foreign body in the right lower quadrant of the abdomen (a). Retained barium with strong artifact on axial (b) and coronal (c) views on abdominal CT.

appendicitis with purulent ascites, and appendectomy was performed. Intraoperative X-ray confirmed that the object was removed after appendectomy. The resected specimen had within it a fragile, white, fecalith (Figure 2(a)). Ascites cultures showed *Pseudomonas aeruginosa*. Histopathological examination showed ulceration, necrosis, and an abscess in the mucosal layer of the appendix and the crystal structure of barium sulfate in the lumen and within the abscess (Figures 2(b)–2(d)). We administered meropenem (1 g/day) from admission until the third postoperative day. Postoperatively, it was revealed to us that he had undergone screening for gastric cancer using barium one month earlier. The postoperative course was uneventful.

3. Discussion

Radiological findings of retained barium are variable [1], and they are frequently confused with metal foreign bodies. Adachi et al. reported an object in the right lower quadrant of the abdomen and, based on the shape and radio-density, led to a preoperative diagnosis of a localized intra-abdominal abscess due to ileocecal perforation secondary to a metallic foreign body such as a dental crown [5]. Similarly, we strongly suspected a foreign metal body in the appendix as the abdominal CT showed that the object had a strong artifact with over 10,000 Hounsfield units. Coronal and sagittal views on CT may aid in diagnosis of barium appendicitis, but differentiation of barium from a metallic object remains difficult. Therefore, a detailed medical history, physical examination, laboratory studies, and radiological imaging are required for early diagnosis of barium appendicitis. In particular, a history of gastrointestinal examination using barium is important. Li et al. reported that barium examination of the gastrointestinal tract has a time-dependent association with appendicitis risk [7].

Barium sulfate is widely used for gastrointestinal imaging and harmful complications are rare. Barium is usually excreted by patients within 3 days after gastrointestinal imaging [3]. However, there are several reports in the literature describing cases of barium appendicitis, with little known about the pathophysiology [2, 3, 8]. The interval before the development of barium appendicitis has been reported to range from a few hours to a few months [1]. Maglinte et al. reported on 31 patients with retained barium in the appendix for longer than 72 hours and followed them for 1 year. They failed to find any association between barium retention and the development of acute appendicitis [9]. This suggests that not all retained barium leads to appendicitis. Therefore, prophylactic appendectomy for retained barium in the appendix is not recommended [6]. On the other

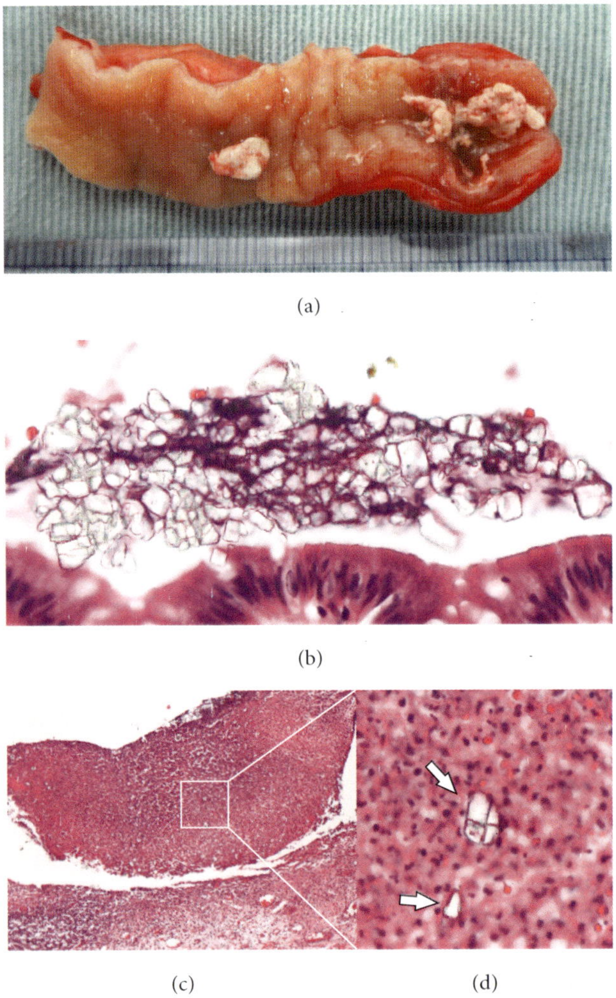

FIGURE 2: Resected specimen shows that the appendix contained a white, fragile fecalith. There was inflammation at the tip of the appendix (a). Crystal structure of barium sulfate on the mucosa (b) and in the infected fluid (c, d). Original magnification 200x (c), 400x (b, d).

hand, when barium appendicitis is definitively diagnosed, appendectomy should be immediately performed as barium appendicitis can lead to perforation [1].

Several authors reported the comparison of clinical outcome between open and laparoscopic appendectomy, and they concluded that laparoscopic appendectomy for acute appendicitis with or without its perforation had beneficial advantages including cost-effectiveness and decrease of wound infection [10–12]. However, we selected open appendectomy but not laparoscopic approach in the present case because we preoperatively could not diagnose barium appendicitis with peritonitis. If preoperative diagnosis of barium appendicitis was given, laparoscopic approach could be considered as an option for the treatment. Hence, early diagnosis of barium appendicitis may be important to make choice of surgical approach.

In conclusion, our experience indicates that barium appendicitis should be taken into consideration for patients with a radiopaque object in right lower quadrant abdomen. Emergency physicians especially should be aware of and alert to possibility of barium appendicitis when facing similar clinical course. Additionally, early diagnosis of barium appendicitis may be important for selection of surgical procedure.

Consent

Written informed consent was obtained from the patient for publication of this case report and any accompanying images.

References

[1] N. Cohen, D. Modai, A. Rosen, A. Golik, and J. Weissgarten, "Barium appendicitis: fact or fancy?: Report of a case and review of the literature," *Journal of Clinical Gastroenterology*, vol. 9, no. 4, pp. 447–451, 1987.

[2] Y.-J. Fang, H.-P. Wang, C.-M. Ho, and K.-L. Liu, "Barium appendicitis," *Surgery*, vol. 146, no. 5, pp. 957–958, 2009.

[3] J. M. Wu and J. T. Liang, "Education and Imaging. Gastrointestinal: barium-induced acute appendicitis," *Journal of gastroenterology and hepatology*, vol. 23, no. 7, part 1, p. 1159, 2008.

[4] N. M. Novotny, K. D. Lillemoe, and M. E. Falimirski, "Barium appendicitis after upper gastrointestinal imaging," *Journal of Emergency Medicine*, vol. 38, no. 2, pp. 148–149, 2010.

[5] M. Adachi, Y. Takahashi, M. Kume, A. Kurenuma, M. Motohashi, and Y. Muramatsu, "Barium-induced appendicitis mimicking accidental ingestion of a dental metal crown in radiological findings," *Clinical Journal of Gastroenterology*, vol. 7, no. 2, pp. 129–131, 2014.

[6] M. K. Sinha, R. K. Sinha, and K. Gaurav, "Retained barium in the appendix or right ureteric colic? A case report of surgeons dilemma," *International Journal of Surgery Case Reports*, vol. 7, pp. 23–25, 2015.

[7] H. Li, L. Yeh, Y. Huang, C. Lin, and C. Kao, "The association between barium examination and subsequent appendicitis: a nationwide population-based study," *The American Journal of Medicine*, vol. 130, no. 1, pp. 54.e5–60.e5, 2017.

[8] S. B. Palder and K. M. Dalessandri, "Barium appendicitis," *Western Journal of Medicine*, vol. 148, no. 4, pp. 462–464, 1988.

[9] D. D. T. Maglinte, M. L. Bush, E. V. Aruta, and G. E. Bullington, "Retained barium in the appendix: diagnostic and clinical significance," *American Journal of Roentgenology*, vol. 137, no. 3, pp. 529–533, 1981.

[10] X. Li, J. Zhang, L. Sang et al., "Laparoscopic versus conventional appendectomy—a meta-analysis of randomized controlled trials," *BMC Gastroenterology*, vol. 10, article 129, 2010.

[11] H.-B. Wei, J.-L. Huang, Z.-H. Zheng et al., "Laparoscopic versus open appendectomy: a prospective randomized comparison," *Surgical Endoscopy and Other Interventional Techniques*, vol. 24, no. 2, pp. 266–269, 2010.

[12] A. Yagmurlu, A. Vernon, D. C. Barnhart, K. E. Georgeson, and C. M. Harmon, "Laparoscopic appendectomy for perforated appendicitis: a comparison with open appendectomy," *Surgical Endoscopy and Other Interventional Techniques*, vol. 20, no. 7, pp. 1051–1054, 2006.

The Association of *Streptococcus gallolyticus* Subspecies *pasteurianus* Bacteremia with the Detection of Premalignant and Malignant Colonic Lesions

Gaurav Chand,[1] Leonid Shamban,[2] Adam Forman,[3] and Prabhat Sinha[4]

[1] *Department of Internal Medicine, Providence Hospital and Medical Center, 16001 W. Nine Mile Road, Southfield, MI 48075, USA*
[2] *Department of Gastroenterology, Genesys Regional Medical Center, One Genesys Parkway, Grand Blanc, MI 48439, USA*
[3] *Department of Hematology and Oncology, Providence Hospital and Medical Center, 16001 W. Nile Mile Road, Southfield, MI 48075, USA*
[4] *Department of Pulmonology and Critical Care, Providence Hospital and Medical Center, 16001 W. Nine Mile Road, Southfield, MI 48075, USA*

Correspondence should be addressed to Gaurav Chand; gauravchand.do@gmail.com

Academic Editor: Daniel C. Damin

Streptococcus gallolyticus subspecies (subsp.) *gallolyticus* (formerly *bovis* biotype I) bacteremia has been associated with colonic adenocarcinoma. The *bovis* species underwent reclassification in 2003. Subtypes of *gallolyticus* are associated with colonic malignancy but are less frequent, resulting in less awareness. A 71-year-old male admitted with worsening lower back pain and fevers. Initial vital signs and laboratory data were within normal limits. MRI revealed lumbosacral osteomyelitis and antibiotics were initiated. Blood cultures showed *Streptococcus* species, prompting a transesophageal echocardiogram (TEE) revealing vegetations on the mitral and aortic valves. The etiology for his endocarditis was unclear. A colonoscopy was suggested, but his clinical instability made such a procedure intolerable. Final cultures revealed *Streptococcus gallolyticus* subsp. *pasteurianus* (previously *bovis* biotype II). After antibiotic completion he underwent aortic grafting with valve replacements. Later, he was readmitted for *Streptococcus* bacteremia. After a negative TEE, colonoscopy revealed a 2.5 × 3 cm cecal tubulovillous adenoma with high-grade dysplasia suspicious for his origin of infection. Clinicians understand the link between *Streptococcus gallolyticus* subsp. *gallolyticus* (*bovis* type I) and malignancy, but the new speciation may be unfamiliar. There are no guidelines for managing *S. gallolyticus* subsp. *pasteurianus* bacteremia; therefore a colonoscopy should be considered when no source is identified.

1. Introduction

Streptococcus bovis biotype I bacteremia has been long associated with infective endocarditis due to an underlying colonic malignancy since its first documented case in 1951 [1]. Previous reports have suggested that *Streptococcus bovis* type I bacteremia has been implicated with concomitant colonic tumors in 25 to 80% of patients [1], as well as the presence of premalignant colonic lesions [2–4]. In the late 1990s and early 2000s, the *Streptococcus bovis* species underwent significant taxonomic changes that resulted in the renaming of *S. bovis* biotype I as *Streptococcus gallolyticus* subsp. *gallolyticus*, biotype II/1 as *S. lutetiensis* (i.e., *S. infantarius* subsp. *infantarius*), and biotype II/2 as *S. gallolyticus* subsp. *pasteurianus* [3, 4]. Multiple reports show that *Streptococcus gallolyticus* subtypes are also associated with colonic malignancy; however, they are less frequent compared to *Streptococcus gallolyticus* subsp. *gallolyticus* [5, 6]. Years later, many clinicians continue to be unfamiliar with the new speciation [7]. Therefore, these organism findings in clinical practice must be highlighted to make clinicians more comfortable with their management. Herein, we report a rarely associated entity of *S. gallolyticus* subsp. *pasteurianus* bacteremia and infective endocarditis with subsequent detection of a tubulovillous adenoma with high-grade dysplasia.

2. Case Report

A 70-year-old Caucasian male presented to the hospital with complaints of progressively worsening low back pain radiating into his bilateral hips ongoing for the past six weeks. Initially, the patient saw a physician in the outpatient setting who evaluated his back pain with a magnetic resonance imaging test (MRI) that revealed degenerative disc disease at the L_5-S_1 level. He was prompted to come to the hospital as his pain significantly worsened over the past ten days resulting in the inability to ambulate. He denied any symptoms of neurological impairment. Additionally, he was noted to be experiencing fevers and chills for the past few weeks, which he attributed to his history of chronic prostatitis.

His past medical history is remarkable for hypertension, hyperlipidemia, chronic prostatitis, and benign prostatic hypertrophy. The patient is retired from the automotive business, lives with his wife, and reported no use of tobacco, alcohol, or illicit drugs. He reported no recent travel. His initial vital signs yielded a blood pressure of 118/74 mmHg, heart rate of 135 beats per minute, respiratory rate of 17 breaths per minute, temperature of 98.5° Fahrenheit (F), and an oxygen saturation of 96 percent on room air. Physical exam revealed a well-nourished male, who was alert and oriented to person, place, time, and situation. Cranial nerves II–XII were grossly intact bilaterally with +5/5 gross bilateral upper extremity strength and +4/5 gross bilateral lower extremity strength. Sensation to noxious and tactile stimuli was intact. Deep tendon reflexes were equal and +1/4 in bilateral lower extremities. The patient experienced significant back pain during the examination, while the rest of his physical exam was unremarkable including his cardiac exam.

Complete blood count results included a white blood cell count, 11.2 K/μL; hemoglobin, 13.1 g/dL; hematocrit, 38.7%; and platelets, 144 K/μL. Chemistry panel showed sodium, 133 mmol/L; potassium, 4.1 mmol/L; chloride, 98 mmol/L; CO_2, 24 mmol/L; blood urea nitrogen, 22 mg/dL; and creatinine, 0.9 mg/dL. An initial computed tomography scan (CT scan) without contrast of the abdomen and pelvis showed nonobstructing renal stones, and a magnetic resonance imaging study (MRI) of the lumbosacral spine showed changes consistent with L_3-L_4 and L_5-S_1 osteomyelitis. Blood cultures were drawn, and the patient was admitted with the diagnosis of lumbosacral osteomyelitis. He was started on broad-spectrum antibiotics. The following day, preliminary blood cultures revealed beta-hemolytic *Streptococcus* bacteremia in two out of two sets, and antibiotics were adjusted to intravenous vancomycin and gentamycin.

During the hospital course, the patient continued to complain of weakness, fatigue, and some chest discomfort despite intravenous antibiotic therapy. A transthoracic echocardiogram exhibited vegetations on mitral and aortic valves, mildly dilated aorta, and a moderate-sized mass on the noncoronary cusp measuring 1.2 by 1.0 centimeters with preserved ejection fraction. These findings prompted a transesophageal echocardiogram that revealed an aortic wall abscess with a mobile tip and vegetations over the mitral valve accompanied by severe mitral valve regurgitation and aortic valve incompetence. Final blood cultures were consistent with *Streptococcus gallolyticus* subsp. *pasteurianus*, and antibiotic therapy was tailored to intravenous ceftriaxone and gentamycin. Due to this discovery, a concern for a colonic etiology arose, as this species is a variant of the previous *Streptococcus bovis* species. However, these results could not be further investigated due the patient's clinical status.

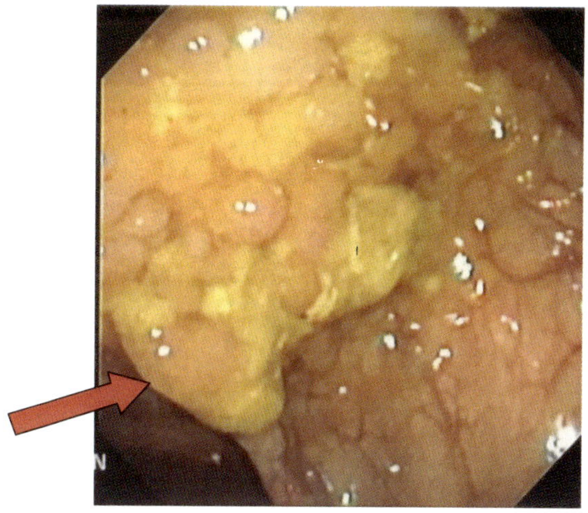

FIGURE 1: Colonoscopy. Colonoscopy findings revealing a 2.5 × 1.0 cm cecal mass.

The patient developed problems with his neck mobility that prompted a CT scan that revealed cervical spine discitis at C_5-C_6 level, which was later confirmed by MRI. Subsequently, the patient underwent three operations over the course of the next two weeks. Neurosurgery had operated on the patient's cervical and lumbosacral discitis in two separate surgeries. Cardiothoracic surgery replaced the patient's mitral and aortic valves and placed an ascending aortic graft due to an aneurysm. Following these surgical procedures and stabilization, the patient was discharged to a subacute rehabilitation facility with a peripherally inserted central catheter for twelve weeks of intravenous ceftriaxone infusion.

After undergoing months of rehabilitation, the patient was readmitted five months from his initial presentation for pyrexia of 100.4°F. Blood cultures were obtained and revealed two out of two sets consistent with gram positive cocci in clusters resembling *Streptococcus*. The patient was reevaluated for osteomyelitis and MRI of the cervical, thoracic, and lumbar spine revealed no acute infection. An endocarditis workup was also unremarkable. The final report for blood cultures showed *Lactococcus garvieae*, and an evaluation for a colonoscopy was undertaken, since there have been few case reports relating colonic pathology as the source of the bacteremia [8, 9]. The patient was advised to have a colonoscopy in the outpatient setting after being discharged from the rehab center, but he did not comply. Colonoscopy revealed a 2.5 by 3.0 centimeter cecal mass (Figure 1), two sessile descending colonic polyps, and mild internal hemorrhoids.

Final pathology yielded a tubulovillous adenoma in the cecum (Figure 2) and hyperplastic polyps in the descending colon.

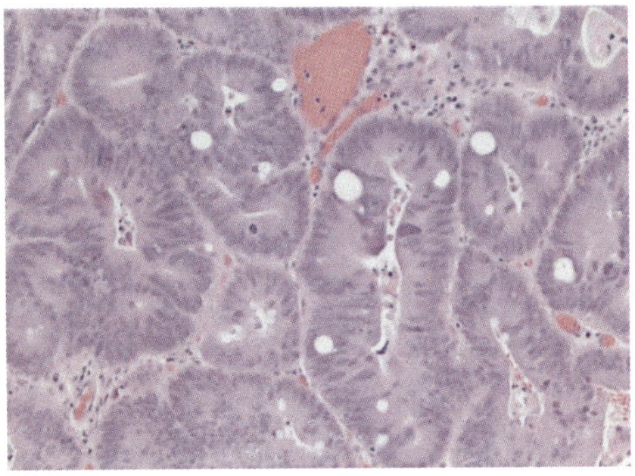

FIGURE 2: Pathology slide. Pathology exhibiting a tubulovillous adenoma with high-grade dysplasia shown under H&E staining at 40x magnification.

TABLE 1: Previous and current classifications of *Streptococcus bovis* and their respective associations with colorectal cancer (CRC).

Previous nomenclature	Current nomenclature	Association with CRC
S. bovis biotype I	*S. gallolyticus* subsp. *gallolyticus*	++++
S. bovis biotype II/1	*S. infantarius* subsp. *infantarius*	++
	S. lutetiensis	++
S. bovis biotype II/2	*S. gallolyticus* subsp. *pasteurianus*	+
	S. gallolyticus subsp. *macedonicus*	–

At this time, the patient was discharged with intravenous vancomycin for three weeks. After completing antibiotic therapy, the patient underwent a right-sided hemicolectomy, and the final surgical pathology showed a tubulovillous adenoma with high-grade dysplasia. Following stabilization during the postoperative period, the patient was discharged in fair condition to a subacute rehabilitation facility.

3. Discussion

In the preceding case, our patient exhibited profound recurrent systemic bacteremia that was eventually attributed to a colonic source. Many clinicians understand the link between *Streptococcus gallolyticus* subsp. *gallolyticus* (*bovis* type I) and malignancy, but the new speciation may be unfamiliar to practitioners. *S. gallolyticus* subsp. *gallolyticus* has a much greater association than *S. gallolyticus* subsp. *pasteurianus* with colonic malignancies as is depicted in Table 1 [10].

In a literature review, the association of *S. gallolyticus* subsp. *gallolyticus* bacteremia was 94% and 71% with clinical infectious endocarditis and underlying colonic malignancy, respectively [11]. However, *S. gallolyticus* subsp. *pasteurianus* bacteremia is less commonly associated with infective endocarditis and occult colonic malignancy at rates of 18% and 17%, respectively [11]. Regardless of the weaker association of *S. gallolyticus* subsp. *pasteurianus* with underlying colonic pathology, we strongly believe that patients exhibiting any *S. bovis* bacteremia (type I or II) should undergo a screening colonoscopy. It has also been noted in previous studies that *S. bovis* is also associated with premalignant colonic lesions, which are often asymptomatic and undetectable by fecal occult blood testing [12].

Interestingly, confounding in this case is the readmission of bacteremia with a different organism, *Lactococcus garvieae*. This organism has been associated in contact with raw fish [9]. However, in our case the origin was not known. It did prompt an inpatient colonoscopy evaluation. There have been few case reports that suggest gastrointestinal risk factors in recent literature such as colonic diverticulosis, duodenal ulcers, and colonic polyps, but the evidence is poor [8, 9]. It is difficult to draw a conclusion that the patient's *Lactococcus garvieae* bacteremia was the result of the colonic pathology. However, there is more literature to support that *S. gallolyticus* subsp. *pasteurianus* bacteremia warrants colonic evaluation.

As there are no guidelines for managing patients with *S. gallolyticus* subsp. *pasteurianus* bacteremia, a colonoscopy should be considered as a part of the evaluation when no definitive source is identifiable. These premalignant lesions may progress to malignant colon cancers over the course of years and addressing these lesions earlier in their clinical course would prove beneficial to the patient in decreasing overall morbidity and mortality. Early detection of premalignant and malignant colonic lesions saves lives, and the discovery of such bacteremia should be investigated with a screening colonoscopy.

References

[1] A. S. Abdulamir, R. R. Hafidh, and F. Abu Bakar, "The association of *Streptococcus bovis/gallolyticus* with colorectal tumors: the nature and the underlying mechanisms of its etiological role," *Journal of Experimental and Clinical Cancer Research*, vol. 30, no. 1, article 11, 2011.

[2] A. Kahveci, E. Ari, H. Arikan, M. Koc, S. Tuglular, and C. Ozener, "*Streptococcus bovis* bacteremia related to colon adenoma in a chronic hemodialysis patient," *Hemodialysis International*, vol. 14, no. 1, pp. 91–93, 2010.

[3] A. S. Abdulamir, R. R. Hafidh, L. K. Mahdi, T. Al-jeboori, and F. Abubaker, "Investigation into the controversial association of Streptococcus gallolyticus with colorectal cancer and adenoma," *BMC Cancer*, vol. 9, article 403, 2009.

[4] A. Murinello, P. Mendonca, C. Ho et al., "Streptococcus gallolyticus bacteraemia associated with colonic adenomatous polyps," *Jornal Português de Gastrenterologia*, vol. 13, no. 3, pp. 152–156, 2006.

[5] J. Corredoira, M. P. Alonso, A. Coira, and J. Varela, "Association between Streptococcus infantarius (formerly *S. bovis* II/1) bacteremia and noncolonic cancer," *Journal of Clinical Microbiology*, vol. 46, no. 4, article 1570, 2008.

[6] A. Boleij, M. M. H. J. Van Gelder, D. W. Swinkels, and H. Tjalsma, "Clinical importance of *Streptococcus gallolyticus*

infection among colorectal cancer patients: systematic review and meta-analysis," *Clinical Infectious Diseases*, vol. 53, no. 9, pp. 870–878, 2011.

[7] B. Romero, M.-I. Morosini, E. Loza et al., "Reidentification of *Streptococcus bovis* isolates causing bacteremia according to the new taxonomy criteria: still an issue?" *Journal of Clinical Microbiology*, vol. 49, no. 9, pp. 3228–3233, 2011.

[8] G. Russo, M. Iannetta, A. D'Abramo et al., "Lactococcus garvieae endocarditis in a patient with colonic diverticulosis: first case report in Italy and review of the literature," *New Microbiologica*, vol. 35, no. 4, pp. 495–501, 2012.

[9] V. Heras Cañas, M. D. Pérez Ramirez, F. Bermudez Jiménez et al., "*Lactococcus garvieae*endocarditis in a native valve identified by MALDI-TOF MS and PCR-based 16s rRNA in Spain: a case report," *New Microbes and New Infections*, vol. 5, pp. 13–15, 2015.

[10] A. A. Khan, *Bacteria and Cancer*, Springer, Dordrecht, The Netherlands, 2012.

[11] N. Takamura, T. Kenzaka, K. Minami, and M. Matsumura, "Infective endocarditis caused by *Streptococcus gallolyticus* subspecies pasteurianus and colon cancer," *BMJ Case Reports*, 2014.

[12] A. Boleij, R. M. J. Schaeps, and H. Tjalsma, "Association between *Streptococcus bovis* and colon cancer," *Journal of Clinical Microbiology*, vol. 47, no. 2, article 516, 2009.

47

Endoscopic Observation of the Growth Process of a Right-Side Sessile Serrated Adenoma/Polyp with Cytological Dysplasia to an Invasive Submucosal Adenocarcinoma

Kaoru Omori,[1] Kanako Yoshida,[1] Sadafumi Tamiya,[2] Tsutomu Daa,[3] and Masahiro Kan[1]

[1] *Department of Gastroenterology and Hepatology, Sato Daiichi Hospital, 77-1 Hokyoji, Usa, Oita 879-0454, Japan*
[2] *Department of Pathology, Kitakyushu Medical Center, 2-1-1 Bashaku, Kitakyushu, Fukuoka 802-0077, Japan*
[3] *Department of Pathology, Graduate School of Medicine, Faculty of Medicine, Oita University, 1-1 Idaigaoka, Yufu, Oita 879-5593, Japan*

Correspondence should be addressed to Masahiro Kan; meitokukai-kan@sato-d1.com

Academic Editor: Daniel C. Damin

A sessile serrated adenoma/polyp (SSA/P) with cytological dysplasia in the right colon, which transformed to an invasive submucosal adenocarcinoma finally, was endoscopically observed in a 76-year-old woman. A whitish soft SSA/P (approximately 25 mm in diameter) was detected in the cecum. Biopsy samples were obtained from the small nodule, and the lesion was eventually diagnosed as an SSA/P with cytological dysplasia, considering endoscopic observations, among which the narrow-band imaging features suggested that the lesion was adenomatous, that is, a round-oval pattern, and hyperplastic, that is, comprising a circular pattern with dots and an invisible capillary vessel. After 11 months, an SSA/P had rapidly developed into a submucosal adenocarcinoma with lymphatic infiltrations, and the most aggressive deep invasion was observed in the central depression. This case suggests that right-side SSA/Ps with cytological dysplasia should be removed immediately, considering the potential for rapid progression to a larger size and eventually to deep and extensive cancer.

1. Introduction

According to the traditional theory of colorectal carcinogenesis involving an adenoma-carcinoma sequence, adenoma is recognized as a precursor lesion of colorectal cancer. In recent years, serrated lesions, including hyperplastic polyps (HPs), traditional serrated adenomas, and sessile serrated adenomas/polyps (SSA/Ps), have been increasingly recognized as being precursor lesions of colorectal cancer [1]. Among these serrated lesions, SSA/Ps have unique characteristics with regard to their clinical and genetic background, such as a proximal dominant location, high frequency of BRAF mutations, and a CpG island methylator phenotype [2]. Therefore, SSA/Ps have been regarded as precursor lesions for colorectal cancer. Although SSA/Ps have been reported to show rapid growth to an early cancer [3], few reports have elucidated the rapid progression speed of SSA/Ps to a large size and associated morphological changes during the transition to an adenocarcinoma sequentially. Here we report a rare case of the endoscopic observation of colon cancer which transformed sequentially from a large right-side SSA/P with cytological dysplasia to an invasive submucosal adenocarcinoma with lymphatic infiltrations, and the most aggressive deep invasion was observed in the central depression.

2. Case Presentation

A 76-year-old woman with diabetes mellitus visited our hospital for routine follow-up. Physical examination revealed no abnormalities. Except for her glucose metabolism, no abnormalities were observed on routine laboratory examinations, including blood biochemistry for serum tumor markers such as carcinoembryonic antigen and carbohydrate antigen 19-9. A laterally spreading soft lesion was detected in the cecum (Figures 1(a)–1(d)). Observation using colonoscopy showed

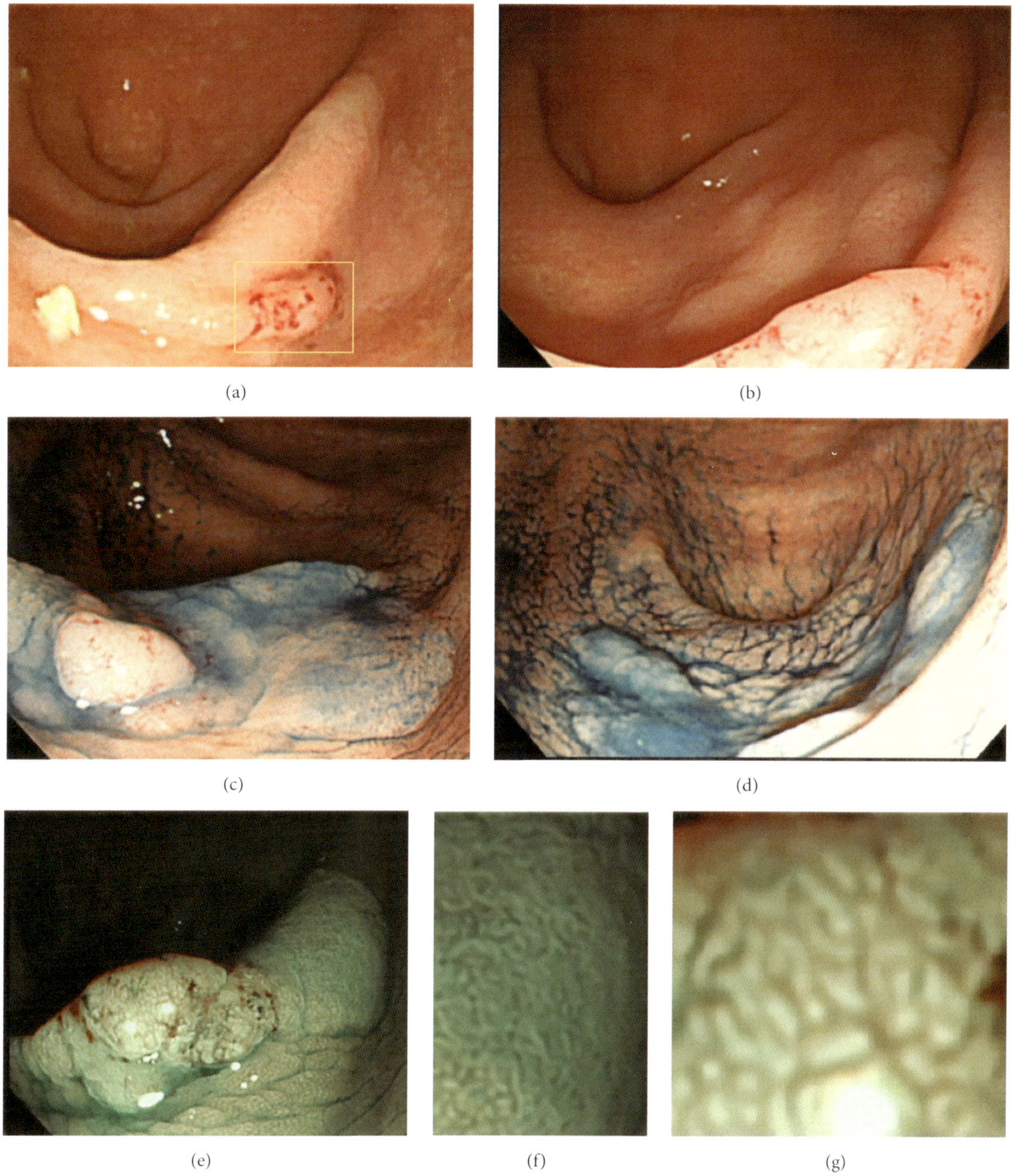

Figure 1: ((a) and (b)) Conventional endoscopic view of a sessile serrated adenoma/polyp (SSA/P) in the cecum. The SSA/P was observed as a whitish laterally spreading soft lesion (approximately 25 mm in diameter) that harbored a small nodule with adhesion of some blood (approximately 5 mm in diameter). ((c) and (d)) Chromoendoscopic view of an SSA/P stained with indigo carmine. The edges and a small nodule of the lesion are emphasized. (e) Endoscopic view of an SSA/P with narrow-band imaging. (f) A pattern with a central dark area surrounded by a clear lighter area, so-called circular pattern with dots, was observed mostly. (g) A central light area surrounded by a dark outer area, so-called round-oval pattern, was observed in a small nodule.

a small nodule with adhesion of some blood (approximately 5 mm in diameter) and a whitish laterally spreading soft lesion (approximately 25 mm in diameter) (Figures 1(a)–1(d)). On narrow-band imaging (NBI), a pattern with a central dark area surrounded by a clear lighter area, that is, a circular pattern with dots, and an invisible capillary vessel, were observed as hyperplastic features, whereas a central light area surrounded by a dark outer area, that is, a round-oval pattern, was observed as an adenomatous feature in a small nodule (Figures 1(e)–1(g)). Therefore, biopsy samples were obtained from the nodule presenting with an adenomatous feature (Figure 2), and the lesion was

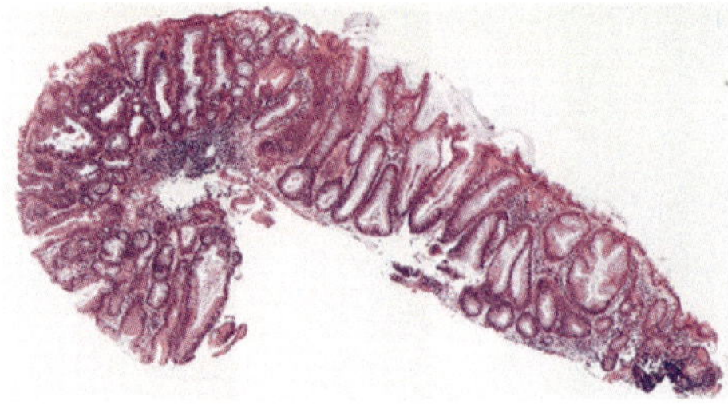

Figure 2: Pathological findings of the biopsy sample obtained from the small nodule (yellow box in Figure 1(a)). Hematoxylin-eosin staining of the sections of the biopsy sample revealed histologic features of a sessile serrated adenoma/polyp with cytological dysplasia at the curved portion (×40).

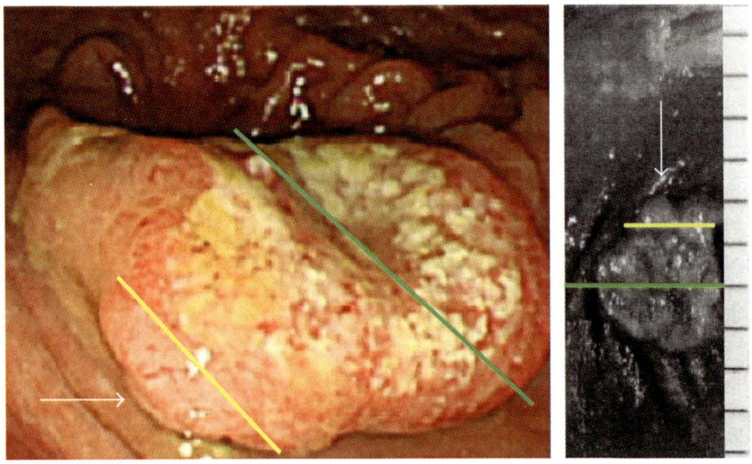

Figure 3: Conventional endoscopic view of a cancer arising from a sessile serrated adenoma/polyp. An elevated lesion with a central depression was observed at the same site in the cecum where a small nodule had been identified previously (white arrow).

eventually diagnosed as an SSA/P with cytological dysplasia, considering the endoscopic observations including the NBI features. The potential risk of progression to cancer was explained to the patient, because of the SSA/P features, that is, location in a right-side colon, being of large size, and being with cytological dysplasia. Endoscopic submucosal dissection was thought to be feasible but was not performed at the patient's request. After 11 months, follow-up colonoscopy was performed. At the same site in the cecum, an elevated lesion with a central depression was observed, where a small nodule had been identified earlier on the basis of the similar appearance and location of the nodule in both the cancer and SSA/P (Figure 3). Biopsy samples were obtained from the central depression site, and the elevated lesion was eventually diagnosed as a moderately differentiated adenocarcinoma. Based on these endoscopic findings, an invasive adenocarcinoma arising from the SSA/P was suspected. Endoscopic resection could not be performed and the lesion was removed surgically. The pathological diagnosis was a moderately differentiated adenocarcinoma extending 2700 μm into the submucosal layer with a mucin pool, lymphatic infiltration (Figures 4(a) and 4(b)), in which the most aggressive deep invasion was observed in a central depression (Figures 4(a) and 4(b)), and a remaining SSA/P with/without cytological dysplasia component that was detected at the periphery of the invasive cancer (Figures 5(a) and 5(b)). Neither recurrence nor metastasis of colon cancer has been detected in the patient till now.

3. Discussion

We report a rare case of an SSA/P with cytological dysplasia progressing to an invasive submucosal adenocarcinoma with lymphatic infiltrations accompanied by distinct morphological changes as observed endoscopically. This case provides information on the risk of malignant transformation of an SSA/P with cytological dysplasia and its management in the right colon. Serrated lesions, including HPs, traditional serrated adenomas, and SSA/Ps, are precursor lesions in the new carcinogenesis pathway for colorectal cancer [1]. SSA/Ps located in the right colon have been considered to be high-risk lesions for progression to colorectal cancer [4]; however, they are sometimes difficult to identify and diagnose correctly by endoscopy because of their flat growth pattern, fuzzy appearance, and presence of abundant mucous [5]. Unmagnified NBI endoscopy enables better visualization of enhanced pit and capillary patterns, which showed fairly good agreement for the high accuracy of real-time histology prediction [6, 7]. Because magnified NBI endoscopy is not widely used, the findings of unmagnified NBI endoscopy

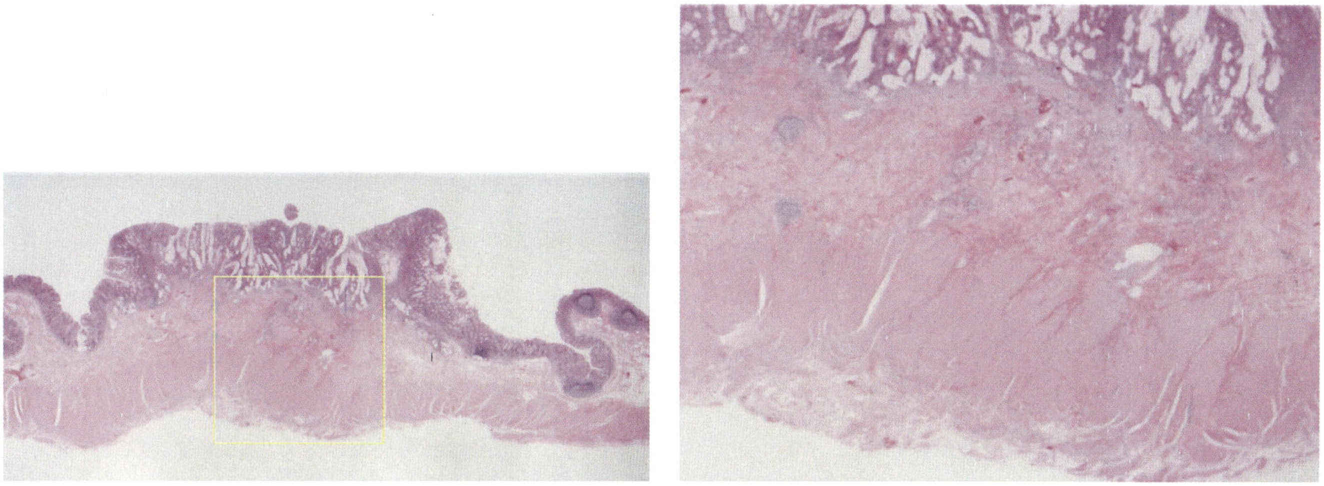

(a) (b)

FIGURE 4: (a) Pathological findings of the resected lesion (approximately 40 mm in diameter). Hematoxylin-eosin staining of the sections of the resected specimen revealed a moderately differentiated adenocarcinoma that extended into the submucosal layer to a depth of 2700 μm with mucin pools and lymphatic infiltrations (green line in Figure 3, ×4). (b) A magnified view of the most aggressive deep infiltration site of submucosal invasion (yellow box in (a), ×40).

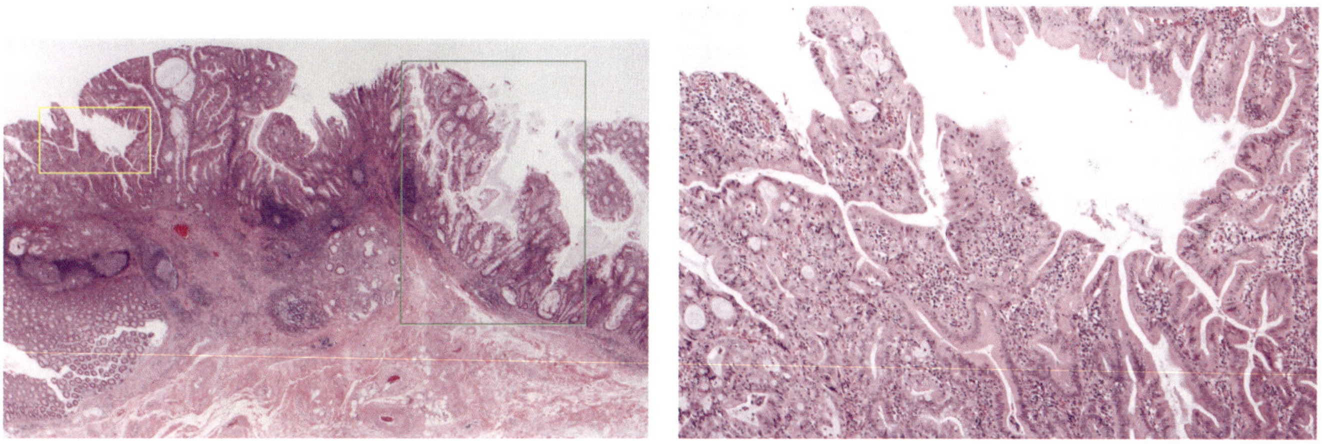

(a) (b)

FIGURE 5: (a) A component of the sessile serrated adenoma/polyp (SSA/P) remained at the periphery of the invasive cancer (yellow line in Figure 3, ×12.5). The green box indicated a component of the SSA/P without cytological dysplasia. (b) A magnified view of a yellow box in (a). Histologically, a transition from the SSA/P with cytological dysplasia to a moderately differentiated adenocarcinoma was identified (×200).

are always important, similar to the usefulness of magnified NBI endoscopy. The lesion was eventually diagnosed as an SSA/P with cytological dysplasia, considering the pathological findings of the biopsy samples and the endoscopic observations, among which the NBI features suggested that the lesion was adenomatous, that is, a round-oval pattern, and hyperplastic, that is, comprising a circular pattern with dots and an invisible capillary vessel [6, 7]. The cancer was found at the same site 11 months later, arising from the SSA/P; the NBI feature of adenocarcinoma has been reported to show an irregular pattern [6]. Histologically, the resected lesion was finally diagnosed as a moderately differentiated adenocarcinoma extending 2700 μm into the submucosal layer with lymphatic infiltrations. SSA/Ps are believed to become serrated pathway cancers via a series of molecular alternations, including BRAF mutation and CpG island methylation, with epigenetic inactivation of the mismatch repair gene MLH1 resulting in microsatellite instability [5]. The first question is why such molecular alternations and transitions to colorectal cancer happened rapidly. The characteristicsof serrated lesions require further research. Although there has been a significant reduction in the incidence of colorectal cancer in the left colon, the incidence and mortality rates for colorectal cancer in the right colon have not decreased in recent years [8]. It is very likely that a significant proportion of these cancers evolve from SSA/Ps that are undetectable during primary colonoscopy [9]. It is believed that up to 20% of all colorectal cancers arise through a serrated lesion pathway [10]. As observed in the present case, where an SSA/P presents a high risk of growing larger relatively quickly and rapidly progressing to an invasive cancer with deep infiltrations within 11 months, although it was previously reported that the progression rate of SSA/P-derived cancers was likely to be variable, some are rapid and some are gradual [11]. To reduce the incidence of colorectal cancers in the right colon, gastroenterologists need to recognize and possibly remove SSA/Ps with cytological dysplasia immediately, considering the potential for rapid progression to a larger size and eventually to deep extensive cancer. As observed in our case, the small nodule of the SSA/P was considered to preserve after progression to an invasive carcinoma on the basis of the similar appearance and location of the nodule in both the cancer and SSA/P. On the other hand, the most aggressive deep infiltration was observed in the central depression of the cancer. Thus, the progression to the invasive cancer may occur in the center of the SSA/P. Considering a previous report, the center in SSA/Ps may always be the most aggressive deep infiltration site, when it transforms to cancer [3]. It was reported that the very limited intramucosal carcinoma arising in an SSA/P showed deep invasion from crypt bases [11]. Thus, the cancer arising in SSA/Ps may be characterized by deep invasion from crypt bases, not by permeation to the surface, resulting in the difficulty of early detection of abnormal endoscopic findings. Therefore, leaving a right-side SSA/P with cytological dysplasia untreated for several months is dangerous in SSA/P-derived cancers. If a right-side SSA/P with cytological dysplasia is not immediately removed, it should certainly be removed within a short period. On the other hand, it is thought that many SSA/Ps do not have the potential risk of invasive cancer progression. To facilitate a precise therapeutic approach, accumulation of additional detailed cases is necessary to further clarify the clinical characteristics of SSA/Ps with the potential risk of invasive cancer progression.

Consent

Informed consent was obtained from the patient.

Authors' Contributions

Masahiro Kan is the paper guarantor. Each author contributed equally to the creation of this paper.

Acknowledgments

The authors are grateful to Dr. Takeshi Okamoto, Institute for Department of Gastroenterology and Hepatology, Yamaguchi University Graduate School of Medicine, Japan, for his support in revising the paper.

References

[1] C. S. Huang, F. A. Farraye, S. Yang, and M. J. O'Brien, "The clinical significance of serrated polyps," *The American Journal of Gastroenterology*, vol. 106, no. 2, pp. 229–240, 2011.

[2] P. Minoo, M. P. Moyer, and J. R. Jass, "Role of BRAF-V600E in the serrated pathway of colorectal tumourigenesis," *The Journal of Pathology*, vol. 212, no. 2, pp. 124–133, 2007.

[3] Y. Oono, K. Fu, H. Nakamura et al., "Progression of a sessile serrated adenoma to an early invasive cancer within 8 months," *Digestive Diseases and Sciences*, vol. 54, no. 4, pp. 906–909, 2009.

[4] F.-J. Lu, D. W. van Niekerk, D. Owen, S. P. L. Tha, D. A. Turbin, and D. L. Webber, "Longitudinal outcome study of sessile serrated adenomas of the colorectum: an increased risk for subsequent right-sided colorectal carcinoma," *The American Journal of Surgical Pathology*, vol. 34, no. 7, pp. 927–934, 2010.

[5] D. Moussata, G. Boschetti, M. Chauvenet et al., "Endoscopic and histologic characteristics of serrated lesions," *World Journal of Gastroenterology*, vol. 21, no. 10, pp. 2896–2904, 2015.

[6] B. J. Kim, M. I. Park, S. J. Park et al., "Differential diagnosis of colorectal polyps with narrow band imaging colonoscopy without magnification," *The Korean Journal of Gastroenterology*, vol. 63, no. 5, pp. 276–282, 2014.

[7] A. Rastogi, J. Keighley, V. Singh et al., "High accuracy of narrow band imaging without magnification for the real-time characterization of polyp histology and its comparison with high-definition white light colonoscopy: a prospective study," *The American Journal of Gastroenterology*, vol. 104, no. 10, pp. 2422–2430, 2009.

[8] H. Brenner, M. Hoffmeister, V. Arndt, C. Stegmaier, L. Altenhofen, and U. Haug, "Protection from right- and left-sided colorectal neoplasms after colonoscopy: population-based study," *Journal of the National Cancer Institute*, vol. 102, no. 2, pp. 89–95, 2010.

[9] G. Michalopoulos and C. Tzathas, "Serrated polyps of right colon: guilty or innocent?" *Annals of Gastroenterology*, vol. 26, no. 3, pp. 212–219, 2013.

[10] W. M. Grady, "CIMP and colon cancer gets more complicated," *Gut*, vol. 56, no. 11, pp. 1498–1500, 2007.

[11] S. Ban, H. Mitomi, H. Horiguchi, H. Sato, and M. Shimizu, "Adenocarcinoma arising in small sessile serrated adenoma/polyp (SSA/P) of the colon: clinicopathological study of eight lesions," *Pathology International*, vol. 64, no. 3, pp. 123–132, 2014.

Urticarial Vasculitis-Associated Intestinal Ischemia

Uni Wong,[1] Harris Yfantis,[2] and Guofeng Xie[3]

[1] *Division of Gastroenterology and Hepatology, University of Maryland Medical Center, Baltimore, MD 21201, USA*
[2] *Department of Pathology, Veterans Affairs Maryland Health Care System, University of Maryland School of Medicine, Baltimore, MD 21201, USA*
[3] *Division of Gastroenterology and Hepatology, Veterans Affairs Maryland Health Care System, University of Maryland School of Medicine, Baltimore, MD 21201, USA*

Correspondence should be addressed to Guofeng Xie; gxie@medicine.umaryland.edu

Academic Editor: Maria Teresa Bardella

Urticarial vasculitis (UV) is a rare small vessel vasculitis. UV is often idiopathic but can also present in the context of autoimmune disorders such as systemic lupus erythematosus, drug reactions, infections, or a paraneoplastic syndrome. Extracutaneous complications include intestinal ischemic injuries, in UV patients with nonspecific gastrointestinal symptoms such as abdominal pain and nausea. Prompt recognition and treatment can minimize morbidity and mortality. This paper describes a case of urticarial vasculitis-associated intestinal ischemia.

1. Introduction

Urticarial vasculitis (UV) is a rare diagnosis with incidence rate of 4.5 per 100,000 person-years [1]. Majority of cases reported are idiopathic, but UV has been associated with autoimmune disorders, infections, drug reactions, and paraneoplastic syndrome [2]. The condition is characterized by cutaneous manifestations of urticaria along with histopathologic findings of leukocytoclastic vasculitis of the small vessels [3–5]. Pathogenesis of UV is thought to be due to formation and attachment of immune complexes in the walls of small blood vessels, resulting in angioedema, ischemia, and/or necrosis. As a result, clinical manifestations of UV can vary, ranging from urticaria with minimal extracutaneous involvement to a more severe form where patients can have minimal urticaria but have life-threatening multiorgan dysfunction [2]. It can be further classified into normocomplementemic and hypocomplementemic where those patients with low complement levels tend to have poorer prognosis [2]. Therefore, prompt recognition and management of UV are vital in minimizing morbidity and potentially life-threatening complications. We present a case where a patient presenting with abdominal pain was found to have intestinal ischemia in setting of urticarial vasculitis.

2. Case Presentation

A 62-year-old African American woman was seen by the gastroenterology consult service for evaluation of diffuse abdominal pain and nausea. Patient was initially seen in the hospital for an infected wound at her left ankle where she recently had a lipoma resected. After getting an incision and drainage of the infected wound, she was treated with clindamycin that was complicated by a skin rash that developed three days later on her bilateral upper and lower extremities. The rash was characterized as erythematous tender papules that were extremely pruritic (Figure 1(a)). She received hydroxyzine and diphenhydramine for symptomatic management. Her antimicrobial therapy was then switched from clindamycin to doxycycline. Patient subsequently developed persistent diffuse abdominal pain, mild hematochezia, and nausea/vomiting. She denied any fever/chills, night sweats, or weight loss. Pertinent review of systems was otherwise unremarkable.

Workup consisted of an abdominal CT scan which revealed thickening and stranding associated with the distal duodenum and proximal jejunum. There was no evidence of large vessel narrowing or significant atherosclerosis on imaging. Skin biopsy showed small vessel vasculitis (vascular damage with intense infiltrates of neutrophils and scattered

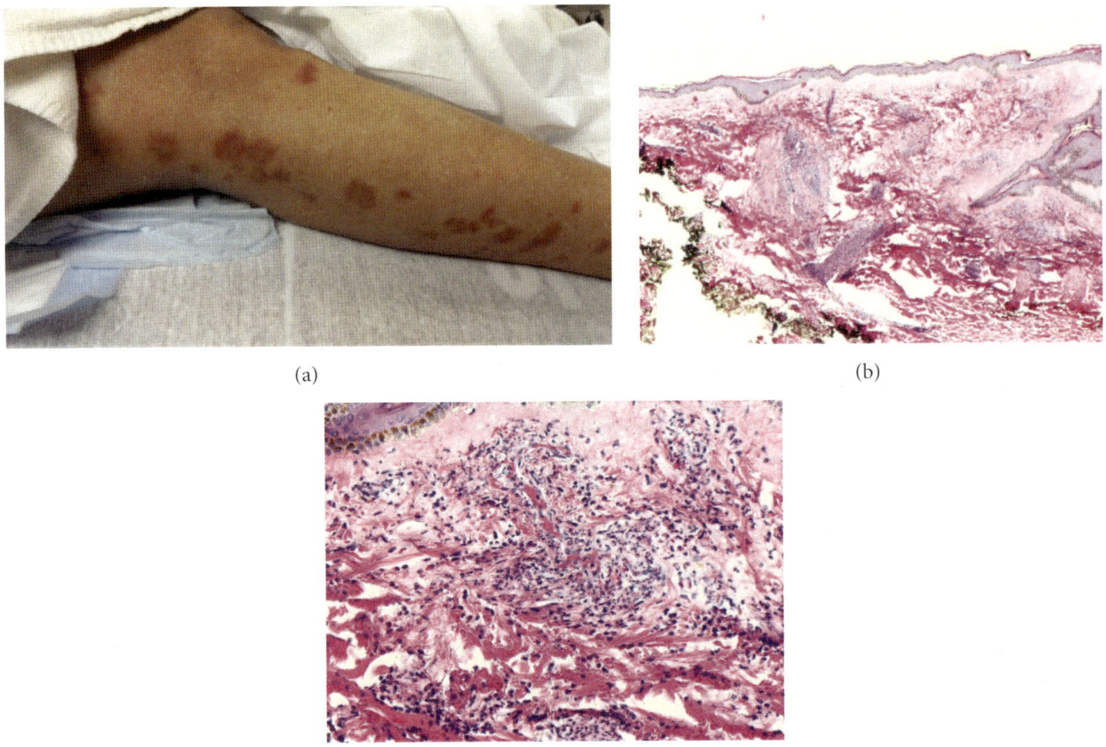

(a) (b) (c)

FIGURE 1: Drug-induced small vessel vasculitis. (a) Skin rash in lower extremities. (b) H&E staining from skin punch biopsy (20x) showing dense infiltrate of neutrophils and eosinophils surrounding vessels with extravasation of red blood cells. (c) H&E staining from the same skin punch biopsy (200x).

eosinophils), consistent with urticarial vasculitis (Figures 1(b) and 1(c)). Serologies obtained to evaluate for concurrent autoimmune disorder, hematological malignancy, or infections including ANA, anti-PR3, anti-TTG, anti-SMA, anti-centromere, anti-gliadin, anti-SSA/SSB, anti-RNP, anti-MPO, anti-dsDNA, c-ANCA and p-ANCA, SPEP/UPEP, HIV, viral hepatitis panel, serum IgG, and cryoglobulin levels were all negative or normal. Complement levels (C3 and C4) were normal. Other infectious workups including C. Diff. and TB were also negative. Esophagogastroduodenoscopy (EGD) performed a week after onset of her GI symptoms revealed severe circumferential ulcerations at the third portion of duodenum (D3) (Figures 2(c) and 2(d)). Histology on endoscopic biopsy showed acute duodenitis with focal necrosis with eosinophils, consistent with intestinal ischemia caused by vasculitis (Figures 2(a) and 2(b)). It should be noted that she had an EGD three months prior to this event for refractory gastroesophageal reflux disease that was completely normal. In addition to her GI symptoms, patient also developed acute renal insufficiency with peak creatinine of 2.9 that eventually resolved before her discharge.

Based on recommendations from dermatology, patient was started on prednisone as well as dapsone for treatment of urticarial vasculitis. Her rash and her GI symptoms improved over the next few weeks, with complete resolution by week 4. A follow-up small bowel enteroscopy performed 2 months later showed a mild to moderate smooth stricture in D3 that was traversed with a pediatric colonoscope and no dilation was required. Repeat endoscopic biopsies showed lamina propria fibrosis, acute and chronic inflammation, and regenerative epithelial changes.

3. Discussion

Urticarial vasculitis is a rare vasculitis with skin urticaria, cutaneous small vessel involvement, and sometimes systemic manifestations [2]. In our patient, given the negative serologies for an autoimmune, infectious, and neoplastic process, the urticarial vasculitis is presumably due to the acute infection with her leg wound or associated with a drug reaction.

Our patient presented with GI symptoms as her initial extracutaneous manifestation of UV. However, urticarial vasculitis can affect various organ systems and patients can present with systemic symptoms including uveitis, episcleritis, angioedema, arthralgia, proteinuria, renal failure, and pulmonary disease [2, 6]. Mehregan et al. found that patients who have low complement level are more likely to have systemic symptoms [6].

Treatment of urticarial vasculitis is based on disease severity. Dapsone, colchicine, indomethacin, or hydroxychloroquine can be used for cutaneous disease in UV [2]. Corticosteroids are often necessary when patients present with extracutaneous manifestations of UV; azathioprine,

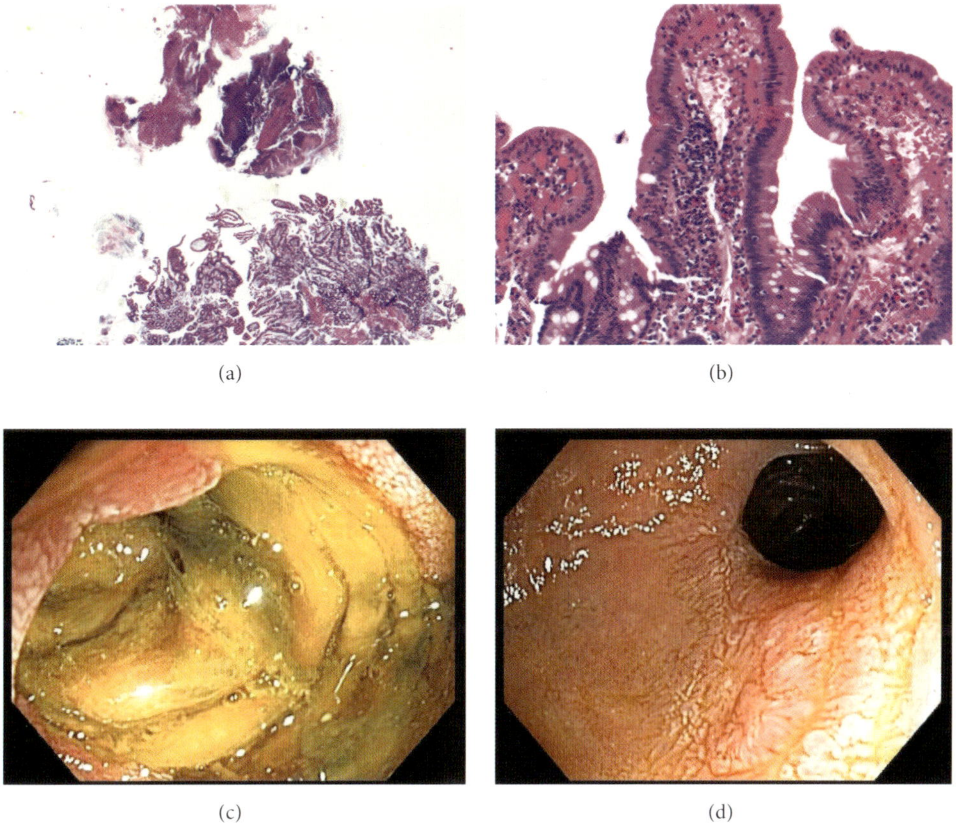

FIGURE 2: Vasculitis-associated duodenitis. (a) H&E staining from duodenal biopsy (40x) showing fibrinopurulent exudate consistent with ulceration/erosion. (b) H&E staining from duodenal biopsy (200x) showing active duodenitis including neutrophils within the surface epithelium and in the lamina propria surrounding small vessels with capillary ectasia and red blood cell extravasation. (c) EGD image of active duodenitis. (d) EGD image of mild to moderate duodenal stricture.

cyclosporine A, cyclophosphamide, and mycophenolate mofetil can be used for those with steroid-refractory disease or severe systemic involvement [2]. In recent years, several authors have reported success in using Omalizumab, an anti-IgE monoclonal antibody, to treat patients who have refractory disease despite steroid and immunosuppressants [7–9].

4. Conclusion

We report a case of urticarial vasculitis-induced intestinal ischemia and emphasize the importance of early recognition of the various types of clinical manifestations of urticarial vasculitis. Prompt management of UV can prevent potentially life-threatening complications.

References

[1] A. Arora, D. A. Wetter, T. M. Gonzalez-Santiago, M. D. P. Davis, and C. M. Lohse, "Incidence of leukocytoclastic vasculitis, 1996 to 2010: a population-based study in Olmsted County, Minnesota," *Mayo Clinic Proceedings*, vol. 89, no. 11, pp. 1515–1524, 2014.

[2] J. Venzor, W. L. Lee, and D. P. Huston, "Urticarial vasculitis," *Clinical Reviews in Allergy & Immunology*, vol. 23, no. 2, pp. 201–216, 2002.

[3] F. C. McDuffie, W. M. Sams Jr., J. E. Maldonado, P. H. Andreini, D. L. Conn, and E. A. Samayoa, "Hypocomplementemia with cutaneous vasculitis and arthritis. Possible immune complex syndrome," *Mayo Clinic Proceedings*, vol. 48, no. 5, pp. 340–348, 1973.

[4] N. A. Soter, "Chronic urticaria as a manifestation of necrotizing venulitis," *The New England Journal of Medicine*, vol. 296, no. 25, pp. 1440–1442, 1977.

[5] R. P. Warin, "Urticarial vasculitis," *British Medical Journal*, vol. 286, no. 6382, pp. 1919–1920, 1983.

[6] D. R. Mehregan, M. J. Hall, and L. E. Gibson, "Urticarial vasculitis: a histopathologic and clinical review of 72 cases," *Journal of the American Academy of Dermatology*, vol. 26, no. 3, part 2, pp. 441–448, 1992.

[7] L. S. Díez, L. M. Tamayo, and R. Cardona, "Omalizumab: therapeutic option in chronic spontaneous urticaria difficult to control with associated vasculitis, report of three cases," *Biomedica*, vol. 33, no. 4, pp. 503–512, 2013.

[8] M. N. Ghazanfar and S. F. Thomsen, "Omalizumab for urticarial vasculitis: case report and review of the literature," *Case Reports in Dermatological Medicine*, vol. 2015, Article ID 576893, 3 pages, 2015.

[9] G. Sussman, J. Hébert, C. Barron et al., "Real-life experiences with omalizumab for the treatment of chronic urticaria," *Annals of Allergy, Asthma and Immunology*, vol. 112, no. 2, pp. 170–174, 2014.

Chronic Hepatitis with Liver Granulomas in a Patient with Granuloma Annulare: A Case Report and Review of the Literature

Majid Alsahafi,[1,2] Mohammed I. AlJasser,[3] Sunil Kalia,[3] H. M. Yang,[4] and Alnoor Ramji[1]

[1]*Division of Gastroenterology, University of British Columbia, Vancouver, BC, Canada*
[2]*Department of Medicine, King Abdulaziz University, Jeddah, Saudi Arabia*
[3]*Department of Dermatology and Skin Science, University of British Columbia, Vancouver, BC, Canada*
[4]*Department of Pathology and Laboratory Medicine, University of British Columbia, Vancouver, BC, Canada*

Correspondence should be addressed to Majid Alsahafi; majidalsahafi@gmail.com

Academic Editor: Hideto Kawaratani

Granuloma annulare (GA) is a benign granulomatous skin disorder of unknown etiology. GA is rarely associated with liver diseases. We report a unique case of chronic hepatitis with liver granulomas in a patient with GA. Despite an extensive workup, no clear etiology for the hepatitis was found. Based on the possible immune pathophysiology of GA and the presence of liver granulomas, the patient was treated with prednisone and azathioprine which resulted in complete normalization of the liver enzymes and concurrent improvement of GA. The association between liver diseases and GA is reviewed.

1. Introduction

Granuloma annulare (GA) is a benign cutaneous granulomatous disorder of unknown etiology. It often presents as annular, red-brown grouped papules which are often asymptomatic or only slightly pruritic. There are four clinical variants of GA: localized, generalized, perforating, and subcutaneous [1]. The pathogenesis of GA remains poorly understood but an immune mediated mechanism has been speculated [2, 3]. GA has been reported in association with several systemic disorders but a causative relationship has not been established [1].

GA is rarely reported in association with liver diseases. Here we report a unique case of a patient with GA, who presented with elevated liver enzymes and a biopsy revealing hepatic granulomas. To our knowledge, a similar association has not been previously reported.

2. Case Presentation

A 57 year-old woman was evaluated for elevated liver enzymes discovered on routine blood work on July 2010. Her blood work showed an alanine transaminase (ALT) at 177 (normal range 15–55 U/L), aspartate aminotransferase (AST) at 86 (normal range 15–45 U/L), and *alkaline phosphatase* (ALP) at 114 (normal range 30–105 U/L) with a normal gamma-glutamyl transferase (GGT) at 44 (normal range < 50 U/L). The patient was asymptomatic. She had no risk factors for viral hepatitis. She drinks alcohol only socially, considered minimal overall. She does not take any medications, including no over-the-counter drugs or herbal supplements. Her past medical history was significant for a 9-year history of generalized GA proven on two skin biopsies for which she receives phototherapy 3 times per week (Figures 1(a) and 1(b)). She has no family history of liver disease. Physical examination was unremarkable except for multiple generalized red-brown annular plaques involving the trunk and extremities (Figure 1(c)).

Laboratory investigations revealed normal complete blood count, renal profile, and *erythrocyte sedimentation rate*. Liver synthetic function tests including international normalized ratio (INR), bilirubin, and albumin were initially normal. Serology for hepatitis C, hepatitis B, cytomegalovirus, and *Epstein-Barr virus* were negative. Workup for autoimmune

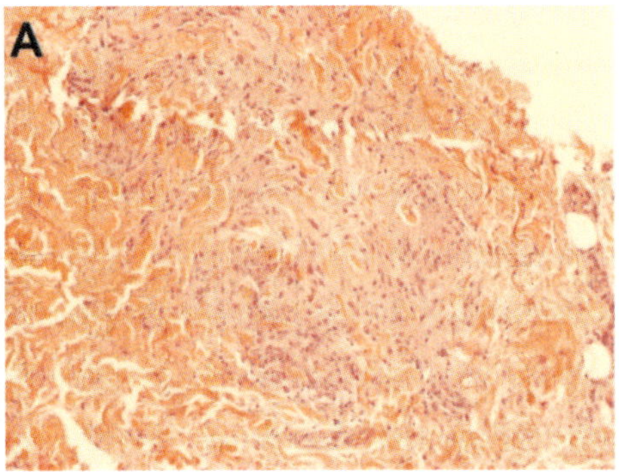

(a)

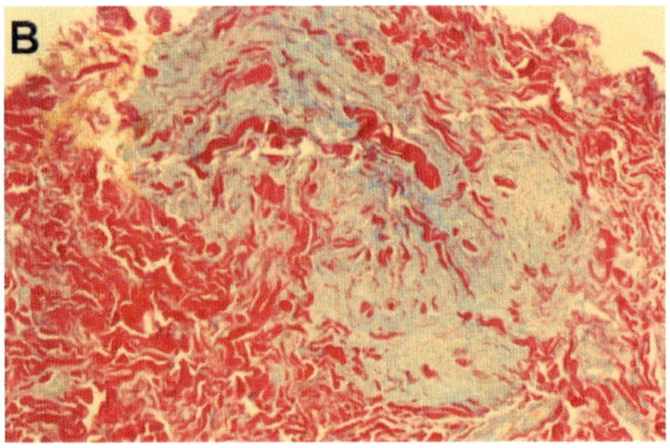

(b)

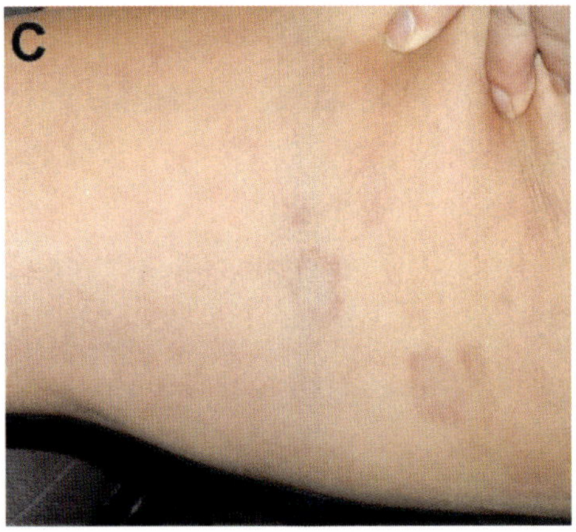

(c)

FIGURE 1: Granuloma annulare. (a) A palisading granuloma with central collagen degeneration (H&E stain, magnification ×100); (b) Alcian blue stain showing increased mucin deposition within the granuloma (Alcian blue stain, magnification ×100); (c) several annular red-brown plaques involving the thigh.

hepatitis revealed negative *antinuclear*, *anti-smooth-muscle*, *anti-liver kidney microsomal*, and *anti-mitochondrial antibodies*. Serum immunoglobulins levels were within the normal limits. Tissue transglutaminase antibodies test was negative. Serum ceruloplasmin and alpha-1-antitrypsin levels were normal. Transferrin saturation was not elevated. Angiotensin converting enzyme was slightly decreased. Abdominal ultrasound revealed a normal size liver with a slight coarse appearance.

On followup, liver enzymes were gradually increasing. On October 2010, ALT and AST were 186 and 260, respectively, while ALP and GGT were 132 and 55, respectively. Subsequently, a liver biopsy was performed and showed a mild nonspecific portal lymphocytic inflammatory infiltrate and aggregates of Kupffer cells containing ceroid pigments in the hepatic lobules and perivenular areas. There no plasma cells, interface hepatitis, or hepatic rosettes to suggest autoimmune hepatitis. Interestingly, granulomas were identified in the hepatic lobules and in the perivenular regions (Figure 2). A repeat workup for viral and autoimmune etiologies was negative.

On February 2011, her liver enzymes became significantly elevated (ALT 667, AST 665, ALP 221, and GGT 308) and the liver function started to decline (bilirubin 46, INR 1.4, and albumin 31). Based on the possible immune pathophysiology of GA and the presence of liver granulomas, a presumptive diagnosis of a similar immune mediated process involving the liver was made. Treatment with prednisone was initiated at 40 mg daily. The repeat blood work showed a rapid improvement of the liver enzymes and function. Interestingly, an improvement of the skin manifestations was also noted. A repeat liver biopsy was done three months after initiating prednisone. It showed a minor degree of nonspecific portal hepatitis with no fibrosis or granulomas. No features of autoimmune hepatitis were identified. The liver enzymes normalized four months after starting prednisone, which was subsequently tapered and discontinued while azathioprine was initiated. The liver enzymes and function tests continued to be normal on followup.

3. Discussion

We reported a unique case of a patient with GA presenting with elevated liver enzymes and findings of hepatic granulomas on pathology. No underlying etiology for the hepatitis was detected despite an extensive workup including two liver biopsies. Based on the possible autoimmune pathogenesis of GA and the fact that corticosteroids are considered one of

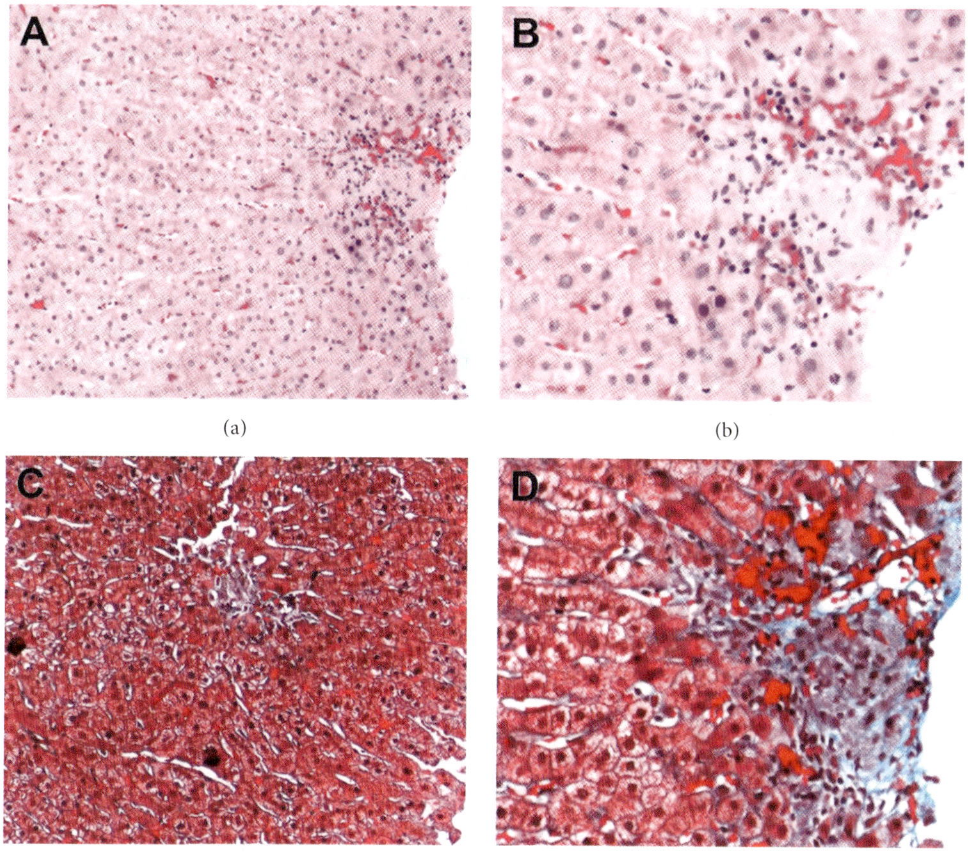

(a) (b) (c) (d)

FIGURE 2: The portal tracts either contain scattered lymphocytes or are entirely devoid of inflammation. In the perivenular areas, Kupffer cells containing ceroid pigments indicative of prior cellular injury and cell turnover are noted. Scattered lymphocytes are also seen in the perivenular zone. Small aggregates of histocytes, "microgranulomata," are identified in the hepatic lobule and in the perivenular region. (a) and (b) 10x and 20x H&E stain; (c) and (d) 10x and 20x trichrome stain.

the treatment options for GA, the patient was treated with prednisone followed by azathioprine which resulted in a rapid and sustained improvement of liver enzymes. Interestingly, an improvement of the skin lesions was also noted which supports the suspicion of a shared autoimmune phenomenon for both conditions. One may argue that the patient may have autoimmune hepatitis. However, the patient did not have any of the characteristic laboratory or histological findings [4]. An atypical presentation of autoimmune hepatitis remains an unlikely possibility. While there are many possible etiologies for liver granulomas such as sarcoidosis, there was no clinical or laboratory suggestion of an alternative etiology in our patient.

GA is rarely reported in association with liver diseases. We performed a literature search in Medline using the search terms "granuloma annulare" in combination with "liver" or "hepatitis." There were no limitations on language or date of publication. We also manually searched the reference lists for the relevant articles. A total of 10 articles were identified, consisting of case reports with one article describing 2 cases. A summary of the findings is shown in Table 1.

GA has been reported in association with hepatitis C [5], hepatitis B [6, 7], and primary biliary cholangitis [8]. In all cases, the diagnosis of liver disease preceded the onset of GA. In one of the two cases in which GA was associated with hepatitis B, HBV DNA was identified in the skin biopsies but the serum HBV DNA was below the detection range ($\leq 10^3$ copies/mL). This patient received treatment with interferon alpha, which resulted in regression of the skin lesions [7]. GA has been also noted to regress following hepatitis C treatment [5]. In contrast, pegylated interferon treatment for chronic hepatitis C was reported in two cases to trigger GA that resolved following end of therapy [9, 10], which suggests an immunogenic mechanism of GA. Hepatitis B vaccination has been associated with new onset GA in two cases [11, 12]. GA developed in sun exposed areas in two liver transplant recipients, 4 and 18 months after liver transplantation [13]. Given the rare coexistence of GA and liver conditions, it is difficult to know whether there is a true association or just coincidence.

Although GA is usually a benign idiopathic condition, it has been associated with different malignant tumors. We found only a single case report of GA occurring in a patient with hepatocellular carcinoma [14]. GA was diagnosed simultaneously with hepatocellular carcinoma. It was impossible to know the nature of the association as the patient died before

Table 1: Summary of the reported association between liver disease and granuloma annulare.

First author	Year of publication	Age	Sex	Association
Koizumi	1990	56	Female	Primary biliary cirrhosis
Wolf	1998	51	Female	Hepatitis B vaccine
Granel	2000	65	Female	Hepatitis C
Derancourt	2000	65	Male	Liver transplant
Derancourt	2000	59	Male	Liver transplant
Criado	2004	58	Female	Hepatitis B vaccine
Kluger	2006	52	Female	Hepatitis C treatment
Ma	2006	63	Female	Hepatitis B
Askin	2009	60	Female	Hepatitis B
Ahmad	2013	49	Male	Hepatitis C treatment
Mestre	2014	68	Male	Hepatocellular carcinoma

receiving treatment for the liver cancer. The occurrence of GA as a paraneoplastic syndrome has been reported with other cancers [15].

We presented a unique case in which liver granuloma were identified in a patient who has GA. A similar association has not been previously reported. Multiple disorders have been associated with liver granulomas [16, 17]. However, a definitive etiology cannot be found in a significant proportion of cases. Interestingly, no granulomas were identified in the second liver biopsy. This may indicate a response to treatment or a patchy involvement resulting in a sampling error. Alternatively, the presence of liver granulomas in a liver biopsy can be a spurious finding and may not necessarily indicate the presence of an underlying granulomatous liver disease [16].

Sarcoidosis, which may mimic GA in its cutaneous form, is a common cause of liver granulomas and has been described in association with GA [18]. While the histopathology findings in our case are not specific, we do not believe that our patient has hepatic sarcoidosis although it is a remote possibility. Hepatic involvement with sarcoidosis is typically associated with a cholestatic rather than a hepatocellular pattern, particularly with the high level of transaminases seen in our case [16]. The patient had no systemic manifestations that suggest sarcoidosis although hepatic sarcoidosis rarely occurs in isolation. The patient had two skin biopsies that were not suggestive of sarcoidosis. While the elevation of serum angiotensin converting enzyme level is a not a very sensitive test for sarcoidosis, it was low in our patient. Similarly, the patient did not have fever, elevated erythrocyte sedimentation rate, or other features suggestive of idiopathic granulomatous hepatitis, which is also characterized by a cholestatic rather than a hepatocellular pattern.

In conclusion, the association between granuloma annulare and liver diseases is rare. We presented a rare case of chronic hepatitis with liver granulomas in association with GA. The patient responded well to prednisone followed by azathioprine treatment. When evaluating a patient with a liver disease, a thorough history and physical examination is essential to asses for potential association with conditions that may have a shared or similar pathophysiology.

References

[1] M. D. Smith, J. B. Downie, and D. DiCostanzo, "Granuloma annulare," *International Journal of Dermatology*, vol. 36, no. 5, pp. 326–333, 1997.

[2] P. Güneş, F. Göktay, A. T. Mansur, F. Köker, and G. Erfan, "Collagen-elastic tissue changes and vascular involvement in granuloma annulare: a review of 35 cases," *Journal of Cutaneous Pathology*, vol. 36, no. 8, pp. 838–844, 2009.

[3] M. V. Dahl, "Speculations on the pathogenesis of granuloma annulare," *Australasian Journal of Dermatology*, vol. 26, no. 2, pp. 49–57, 1985.

[4] M. P. Manns, A. J. Czaja, J. D. Gorham et al., "Diagnosis and management of autoimmune hepatitis," *Hepatology*, vol. 51, no. 6, pp. 2193–2213, 2010.

[5] B. Granel, J. Serratrice, J. Rey et al., "Chronic hepatitis C virus infection associated with a generalized granuloma annulare," *Journal of the American Academy of Dermatology*, vol. 43, no. 5, pp. 918–919, 2000.

[6] Ü. Askin, M. Durdu, and E. Senel, "Generalized granuloma annulare in a patient with myelocytic leukemia and chronic hepatitis B virus infection," *Indian Journal of Dermatology, Venereology and Leprology*, vol. 75, no. 3, pp. 287–289, 2009.

[7] H. J. Ma, W. Y. Zhu, and X. Z. Yue, "Generalized granuloma annulare associated with chronic hepatitis B virus infection," *Journal of the European Academy of Dermatology and Venereology*, vol. 20, no. 2, pp. 186–189, 2006.

[8] H. Koizumi, T. Matsumura, M. Kumakiri, and A. Ohkawara, "Generalized granuloma annulare with primary biliary cirrhosis," *Nippon Hifuka Gakkai zasshi*, vol. 100, no. 8, pp. 871–878, 1990.

[9] U. Ahmad, X. Li, T. Sodeman, and I. Daboul, "Hepatitis c virus treatment with Pegylated interferon-Alfa therapy leading to generalized interstitial granuloma annulare and review of the literature," *American Journal of Therapeutics*, vol. 20, no. 5, pp. 585–587, 2013.

[10] N. Kluger, P. Moguelet, D. Chaslin-Ferbus, K. Khosrotherani, and S. Aractingi, "Generalized interstitial granuloma annulare induced by pegylated interferon-alpha," *Dermatology*, vol. 213, no. 3, pp. 248–249, 2006.

[11] F. Wolf, P. Grézard, F. Bérard, G. Clavel, and H. Perrot, "Generalized granuloma annulare and hepatitis B vaccination," *European Journal of Dermatology*, vol. 8, no. 6, pp. 435–436, 1998.

[12] P. R. Criado, R. de Oliveira Ramos, C. Vasconcellos, R. F. J. Criado, and N. Y. S. Valente, "Two case reports of cutaneous adverse reactions following hepatitis B vaccine: lichen planus and granuloma annulare," *Journal of the European Academy of Dermatology and Venereology*, vol. 18, no. 5, pp. 603–606, 2004.

[13] C. Derancourt, M. Senser, L. Atallah, M.-C. Becker, and R. Laurent, "Granuloma annulare of the photoexposed areas in two liver transplant recipients," *Annales de Dermatologie et de Venereologie*, vol. 127, no. 8-9, pp. 723–727, 2000.

[14] T. Mestre, A. M. Rodrigues, and J. Cardoso, "Disseminated granuloma annulare and hepatocellular carcinoma: association or coincidence?" *Case Reports*, vol. 2014, Article ID bcr2014205883, 2014.

[15] P. R. Cohen, "Granuloma annulare associated with malignancy," *Southern Medical Journal*, vol. 90, no. 10, pp. 1056–1059, 1997.

[16] S. L. Flamm, "Granulomatous liver disease," *Clinics in Liver Disease*, vol. 16, no. 2, pp. 387–396, 2012.

[17] U. Drebber, H.-U. Kasper, J. Ratering et al., "Hepatic granulomas: histological and molecular pathological approach to differential diagnosis–a study of 442 cases," *Liver International*, vol. 28, no. 6, pp. 828–834, 2008.

[18] E. W. Ehrich, J. L. McGuire, and Y. H. Kim, "Association of granuloma annulare with sarcoidosis," *Archives of Dermatology*, vol. 128, no. 6, pp. 855–856, 1992.

Postmenopausal Deep Infiltrating Endometriosis of the Colon: Rare Location and Novel Medical Therapy

Benjamin M. Snyder,[1] Joseph W. Beets,[2] Bruce A. Lessey,[3] Samuel R. W. Horton,[4] and Gary A. Abrams[2]

[1] *University of South Carolina School of Medicine Greenville, Greenville, SC, USA*
[2] *Department of Gastroenterology/Liver Center, Greenville Health System, University of South Carolina School of Medicine Greenville, Greenville, SC, USA*
[3] *Department of Obstetrics and Gynecology, Greenville Health System, University of South Carolina School of Medicine Greenville, Greenville, SC, USA*
[4] *Department of Pathology, Greenville Health System, University of South Carolina School of Medicine Greenville, Greenville, SC, USA*

Correspondence should be addressed to Benjamin M. Snyder; bmsnyder@email.sc.edu

Academic Editor: Daniel C. Damin

We report an uncommon case of deep infiltrating endometriosis of the colon presenting as iron deficiency anemia nine years after hysterectomy with bilateral salpingo-oophorectomy. The endometrial implant was found at the hepatic flexure, an exceedingly rare location for endometriosis invasion with no cases distinctly reported in the literature. Additionally, the presentation of gastrointestinal endometriosis as iron deficiency anemia is not well documented in the literature. Instead of surgery, we prescribed a novel medical therapeutic approach using conjugated estrogen-bazedoxifene to antagonize the proliferative effects of estrogen on endometrial tissue. After five months of therapy and repeat colonoscopy, no evidence of endometrial tissue remained in the hepatic flexure.

1. Introduction

Endometriosis is a common disorder in women of reproductive age occurring in 8–10% [1]. However, endometriosis has not been significantly studied in postmenopausal women. The development of endometriosis after menopause is a rare phenomenon, and it has often been reported in the setting of hormone replacement therapy (HRT) [2] and treatment with tamoxifen [3, 4]. While postmenopausal endometriosis is uncommon, deep infiltrating endometriosis involving the colon in postmenopausal women has been noted only in the case report literature [5–9]. We describe a case of a postmenopausal woman presenting with iron deficiency anemia due to colonic endometrial infiltration and a novel therapeutic approach.

2. Case Report

A 60-year-old Caucasian woman was referred to gastroenterology department due to three years of persistent iron deficiency anemia (IDA) resistant to oral iron supplementation with patient-reported blood in the stool. Her history was significant for endometriosis in early reproductive years and uterine fibroids treated by hysterectomy with bilateral salpingo-oophorectomy nine years before her current presentation. She was given oral estradiol therapy as part of hormone replacement therapy (HRT). She underwent an esophagogastroduodenoscopy (EGD) that was of normal result and a colonoscopy that revealed moderately severe diverticulosis and a nodular ulcerated lesion at the hepatic flexure (Figure 1) that was partially removed by hot snare cauterization (Figure 2). This was not a complete resection and allowed for better tissue sampling. The nodule appeared

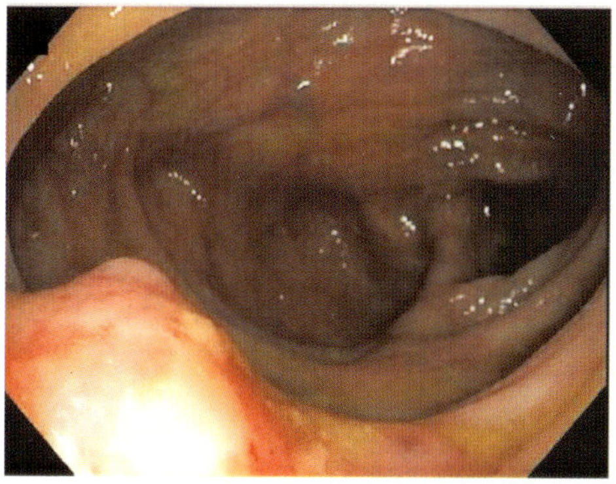

FIGURE 1: The nodule was visualized at the hepatic flexure with mild ulceration and bleeding at the surface. Ulceration and blood loss were the presumed explanation for the patient's chronic iron deficiency.

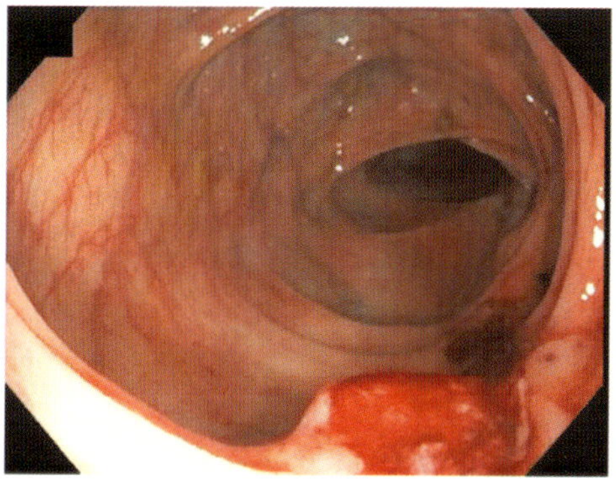

FIGURE 2: The nodule was partially removed by cold snare polypectomy but was not amenable to complete removal under endoscopy.

deeper than what could be visualized by endoscopy and was biopsied multiple times. India ink was used to tattoo the location of the nodule for a follow-up examination.

Histological analysis of the biopsies noted mural endometriosis and adenomatous tissue within the endometrial tissue and surrounding mucosa (Figure 3). The endometrial tissue infiltrated the full thickness of the biopsy specimen, which extended through the submucosa. The presence of endometrial tissue through the depth of the biopsy, extending into the mucosa, is indicative of complete thickness penetration of the colonic wall. Though the patient experienced no other symptoms of endometriosis, deep infiltrating endometriosis was a likely explanation for her IDA. Gynecology was consulted, and the patient's estradiol therapy was discontinued. Given that the subject had few physical symptoms of her disease but had previously suffered vasomotor symptoms of menopause, medical treatment was an appropriate approach for her condition. A course of conjugated estrogen-bazedoxifene (CE/BZA) (Duavee: 0.45–20 mg, Pfizer, New York, NY) was selected instead of surgery. CE/BZA is commonly used in women with a uterus who desire HRT, as it prevents estrogen from stimulating endometrial tissues using the selective estrogen receptor modulator, bazedoxifene.

Approximately three months after her original visit to gastroenterology department and consultation with hematology, the patient received two intravenous iron infusions one week apart in conjunction with the course of CE/BZA therapy. Follow-up colonoscopy, eight months after the initial colonoscopy and five months of CE/BZA therapy, demonstrated scarring from the initial procedure and no residual nodule at the hepatic flexure (Figure 4). Biopsies taken identified fragments of tubular adenoma without any evidence of remaining endometriosis suggesting complete regression. Follow-up labs revealed normalization of iron studies, anemia, and microcytosis. Iron infusion and complete regression of endometrial tissue and reversal of minor blood loss from associated ulceration are the presumptive explanation for resolution of this patient's iron deficiency anemia.

3. Discussion

Deep endometriosis (also called deep infiltrating endometriosis) is a form of endometriosis that invades any vital structures such as bowel, ureters, or bladder [10]. Intestinal involvement of endometriosis has been estimated to exist in between 3.8% and 37% of patients with an endometriosis diagnosis [11]. The most common sites of bowel endometriosis are rectum, ileum, appendix, and cecum from most to least prevalent, while some cases of gastric and transverse colonic involvement have been reported [11]. Endometriosis is often difficult to diagnose due to the generalized nature of symptoms: pelvic pain, dysmenorrhea, dyspareunia, and dysuria/dyschezia [12]. Symptoms associated with bowel endometriosis are abdominal pain relieved with defection, change in frequency or appearance of stool, and abnormal rectal bleeding, but most of these symptoms are seen only in cases of mucosal involvement [13]. Additionally, it is difficult to diagnose bowel endometriosis even with colonoscopy as most cases do not infiltrate beyond the serosa and very few infiltrate the mucosa [14]. With a wide range of presentations and the often asymptomatic disease course, until it significantly progressed, deep infiltrating endometriosis is a complicated disease to diagnose and treat.

The treatment of endometriosis has primarily focused on alleviating symptoms and restoring fertility in women of reproductive age [15–17], but to this point, no curative therapy exists. To date, research has primarily focused on the surgical treatment of deep endometriosis with fewer resources being devoted to understanding the medical management of the disease. Specifically, research in postmenopausal endometriosis has purported to indicate the necessity of resection due to the risk of malignancy [18, 19]. However, recurrence of the disease is possible even with surgical intervention, and there is a risk of significant complications as a result of surgical resection especially in bowel endometriosis [20]. There has been a rise in invasive bowel resection for treatment of colorectal endometriosis in recent years, and some authors have begun to question the efficacy of such a practice in favor of less invasive interventions such as ablation or medical management [21–23]. Complete excision of endometriosis of the bowel, more

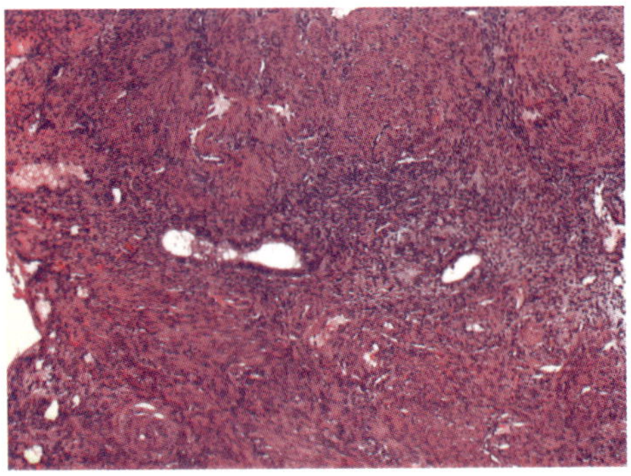

(a)

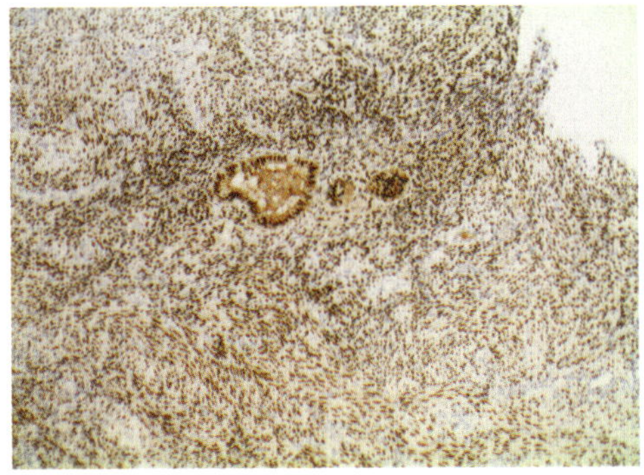

(b)

Figure 3: (a) Staining of the colonic nodule shows active proliferative endometrial glands and stromal tissue (hematoxylin and eosin, 40x). (b) Immunohistochemistry demonstrates diffusely positive staining for the estrogen receptor in a pattern consistent with endometrial tissue (100x).

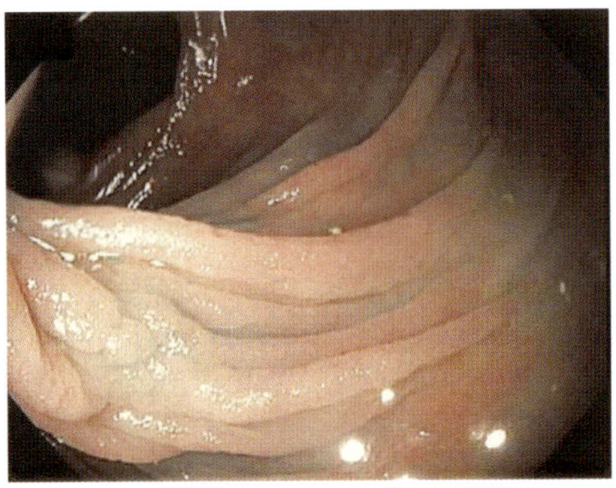

Figure 4: Approximately eight months after cold snare polypectomy and treatment with conjugated estrogen/bazedoxifene, no evidence of the nodule remained at the marked site at the hepatic flexure of the colon.

than ablation, has been shown to reduce some symptoms such as dyspareunia, but overall symptoms are decreased nearly identically with ablation or excision [24]. The difficulty of completely eliminating endometriosis of the bowel and permanently reducing symptoms is the preferential association of endometriosis tissue with the enteric nervous system, which also accounts for the set of symptoms seen in deep infiltrating endometriosis of the bowel [13, 25, 26]. Additionally, macronodules of endometriosis may be readily visible during surgery, but micronodules are identified in histology making complete excision of endometriosis unlikely [27]. As discussed here, many complicating factors are associated with surgical intervention in deep infiltrating endometriosis in a postmenopausal population. A more patient-oriented approach evaluates specific patient factors as in this case, demonstrating a less invasive method, that is, ablation followed by CE/BZA therapy in this case.

Medical management of endometriosis and especially postmenopausal endometriosis is evolving. The currently postulated mechanisms of premenopausal endometriosis include retrograde menstruation, coelomic metaplasia, immune deficiencies, and Mullerian remnants, but these do not adequately account for all cases in women of reproductive age [17]. Postmenopausal endometriosis cannot be fully explained by the postulated mechanisms, but high levels of ectopic estrogen production from nonovarian tissue can activate endometrial tissue [28]. Aromatase has been shown to have a role in the pathogenesis of endometriosis and has long been a proposed target for treatment [29]. Few cases of the treatment of postmenopausal endometriosis with aromatase inhibitors (AI) have been reported; however they suggest that significant symptom reduction is possible with AIs [18]. One case even notes the positive effects of AIs on abdominal endometriosis and suggests a potential role for AIs in the treatment of postmenopausal deep infiltrating endometriosis [30]. Although there are articles demonstrating the usefulness of AIs in postmenopausal endometriosis, empiric research is lacking.

CE/BZA was approved in 2013 for treatment of the vasomotor symptoms associated with menopause as well as the treatment of postmenopausal osteoporosis by a non-hormone replacement therapy/menopausal hormone therapy mechanism [31]. CE/BZA is a combination of conjugated estrogen and bazedoxifene, a selective estrogen receptor modulator (SERM) that induces degradation of estrogen receptors in breast and endometrial tissue [32]. Original clinical trials validated the efficacy of CE/BZA in reduction of menopausal vasomotor symptoms and protection against osteoporosis, while demonstrating the protective effects of bazedoxifene on breast and endometrial tissue in the presence of estrogen [33]. Research has also shown that CE/BZA can cause regression of endometriosis in a murine model [34, 35]. It was by this mechanism hypothesized that CE/BZA would be an ideal option for medical management in this postmenopausal patient thereby inducing regression of endometrial tissue while providing the protective bone effects of estrogen and preventing vasomotor symptoms of menopause.

In conclusion, this case highlights an unusual presentation of iron deficiency anemia due to a rare colonic location of deep infiltrating endometriosis in a postmenopausal woman successfully treated medically with a novel and less invasive approach (CE/BZA) that provides mechanisms for both symptom control and disease regression.

Consent

Informed consent was obtained from the patient discussed in this case report.

Disclosure

Gary A. Abrams is the article guarantor. The source is Greenville Memorial Hospital, Greenville, SC.

Acknowledgments

Funding for this submission is provided by the Department of Medicine at Greenville Memorial Hospital.

References

[1] P. Acién and I. Velasco, "Endometriosis: A Disease That Remains Enigmatic," *ISRN Obstetrics and Gynecology*, vol. 2013, pp. 1–12, 2013.

[2] Sung Woo Choi, Hye Nam Lee, Seok Jin Kang, and Hyung Ok Kim, "A case of cutaneous endometriosis developed in postmenopausal woman receiving hormonal replacement," *Journal of the American Academy of Dermatology*, vol. 41, no. 2, pp. 327–329, 1999.

[3] C. H. Buckley, "Tamoxifen-associated postmenopausal endometriosis," *Histopathology*, vol. 31, no. 3, p. 296, 1997.

[4] I. Cohen, M. M. Altaras, S. Lew, R. Tepper, Y. Beyth, and G. Ben-Baruch, "Ovarian Endometrioid Carcinoma and Endometriosis Developing in a Postmenopausal Breast Cancer Patient during Tamoxifen Therapy: A Case Report and Review of the Literature," *Gynecologic Oncology*, vol. 55, no. 3, pp. 443–447, 1994.

[5] B. Deval, A. Rafii, M. F. Dachez, R. Kermanash, and M. Levardon, "Sigmoid endometriosis in a postmenopausal woman," *American Journal of Obstetrics & Gynecology*, vol. 187, no. 6, pp. 1723–1725, 2002.

[6] K. Izuishi, T. Sano, A. Shiota, H. Mori, and K. Ebara, "Small bowel obstruction caused by endometriosis in a postmenopausal woman," *Asian Journal of Endoscopic Surgery*, vol. 8, no. 2, pp. 205–208, 2015.

[7] V. E. Klenov, T. A. Potretzke, J. K. Sehn, and P. H. Thaker, "Postmenopausal invasive endometriosis requiring supralevator pelvic exenteration," *Obstetrics & Gynecology*, vol. 126, no. 6, pp. 1215–1218, 2015.

[8] J. G. Petros, N. Spirito, and R. Gosshein, "Endometriosis causing colon obstruction in two postmenopausal women," *Mount Sinai Journal of Medicine*, vol. 59, no. 4, pp. 362–365, 1992.

[9] P. Popoutchi, C. R. dos Reis Lemos, J. C. R. Silva, A. A. Nogueira, O. Feres, and J. J. R. da Rocha, "Postmenopausal intestinal obstructive endometriosis: Case report and review of the literature," *São Paulo Medical Journal*, vol. 126, no. 3, pp. 190–193, 2008.

[10] P. Vercellini, G. Frontino, G. Pietropaolo, U. Gattei, R. Daguati, and P. G. Crosignani, "Deep endometriosis: Definition, pathogenesis, and clinical management," *The Journal of Minimally Invasive Gynecology* , vol. 11, no. 2, pp. 153–161, 2004.

[11] V. Remorgida, S. Ferrero, E. Fulcheri, N. Ragni, and D. C. Martin, "Bowel endometriosis: presentation, diagnosis, and treatment," *Obstetrical & Gynecological Survey* , vol. 62, no. 7, pp. 461–470, 2007.

[12] J. Nassif, P. Trompoukis, S. Barata, A. Furtado, B. Gabriel, and A. Wattiez, "Management of deep endometriosis," *Reproductive BioMedicine Online*, vol. 23, no. 1, pp. 25–33, 2011.

[13] V. Remorgida, N. Ragni, S. Ferrero, P. Anserini, P. Torelli, and E. Fulcheri, "The involvement of the interstitial Cajal cells and the enteric nervous system in bowel endometriosis," *Human Reproduction*, vol. 20, no. 1, pp. 264–271, 2005.

[14] M. Milone, A. Mollo, M. Musella et al., "Role of colonoscopy in the diagnostic work-up of bowel endometriosis," *World Journal of Gastroenterology*, vol. 21, no. 16, pp. 4997–5001, 2015.

[15] C. Mohr, F. R. Nezhat, C. H. Nezhat, D. S. Seidman, and C. R. Nezhat, "Fertility considerations in laparoscopic treatment of infiltrative bowel endometriosis.," *JSLS : Journal of the Society of Laparoendoscopic Surgeons / Society of Laparoendoscopic Surgeons*, vol. 9, no. 1, pp. 16–24, 2005.

[16] A. Moini, L. Bahar, M. Ashrafinia, B. Eslami, R. Hosseini, and N. Ashrafinia, "Fertility outcome after operative laparoscopy versus no treatment in infertile women with minimal or mild endometriosis," *International Journal of Fertility & Sterility*, vol. 5, no. 4, pp. 235–240, 2012.

[17] P. Vercellini, P. Viganò, E. Somigliana, and L. Fedele, "Endometriosis: pathogenesis and treatment," *Nature Reviews Endocrinology*, vol. 10, no. 5, pp. 261–275, 2014.

[18] N. P. Polyzos, H. M. Fatemi, A. Zavos et al., "Aromatase inhibitors in post-menopausal endometriosis," *Reproductive Biology and Endocrinology*, vol. 9, article no. 90, 2011.

[19] L. H. Thomsen, T. H. Schnack, K. Buchardi et al., "Risk factors of epithelial ovarian carcinomas among women with endometriosis: a systematic review," *Acta Obstetricia et Gynecologica Scandinavica*, vol. 96, no. 6, pp. 761–778, 2017.

[20] C. Meuleman, C. Tomassetti, A. D'Hoore et al., "Surgical treatment of deeply infiltrating endometriosis with colorectal involvement," *Human Reproduction Update*, vol. 17, no. 3, pp. 311–326, 2011.

[21] M. S. Abrão, F. Petraglia, T. Falcone, J. Keckstein, Y. Osuga, and C. Chapron, "Deep endometriosis infiltrating the recto-sigmoid: Critical factors to consider before management," *Human Reproduction Update*, vol. 21, no. 3, pp. 329–339, 2015.

[22] P. Acién, C. Núñez, F. Quereda, I. Velasco, M. Valiente, and V. Vidal, "Is a bowel resection necessary for deep endometriosis with rectovaginal or colorectal involvement?" *International Journal of Women's Health*, vol. 5, no. 1, pp. 449–455, 2013.

[23] P. Vercellini, P. G. Crosignani, E. Somigliana, N. Berlanda, G. Barbara, and L. Fedele, "Medical treatment for rectovaginal endometriosis: what is the evidence?" *Human Reproduction*, vol. 24, no. 10, pp. 2504–2514, 2009.

[24] M. Healey, C. Cheng, and H. Kaur, "To excise or ablate endometriosis? A prospective randomized double-blinded trial after 5-year follow-up," *Journal of Minimally Invasive Gynecology*, vol. 21, no. 6, pp. 999–1004, 2014.

[25] V. Anaf, I. E. Nakadi, P. Simon et al., "Preferential infiltration of large bowel endometriosis along the nerves of the colon," *Human Reproduction*, vol. 19, no. 4, pp. 996–1002, 2004.

[26] G. Wang, N. Tokushige, P. Russell, S. Dubinovsky, R. Markham, and I. S. Fraser, "Hyperinnervation in Intestinal Deep Infiltrating Endometriosis," *Journal of Minimally Invasive Gynecology*, vol. 16, no. 6, pp. 713–719, 2009.

[27] A. Badescu, H. Roman, M. Aziz et al., "Mapping of bowel occult microscopic endometriosis implants surrounding deep endometriosis nodules infiltrating the bowel," *Fertility and Sterility*, vol. 105, no. 2, pp. 430–434, 2016.

[28] C. L. Bendon and C. M. Becker, "Potential mechanisms of postmenopausal endometriosis," *Maturitas*, vol. 72, no. 3, pp. 214–219, 2012.

[29] K. M. Zeitoun and S. E. Bulun, "Aromatase: a key molecule in the pathophysiology of endometriosis and a therapeutic target," *Fertility and Sterility*, vol. 72, no. 6, pp. 961–969, 1999.

[30] I. E. Sasson and H. S. Taylor, "Aromatase inhibitor for treatment of a recurrent abdominal wall endometrioma in a postmenopausal woman," *Fertility and Sterility*, vol. 92, no. 3, pp. 1170–e4, 2009.

[31] T. Goldberg and B. Fidler, "Conjugated Estrogens/Bazedoxifene(Duavee) A Novel Agent for the Treatment of Moderate-to-Severe Vasomotor Symptoms Associated with Menopause and the Prevention of Postmenopausal Osteoporosis," *P&T*, vol. 40, no. 3, pp. 178–182, 2015.

[32] R. Kagan, S. R. Goldstein, J. H. Pickar, and B. S. Komm, "Patient considerations in the management of menopausal symptoms: Role of conjugated estrogens with bazedoxifene," *Therapeutics and Clinical Risk Management*, vol. 12, pp. 549–562, 2016.

[33] D. F. Archer, E. W. Freeman, B. S. Komm et al., "Pooled Analysis of the Effects of Conjugated Estrogens/Bazedoxifene on Vasomotor Symptoms in the Selective Estrogens, Menopause, and Response to Therapy Trials," *Journal of Women's Health*, vol. 25, no. 11, pp. 1102–1111, 2016.

[34] H. Naqvi, S. Sakr, T. Presti, G. Krikun, B. Komm, and H. S. Taylor, "Treatment with bazedoxifene and conjugated estrogens results in regression of endometriosis in a murine model," *Biology of Reproduction*, vol. 90, no. 6, article no. 121, 2014.

[35] S. Sakr, H. Naqvi, B. Komm, and H. S. Taylor, "Endometriosis impairs bone marrow-derived stem cell recruitment to the uterus whereas bazedoxifene treatment leads to endometriosis regression and improved uterine stem cell engraftment," *Endocrinology*, vol. 155, no. 4, pp. 1489–1497, 2014.

51

Fatal Systemic Vasoconstriction in a Case of Metastatic Small-Intestinal NET

Jochen Stenzel,[1] Sebastian Noe,[2] Konstantin Holzapfel,[3] Franziska Erlmeier,[4] and Florian Eyer[1]

[1] *Department of Clinical Toxicology, Klinikum rechts der Isar, Technical University of Munich, Ismaningerstrasse 22, 81675 Munich, Germany*
[2] *Department of Internal Medicine II (Gastroenterology), Klinikum rechts der Isar, Technical University of Munich, Ismaningerstrasse 22, 81675 Munich, Germany*
[3] *Department of Diagnostic and Interventional Radiology, Klinikum rechts der Isar, Technical University of Munich, Ismaningerstrasse 22, 81675 Munich, Germany*
[4] *Institute of Pathology, Klinikum rechts der Isar, Technical University of Munich, Ismaningerstrasse 22, 81675 Munich, Germany*

Correspondence should be addressed to Jochen Stenzel; j.stenzel@tum.de

Academic Editor: Gregory Kouraklis

An increased release of serotonin secreted by ileal NETs is thought to be the major factor causing the carcinoid syndrome. However, in acutely arising carcinoid crisis also other vasoactive factors may lead to hazardous fluctuations in blood pressure and bronchial constriction. In rare cases, systemic vasoconstriction can be observed, probably caused by catecholamines or similar acting substances. Here, we report a fatal case of fulminant systemic vasoconstriction possibly caused by catecholamines in a patient with metastasized ileal NET. The vasospasm was detected by CT-angiography, and hemodynamic monitoring revealed a high systemic vascular resistance. Epinephrine, norepinephrine, and chromogranin A levels in plasma were elevated as was the urinary 5-hydroxyindoleacetic acid (5-HIAA). The cause of death was heart failure due to severe circulatory insufficiency. The progression of the tumor disease was confirmed by autopsy.

1. Introduction

Neuroendocrine tumors (NET) of the gastroenteropancreatic system are low-grade malignant neoplasms derived from local neuroendocrine cells [1].

Their clinical presentation largely depends on primary tumor site and whether or not significant amounts of hormones are produced and secreted. The predominantly secreted hormonally active substances, such as polypeptides, biogenic amines, and prostaglandins, vary, depending on tumor localization [2–5]. NETs of the ileum primarily release serotonin (5-hydroxytryptophan (5-HT)) and metastasize to the lymph nodes and liver resulting in a reduced presystemic metabolism of hormonal active substances by the liver [2, 6, 7].

An excessive release of these active substances caused by different triggers like surgery/anaesthesia, interventional diagnostic and therapy, radionuclide therapy, medication, and examination can lead to carcinoid crisis characterized by dramatic blood pressure fluctuation, arrhythmias, bronchospasm, and mental disturbances [8–13]. Commonly, hypotension is the expected hemodynamic change; however a small group of carcinoid patients experiences hypertension during carcinoid crisis [14, 15]. The occurrence of localized or generalized vasospasms associated with NETs has been described in case reports only [16–18]; see also Table 2.

Here, we report a fatal case of a metastasized syndromic NET of the terminal ileum with systemic vasospasm resulting in secondary low-output syndrome and consecutive multiorgan failure. CT-angiography, advanced hemodynamic monitoring, and determination of catecholamines, chromogranin A in plasma, and 5-hydroxyindoleacetic acid (5-HIAA) in urine were performed. The cause of death was determined post-mortem by autopsy.

Table 1: Hemodynamic parameters.

Hours after admission to ICU*	99,4	100,9	104,5	115,9	117	118	119,4	120	138,5	139,2	141,1	141.7
CI*	2.13	2.09	2.14	1.36	1.36	1.1	1.8		1.73	1.6	1.18	2.18
SVRI**	4247	3523	1526	3092	2200	7500	2916	3500	3034	3875	2857	2505

*Admission hour $h = 0$ (reference values: *3.0–5.0 l/min/m^2; **1700–2400 dyn∗s∗cm^{-5}∗m^2).

Table 2: Similar case reports in literature.

Clinical presentation	Site of tumor	Publication
Coronary vasospasm	Liver metastases of unknown origin	[16, 17]
	Carcinoid tumor, originated from ileum	[18]
Systemic vasoconstriction	Pulmonary NET	[19]
Catecholamine producing	Ileal NET	[20]
	GEP NET with diffuse liver metastases	[21]

2. Case Report

In 2011, a liver biopsy of hepatic lesions of a 51-year-old female revealed liver metastases from a well-differentiated small intestine NET (G1, Ki 67 max. 3%).

A DOTA-TOC-PET/CT demonstrated metastatic disease with a suspected ileal primary; see Figure 3. After hemihepatectomy and resection of the primary tumor in the ileum, histopathology of the terminal ileum showed a serotonin-producing, well-differentiated NET. Flush-symptoms were controlled under treatment with somatostatin analogues. With reappearance of the symptoms after almost one year, another DOTA-NOC-PET-CT showed distinct ubiquitary tumor progress. It was therefore decided to perform a peptide radioreceptor radionuclide therapy (PRRT) in 2013. About 4 days after the beginning of the PRRT, her general condition deteriorated dramatically. The patient was transferred to our ICU due to impaired consciousness, progressive delirium, and increase of inflammatory parameters (CRP 16 mg/dL, WBC 23.6 G/L) for suspected urosepsis originating from a chronic second grade hydronephrosis. After admission the patient showed hypertensive blood pressure values measured via a femoral artery catheter in contrast to hypotensive noninvasive blood pressure determinations. Blood culture revealed Klebsiella pneumoniae sensitive to empiric antibiotics. However, despite decreasing inflammation parameters, the patient's condition deteriorated with progression of liver and renal failure, delirium, and bloody diarrhoea. A pattern reminiscent of dermal livedo reticularis appeared (Figure 1) and a thoracic-abdominal contrast CT-scan revealed a massive and generalized arterial vasoconstriction with infarction of the kidneys, liver, and spleen (Figures 2 and 4). Massively elevated systemic vascular resistance index (SVRI) and a reduced cardiac index (CI) were measured using an advanced hemodynamic monitoring (PICCO®, Pulsion Medical Systems SE); see Table 1. Markers of myocardial necrosis along with NT-proBNP (max. 1287 pg/ml) steadily increased because of progressive cardiac failure. In contrast, an echocardiography performed in 2013 showed a normal left/right ventricular function and a first grade mitral and tricuspid regurgitation. Peripheral hydropic decompensation with extensive bilateral pleural effusions, oliguria, absence of hypotension, arterial hypoxemia, and ultimately the end stage condition of the patient thwarted aggressive volume therapy.

An excess of vasoactive amines secreted by the NET was now regarded as the most likely reason for clinical deterioration. Massively elevated chromogranin A in plasma and, notably, elevated catecholamine plasma levels (in pg/ml) supported this hypothesis: epinephrine 2318.3 (50–100 pg/ml), norepinephrine 1339.3 (<400 pg/mL), metanephrine 170.2 (<90 pg/mL), normetanephrine 349,5 (<180 pg/mL), and chromogranin A (in ng/ml, <84.7 ng/ml) 896 (11/2011), 717 (06/2012), 1.120 (01/2013), and 16.310 6 days before and 33.580 6 days after ICU admission. In contrast, the 5-HIAA levels in urine were elevated but remained stable: 66.2 mg/12 h on day 6 after admission and 153 mg/24 h 452 days before admission (1–10 mg/24 h); see Table 3.

Octreotide dose was increased and administered intravenously combined with orally administered cyproheptadine. Treatment attempts with nimodipine, phentolamine, and dobutamine aiming at reducing SVRI and cardiac afterload and thereby improving the CI were largely ineffective. Respiratory insufficiency worsened but intubation and mandatory ventilation were not performed in agreement with the family due to the underlying progressive malignancy. The patient finally died 7 days after ICU admission.

At autopsy the affected organs included the heart (disseminated pericardial, intramural, and endocardial metastases with involvement of the papillary muscles; histologically, approximately 60% vital tumor mass persisted after therapy; angioinvasion; no endocardial fibrosis), lungs (disseminated metastases and perivascular), stomach, pancreas, soft tissues, thyroid gland, ovaries, and bones. Histologically, a partial treatment response was found. The final TNM UICC classification was aT3 (m), aN1 (2/2), aM1 (PUL, HEP, PER, OTH, OSS, and LYM), aL1, aV1, and aPn1; grading G1. The cause of death was determined as heart failure due to severe circulatory insufficiency.

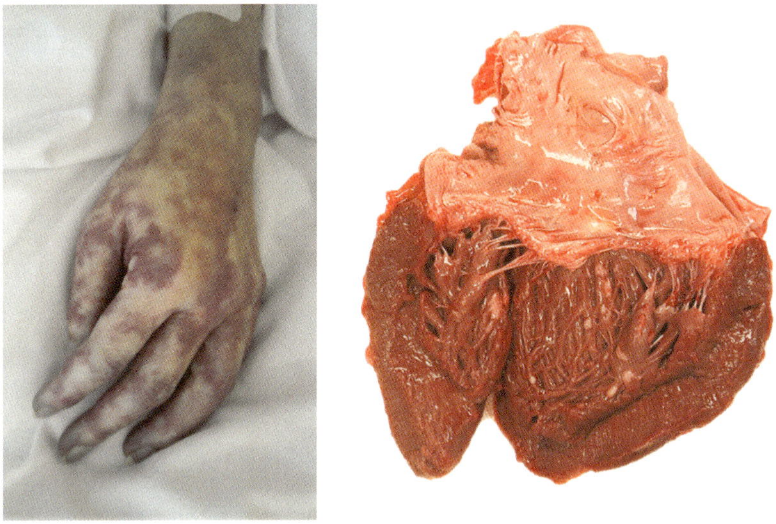

(a) (b)

Figure 1: (a) Skin with regional vasospasm; (b) opened heart, showing multiple small white metastases of a midgut NET.

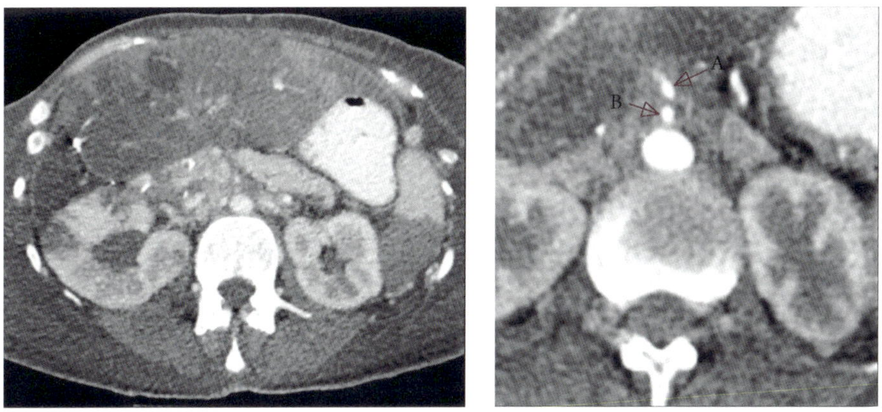

(a) (b)

Figure 2: Abdominal CT-scan. (a) Centralized perfusion with constricted peripheral intestinal arteries. (b) Reduced diameters of abdominal arteries. (A) Truncus coeliacus: 3 mm. (B) A. mesenterica sup.: 3 mm; aorta 15 mm.

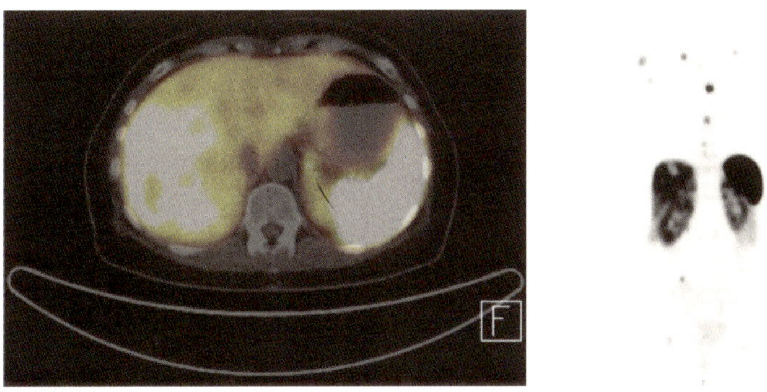

(a) (b)

Figure 3: Somatostatin receptor imaging with CT-scan (PET-CT) (a) showing extensive liver metastasis in the right liver lobe in 12/2011 and (b) additionally showing hydronephrosis.

TABLE 3: Hormone levels in blood and urine.

	Days before and after admission (admission = d 0)							
	d −476	d −452	d −364	d −266	d −58	d −56	d −6	d 6
Chromogranin A (plasma*,**)	896**		748**	717**	1120*		16310*	33580*
5-HIES (urine/24 h, 1–10 mg/24 h)		153				121		132,4$^{\#}$

**CIS Bio Radioimmunoassay (normal levels < 84.7 ng/ml). *Brahms Immunoassay/Thermofisher (normal levels < 110 ng/ml). $^{\#}$Urine was collected over a 12-hour period.

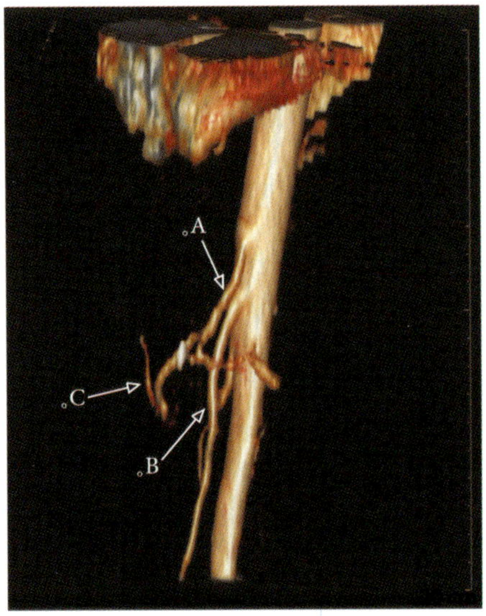

FIGURE 4: 3D reconstruction of the abdominal arteries showing the rarefication of the peripheral hepatic arteries. (A) Truncus coeliacus. (B) A. mesenterica sup. (C) Branch of the constricted hepatic artery.

3. Discussion

The dramatic deterioration in our patient was caused by a progressive cardiac failure with increased vascular resistance and low cardiac index leading to a secondary low-output syndrome.

The massive increase of chromogranin A suggested a carcinoid crisis, although presenting with an atypical systemic vasoconstriction instead of more commonly found vasodilatation and might have possibly been triggered by the preceding PRRT.

Excluding cardiac valvular lesions, the main symptoms of the typical carcinoid syndrome with cutaneous flushing, venous telangiectasia, diarrhoea, and bronchospasm were present for about 2 years in our patient. Functional midgut NETs mainly secret serotonin leading to the typical carcinoid syndrome. Depending on the location of the NET (foregut, hindgut, and pulmonary) other hormones can predominate in systemic circulation resulting in an atypical carcinoid syndrome with variant clinical symptoms [22]. Carcinoid crisis is the life-threatening form of the carcinoid syndrome typically accompanied by severe hypotension. It can be triggered during tumor surgery by manipulation at tumor and metastatic sites or anaesthesia and has, yet more rarely, been described after chemotherapy, hepatic arterial embolization, or radionuclide therapy [23–25]. In a minority of patients, hypertension emerges during carcinoid crisis. This phenomenon was sparsely reported so far. In 1968 Rosenberg published a case report with additional 22 cases of previous literature with hypertensive carcinoid crisis [14]. Warner et al. reported another 2 cases and a review of literature. Based on these observations, (pre)treatment with octreotide is recommended for therapeutic interventions in functional midgut NET. Although some drugs have been successfully used in certain cases, for example, cyproheptadine, ketanserin, 5-HT receptor antagonists, corticosteroids, and H1- and H2-receptor antagonists [15], somatostatin analogues are considered most effective and are recommended as first-line therapy [8, 9, 26].

Still, there are differing opinions regarding octreotide pretreatment against carcinoid crisis before invasive procedures. A retrospective study evaluating the perioperative high-dose octreotide infusion showed a minimized incidence of carcinoid crisis [26]. In contrast, in a meta-analysis, the efficacy of somatostatin analogues to prevent carcinoid crisis could not be confirmed [8].

Pharmacological interventions to overcome the systemic vasoconstriction ultimately failed, despite the use of potent vasodilators. Treatment with nimodipine applied in the early phase of the ICU course seemed to be more effective compared to phentolamine. Intravenous octreotide applied in a dose of 500 μg/24 h continuously iv was also ineffective (recommended dose for carcinoid crisis 50–600 μg/day iv). There are reports of the successful administration of 150 μg/h iv continuously over several days or of a bolus dose of up to 1,5 mg iv [9].

Both sepsis and previous PRRT might have served as a trigger but despite effective sepsis therapy the patient's condition worsened. Furthermore, a high SVRI along with a low CI strongly indicates the development of a cardiogenic shock; see Table 1 [27].

The renal function was normal before PRRT with a creatinine of 0.8 mg/dL and slightly impaired after ICU admission (creatinine 1.6 mg/dL, maximum 2.0 mg/dl). In the long term, PRRT can worsen renal function [28]. We postulate that the acute hemodynamic changes in short term are significantly more likely the cause of the acute renal failure in our patient.

Myocardial tumor infiltration may have additionally contributed to the development of cardiac failure, but the cardiac metastases with a maximum diameter of only 1.5 cm were not pronounced enough to explain the finding sufficiently. Cardiac metastases of a midgut NET are rare but may occur [29].

Interestingly, none of the diagnostic imaging—including echocardiography, MRT, and PET-CT performed one and two months previously—showed any signs of cardiac tumor manifestation. Markers of myocardial necrosis along with NT-proBNP steadily increased during the clinical course of our patient and indicated progressive cardiac failure. However, the pathomechanism compared to coronary heart disease may be reversed in case of primarily exceeding humoral vasoconstrictive factors. The development of heart failure occurred secondary to the pronounced increased vascular resistance with the need of an augmented heart work against a high afterload.

In our case, only a minimal increase of 5-HIAA levels in urine was observed and this might indicate a less pronounced serotonin excess. However, the value was derived from a 12-hour period urine collection and an oliguric kidney injury was present; see Table 3.

It has suggested that serotonin may lead to ergotism, a similar condition of systemic vasoconstriction [19]. Serotonin is able to release noradrenaline in several adrenergic innervated tissues [30] and can amplify the effect of epinephrine, norepinephrine, and angiotensin II [31].

Midgut NETs are able to excrete catecholamines [32]. A single determination of serum catecholamines in our patient showed remarkably elevated catecholamine levels in blood. Epinephrine levels were twice as high as those, for example, observed in stress cardiomyopathy [33].

By immunohistochemically staining of catecholamine-synthesizing enzymes it has been shown that the enzyme pathway for catecholamines in midgut NETs is similar to that in pheochromocytomas [34].

4. Conclusion

Serotonin is mainly assumed to be responsible for the carcinoid crisis. Based on the clinical presentation of our patient with a concomitant excess of catecholamines, we suggest that catecholamines at last contributed to the occurrence of the observed generalized systemic vasoconstriction, ultimately leading to acute heart failure.

Abbreviations

CI:	Cardiac index
DOTA-NOC:	[^{68}Ga-DOTA^{0}-1NaI^{3}]octreotide
DOTA-TOC:	[^{68}Ga-DOTA^{0}-Phe^{1}-Tyr^{3}]octreotide
5-HIAA:	5-Hydroxyindoleacetic acid
5-HT:	5-Hydroxytryptophan
NET:	Neuroendocrine tumor
NT-proBNP:	N-terminal of the prohormone brain natriuretic peptide
PRRT:	Peptide radioreceptor radionuclide therapy
SVRI:	Systemic vascular resistance index.

Acknowledgments

The authors would like to thank Professor Günther Klöppel, Technical University of Munich, Institute of Pathology, Germany, for the very helpful contribution throughout the course of this work.

References

[1] M. Schott, G. Klöppel, A. Raffel, A. Saleh, W. T. Knoefel, and W. A. Scherbaum, "Neuroendocrine neoplasms of the gastrointestinal tract," *Deutsches Ärzteblatt International*, vol. 108, no. 18, pp. 305–312, 2011.

[2] H. De Vries, R. C. J. Verschueren, P. H. B. Willemse, I. P. Kema, and E. G. E. De Vries, "Diagnostic, surgical and medical aspect of the midgut carcinoids," *Cancer Treatment Reviews*, vol. 28, no. 1, pp. 11–25, 2002.

[3] M. Berretta, A. Cappellani, M. Di Vita et al., "Biomarkers in neuroendocrine tumors," *Frontiers in Bioscience*, vol. 2, no. 1, pp. 332–342, 2010.

[4] P. Ferolla, A. Faggiano, G. Mansueto et al., "The biological characterization of neuroendocrine tumors: the role of neuroendocrine markers," *Journal of Endocrinological Investigation*, vol. 31, no. 3, pp. 277–286, 2008.

[5] M. H. Kulke and R. J. Mayer, "Carcinoid tumors," *The New England Journal of Medicine*, vol. 340, no. 11, pp. 858–868, 1999.

[6] P. R. V. Johnson, "Gastroenteropancreatic neuroendocrine (carcinoid) tumors in children," *Seminars in Pediatric Surgery*, vol. 23, no. 2, pp. 91–95, 2014.

[7] L. K. Kvols, "Therapeutic considerations for the malignant carcinoid syndrome," *Acta Oncologica*, vol. 28, no. 3, pp. 433–438, 1989.

[8] L.-J. Guo and C.-W. Tang, "Somatostatin analogues do not prevent Carcinoid crisis," *Asian Pacific Journal of Cancer Prevention*, vol. 15, no. 16, pp. 6679–6683, 2014.

[9] N. Seymour and S. C. Sawh, "Mega-dose intravenous octreotide for the treatment of carcinoid crisis: A systematic review," *Canadian Journal of Anesthesia*, vol. 60, no. 5, pp. 492–499, 2013.

[10] M. E. Kahil, H. Brown, and H. L. Fred, "The Carcinoid Crisis," *Archives of Internal Medicine*, vol. 114, no. 1, pp. 26–28, 1964.

[11] A. S. Anderson, D. Krauss, and R. Lang, "Cardiovascular complications of malignant carcinoid disease," *American Heart Journal*, vol. 134, no. 4, pp. 693–702, 1997.

[12] M. A. O. Kinney, M. E. Warner, D. M. Nagorney et al., "Perianaesthetic risks and outcomes of abdominal surgery for metastatic carcinoid tumours," *British Journal of Anaesthesia*, vol. 87, no. 3, pp. 447–452, 2001.

[13] J. W. Kleine, Y. H. Khouw, and M. G. Heeres, "Anaesthesia and the carcinoid syndrome," *Anaesthesia*, vol. 34, no. 7, pp. 674-674, 1979.

[14] E. B. Rosenberg, "The Carcinoid Syndrome and Hypertension," *Archives of Internal Medicine*, vol. 121, no. 1, pp. 95-96, 1968.

[15] R. R. P. Warner, S. Mani, J. Profeta, and E. Grunstein, "Octreotide treatment of carcinoid hypertensive crisis," *Mount Sinai Journal of Medicine*, vol. 61, no. 4, pp. 349–355, 1994.

[16] C. Bourgault, S. Bergeron, P. Bogaty, and P. Poirier, "A most unusual acute coronary syndrome," *Canadian Journal of Cardiology*, vol. 22, no. 5, pp. 429–432, 2006.

[17] E. J. Topol and N. J. Fortuin, "Coronary artery spasm and cardiac arrest in carcinoid heart disease," *The American Journal of Medicine*, vol. 77, no. 5, pp. 950–952, 1984.

[18] K.-G. Petersen, W.-R. Seemann, R. Plagwitz, and L. Kerp, "Evidence for coronary spasm during flushing in the carcinoid syndrome," *Clinical Cardiology*, vol. 7, no. 8, pp. 445–448, 1984.

[19] C. Karadeniz, F. Köse, H. Abali et al., "Severe systemic vasoconstriction starting with acute limb ischemia leading to death in a patient with well-differentiated pulmonary neuroendocrine carcinoma: a new paraneoplastic syndrome?" *Acta Oncologica*, vol. 51, no. 1, pp. 124–127, 2012.

[20] M. Goedert, U. Otten, K. Suda et al., "Dopamine, norepinephrine and serotonin production by an intestinal carcinoid tumor," *Cancer*, vol. 45, no. 1, pp. 104–107, 1980.

[21] H. H. Whitman III, E. K. Fishman, K. Öberg, J. M. Wildman, and A. L. Long, "Catecholamine-secreting metastatic carcinoid as differential diagnosis in pheochromocytoma: Clinical, laboratory, and imaging clues in the search for the lurking neuroendocrine tumor (NET)," *Annals of the New York Academy of Sciences*, vol. 1073, pp. 59–78, 2006.

[22] K. J. Woodside, C. M. Townsend Jr., and B. Mark Evers, "Current management of gastrointestinal carcinoid tumors," *Journal of Gastrointestinal Surgery*, vol. 8, no. 6, pp. 742–756, 2004.

[23] M. V. Davì, L. Bodei, G. Francia et al., "Carcinoid crisis induced by receptor radionuclide therapy with 90Y-DOTATOC in a case of liver metastases from bronchial neuroendocrine tumor (atypical carcinoid)," *Journal of Endocrinological Investigation*, vol. 29, no. 6, pp. 563–567, 2006.

[24] H. Al Kharrat and H. Taubin, "Carcinoid crisis induced by external manipulation of liver metastasis," *Journal of Clinical Gastroenterology*, vol. 36, no. 1, pp. 87-88, 2003.

[25] D. J. A. Vaughan and M. D. Brunner, "Anesthesia for patients with carcinoid syndrome," *International Anesthesiology Clinics*, vol. 35, no. 4, pp. 129–142, 1997.

[26] E. A. Woltering, A. E. Wright, M. A. Stevens et al., "Development of effective prophylaxis against intraoperative carcinoid crisis," *Journal of Clinical Anesthesia*, vol. 32, pp. 189–193, 2016.

[27] G. Cotter, Y. Moshkovitz, E. Kaluski et al., "The role of cardiac power and systemic vascular resistance in the pathophysiology and diagnosis of patients with acute congestive heart failure," *European Journal of Heart Failure*, vol. 5, no. 4, pp. 443–451, 2003.

[28] D. Hörsch, S. Ezziddin, A. Haug et al., "Effectiveness and side-effects of peptide receptor radionuclide therapy for neuroendocrine neoplasms in Germany: A multi-institutional registry study with prospective follow-up," *European Journal of Cancer*, vol. 58, pp. 41–51, 2016.

[29] H. Jann, T. Wertenbruch, U. Pape et al., "A matter of the heart: Myocardial metastases in neuroendocrine tumors," *Hormone and Metabolic Research*, vol. 42, no. 13, pp. 967–976, 2010.

[30] T. Kimura and S. Satoh, "Presynaptic inhibition by serotonin of cardiac sympathetic transmission in dogs," *Clinical and Experimental Pharmacology and Physiology*, vol. 10, no. 5, pp. 535–542, 1983.

[31] O. Yildiz, J. R. Smith, and R. E. Purdy, "Serotonin and vasoconstrictor synergism," *Life Sciences*, vol. 62, no. 19, pp. 1723–1732, 1998.

[32] I. P. Kema, E. G. E. De Vries, M. J. H. Slooff, B. Biesma, and F. A. J. Muskiet, "Serotonin, catecholamines, histamine, and their metabolites in urine, platelets, and tumor tissue of patients with carcinoid tumors," *Clinical Chemistry*, vol. 40, no. 1, pp. 86–95, 1994.

[33] I. S. Wittstein, D. R. Thiemann, J. A. C. Lima et al., "Neurohumoral features of myocardial stunning due to sudden emotional stress," *New England Journal of Medicine*, vol. 352, no. 6, pp. 539–548, 2005.

[34] W. G. Meijer, S. C. V. M. Copray, H. Hollema et al., "Catecholamine-synthesizing enzymes in carcinoid tumors and pheochromocytomas," *Clinical Chemistry*, vol. 49, no. 4, pp. 586–593, 2003.

Association of Chronic Pancreatitis and Malignant Main Duct IPMN: A Rare but Difficult Clinical Problem

Zoltán Berger,[1] Hernán De La Fuente,[2] Manuel Meneses,[3] Fernanda Matamala,[4] Makarena Sepúlveda,[5] and Claudia Rojas[5]

[1]*Departamento Medicina, Sección Gastroenterología, Hospital Clínico Universidad de Chile, Santiago, Chile*
[2]*Clínica Santa María, Santiago, Chile*
[3]*Fundación Arturo López Pérez, Santiago, Chile*
[4]*Universidad Andres Bello, Santiago, Chile*
[5]*Universidad de los Andes, Santiago, Chile*

Correspondence should be addressed to Zoltán Berger; berger.zoltan@gmail.com

Academic Editor: Gregory Kouraklis

We report the case of a 70-year-old woman who consulted for recurrent short episodes of mild-to-moderate abdominal pain. Dilated main pancreatic duct was seen on CAT scan and magnetic resonance, with multiple calcifications and intraductal stones, typical in CP. However, for a more pronounced cystic dilatation in the pancreatic head, we could not exclude the coexistence of a main duct IPMN. ERCP was performed, with pancreatic sphincterotomy and extraction of pancreatic stones, but, at the same time, mucin extrusion was seen from the dilated duct through the papilla. Pancreatoduodenectomy was performed. Surgery and histology confirmed malignant IPMN with the typical image of chronic pancreatitis and intraductal stones in the vicinity. The patient is doing well 4 years after the surgery, without recurrence of the malignant disease, with changes of chronic pancreatitis in the pancreatic remnant. This paper discusses the possible relationships between the two entities and emphasizes the need of differential diagnosis.

1. Introduction

Chronic pancreatitis is a chronic inflammatory disease of the pancreas, frequently with a benign clinical course. The diagnosis of the advanced forms is generally easy thanks to characteristic morphologic findings: irregularly dilated main pancreatic duct with intraductal stones, calcifications, and frequent dilation of branch ducts [1]. CP can also be complicated by pseudocysts, sometimes communicated to the main duct.

In contrast, intraductal papillary mucinous neoplasia (IPMN) is a mucin-producing tumor of ductal origin, with variable probability of malignant transformation. In the case of main duct IPMN, high-grade dysplasia and even invasive cancer are already present in 50–70% of lesions when diagnosed [2, 3] and this frequency is increasing. Differential diagnosis is based on CAT scan and magnetic resonance images (MRI): presence of pancreatic stones, diffuse dilatation of the main duct with "chain of lakes" images, and dilated branch ducts argue in favor of CP, while more circumscribed and larger cystic lesions, particularly with mural nodules, are frequent in the main duct IPMN. The therapy of the two diseases is quite different: conservative treatment or minimally invasive endoscopic procedures in CP and radical surgical resolution in main duct IPMN, with a relatively good prognosis of about 70% survival at 5 years [2].

However, differential diagnosis can be difficult, particularly if calcifications are present in the dilated duct.

We report the case of our patient, in whom CP and main duct IPMN were simultaneously detected and treated successfully by surgery.

2. Case Report

A 70-year-old female patient consulted medical doctor for recurrent moderate abdominal pain in the last few months.

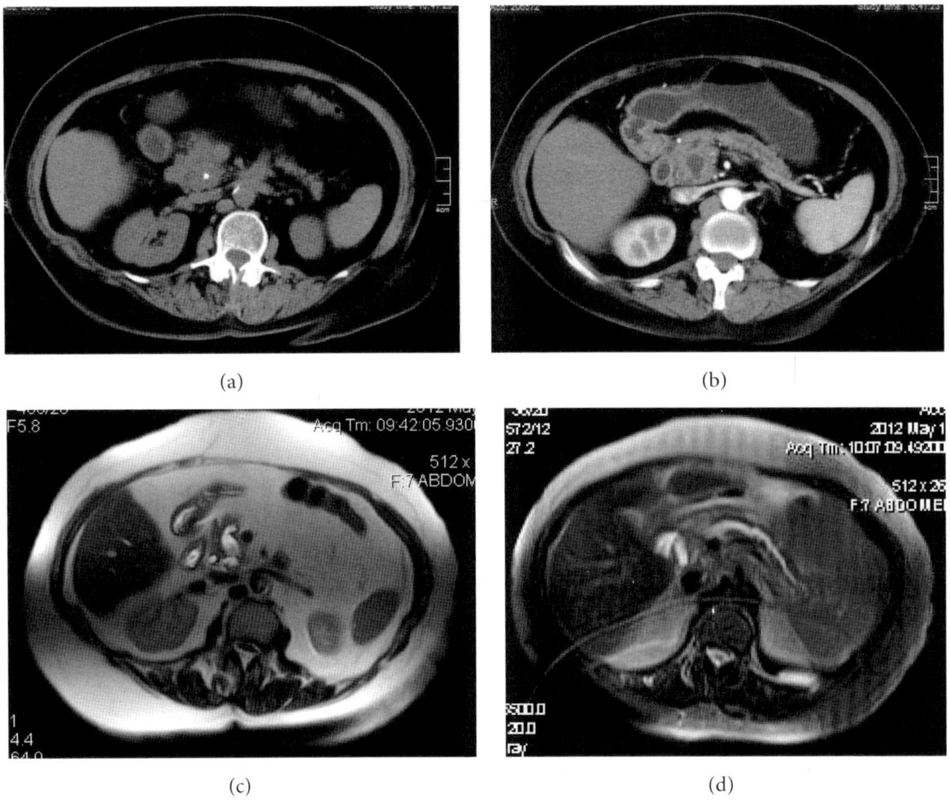

Figure 1: CAT scan ((a) and (b)) and magnetic resonance ((c) and (d)) images before the surgery. (a) Pancreatic head increased in size, with focal calcification, without mass lesion. (b) Dilated pancreatic duct in the whole pancreas, with major diameter, and fusiform dilatation in the pancreatic head. Slight atrophy of pancreatic parenchyma. (c) Fusiform dilated main pancreatic duct in the pancreatic head, with small filling defect suspected. (d) Dilated main pancreatic duct in pancreatic body and tail, with slight atrophy of parenchyma.

She had had a cholecystectomy 30 years ago; later on, without significant illness in medical history, she was a teetotaler and she smoked 2 cigarettes per day during 10 years but stopped completely during the 6 last months. Routine blood tests were in the normal range. Abdominal ultrasound did not visualize the pancreas well due to bloating. A CAT scan was performed, finding multiple calcifications and irregularly dilated main pancreatic duct, predominantly in the pancreatic head (Figures 1(a) and 1(b)), where the dilatation had some cystic aspect and was disproportionally more pronounced than in the pancreatic body and tail. The same alterations were confirmed by MRI (Figures 1(c) and 1(d)), without intramural nodules in the dilated main duct. Based on the two imaging methods, we could not distinguish between chronic calcifying pancreatitis and mucin-producing neoplasia, that is, main duct IPMN. ERCP was performed, and contrast injection revealed a cystic dilation of main pancreatic duct in the head (Figure 2(a)). The duct of Wirsung was less dilated in the body. Through pancreatic papillotomy, typical whitish pancreatic stone passed into the duodenal lumen (Figure 2(b)). However, after having continued the contrast injection, mucin passage was seen producing the typical fish eye appearance in the major and also the minor papilla (Figures 2(c) and 2(d)). Simultaneous existence of CP with pancreatic stones and main duct IPMN was our final diagnosis. Given the high probability of malignancy in the dominant cystic lesion, surgery was decided and performed. Surgery revealed a cystic tumor that was found in a fibrotic pancreas. Pancreatoduodenectomy was performed with preservation of pylorus and pancreaticogastrostomy. Some whitish pancreatic stones were extracted. No lymph node metastasis was seen. Histological (Figure 3) findings confirmed the existence of a mucinous tumor emerging from the main pancreatic duct, with multiple foci of high grade dysplasia and even with evident transformation into an infiltrative malignant lesion (Figure 3). No lymph node metastasis or vascular involvement was found. Fibrosis, acinar cell degeneration, and tubular complexes [4] were seen in the surrounding tumor-free pancreatic tissue. The patient is still doing well 4 years after the intervention, without suspicion of any tumor recurrence.

3. Discussion

IPMN is recognized with increasing frequency, thanks to the general accessibility of imaging methods, as an incidental finding in the vast majority of cases. These mucinous benign tumors generally originate in the branch ducts. Main duct IPMN is far less frequent but a much more severe entity for its high probability of malignant transformation. Furthermore,

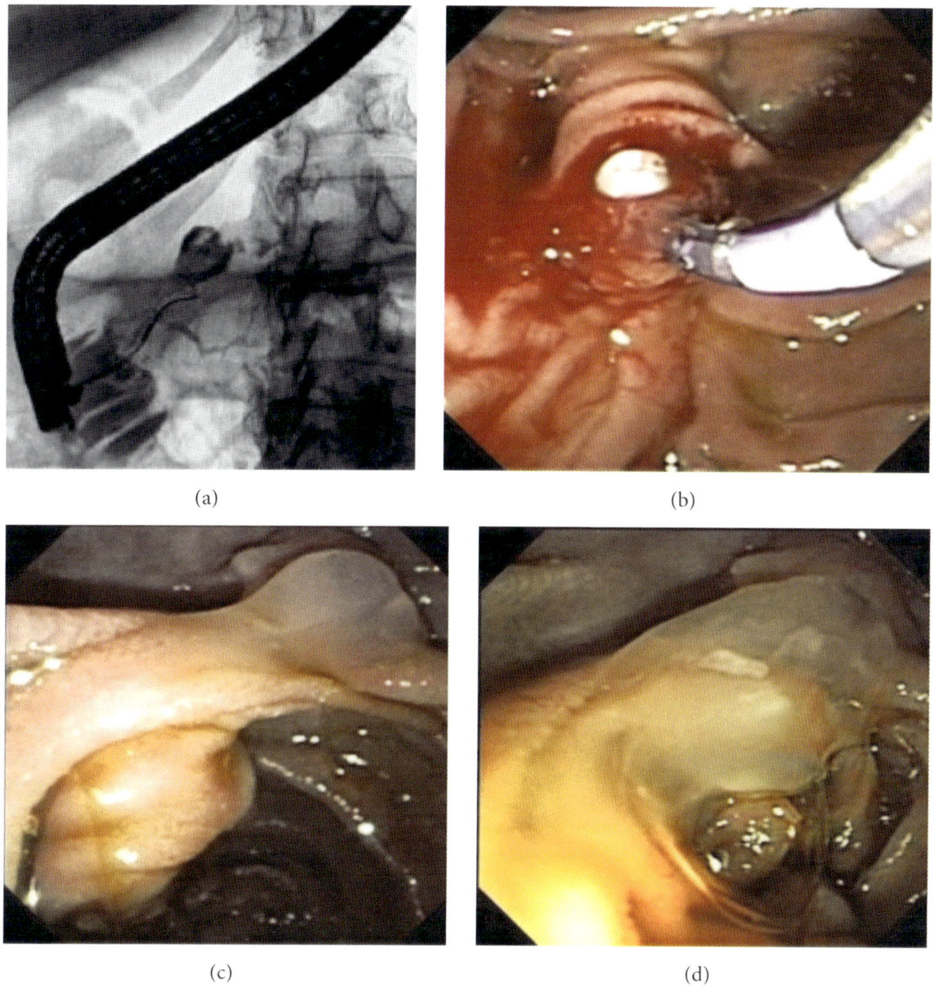

FIGURE 2: ERCP. (a) ERCP: incomplete contrast injection in the pancreatic duct. Cystic dilatation of the main pancreatic duct in the head of pancreas; initial opacification of less dilated duct in the body. Note normal caliber duct in uncinated process. (b) Pancreatic papillotomy, followed by passage of white pancreatic stone. No mucin was seen at this moment. (c) "Fish eye" sign; mucin spurring from the minor papilla. (d) Flow of mucin from the minor papilla.

in some cases, it is difficult to distinguish between CP and IPMN and the two entities can coexist in the same pancreas [5–9].

The presence of histological alterations of focal chronic pancreatitis near to any pancreatic tumor is a usual finding, but calcification is only exceptionally present. If calcification is seen, one can hypothesize 3 possibilities. (1) The first hypothesis is calcification of the tumor, frequent as a central scare in benign serous cystadenomas and peripheral in malignant mucinous cystadenoma. However, in these cases, the calcification is present in the tumor and not in the focal chronic pancreatitis. (2) The second hypothesis is calcification, where intraductal stones can be part of a preexistent chronic pancreatitis and the main duct IPMN can develop in a previously ill pancreas. In effect, the risk of pancreatic adenocarcinoma is higher in CP, but it is a ductal adenocarcinoma and not an IPMN with malignant transformation. (3) The third hypothesis is that IPMN, like all pancreatic tumors, can produce a focal CP, probably by partial obstruction. However, obstructive CP generally does not present stones. Zapiach et al. [5] analyzed possible mechanisms of calcification seen in their 10 patients and they found this last mechanism as a possible explanation: long-lasting partial ductal obstruction could be the cause of the stone formation in this special form of human obstructive pancreatitis. Our case seems to be in line with this hypothesis: the medical history of our patient was relatively short; some months, she had no symptoms of chronic pancreatitis earlier and she had none of the known etiological factors of the disease. Probably the slowly growing main duct IPMN was the cause of her obstructive pancreatitis with subsequent stone formation.

Our case, while not unique, seems to be rare, given the simultaneous presence of radiological signs of CP with intraductal stones and a malignant IPMN. Endoscopic therapy, extraction of stones, could have been a good therapeutic option for the recurrent pain produced by CP. On the other hand, the only curative possibility for a main duct IPMN is radical surgery [10]. Although malignant, as in our case, the prognosis is quite different from ductal adenocarcinoma,

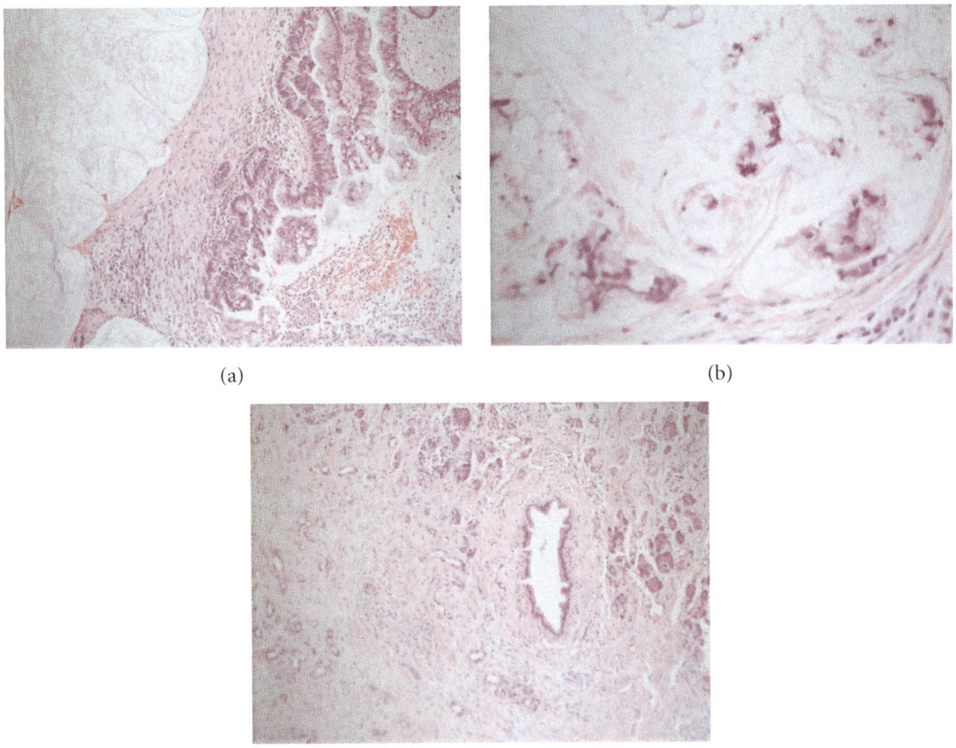

(a) (b) (c)

Figure 3: Histologic findings. Hematoxylin-eosin, 100x. (a) Neoplastic epithelium of a pancreatic duct, with formation of papillary structures (on the right). Abundant mucin formation on the left side. (b) Mucinous uniform cells with epithelial atypia and invasion of the neighborhood. (c) Tumor-free pancreatic tissue. Distortion of the normal architecture; moderate-to-severe fibrosis is seen with inflammatory cell infiltration. We can observe dilated ductal elements and atrophy of acinar cells.

with >70% of 5-year survival. In our case, ERCP findings were also equivocal, even including pancreatic stone extraction, but finally the mucin extrusion from the papillary orifice after manipulation in the pancreatic duct permitted the final preoperative diagnosis and the correct choice of surgical therapy.

Our case emphasizes again the possibility that IMPN and chronic pancreatitis may coexist in the same patient. Morphologic signs of CP, even the presence of intraductal stones, are not enough to exclude the simultaneous presence of main duct IPMN. If radiological findings are not clear enough [11] and the suspicion of a focal lesion persists, every possible effort must be made to reach a precise diagnosis, since the distinction between these two entities is of vital importance for the patient. In our case, we considered a high probability of CP without IPMN on the basis of CT and MRI. ERCP was thus chosen as first procedure with diagnostic and therapeutic purposes. However, EUS and fine-needle biopsy could be also the first, less invasive step. The finding of mucin defined the nature of the lesion without any other procedure, but in some cases EUS, fine-needle biopsy, and ERCP could be necessary to establish the final diagnosis.

References

[1] D. L. Conwell, L. S. Lee, D. Yadav et al., "American Pancreatic Association practice guidelines in chronic pancreatitis evidence-based report on diagnostic guidelines," *Pancreas*, vol. 43, no. 8, pp. 1143–1162, 2014.

[2] M. Tanaka, C. Fernández-Del Castillo, V. Adsay et al., "International consensus guidelines 2012 for the management of IPMN and MCN of the pancreas," *Pancreatology*, vol. 12, no. 3, pp. 183–197, 2012.

[3] E. Paal, L. D. R. Thompson, R. M. Przygodzki, G. L. Bratthauer, and C. S. Heffess, "A clinicopathologic and immunohistochemical study of 22 intraductal papillary mucinous neoplasms of the pancreas, with a review of the literature," *Modern Pathology*, vol. 12, no. 5, pp. 518–528, 1999.

[4] D. E. Bockman, W. R. Boydston, and M. C. Anderson, "Origin of tubular complexes in human chronic pancreatitis," *The American Journal of Surgery*, vol. 144, no. 2, pp. 243–249, 1982.

[5] M. Zapiach, D. Yadav, T. C. Smyrk et al., "Calcifying obstructive pancreatitis: a study of intraductal papillary mucinous neoplasm associated with pancreatic calcification," *Clinical Gastroenterology and Hepatology*, vol. 2, no. 1, pp. 57–63, 2004.

[6] A. Petrou, A. Papalambros, N. Brennan et al., "Intraductal papillary mucinous neoplasm (IPMN) and chronic pancreatitis: overlapping pathological entities? Two case reports," *Journal of the Pancreas*, vol. 12, no. 1, pp. 50–54, 2011.

[7] W. Kimura, "Pancreatic lithiasis and intraductal papillary-mucinous neoplasm with special reference to the pathogenesis

of lithiasis," *Journal of Hepato-Biliary-Pancreatic Sciences*, vol. 17, no. 6, pp. 776–781, 2010.

[8] E. Kalaitzakis, B. Braden, P. Trivedi, Y. Sharifi, and R. Chapman, "Intraductal papillary mucinous neoplasm in chronic calcifying pancreatitis: egg or hen?" *World Journal of Gastroenterology*, vol. 15, no. 10, pp. 1273–1275, 2009.

[9] M. Abu-Hilal, R. Salvia, A. Casaril et al., "Obstructive chronic pancreatitis and/or intraductal papillary mucinous neoplasms (IPMNs): a 21-year long case report," *Journal of the Pancreas*, vol. 7, no. 2, pp. 218–221, 2006.

[10] S. Crippa, I. Pergolini, C. Rubini et al., "Risk of misdiagnosis and overtreatment in patients with main pancreatic duct dilatation and suspected combined/main-duct intraductal papillary mucinous neoplasms," *Surgery*, vol. 159, no. 4, pp. 1041–1049, 2016.

[11] J. H. Kim, S. S. Hong, Y. J. Kim, J. K. Kim, and H. W. Eun, "Intraductal papillary mucinous neoplasm of the pancreas: differentiate from chronic pancreatits by MR imaging," *European Journal of Radiology*, vol. 81, no. 4, pp. 671–676, 2012.

A Challenging Case of Severe Ulcerative Colitis following the Initiation of Secukinumab for Ankylosing Spondylitis

Dean Ehrlich,[1] Nimah Jamaluddin,[1] Joseph Pisegna,[1,2] and David Padua[1,2]

[1] *Division of Digestive Diseases, Department of Medicine, David Geffen School of Medicine at UCLA, Los Angeles, CA, USA*
[2] *Division of Gastroenterology, Hepatology and Parenteral Nutrition, VA Greater Los Angeles Healthcare System, Los Angeles, CA, USA*

Correspondence should be addressed to David Padua; dpadua@mednet.ucla.edu

Academic Editor: Hirotada Akiho

Secukinumab is an interleukin-17 inhibitor used for the treatment of ankylosing spondylitis (AS), psoriasis, and psoriatic arthritis. The risk of exacerbating underlying inflammatory bowel disease (IBD) in patients being treated with secukinumab for other conditions is controversial. We document a patient with AS and previously undiagnosed IBD, found to be in a severe ulcerative colitis flare shortly after receiving the loading dose of secukinumab. There are no guidelines regarding biologic salvage therapy for IBD in the setting of active treatment with another biologic agent. After waiting one half-life of secukinumab, our patient had an excellent response to initiation of infliximab.

1. Introduction

Secukinumab is an interleukin-17 (IL-17) monoclonal antibody inhibitor approved for the treatment of ankylosing spondylitis, psoriatic arthritis, and psoriasis [1]. Data previously showed that secukinumab has no efficacy in Crohn's Disease [2]; however, the risk of exacerbating underlying Crohn's Disease or Ulcerative Colitis in patients being treated with secukinumab for other conditions is controversial.

2. Case

We present the case of a 42-year-old male with a past medical history of ankylosing spondylitis (AS) and anterior uveitis who came to the hospital with nonbloody diarrhea. For the ten days prior to presentation, the patient reported over twenty loose nonbloody bowel movements per day, with associated nocturnal symptoms, tenesmus, fevers, chills, night sweats, and five-pound weight loss. For the two years prior to the onset of these symptoms, he had five bowel movements per day, with intermittent bloody stool, tenesmus, and 20-pound weight loss but never had a workup for inflammatory bowel disease (IBD) including a prior colonoscopy. He was a resident of Los Angeles with no recent travel outside the continental United States and no unusual exposures. He denied relevant family history of inflammatory disorders. He had attributed these chronic gastrointestinal symptoms to a prior diagnosis of external hemorrhoids.

His ankylosing spondylitis (HLA-B27 positive) was active with severe daily stiffness and thoracolumbar back pain but had no symptoms of anterior uveitis for several years. For AS, he was prescribed naproxen and methotrexate. He had previously been trialed on etanercept and then adalimumab, which were both discontinued due to rash. Six weeks prior to admission, he was started on secukinumab and received all five loading doses without change in his AS symptoms. He stopped taking naproxen 10 days prior to admission when the diarrhea began.

On admission, his exam was notable for a temperature of 102.3°F and the absence of any eye, oral, skin, or rectal abnormalities. His abdomen was soft but diffusely tender. Labs were notable for 13.99 (M/uL) white blood cells, hemoglobin 10.6 (g/dL), platelets 501 (k/uL), ESR 78 (mm/hr), CRP 18.9 (mg/dL), albumin 3.2 (g/dL), and fecal calprotectin 359 (mcg/g). He had a normal complete metabolic panel and TSH, with negative HIV, blood cultures, and stool infectious workup, including C. diff toxin. A CT abdomen and pelvis with contrast showed pancolitis. A flexible sigmoidoscopy

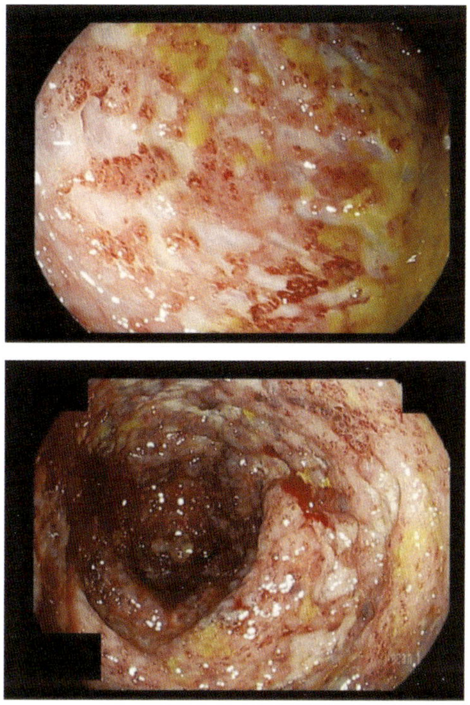

FIGURE 1: Endoscopic evaluation on presentation. Severe colitis seen throughout the colon.

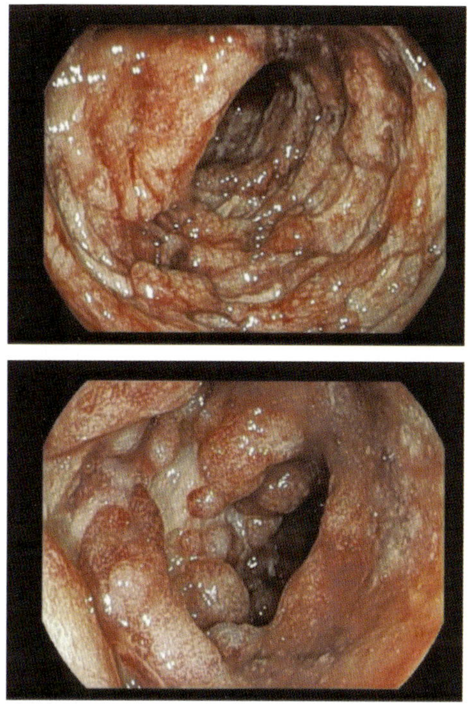

FIGURE 2: Endoscopic evaluation after failed trial on oral steroids. Severe colitis seen up to 40 cm; further evaluation was limited given degree of inflammation.

performed shortly after admission showed severe colitis with deep ulcerations, absent vascular pattern, and friable mucosa in the transverse and sigmoid colon (Figure 1). There was mild colitis in the rectum with patchy erythema. Pathology from the transverse and distal colon showed focal neutrophilic cryptitis, crypt microabscesses, and missing crypts, consistent with inflammatory bowel disease. Histology was negative for CMV colitis. Magnetic resonance enterography showed no evidence of small bowel disease.

A new diagnosis of an ulcerative colitis (UC) flare (Mayo Score 12) was made. The patient was treated with intravenous solumedrol (60 mg per day) and had a brief period of improvement. However, he did not tolerate a transition to oral prednisone (60 mg per day) and suffered a syncopal event from blood loss. A repeat flexible sigmoidoscopy demonstrated edematous mucosa with loss of vascularity and scattered ulcers from anus to 15 cm and deep large ulcers with friable mucosa and spontaneous bleeding from 15 cm to 40 cm (Figure 2).

Surgical consultation was requested after the patient failed the oral steroid trial; however, the patient was hesitant to undergo total proctocolectomy and declined surgical intervention. Biologic salvage therapy was considered, but the timing of initiating a biologic agent was troublesome knowing that he was already on a long acting immunosuppressant (secukinumab) and appreciating the risks of severe immunosuppression. He was put back on intravenous solumedrol; however, his symptoms only mildly improved. After discussion with the patient, the decision was made to start infliximab one month after the last secukinumab infusion along with an oral steroid taper. The patient responded

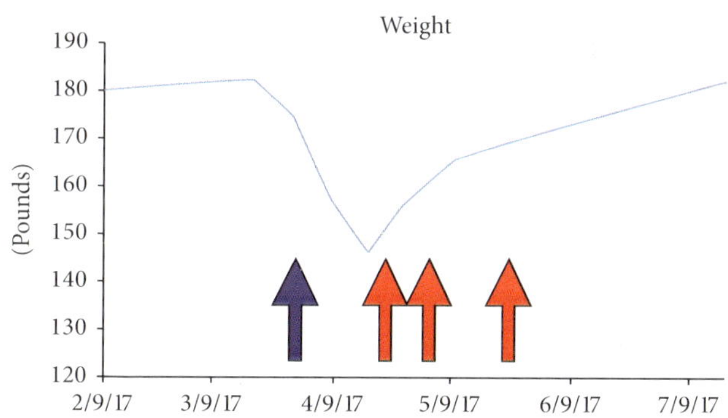

FIGURE 3: Charted weights. Significant weight loss seen on presentation (blue arrow). Red arrows: indication dates of infliximab administration with the corresponding weight gain.

well after two doses of infliximab (10 mg/kg) with improved bloody diarrhea to three times per day and 15-pound weight gain within the first month (Figure 3). The patient has received a total three doses of infliximab. We plan for the patient to receive maintenance infliximab therapy every eight weeks.

3. Discussion

This case documents the association of initiating secukinumab, an IL-17 inhibitor, with a severe flare of ulcerative colitis in a patient with previously undiagnosed IBD.

The question of whether secukinumab impacts inflammatory bowel disease first arose in 2012 when a study on the treatment of Crohn's Disease with secukinumab demonstrated poorer outcomes and more adverse events in treated patients than those given a placebo [2]. However, in larger trials on the use of secukinumab in treating AS, there were only six reports of inflammatory bowel disease as adverse events, just two of which were considered serious [3, 4]. Then in October 2016, a review of 14 studies, in which patients were treated with secukinumab for AS, psoriasis, or psoriatic arthritis, made the claim that there was *no* increased risk of IBD due to secukinumab. The review stated that the incidence of IBD in patients treated with secukinumab was similar to rates of IBD seen in the literature in patients with AS, psoriasis, and psoriatic arthritis [5].

The acute management of this patient was challenging because of the recent administration of secukinumab which has a half-life of 22–31 days [1]. The addition of another active biologic agent to treat the IBD flare may have subjected the patient to excessive immunosuppression and placed him at increased risk for a negative outcome. There are no guidelines for management of the waiting period between biologic agents in IBD. In the psoriasis literature, there is some consensus on giving the first dose of a new biologic at the time the next dose of the old biologic would be due; however, this is based on expert opinion [6, 7]. In Crohn's Disease literature, safe administration of adding natalizumab or vedolizumab to infliximab therapy has been described in refractory cases [8, 9]. However, there is no data on using infliximab as an overlapping induction agent in the setting of recent secukinumab use and severe UC. We opted to wait 30 days before starting infliximab (roughly one half-life of secukinumab), which also coincided with the next due dose of secukinumab. Our surgical team was also closely following the patient if his health had declined any further.

An important consideration for this case is that the patient may have had underlying undiagnosed IBD (based on symptom history) and therefore secukinumab may have triggered an IBD flare, rather than a de novo case of IBD. While there is no way to determine whether the patient had previously undiagnosed IBD, even the triggering of an IBD flare by secukinumab has been rarely reported and would be an especially important finding because of the recent literature which specifically refutes this association as a concern for patients with IBD taking secukinumab [5]. Another consideration is that NSAIDs may have triggered the IBD flare; however, the patient had been taking NSAIDs for months to years without issue.

The pathogenesis of UC triggered by secukinumab is largely unknown. Given the delicate balance of the immune response in the setting of inflammatory bowel disease, it is often difficult to predict the effects of cytokine blockade on disease progression. Il-17 antagonists showed promise in preclinical trials. However, not all studies were positive. In 2004, Ogawa et al. reported on a mouse model of colitis that a neutralizing Il-17 monoclonal antibody worsened colitis via increases in CD4-positive helper T cells and CD11b-positive granulocytes-monocytes infiltration and increases in tumor necrosis factor-alpha, interferon-gamma, and IL-6 [10]. It is possible that these mechanisms were at play in our patient. The combination of his potential genetics and secukinumab exposure may have elicited this severe colitis response. Per Hueber et al., in Crohn's Disease genetic polymorphisms (i.e., TL1A) likely play a role in the response to secukinumab [2]. It is unclear whether our patient had this polymorphism; however, this may be important for future risk stratification of patients.

This case presents an interesting study in the potential side effects evoked by IL-17 antagonists. Given the potential risk of IBD exacerbation with these agents, providers should consider evaluating for underlying IBD prior to their initiation. As more targeted therapies come to the market to treat various inflammatory conditions, it will be important to monitor these side effects and develop strategies to ameliorate the adverse events.

Consent

The patient consented to publication of the case details.

Authors' Contributions

Dean Ehrlich, Nimah Jamaluddin, Joseph Pisegna, and David Padua were all involved in the writing and editing of this manuscript. David Padua is the article guarantor.

Acknowledgments

This work received grant support from Department of Veterans Affairs RR&D Merit Review (Joseph Pisegna) I01 RX000194 and Human Studies CORE through CURE: Digestive Diseases Research Center supported by NIH Grant P30DK41301 (Joseph Pisegna, David Padua).

References

[1] *Secukinumab [package insert]. Novartis Pharmaceuticals*, East Hanover, New Jersey, USA, 2015, https://www.pharma.us.novartis.com/sites/www.pharma.us.novartis.com/files/cosentyx.pdf.

[2] W. Hueber, B. E. Sands, S. Lewitzky et al., "Secukinumab, a human anti-IL-17A monoclonal antibody, for moderate to severe Crohn's disease: unexpected results of a randomised, double-blindplacebo-controlled trial," *Gut*, vol. 61, no. 12, pp. 1693–1700, 2012.

[3] D. Baeten, J. Sieper, J. Braun et al., "Secukinumab, an interleukin-17A inhibitor, in ankylosing spondylitis," *The New England Journal of Medicine*, vol. 373, no. 26, pp. 2534–2548, 2015.

[4] X. Baraliakos, A. Kivitz, A. Deodhar et al., "THU0397 Secukinumab provides sustained improvements in the signs and symptoms of active ankylosing spondylitis: 3-year results from a phase 3 extension trial (MEASURE 1)," in *Proceedings of the Annual European Congress of Rheumatology, 14–17 June, 2017*, pp. 357.2-358.

[5] S. Schreiber, B. Sands, A. Deodhar et al., "OP0113 No Increased Incidence of Inflammatory Bowel Disease among Secukinumab-Treated Patients with Moderate To Severe Psoriasis, Psoriatic Arthritis, or Ankylosing Spondylitis: Data from 14 Phase 2 and Phase 3 Clinical Studies," *Annals of the Rheumatic Diseases*, vol. 75, no. Suppl 2, pp. 97-98, 2016.

[6] F. Kerdel and M. Zaiac, "An evolution in switching therapy for psoriasis patients who fail to meet treatment goals," *Dermatologic Therapy*, vol. 28, no. 6, pp. 390–403, 2015.

[7] U. Mrowietz, E. M. G. J. De Jong, K. Kragballe et al., "A consensus report on appropriate treatment optimization and transitioning in the management of moderate-to-severe plaque psoriasis," *Journal of the European Academy of Dermatology and Venereology*, vol. 28, no. 4, pp. 438–453, 2014.

[8] R. Hirten, R. S. Longman, B. P. Bosworth, A. Steinlauf, and E. Scherl, "Vedolizumab and infliximab combination therapy in the treatment of Crohn's disease," *American Journal of Gastroenterology*, vol. 110, no. 12, pp. 1737-1738, 2015.

[9] B. E. Sands, R. Kozarek, J. Spainhour et al., "Safety and tolerability of concurrent natalizumab treatment for patients with Crohn's disease not in remission while receiving infliximab," *Inflammatory Bowel Diseases*, vol. 13, no. 1, pp. 2–11, 2007.

[10] A. Ogawa, A. Andoh, Y. Araki, T. Bamba, and Y. Fujiyama, "Neutralization of interleukin-17 aggravates dextran sulfate sodium-induced colitis in mice," *Clinical Immunology*, vol. 110, no. 1, pp. 55–62, 2004.

54

Metastatic Cutaneous Melanoma of the Gallbladder

Dhruvan Patel,[1] Shazia Sohrawardy,[2] Yub Raj Sedhai,[1] Soney Basnyat,[3] Anisha Daxini,[4] Aparna Basu,[5] Vivek R. Mehta,[6] Aasim Mohammed,[1] and Steven Lichtenstein[7]

[1]*Internal Medicine, Mercy Catholic Medical Center, Darby, PA, USA*
[2]*Philadelphia College of Osteopathic Medicine, Philadelphia, PA, USA*
[3]*Nepal Medical College Teaching Hospital, Kathmandu, Nepal*
[4]*JJM Medical College, Davangere, India*
[5]*Hematology & Oncology, Henry Ford Medical Center, Detroit, MI, USA*
[6]*Rheumatology, Albany Medical Center, Albany, NY, USA*
[7]*Division of Gastroenterology & Hepatology, Mercy Health System, Philadelphia, PA, USA*

Correspondence should be addressed to Yub Raj Sedhai; dr.sedhai@gmail.com

Academic Editor: Daniel C. Damin

Metastatic melanoma is an aggressive disease that can spread to many organs of the body. In rare cases, it can spread to the gallbladder causing secondary lesions, yet presenting with little to no symptoms. Therefore, most cases of metastatic melanoma lesions to the gallbladder go undiagnosed. Here, we present the case of a 41-year-old male with a four-month history of melanoma of the face, with a postresection status, who presented with right upper quadrant abdominal pain. Doppler ultrasound and computed tomography confirmed the presence of a mass on the gallbladder. Laparoscopic excision along with liver wedge resection was performed. Pathology staining revealed the presence of a malignant metastatic melanoma lesion of the gallbladder.

1. Introduction

Cutaneous melanoma is a very aggressive disease, arising from the proliferation of melanocytes, a type of dendritic cell found in the epidermis, uvea, meninges, intestinal tract, upper respiratory tract, and along regional lymph nodes [1–3]. While it comprises less than 5% of all skin cancer cases, it has an extremely high morbidity and mortality due to its high tendency to metastasize throughout the body [1–4]. The most common sites of distant metastases are the lungs, brain, liver, and GI tract [1–3]. Only 2–4% of patients affected by cutaneous melanoma are diagnosed with gastrointestinal metastases and the most common sites are the small bowel, colon, and stomach [1, 2]. Metastatic involvement of the gallbladder is extremely rare and, when present, is often part of a widespread complex of metastases with a very poor prognosis [1, 4, 5]. Interestingly, autopsy reports suggest gallbladder involvement in 4–20% of all cutaneous melanoma metastasis patients; however, they are associated with minimal to no symptoms, making diagnosis difficult during its lifetime [5–7].

Here, we report a rare case of melanoma metastasis to the gallbladder as the first site of recurrence following cutaneous melanoma treatment. The patient presented with right upper quadrant abdominal pain and was successfully treated with cholecystectomy and liver wedge resection surgery.

2. Case Report

Written consent for publication of this case was obtained from the patient. We present a 41-year-old male with a medical history of cutaneous melanoma of the face who presented to the hospital with abdominal pain. Three months prior to this admission, the patient was diagnosed with an ulcerated nodular malignant melanoma of his right temple, Breslow thickness 12 mm, invasive to Clark anatomic level IV. The patient underwent wide local excision of the lesion, with a negative sentinel node biopsy (Stage IIC, T4N0M0).

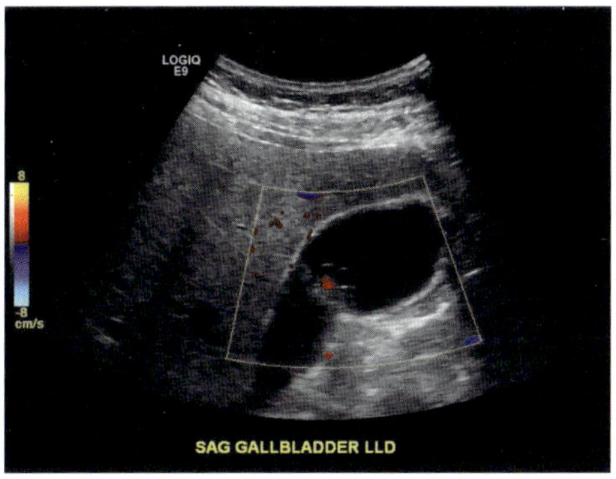

FIGURE 1: Ultrasound Doppler showing gallbladder mass with high blood flow.

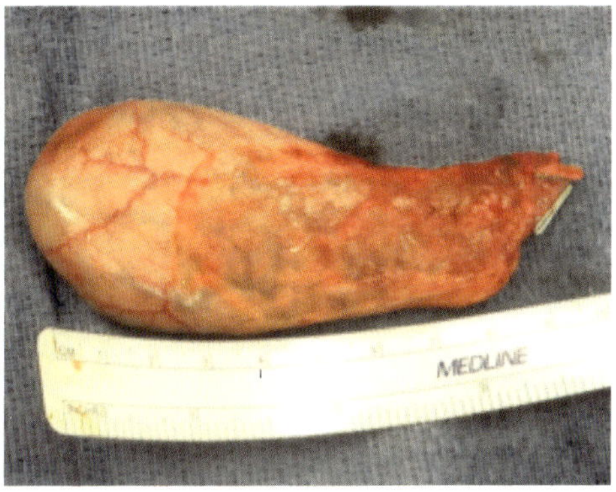

FIGURE 2: Surface of resected gallbladder.

Following excision of his facial lesion, he was started on interferon therapy 5 days a week. A one-month follow-up included a normal physical exam, normal complete blood count, and normal complete metabolic panel. Positron emission tomography (PET-CT) was also obtained at the same time and was negative for any metastatic lesions.

Three months after follow-up, the patient presented to the hospital with a 3-week history of right upper quadrant (RUQ) abdominal pain, nausea, alternating bowel movements, and a 15-pound weight loss. Physical exam revealed RUQ tenderness but was otherwise unremarkable. Laboratory testing showed his bilirubin, AST, and ALT to be 0.3 mg/dL, 62 U/L, and 96 U/L, respectively. An abdominal computed tomography showed a gallbladder lesion. Doppler ultrasound confirmed a 1.1 × 1 cm gallbladder lesion with high blood flow (Figure 1). Following this, an ultrasound-guided gallbladder biopsy was attempted but was unsuccessful because of an inability to locate the lesion precisely. Due to the high suspicion of metastasis, the patient underwent a laparoscopic cholecystectomy along with a hepatic wedge resection (Figure 2). This resection revealed no external evidence of a metastatic gallbladder lesion, both intraoperatively or on back table inspection. A frozen section of the gallbladder was also found to be negative for melanoma metastasis. There was no evidence of pigmentation within the abdomen. Despite all of this, pathology confirmed the suspicion of metastatic melanoma of the gallbladder through a positive immunohistochemistry stain, showing a BRAF V600K mutation (Figure 3). Our operative report justifies the presence of an intraluminal gallbladder mass, which can be easily missed on external appearance or on frozen section.

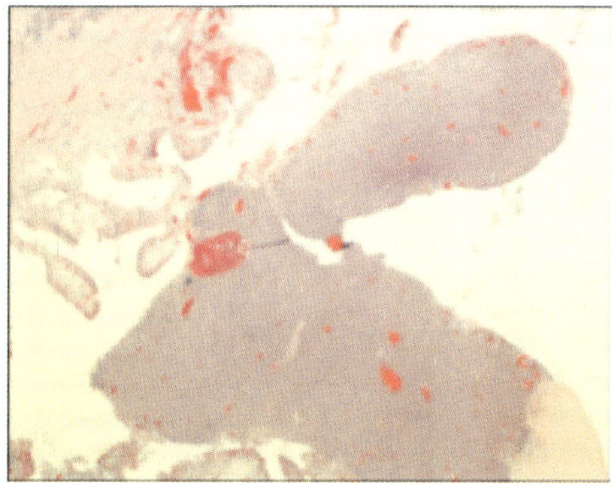

FIGURE 3: Pathology of gallbladder mass showing metastatic melanoma.

After surgery, the patient did not require adjuvant therapy, such as high-dose interferon or dabrafenib/trametinib, for his localized metastatic lesion, in accordance with the most recent guidelines for malignant melanoma [1, 5]. A follow-up PET-CT was obtained 1 month after surgery and showed no evidence of the disease recurrence. At the most recent follow-up, clinic evaluation 6 months after surgery, the patient was well without any evidence of recurrence.

3. Discussion

Melanocytes are a dendritic-type cell, which provides melanin to keratinocytes and can be found in most organ viscera, depending on neural crest migration during embryogenesis [1, 8]. Melanoma is a malignant tumor of melanocytes and represents <5% of all skin cancers [5, 9]. However, it has a high potential for widespread metastatic disease and thus is associated with high mortality. The incidence of melanoma is growing faster than any other potentially preventable cancer in the United States with an approximately 1.9 percent growth annually between 2000 and 2009 [10]. Globally, 132,000 new cases of melanoma will arise this year with 48,000 deaths per year [2].

Melanoma usually follows a benign course of early radial growth. The potential for metastasis greatly increases once the cutaneous lesion begins to spread vertically, penetrating blood and lymph vessels [1, 11, 12]. Tumor cells can spread to the local lymph nodes draining the region of the primary lesion. It can also travel hematogenously to distant sites, such as the soft tissues (50–75%), lung (70–87%), liver (54–77%), and brain [9, 11, 13]. Many authors have also postulated dissemination of tumor cells via bile, contributing to liver and GI tract invasion. Only 2–4% of patients affected by cutaneous melanoma are diagnosed with gastrointestinal metastases [8]. The most common sites for GI invasion are the small bowel (35–65%), colon (5–9%), and stomach (5–7%) [1, 2].

Cutaneous metastatic melanoma to the gallbladder is rarely found during a patient's life [9, 11, 14]. When found, it usually presents as part of a widespread metastatic disease. It is important to note that though travel to the gallbladder is rare, gallbladder melanoma accounts for 50–67% of all gallbladder tumors [11, 12, 15]. The prognosis is extremely poor for metastatic gallbladder melanoma with an average survival of 8.4 months and a 5-year survival of only 15% [9, 15, 16]. However, the prognosis of metastatic gallbladder melanoma drastically increases when the gallbladder lesion is a single focus of metastasis with no other lesions and is surgically removed [9, 13, 16]. Gallbladder metastases are relatively asymptomatic, which is why most cases are discovered during autopsy: Das Gupta et al. conducted an autopsy study on 125 patients and found that 15% (19 patients) presented with metastatic lesions to the gallbladder [6, 9, 11, 14]. In rare cases, melanoma metastasis to the gallbladder will present with symptoms such as abdominal pain, as was seen in our patient, or as an acute cholecystitis [11, 15]. Patient clinical presentation may include jaundice from obstruction of the bile duct by the tumor mass, hemobilia, biliary fistulas, vomiting, nausea, and weight loss [5, 7, 14].

The rarity of the metastasis combined with its asymptomatic nature means the widespread disease has usually occurred by the time of diagnosis [5, 9, 13]. Addressing this involves maintaining a high level of suspicion in patients who present with biliary symptoms and have a known history of cutaneous melanoma [2, 8]. Doppler ultrasonography remains to be the method of choice for determining the presence of a gallbladder malignancy by detecting high blood flow regions [7, 13, 15]. In cases of gallbladder melanoma, ultrasonography will show single or multiple infiltrative lesions (at least 1 cm in diameter) attached to the inner mucosal wall [3]. Computed tomography can also be utilized and has 60–70% sensitivity in detecting metastases [2]. Positron emission tomography can be utilized secondarily in detecting the extent of spread [1, 2]. Finally, biopsy of the gallbladder lesion and immunohistochemical staining are used to confirm the diagnosis [2].

Surgery, as a treatment modality for metastatic melanoma to the gallbladder, remains questionable since most cases of gallbladder melanoma are a part of widespread disease [1]. Metastasectomy remains to be the mainstay approach, for its palliative and symptom-reducing effects and for cases of a single localized lesion to the gall bladder like in our patient [7, 9, 15]. Surgery also functions to prevent further dissemination from the gallbladder via bile [1]. Dong et al. found that the 1-year survival in surgically resected patients can be up to 100%, but without surgery it is documented at as low as 0% [9]. A liver wedge resection, targeting nearby regions of the liver pedicle, should also be performed in cases of probable contiguous spread of neoplastic cells [8].

Management of the patient can also involve chemoimmunotherapy, especially in the case of a nonlocalized lesion [1, 2]. Its utility as adjuvant therapy remains unclear [1–3]. Chemoimmunotherapy has garnered recent interest as an effective treatment modality. Among them is the use of high-bolus interleukin-2 (IL-2) which has been found to induce remission in 15% of patients; however, its use is limited due to toxicity [2, 8]. BRAF inhibitors along with immune therapy have been utilized in generating an immune response to the tumors [2, 8]. The use of MEK inhibitors concurrently with BRAF inhibitors has been shown to lower adverse reactions, prolong disease-free survival, and delay the resistance that has been seen in BRAF inhibitor use alone [1].

Melanoma undergoes extensive and rapid growth and causes widespread damage with very high morbidity and mortality. We have presented this case to address the need for a prompt workup with a potential diagnosis of metastasis, especially in patients with a known history of cutaneous melanoma. The key to prolonging survival is to consider metastases early and begin aggressive treatment. Most cases of gallbladder metastases present with no symptoms. Workup should begin with imaging, along with immunohistochemical staining for confirmation. Adequate treatment may be achieved with laparoscopic cholecystectomies and/or chemoimmunotherapy.

References

[1] I. Giannini, D. A. Cutrignelli, L. Resta, A. Gentile, and L. Vincenti, "Metastatic melanoma of the gallbladder: report of two cases and a review of the literature," *Clinical and Experimental Medicine*, vol. 16, no. 3, pp. 295–300, 2016.

[2] H. Ettahri, F. Elomrani, M. Elkabous et al., "Duodenal and gallbladder metastasis of regressive melanoma: a case report and review of the literature," *Journal of Gastrointestinal Oncology*, vol. 6, no. 5, pp. E77–E81, 2015.

[3] M. F. Haskaraca, M. Ozsoy, İ. Özsan, and K. Kurt, "Primary malignant melanoma of the gallbladder: a case report and review of the literature," *Case Reports in Surgery*, vol. 2012, Article ID 693547, 4 pages, 2012.

[4] P. Cellerino, F. Corsi, E. Morandi, D. Foschi, and E. Trabucchi, "Metastatic melanoma of the gallbladder," *European Journal of Surgical Oncology*, vol. 26, no. 8, pp. 815–816, 2000.

[5] M. K. Samplaski, E. L. Rosato, A. K. Witkiewicz, M. J. Mastrangelo, and A. C. Berger, "Malignant melanoma of the gallbladder: a report of two cases and review of the literature," *Journal of Gastrointestinal Surgery*, vol. 12, no. 6, pp. 1123–1126, 2008.

[6] S. C. Katz, W. B. Bowne, J. D. Wolchok, K. J. Busam, D. P. Jaques, and D. G. Coit, "Surgical management of melanoma of the gallbladder: a report of 13 cases and review of the literature," *American Journal of Surgery*, vol. 193, no. 4, pp. 493–497, 2007.

[7] J.-P. A. Martel, C. A. McLean, and R. N. Rankin, "Best cases from the AFIP: melanoma of the gallbladder," *Radiographics*, vol. 29, no. 1, pp. 291–296, 2009.

[8] D. Christou, N. Katodritis, M. P. Decatris et al., "Melanoma of the gallbladder: appropriate surgical management and review of the literature," *Clinical Case Reports*, vol. 2, no. 6, pp. 313–318, 2014.

[9] X. D. Dong, P. DeMatos, V. G. Prieto, and H. F. Seigier, "Melanoma of the gallbladder: a review of cases seen at Duke University Medical Center," *Cancer*, vol. 85, no. 1, pp. 32–39, 1999.

[10] N. Howlader, A. M. Noone, M. Krapcho et al., Eds., *SEER Cancer Statistics Review, 1975–2009 (Vintage 2009 Populations)*, National Cancer Institute, Bethesda, Md, USA, 2012 http://seer.cancer.gov/csr/1975_2009_pops09/.

[11] T. Das Gupta and R. Brasfield, "Metastatic melanoma: a clinicopathological study," *Cancer*, vol. 17, pp. 1323–1339, 1964.

[12] Y. Takayama, Y. Asayama, K. Yoshimitsu et al., "Metastatic melanoma of the gallbladder," *Computerized Medical Imaging and Graphics*, vol. 31, no. 6, pp. 469–471, 2007.

[13] J. Gogas, D. Mantas, H. Gogas, E. Kouskos, C. Markopoulos, and S. Vgenopoulou, "Metastatic melanoma in the gallbladder: report of a case," *Surgery Today*, vol. 33, no. 2, pp. 135–137, 2003.

[14] S. Vernadakis, G. Rallis, N. Danias et al., "Metastatic melanoma of the gallbladder: an unusual clinical presentation of acute cholecystitis," *World Journal of Gastroenterology*, vol. 15, no. 27, pp. 3434–3436, 2009.

[15] M. Guida, A. Cramarossa, A. Gentile et al., "Metastatic malignant melanoma of the gallbladder: a case report and review of the literature," *Melanoma Research*, vol. 12, no. 6, pp. 619–625, 2002.

[16] H. Matsubayashi, Y. Kiyohara, K. Sasaki et al., "Metastatic malignant melanoma of the gallbladder diagnosed by cytology of endoscopic naso-gallbladder drainage fluid," *Journal of Digestive Diseases*, vol. 13, no. 3, pp. 190–194, 2012.

Solid Pseudopapillary Neoplasm of the Pancreas in Young Male Patients: Three Case Reports

Akira Aso,[1,2] Eikichi Ihara,[2] Kazuhiko Nakamura,[2] Irina Sudovykh,[3] Tetsuhide Ito,[2] Masafumi Nakamura,[4] Tetsuo Ikeda,[5] Nobuyoshi Takizawa,[6] Yoshinao Oda,[6] and Shuji Shimizu[1]

[1] *International Medical Department, Kyushu University Hospital, Fukuoka, Japan*
[2] *Department of Medicine and Bioregulatory Science, Graduate School of Medical Sciences, Kyushu University, Fukuoka, Japan*
[3] *Endoscopic Therapeutics Department, Kyushu University Hospital, Fukuoka, Japan*
[4] *Department of Surgery and Oncology, Graduate School of Medical Sciences, Kyushu University, Fukuoka, Japan*
[5] *Department of Surgery and Science, Graduate School of Medical Sciences, Kyushu University, Fukuoka, Japan*
[6] *Department of Anatomic Pathology, Graduate School of Medical Sciences, Kyushu University, Fukuoka, Japan*

Correspondence should be addressed to Eikichi Ihara; eikichi@intmed3.med.kyushu-u.ac.jp

Academic Editor: Chia-Tung Shun

A preoperative diagnosis of solid pseudopapillary neoplasms (SPNs) in young male patients is difficult to achieve using radiological images. We herein present three cases of young male patients with relatively small SPNs. Endoscopic ultrasound (EUS) showed well-encapsulated, smooth-surfaced, heterogeneous solid lesions in all patients, and all preoperative diagnoses were achieved by EUS-guided fine needle aspiration (EUS-FNA). The final pathological diagnosis after surgery was an SPN with a Ki-67 labeling index of <2%. SPNs should be considered even in young male patients. EUS with EUS-FNA could be a useful diagnostic modality for SPNs even in young male patients.

1. Introduction

Solid pseudopapillary neoplasms (SPNs) are rare, low-grade, epithelial neoplasms that are usually discovered incidentally in young female patients [1, 2]. A preoperative diagnosis is difficult to achieve because the clinical imaging findings of SPNs are vary widely. Some SPNs present as solid tumors, while others are observed as cystic lesions and are therefore usually diagnosed postoperatively. SPNs in young male patients are extremely rare. Because of the limited information for such patients, it is currently difficult to predict the likelihood of SPNs in young males. Additionally, SPNs seem to have higher malignant potential in male than in female patients [3, 4]. Thus, it is important to accumulate clinical information about SPNs in young male patients. We herein present three cases of SPNs in young male patients.

2. Patients and Methods

A total of 4867 patients underwent endoscopic ultrasound (EUS) at Kyushu University Hospital from April 2009 to June 2015. We retrospectively reviewed the clinical data of these patients. Among them, only three male patients were diagnosed with SPNs, and we present these three cases in this report. The SPNs were preoperatively diagnosed by EUS-guided fine needle aspiration (EUS-FNA) using a curvilinear echoendoscope (GF-UCT240-AL5; Olympus Medical Systems Co., Tokyo, Japan) through the stomach wall with a 22-gauge EchoTip Ultra needle (Wilson-Cook Medical Inc., Tokyo, Japan). After examination by on-site cytopathologists to evaluate the sample quality, the final diagnosis was determined by an experienced histopathologist at Kyushu University.

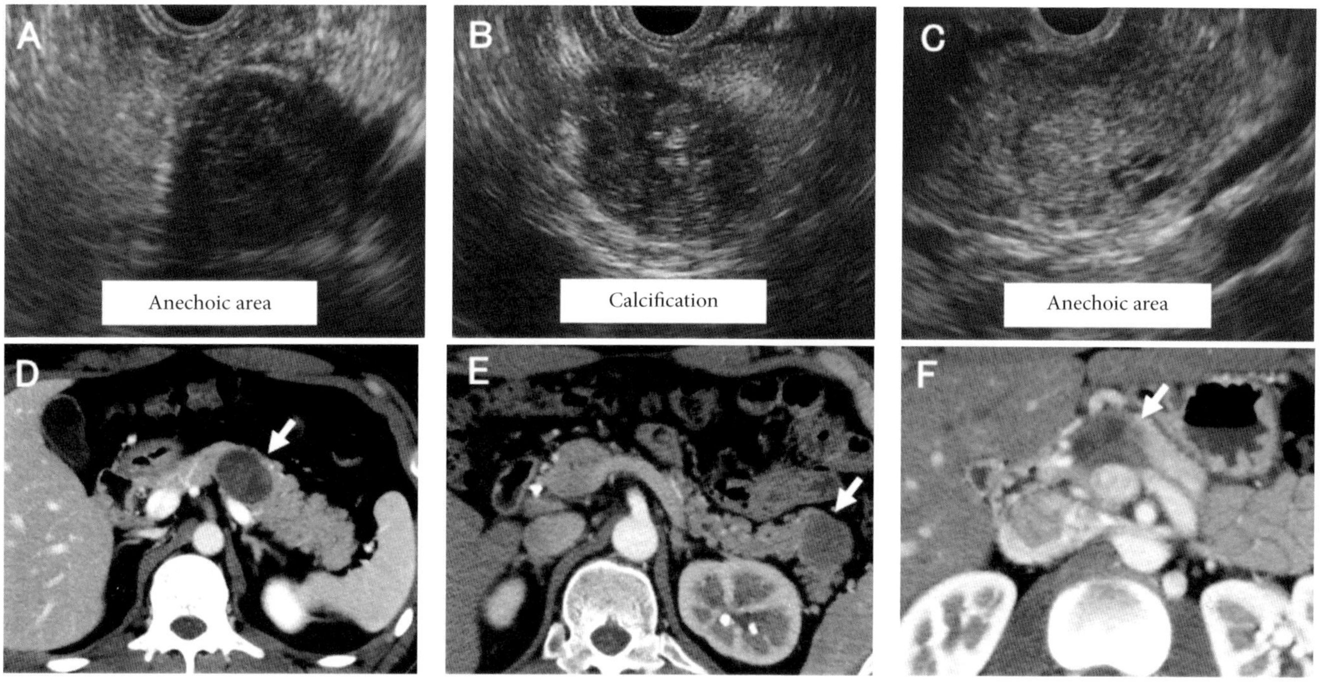

FIGURE 1: Endoscopic ultrasound and computed tomography findings of three young male patients with solid pseudopapillary neoplasms. The endoscopic ultrasound and computed tomography findings of three young male patients with solid pseudopapillary neoplasms are shown. Solid and hypoechoic masses with anechoic areas were observed in (A) Case 1 and (C) Case 3. Internal calcification was observed in (B) Case 2 by endoscopic ultrasound. Computed tomography showed low-density tumors with slight enhancement at the margin in all three cases.

3. Case Reports

3.1. Case 1. Case 1 involved a 34-year-old male patient who was referred to our hospital for evaluation of epigastric pain. EUS revealed a well-encapsulated, smooth-surfaced, heterogeneous solid lesion at the body of the pancreas. The lesion measured 24 mm in diameter and contained hypoechoic/anechoic areas (Figure 1(A)). Hematoxylin-eosin staining of the biopsy specimens revealed that the tumor cells exhibited acidophilic cytoplasm with small, round nuclei and formed pseudopapillary structures. Immunohistochemical analysis revealed that the tumor cells were positive for β-catenin, vimentin, CD10, and progesterone receptor (Figure 2).

3.2. Case 2. Case 2 involved a 30-year-old male patient with acute abdominal pain. EUS showed a solid hypoechoic lesion in the tail of the pancreas. The lesion measured 20 mm in diameter and had a clear margin, regular borderline, and internal calcifications (Figure 1(B)). The pathological results were similar to those obtained by examination of the EUS-FNA samples in Case 1.

3.3. Case 3. Case 3 involved an 18-year-old male patient who was referred to our hospital for further evaluation of an abdominal mass incidentally detected by abdominal ultrasound. EUS showed a solid hypoechoic lesion at the body of the pancreas. The lesion measured 27 mm in diameter and contained small anechoic areas, a clear margin, and regular borderline (Figure 1(C)). The pathological results were similar to those obtained by examination of the EUS-FNA samples in Case 1.

The patients' clinical characteristics and EUS findings are shown in Table 1. The EUS findings were atypical but prompted us to consider the possibility of SPNs. However, other pancreatic tumors, especially neuroendocrine tumors (NETs), needed to be ruled out. Computed tomography (CT) in each case showed a solid tumor with slight enhancement at the margin, which is a not typical feature of SPNs (Figures 1(D)–1(F)). Magnetic resonance imaging (MRI) also did not provide additional useful information for achieving a definitive diagnosis. Consequently, we made a preoperative pathological diagnosis of SPN by EUS-FNA, and surgery was performed in all three patients. The final pathological diagnosis after surgery was an SPN with a Ki-67 labeling index of <2% in all three patients. All three patients remained free of disease during the follow-up period (Case 1, 26 months; Case 2, 12 months; Case 3, 18 months).

4. Discussion

An SPN is a very rare pancreatic tumor and is often recognized as a solid pancreatic mass. SPNs reportedly account for 1% to 2% of all pancreatic tumors [1]. They mostly affect young female patients; only 12.2% of patients with SPNs are male [2], most of whom are middle-aged. Therefore, SPNs in young male patients are extremely rare, and achieving a preoperative diagnosis of SPNs in our young male patients was difficult because previous data regarding typical imaging findings of SPNs are limited. We focused on the EUS findings of our three

Table 1

	Case 1	Case 2	Case 3
Age	34	30	18
Tumor size (mm)	24	20	27
Location	Body	Tail	Body
Echo level	Hypoechoic	Hypoechoic	Hypoechoic
Demarcation of tumor edge	Well-demarcated	Well-demarcated	Poorly demarcated
Internal echo pattern	Heterogenous	Heterogenous	Heterogenous
Cystic component	Presence	Absence	Presence
Calcification	Absence	Presence	Absence
Vascularity	Hypovascular	Hypovascular	Hypovascular
Dilation of MPD	Absence	Absence	Absence
Stenosis of MPD	Absence	Absence	Absence
Vessel invasion	Absence	Absence	Absence

MPD, main pancreatic duct.

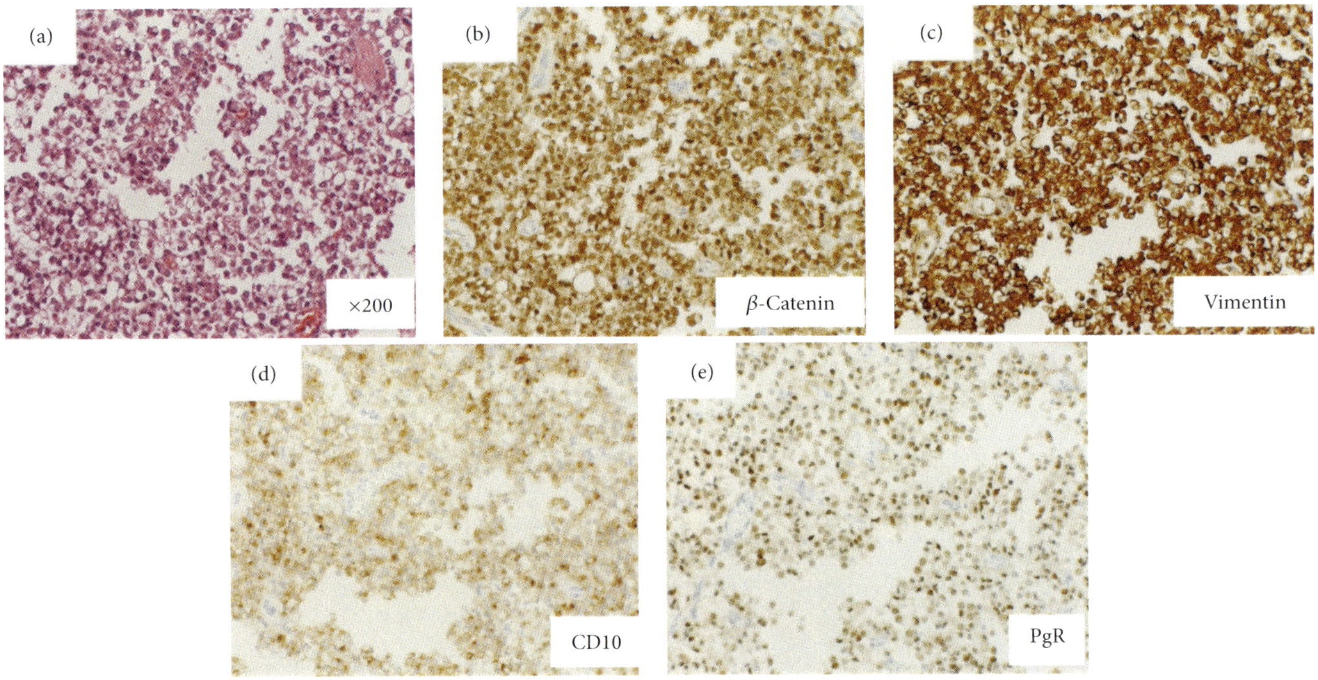

Figure 2: Histopathological results of biopsy samples obtained by endoscopic ultrasound-guided fine needle aspiration in Case 1. Histopathological analyses of the biopsy samples obtained by endoscopic ultrasound-guided fine needle aspiration in Case 1 are shown. (a) Hematoxylin-eosin staining revealed that the tumor cells exhibited acidophilic cytoplasm with small, round nuclei and formed pseudopapillary structures. Immunohistochemical analysis demonstrated that the tumor cells were positive for (b) β-catenin, (c) vimentin, (d) CD10, and (e) progesterone receptor.

young male patients with relatively small SPNs and found that all SPNs were heterogeneous, hypoechoic, hypovascular, solid lesions.

Although most patients with SPNs have a good prognosis and favorable outcome with 5-year survival rates of almost 90% [1, 5], approximately 15% of SPNs have the potential for malignant transformation [5]. Specifically, one study showed that distant metastases occurred in 10% to 15% of patients with SPNs with lymph node metastasis in 2% [1]. The natural history of SPNs in male patients remains unclear, but it has been suggested that the biological malignant potential of SPNs is higher in males than in females [3, 4]. Therefore, surgical treatment should be considered when an SPN is diagnosed, especially in male patients. The number of patients diagnosed with SPNs has recently increased with the more widespread use of imaging modalities including ultrasound, CT, and MRI. These techniques have provided greater opportunities to incidentally detect relatively small lesions suspected to be SPNs.

Despite recent innovations in imaging modalities such as contrast-enhanced CT and MRI, differential diagnoses of pancreatic tumors are difficult to achieve, especially for relatively small lesions. Among several imaging modalities, EUS is generally accepted to be one of the best methods with which to detect and evaluate solid pancreatic lesions because of its high resolution [6]. Even by EUS, however, a definitive diagnosis of SPNs remains difficult to achieve for the following reasons. First, the EUS findings of SPNs are complex and often variable depending on the extent of hemorrhagic degeneration [7, 8]. Second, the EUS appearance of SPNs in male patients tends to be a small, solid lesion without a cystic component, and small SPNs frequently tend to present as pure solid masses with a sharp margin. Third, the EUS findings of SPNs of <3 cm seem to differ from those of SPNs of >3 cm [9]. All SPNs in the three young male patients in the present report were solitary, heterogeneous, hypoechoic, hypovascular, and solid on EUS. Besides these common features, small cystic changes were observed in Cases 1 and 3, while internal calcification was identified in Case 2. Differentiation of SPNs from NETs by radiological findings is generally difficult because both are sometimes accompanied by cystic degeneration and calcification, and even the pathological appearances may be similar between SPNs and NETs. We propose that the internal echo pattern could be the key EUS finding that is most useful for differentiating SPNs from NETs. It seems that a heterogeneous pattern is more prominent in SPNs than in NETs (Table 1), although further studies are needed to clarify this point.

After a lesion suspected to be an SPN has been identified by EUS, a definitive diagnosis of SPN must be made histologically. EUS-FNA is a diagnostic method that should be considered for this purpose because it is a well-established modality in the diagnosis of solid pancreatic tumors. The addition of EUS-FNA to currently used diagnostic modalities including CT or CT/EUS has been reported to significantly increase the diagnostic yield [10]. Consistent with this, a preoperative histological diagnosis of SPN could be made by EUS-FNA in all three cases in the present report.

In conclusion, we have herein presented three cases of relatively small SPNs in young male patients, mainly focusing on the EUS findings of these tumors. SPNs should be considered even in young male patients. EUS with EUS-FNA could be a useful diagnostic modality for SPNs, even in young males.

Authors' Contributions

A. Aso performed the endoscopic examinations and collected the data. A. Aso, Irina Sudovykh, and E. Ihara mainly wrote the paper. K. Nakamura and T. Ito provided clinical and technical advice. M. Nakamura and T. Ikeda performed the surgical treatments. S. Shimizu reviewed the manuscript and provided comments. N. Takizawa and Y. Oda performed the pathological analysis. All authors approved the final manuscript for publication.

Acknowledgments

The authors would like to thank all medical team and staff members at Kyushu University Hospital.

References

[1] J. K. Law, A. Ahmed, V. K. Singh et al., "A systematic review of solid-pseudopapillary neoplasms: are these rare lesions?" *Pancreas*, vol. 43, no. 3, pp. 331–337, 2014.

[2] T. Papavramidis and S. Papavramidis, "Solid pseudopapillary tumors of the pancreas: review of 718 patients reported in english literature," *Journal of the American College of Surgeons*, vol. 200, no. 6, pp. 965–972, 2005.

[3] M. C. C. Machado, M. A. C. Machado, T. Bacchella, J. Jukemura, J. L. Almeida, and J. E. M. Cunha, "Solid pseudopapillary neoplasm of the pancreas: distinct patterns of onset, diagnosis, and prognosis for male versus female patients," *Surgery*, vol. 143, no. 1, pp. 29–34, 2008.

[4] M. Y. C. Lin and B. E. Stabile, "Solid pseudopapillary neoplasm of the pancreas: a rare and atypically aggressive disease among male patients," *The American Surgeon*, vol. 76, no. 10, pp. 1075–1078, 2010.

[5] J. H. Baek, J. M. Lee, S. H. Kim et al., "Small (≤3 cm) solid pseudopapillary tumors of the pancreas at multiphasic multidetector CT," *Radiology*, vol. 257, no. 1, pp. 97–106, 2010.

[6] A. Aso, E. Ihara, T. Osoegawa et al., "Key endoscopic ultrasound features of pancreatic ductal adenocarcinoma smaller than 20 mm," *Scandinavian Journal of Gastroenterology*, vol. 49, no. 3, pp. 332–338, 2014.

[7] X. Yao, Y. Ji, M. Zeng, S. Rao, and B. Yang, "Solid pseudopapillary tumor of the pancreas: cross-sectional imaging and pathologic correlation," *Pancreas*, vol. 39, no. 4, pp. 486–491, 2010.

[8] M. Yoshioka, K. Egami, S. Maeda et al., "The clinicopathological characteristic and surgical management of Solid pseudopapillary tumor: report of own six cases and a review of 302 cases in Japanese literature," *Tan to Sui*, vol. 22, pp. 45–52, 2001.

[9] N. Jani, J. Dewitt, M. Eloubeidi et al., "Endoscopic ultrasound-guided fine-needle aspiration for diagnosis of solid pseudopapillary tumors of the pancreas: a multicenter experience," *Endoscopy*, vol. 40, no. 3, pp. 200–203, 2008.

[10] J. K. Law, A. Stoita, W. Wever et al., "Endoscopic ultrasound-guided fine needle aspiration improves the pre-operative diagnostic yield of solid-pseudopapillary neoplasm of the pancreas: an international multicenter case series (with video)," *Surgical Endoscopy*, vol. 28, no. 9, pp. 2592–2598, 2014.

Permissions

All chapters in this book were first published in CRGM, by Hindawi Publishing Corporation; hereby published with permission under the Creative Commons Attribution License or equivalent. Every chapter published in this book has been scrutinized by our experts. Their significance has been extensively debated. The topics covered herein carry significant findings which will fuel the growth of the discipline. They may even be implemented as practical applications or may be referred to as a beginning point for another development.

The contributors of this book come from diverse backgrounds, making this book a truly international effort. This book will bring forth new frontiers with its revolutionizing research information and detailed analysis of the nascent developments around the world.

We would like to thank all the contributing authors for lending their expertise to make the book truly unique. They have played a crucial role in the development of this book. Without their invaluable contributions this book wouldn't have been possible. They have made vital efforts to compile up to date information on the varied aspects of this subject to make this book a valuable addition to the collection of many professionals and students.

This book was conceptualized with the vision of imparting up-to-date information and advanced data in this field. To ensure the same, a matchless editorial board was set up. Every individual on the board went through rigorous rounds of assessment to prove their worth. After which they invested a large part of their time researching and compiling the most relevant data for our readers.

The editorial board has been involved in producing this book since its inception. They have spent rigorous hours researching and exploring the diverse topics which have resulted in the successful publishing of this book. They have passed on their knowledge of decades through this book. To expedite this challenging task, the publisher supported the team at every step. A small team of assistant editors was also appointed to further simplify the editing procedure and attain best results for the readers.

Apart from the editorial board, the designing team has also invested a significant amount of their time in understanding the subject and creating the most relevant covers. They scrutinized every image to scout for the most suitable representation of the subject and create an appropriate cover for the book.

The publishing team has been an ardent support to the editorial, designing and production team. Their endless efforts to recruit the best for this project, has resulted in the accomplishment of this book. They are a veteran in the field of academics and their pool of knowledge is as vast as their experience in printing. Their expertise and guidance has proved useful at every step. Their uncompromising quality standards have made this book an exceptional effort. Their encouragement from time to time has been an inspiration for everyone.

The publisher and the editorial board hope that this book will prove to be a valuable piece of knowledge for researchers, students, practitioners and scholars across the globe.

List of Contributors

Piotr Pardak and Ewa Walczak
Department of Internal Medicine, Institute of Rural Health, 20-090 Lublin, Poland

RafaB S. Filip
Department of Clinical Endoscopy, Institute of Rural Health, 20-090 Lublin, Poland
Department of Public Health and Social Medicine, University of Rzeszów, 35-959 Rzeszów, Poland

Ravish Parekh and Nirmal Kaur
Inflammatory Bowel Disease Center, Henry Ford Health System, 39450West Twelve Mile Roud, Novi, MI 48377, USA

Noritaka Minagawa and Takayuki Torigoe
Department of Surgery 1, School of Medicine, University of Occupational and Environmental Health, 1-1 Iseigaoka, Yahata-nishi-ku, Kitakyushu 807-8555, Japan

Yoshifumi Nakayama, Toshihito Uehara and Masaki Akiyama
Department of Surgery 1, School of Medicine, University of Occupational and Environmental Health, 1-1 Iseigaoka, Yahata-nishi-ku, Kitakyushu 807-8555, Japan
Department of Gastroenterological and General Surgery, Wakamatsu Hospital of University of Occupational and Environmental Health, 1-17-1 Hamamachi, Wakamatsu-ku, Kitakyushu 808-0024, Japan

Naohiro Fujimoto
Department of Urology, School of Medicine, University of Occupational and Environmental Health, 1-1 Iseigaoka, Yahata-nishi-ku, Kitakyushu 807-8555, Japan

Justin Cochrane
Junior Faculty Spokane Teaching Health Center (Internal Medicine Residency), Providence Sacred Heart Medical Center, Spokane, WA 99204, USA

Greg Schlepp
Spokane Digestive Disease Center, Spokane, WA 99204, USA

Satya Allaparthi, Mohammed Sageer and Mark J. Sterling
Lahey Clinic, Burlington, MA 01805, USA

Guillermo López-Medina, Manuel Gallo, Alejandro Prado and Iliana Vicuña-Honorato
Hospital Angeles Clinica Londres, Durango No. 50, Roma Norte, Cuauhtémoc, 06700 Ciudad de México, DF, Mexico

Roxana Castillo Díaz de León
Hospital Angeles Mocel, Gregorio V. Gelati No. 29, San Miguel Chapultepec, Miguel Hidalgo, 11850 Ciudad de México, DF, Mexico

Carina Santos, Francisco Morgado, Celestina Blanco, João Parreira, João Costa, Lara Rodrigues, Luís Marfull and Patrícia Cardoso
Department of Internal Medicine, Radiology, University Hospital Center "Sousa Martins", Guarda, Portugal

Cyriac Abby Philips, Chetan Ramesh Kalal, Amrish Sahney and KN Chandan Kumar
Department of Hepatology, Institute of Liver and Biliary Sciences, D-1, Vasant Kunj, New Delhi 110070, India

Chhagan Bihari and Archana Rastogi
Department of Pathology, Institute of Liver and Biliary Sciences, D-1, Vasant Kunj, New Delhi 110070, India

Ali Zakaria, Bayan Al Share, Issam Turk, Samira Ahsan and Waseem Farra
Department of Internal Medicine, Division of Pulmonology, Providence-Providence Park Hospital, Michigan State University College of Human Medicine, Southfield, MI, USA

Venkata S. Tammana, Rehana Begum, Patricia Oneal, Hemamalini Karpurapu, Amruta Muley, Sri Lakshmi Hyndavi Yeruva and Eyasu Mekonen
Department of Internal Medicine, Howard University Hospital, 2041 Georgia Avenue, NW, Washington, DC 20060, USA

Jacquelyn Dunmore-Griffith
Department of Radiation Oncology, Howard University Hospital, Washington, DC, USA

Nabhani Hasan
Department of Radiology, Howard University Hospital, Washington, DC, USA

Yu Ishimine, Akira Goto, Suguru Nakagaki, Takashi Yabana, Takeya Adachi and Yoshihiro Kondo
Department of Gastroenterology, Otaru General Hospital, 1-2-1Wakamatu, Otaru 047-8550, Japan

Yoshito Watanabe
Department of Surgery, Otaru General Hospital, 1-2-1Wakamatu, Otaru 047-8550, Japan

Hidetaka Yajima
Department of Gastroenterology, Rheumatology, and Clinical Immunology, Sapporo Medical University, S1W17, Chuo-ku, Sapporo 060-8556, Japan

Kiyoshi Kasai
Department of Laboratory Medicine, Otaru General Hospital, 1-2-1Wakamatu, Otaru 047-8550, Japan

Jason Deforest Jones and Rishi Pawa
Division of Gastroenterology, Department of Internal Medicine, Wake Forest School of Medicine, Winston-Salem, NC, USA

Amir Kashani and Laith H. Jamil
Department of Gastroenterology, Cedars-Sinai Medical Center, 8700 Beverly Boulevard, Los Angeles, CA 90048, USA

Nicholas N. Nissen
Hepatobiliary and Pancreatic Surgery, Cedars-Sinai Medical Center, 8700 Beverly Boulevard, Los Angeles, CA 90048, USA

Maha Guindi
Department of Pathology and Laboratory Medicine, Cedars-Sinai Medical Center, 8700 Beverly Boulevard, Los Angeles, CA 90048, USA

Naomi Hauser, Devon McKenzie, Xavier Fonseca and Jose Orsini
Department of Medicine, New York University School of Medicine, Woodhull Medical and Mental Health Center, Brooklyn, NY 11206, USA

Nobuhiro Takeuchi
Department of Gastroenterology, Kawasaki Hospital, Kobe, Hyogo 652-0042, Japan

Kazuyoshi Naba
Department of Laboratory Medicine, Kawasaki Hospital, Kobe, Hyogo 652-0042, Japan

Joel Johansson and Mattias Ekstedt
Department of Gastroenterology and Department of Clinical and Experimental Medicine, Linköping University, 58185 Linköping, Sweden

Bergthor Björnsson and Per Sandström
Department of Surgery, County Council of Östergötland, 58185 Linköping, Sweden
Division of Surgery, Department of Clinical and Experimental Medicine, Faculty of Health Sciences, Linköping University, 581 85 Linköping, Sweden

Simone Ignatova
Department of Pathology, Linköping University Hospital, 581 85 Linköping, Sweden

Asad Khan
SUNY Upstate Medical University, Syracuse, NY 13210, USA

Sejal Patel
Department of Radiology, SUNY Upstate Medical University, Syracuse, NY 13210, USA

Daniel J. Zaccarini
Department of Pathology, SUNY Upstate Medical University, Syracuse, NY 13210, USA

Mary McGrath
Department of Nuclear Medicine, SUNY Upstate Medical University, Syracuse, NY 13210, USA

Manuela Cesaretti, Manuela Trotta and Irene Leale
Dipartimento di Scienze Chirurgiche e Diagnostiche Integrate (DISC), Università degli Studi di Genova, 8 Largo Benzi, 16132 Genoa, Italy

Giovanni Bruno Camerini and Giacomo Borgonovo
Dipartimento di Scienze Chirurgiche e Diagnostiche Integrate (DISC), Università degli Studi di Genova, 8 Largo Benzi, 16132 Genoa, Italy
Ospedale Policlinico San Martino, 10 Largo Benzi, 16132 Genoa, Italy

Giuseppe Antonio Minetti and Giuseppe Cittadini
Department of Radiology, Ospedale Policlinico San Martino, 10 Largo Benzi, 16132 Genoa, Italy

Fabrizio Montecucco
Ospedale Policlinico San Martino, 10 Largo Benzi, 16132 Genoa, Italy
First Clinic of Internal Medicine, Department of Internal Medicine, University of Genoa, 6 Viale Benedetto XV, 16132 Genoa, Italy
Centre of Excellence for Biomedical Research (CEBR), University of Genoa, 9 Viale Benedetto XV, 16132 Genoa, Italy

Yana Cavanagh, Neal Carlin and Sohail Shaikh
Department of Gastroenterology, New York Medical College at St. Joseph's Regional Medical Center, Paterson, NJ, USA

Ruhin Yuridullah
Department of Medicine, New York Medical College at St. Joseph's Regional Medical Center, Paterson, NJ, USA

Maria Paparoupa, Viola Schmidt, Huy Ho and Frank Schuppert
Department of Gastroenterology, Endocrinology, Diabetology and General Medicine, Klinikum Kassel, M¨onchebergstraße 41-43, 34125 Kassel, Germany

Helgard Weckauf
Institute of Pathology, Klinikum Kassel, Mönchebergstraße 41-43, 34125 Kassel, Germany

Daniyeh Khurram, Leonid Shamban, Robert Kornas and Maryann Paul
Department of Internal Medicine, Providence Hospital and Medical Center, 16001W. Nile Mile Road, Southfield, MI 48075, USA

Jason S. Radowsky, Joseph S. Lee and Andrew T. Schlussel
Department of General Surgery, Brian Allgood Army Community Hospital, Yongsan 96205, Republic of Korea

Tolga Dinc, Selami Ilgaz Kayilioglu, Ahmet Erdogan, Erdinc Cetinkaya, Ozgur Akgul and Faruk Coskun
Ankara Numune Training and Research Hospital, Department of General Surgery, 06100 Ankara, Turkey

Mouhanna Abu Ghanimeh
Henry Ford Health System, 2799WGrand Blvd, Gastroenterology K-7 Room E-744, Detroit, MI 48202, USA

Omar Abughanimeh
Internal Medicine, Graduate Medical Education, School of Medicine, University of Missouri-Kansas City, 2411 Holmes Street, M2-302, Kansas City, MO 64108, USA

Khalil Abuamr, Osama Yousef and Esmat Sadeddin
Gastroenterology, School of Medicine, University of Missouri-Kansas City, 2411 Holmes Street, Kansas City, MO 64108, USA

BenteM. de Kok, Fleur I. de Korte and Frank M. Zijta
Department of Radiology, Haaglanden Medical Centre, Lijnbaan 32, 2512 VAThe Hague, Netherlands

Lars E. Perk
Department of Gastroenterology, Haaglanden Medical Centre, Lijnbaan 32, 2512 VAThe Hague, Netherlands

Valeska Terpstra
Department of Pathology, Haaglanden Medical Centre, Lijnbaan 32, 2512 VAThe Hague, Netherlands

J. Sven D. Mieog
Department of Surgery, Leiden University Medical Centre, Albinusdreef 2, 2333 ZA, Leiden, Netherlands

NoritakaMinagawa, Takayuki Torigoe and Keiji Hirata
Department of Surgery 1, School of Medicine, University of Occupational and Environmental Health, 1-1 Iseigaoka, Yahata-nishi-ku, Kitakyushu 807-8555, Japan

Yoshifumi Nakayama, Masaki Akiyama and Yusuke Sawatsubashi
Department of Surgery 1, School of Medicine, University of Occupational and Environmental Health, 1-1 Iseigaoka, Yahata-nishi-ku, Kitakyushu 807-8555, Japan
Department of Gastroenterological and General Surgery, Wakamatsu Hospital of University of Occupational and Environmental Health, 1-17-1 Hamamachi, Wakamatsu-ku, Kitakyushu 808-0024, Japan

Roisin Stack, Joseph McLoughlin and Barbara M. Ryan
Department of Gastroenterology, Tallaght Hospital and Trinity College, Dublin, Ireland

Amy Gillis
Department of Surgery, Tallaght Hospital and Trinity College, Dublin, Ireland

Samuel Torres-Landa, Edgar Alejandro-Medrano, Bárbara Ramos-Ávalos and Gonzalo Torres-Villalobos
Department of Experimental Surgery, Instituto Nacional de Ciencias Médicas y Nutrición Salvador Zubirán, Vasco de Quiroga No. 15, Colonia Belisario Domínguez Sección XVI, 14080 Mexico City, Mexico

Janette Furuzawa-Carballeda
Department of Immunology and Rheumatology, Instituto Nacional de Ciencias Médicas y Nutrición Salvador Zubirán, Vasco de Quiroga No. 15, Colonia Belisario Domínguez Sección XVI, 14080 Mexico City, Mexico

Enrique Coss-Adame and Miguel A. Valdovinos
Department of Gastroenterology, Instituto Nacional de Ciencias M´edicas y Nutrición Salvador Zubirán, Vasco de Quiroga No. 15, Colonia Belisario Domínguez Sección XVI, 14080 Mexico City, Mexico

BraulioMartínez-Benítez
Department of Pathology, Instituto Nacional de Ciencias Médicas y Nutrición Salvador Zubirán, Vasco de Quiroga No. 15, Colonia Belisario Domínguez Sección XVI, 14080 Mexico City, Mexico

Rachel Hudacko
Orange Pathology Associates, PC, Department of Pathology, Orange Regional Medical Center, 707 East Main St., Middletown, NY 10940, USA

Lance Siegel
Horizon Family Medical Group, Department of Gastroenterology, Orange Regional Medical Center, 707 East Main St., Middletown, NY 10940, USA

Manabu Kaneko, Shin Sasaki, Kosuke Ozaki, Kazuhiro Ishimaru, Emi Terai, Hiroshi Nakayama and Toshiyuki Watanabe
Department of Surgery, Omori Red Cross Hospital, 4-30-1 Chuo, Ota-ku, Tokyo 143-8527, Japan

Shuzo Teruya
Department of Internal Medicine, Division of Rheumatology, Omori Red Cross Hospital, 4-30-1 Chuo, Ota-ku, Tokyo 143-8527, Japan

Zahava C. Farkas and Khwaja F. Haq
Department of Medicine, New York Medical College at Westchester Medical Center, Valhalla, NY, USA

Priyanka Chugh, Shalom Frager and Roxana Bodin
Division of Gastroenterology and Hepatobiliary Disease, New York Medical College at Westchester Medical Center, Valhalla, NY, USA

Muhammad Ali Khan
Division of Gastroenterology and Hepatobiliary Disease, University of Tennessee Health Science Center, Memphis, TN, USA

Shantanu Solanki
Internal Medicine, New York Medical College at Westchester Medical Center, Valhalla, NY, USA

Edward Esses
Department of Radiology, New York Medical College at Westchester Medical Center, Valhalla, NY, USA

Gregory Veillette
Department of Hepatobiliary Surgery, New York Medical College at Westchester Medical Center, Valhalla, NY, USA

Mohammad Saud Khan, Zubair Khan, Toseef Javaid, Abdelmoniem Moustafa and Abhinav Tiwari
Department of Internal Medicine, University of Toledo Medical Center, Toledo, OH, USA

Jamal Akhtar and Amos Lal
Department of Internal Medicine, Saint Vincent Hospital, Worcester, MA, USA

Mohammad Taleb
Division of Pulmonary, Critical Care and Sleep Medicine, University of Toledo Medical Center, Toledo, OH, USA

Sandra Mabel Camacho-Gomez and Neelesh Ajit Tipnis
Department of Pediatrics, University of Mississippi Medical Center, 2500 North State Street, Jackson, MS 39216, USA

Anas Bernieh and Ali G. Saad
Department of Pathology, University of Mississippi Medical Center, 2500 North State Street, Jackson, MS 39216, USA

Abhishek Bhurwal, Muhammad Masoodul Haq and Sunil Sapru
Department of Internal Medicine, Saint Barnabas Medical Center, RWJBarnabas Health, West Orange, NJ, USA

Matthew Tortora
Department of Pathology, Saint Barnabas Medical Center, RWJBarnabas Health, West Orange, NJ, USA

Dhanasekaran Ramasamy
Department of Internal Medicine, Division of Gastroenterology, Saint Barnabas Medical Center, RWJBarnabas Health, West Orange, NJ, USA

Raghav Bansal, Soohwan Chun, Joel Baum and Melik Tiba
Division of Gastroenterology and Hepatology, Icahn School of Medicine at Mount Sinai, Elmhurst Hospital Center, Elmhurst, NY, USA

Mohamed Barakat
Department of Internal Medicine, Icahn School of Medicine at Mount Sinai, Queens Hospital Center, Jamaica, NY, USA

Sonam Rosberger
Department of Radiology, Icahn School of Medicine at Mount Sinai, Elmhurst Hospital Center, Elmhurst, NY, USA

H. Kuriry and A.M. Swied
Gastroenterology Division, Department of Medicine 1443, King Abdulaziz Medical City, Riyadh 11426, Saudi Arabia

R. Alenezi
Department of Medicine 1443, King Abdulaziz Medical City, Riyadh 11426, Saudi Arabia

A. Alghamdi
Gastroenterology Division, Department of Medicine, King Fahad Medical City, Riyadh 11525, Saudi Arabia

Adrienne Lenhart, AlirezaMeighani and Omar Sadiq
Department of Internal Medicine, Henry Ford Hospital, Detroit, MI 48202, USA

Mona Hassan and Yousuf Siddiqui
Division of Gastroenterology and Hepatology, Henry Ford Hospital, Detroit, MI 48202, USA

Rajat Garg
Department of Internal Medicine, St. John Hospital and Medical Center, Detroit, MI, USA

Louis D. Saravolatz
Department of Medicine, St. John Hospital and Medical Center, Detroit, MI, USA

Mohammed Barawi
Division of Gastroenterology and Hepatology, St. John Hospital and Medical Center, Detroit, MI, USA

Seiji Kawano and Hiroyuki Okada
Department of Gastroenterology and Hepatology, Okayama University Graduate School of Medicine, Dentistry and Pharmaceutical Sciences, Okayama 700-8558, Japan

Masaya Iwamuro
Department of Gastroenterology and Hepatology, Okayama University Graduate School of Medicine, Dentistry and Pharmaceutical Sciences, Okayama 700-8558, Japan
Department of General Medicine, Okayama University Graduate School of Medicine, Dentistry and Pharmaceutical Sciences, Okayama 700-8558, Japan

Sayo Kobayashi
Department of Internal Medicine, Fukuyama City Hospital, Fukuyama 721-8511, Japan

Nobuya Ohara
Department of Pathology, Okayama University Graduate School of Medicine, Dentistry and Pharmaceutical Sciences, Okayama 700-8558, Japan
Department of Pathology, Kagawa Rosai Hospital, Marugame 763-8502, Japan

Yoshiro Kawahara
Department of Endoscopy, Okayama University Hospital, Okayama 700-8558, Japan

HassanM. Ghoz, ShamlanM. Sheikh and Kanika Khandelwal
Division of Internal Medicine, Steward Carney Hospital, Tufts School of Medicine, Dorchester, MA, USA

Joseph Fiore
Division of Gastroenterology and Hepatology, Steward Carney Hospital, Tufts School of Medicine, Dorchester, MA, USA

Nicholas James
Division of Pulmonology and Critical Care, Steward Carney Hospital, Tufts School of Medicine, Dorchester, MA, USA

Joel Weinstock
Division of Gastroenterology and Hepatology, Tufts Medical Center, Tufts School of Medicine, Boston, MA, USA

Weam El Hajj and Antoine Abou Rached
Department of Internal Medicine, Gastroenterology Division, Faculty of Medical Sciences, Lebanese University, Hadath Campus, Hadath, Beirut 2903 1308, Lebanon

Gilbert Nakad
Department of General Surgery, Faculty of Medical Sciences, Lebanese University, Hadath Campus, Hadath, Beirut 2903 1308, Lebanon

Venkata Rajesh Konjeti and Sravanthi Paluri
Virginia Commonwealth University, Richmond, VA, USA

Gerald M. Hefferman
Alpert Medical School of Brown University, Providence, RI, USA

Prerna Ganjoo
Nephrology Associates, East Providence, RI, USA

Cherng Harng Lim, Hsu-Heng Yen and Wei-Wen Su
Division of Gastroenterology and Hepatology, Department of Internal Medicine, Changhua Christian Hospital, Changhua City, Taiwan

Cherng-Jyr Lim
Department of Emergency Medicine, Cathay General Hospital, Changhua City, Taiwan

Hao-Chien Tsai and Shi-Ting Chen
Nursing Department, Changhua Christian Hospital, Changhua City, Taiwan

Oluwaseun Shogbesan, Abdullateef Abdulkareem and Anthony Donato
Department of Internal Medicine, Reading Health System, Spruce Street and 6th Avenue, West Reading, PA 19610, USA

Andrew Rettew
Department of Hematology and Oncology, Banner University Medical Center, Tuscon, AZ, USA

Bilal Shaikh
St Francis Medical Center, Cape Girardeau, MO, USA

Susumu Saigusa and Chikao Miki
Department of Surgery, Iga City General Hospital, 831 Shijuku-cho, Iga, Mie 518-0823, Japan

Masaki Ohi, Minako Kobayashi and Yasuhiro Inoue
Department of Gastrointestinal and Pediatric Surgery, Mie University Hospital, 2-174 Edobashi, Tsu, Mie 514-8507, Japan

Satoshi Oki and Takashi Ichikawa
Department of Gastrointestinal and Pediatric Surgery, Mie University Hospital, 2-174 Edobashi, Tsu, Mie 514-8507, Japan
Department of Surgery, Wakaba Hospital, 28-13 Minami-Chuo, Tsu, Mie 514-0832, Japan

Gaurav Chand
Department of Internal Medicine, Providence Hospital and Medical Center, 16001W. Nine Mile Road, Southfield, MI 48075, USA

Leonid Shamban
Department of Gastroenterology, Genesys Regional Medical Center, One Genesys Parkway, Grand Blanc, MI 48439, USA

Adam Forman
Department of Hematology and Oncology, Providence Hospital and Medical Center, 16001W. Nile Mile Road, Southfield, MI 48075, USA

Prabhat Sinha
Department of Pulmonology and Critical Care, Providence Hospital and Medical Center, 16001W. Nine Mile Road, Southfield, MI 48075, USA

Kaoru Omori, Kanako Yoshida and Masahiro Kan
Department of Gastroenterology and Hepatology, Sato Daiichi Hospital, 77-1 Hokyoji, Usa, Oita 879-0454, Japan

Sadafumi Tamiya
Department of Pathology, Kitakyushu Medical Center, 2-1-1 Bashaku, Kitakyushu, Fukuoka 802-0077, Japan

Tsutomu Daa
Department of Pathology, Graduate School of Medicine, Faculty of Medicine, Oita University, 1-1 Idaigaoka, Yufu, Oita 879-5593, Japan

Uni Wong
Division of Gastroenterology and Hepatology, University of Maryland Medical Center, Baltimore, MD 21201, USA

Harris Yfantis
Department of Pathology, Veterans Affairs Maryland Health Care System, University of Maryland School of Medicine, Baltimore, MD 21201, USA

Guofeng Xie
Division of Gastroenterology and Hepatology, Veterans Affairs Maryland Health Care System, University of Maryland School of Medicine, Baltimore, MD 21201, USA

Alnoor Ramji
Division of Gastroenterology, University of British Columbia, Vancouver, BC, Canada

Majid Alsahafi
Division of Gastroenterology, University of British Columbia, Vancouver, BC, Canada
Department of Medicine, King Abdulaziz University, Jeddah, Saudi Arabia

Mohammed I. AlJasser and Sunil Kalia
Department of Dermatology and Skin Science, University of British Columbia, Vancouver, BC, Canada

H. M. Yang
Department of Pathology and Laboratory Medicine, University of British Columbia, Vancouver, BC, Canada

Benjamin M. Snyder
University of South Carolina School of Medicine Greenville, Greenville, SC, USA

Joseph W. Beets and Gary A. Abrams
Department of Gastroenterology/Liver Center, Greenville Health System, University of South Carolina School of Medicine Greenville, Greenville, SC, USA

Bruce A. Lessey
Department of Obstetrics and Gynecology, Greenville Health System, University of South Carolina School of Medicine Greenville, Greenville, SC, USA

Samuel R. W. Horton
Department of Pathology, Greenville Health System, University of South Carolina School of Medicine Greenville, Greenville, SC, USA

Jochen Stenzel and Florian Eyer
Department of Clinical Toxicology, Klinikum rechts der Isar, Technical University of Munich, Ismaningerstrasse 22, 81675 Munich, Germany

Sebastian Noe
Department of Internal Medicine II (Gastroenterology), Klinikum rechts der Isar, Technical University of Munich, Ismaningerstrasse 22, 81675 Munich, Germany

Konstantin Holzapfel
Department of Diagnostic and Interventional Radiology, Klinikum rechts der Isar, Technical University of Munich, Ismaningerstrasse 22, 81675 Munich, Germany

Franziska Erlmeier
Institute of Pathology, Klinikum rechts der Isar, Technical University of Munich, Ismaningerstrasse 22, 81675Munich, Germany

Zoltán Berger
Departamento Medicina, Sección Gastroenterología, Hospital Clínico Universidad de Chile, Santiago, Chile

Hernán De La Fuente
Clínica Santa María, Santiago, Chile

Manuel Meneses
Fundación Arturo López Pérez, Santiago, Chile

Fernanda Matamala
Universidad Andres Bello, Santiago, Chile

Makarena Sepúlveda and Claudia Rojas
Universidad de los Andes, Santiago, Chile

Dean Ehrlich and Nimah Jamaluddin
Division of Digestive Diseases, Department of Medicine, David Geffen School of Medicine at UCLA, Los Angeles, CA, USA

Joseph Pisegna and David Padua
Division of Digestive Diseases, Department of Medicine, David Geffen School of Medicine at UCLA, Los Angeles, CA, USA
Division of Gastroenterology, Hepatology and Parenteral Nutrition, VA Greater Los Angeles Healthcare System, Los Angeles, CA, USA

Dhruvan Patel, Yub Raj Sedhai and Aasim Mohammed
Internal Medicine, Mercy Catholic Medical Center, Darby, PA, USA

Shazia Sohrawardy
Philadelphia College of Osteopathic Medicine, Philadelphia, PA, USA

Soney Basnyat
Nepal Medical College Teaching Hospital, Kathmandu, Nepal

Anisha Daxini
JJM Medical College, Davangere, India

Aparna Basu
Hematology&Oncology, Henry Ford Medical Center, Detroit, MI, USA

Vivek R. Mehta
Rheumatology, Albany Medical Center, Albany, NY, USA

Steven Lichtenstein
Division of Gastroenterology and Hepatology, Mercy Health System, Philadelphia, PA, USA

Shuji Shimizu
International Medical Department, Kyushu University Hospital, Fukuoka, Japan

Akira Aso
International Medical Department, Kyushu University Hospital, Fukuoka, Japan
Department of Medicine and Bioregulatory Science, Graduate School of Medical Sciences, Kyushu University, Fukuoka, Japan

Eikichi Ihara, Kazuhiko Nakamura and Tetsuhide Ito
Department of Medicine and Bioregulatory Science, Graduate School of Medical Sciences, Kyushu University, Fukuoka, Japan

Irina Sudovykh
Endoscopic Therapeutics Department, Kyushu University Hospital, Fukuoka, Japan

Masafumi Nakamura
Department of Surgery and Oncology, Graduate School of Medical Sciences, Kyushu University, Fukuoka, Japan

Tetsuo Ikeda
Department of Surgery and Science, Graduate School of Medical Sciences, Kyushu University, Fukuoka, Japan

Nobuyoshi Takizawa and Yoshinao Oda
Department of Anatomic Pathology, Graduate School of Medical Sciences, Kyushu University, Fukuoka, Japan

Index

O

P

R

S

T

U

V

Z